MEDICAL RADIOLO[G]

Diagnostic Imaging and Radiation Oncology – Softco

D1549581

Mike Mackenzie

01706 341100

07810 892 667

Springer
Berlin
Heidelberg
New York
Barcelona
Hong Kong
London
Milan
Paris
Singapore
Tokyo

Radiology of Trauma

With Contributions by

A.L. Baert·J. Brossmann·C.H. Buitrago-Téllez·A. Chavan·U. Dietrich·F.J. Ferstl
A. Fink·M. Freund·M. Galanski·S. Gryspeerdt·F. Häckl·K.D. Hagspiel·M. Heller
K.-F. Kreitner·M. Langer·R. Low·V. Metz·C. Muhle·R.H. Oyen S. Palmié·M. Reuter
H. Schwarzenberg·L. Van Hoe·F. Zanella

Edited by

M. Heller and A. Fink

Foreword by

Albert L. Baert

With 450 Figures in 843 Separate Illustrations, 1 in Colour

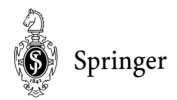

Springer

Professor Dr. med. Martin Heller
Dr. med. Andreas Fink

Klinik für Diagnostische Radiologie
Klinikum an der Christian-Albrechts-Universität zu Kiel
Arnold-Heller-Straße 9
24105 Kiel
Germany

MEDICAL RADIOLOGY · Diagnostic Imaging and Radiation Oncology

Continuation of
Handbuch der medizinischen Radiologie
Encyclopedia of Medical Radiology

ISSN 0942-5373
ISBN 3-540-66338-X Springer-Verlag Berlin Heidelberg New York

Library of Congress Cataloging-in-Publication Data applied for

Die Deutsche Bibliothek – CIP-Einheitsaufnahme
Radiology of trauma / with contributions by A. L. Baert ... Ed. by M. Heller and A. Fink. Foreword by Albert L. Baert.
– Berlin; Heidelberg; New York; Barcelona; Hong Kong; London; Milan; Paris; Singapore; Tokyo: Springer, 2000.
(Medical radiology). ISBN 3-540-66338-X

© Springer-Verlag Berlin · Heidelberg 2000
Printed in Germany

Cover-Design: Joan Greenfield, New York

Typesetting: Best-set Typesetter Ltd., Hong Kong

SPIN: 10741721   21/3135/SPS – 5 4 3 2 1 – Printed on acid-free paper

Foreword

Trauma is a very common condition in medical practice and a frequent cause of death, morbidity and disability. Although most radiologists will spend a considerable amount of their time dealing with trauma patients, this topic has not acquired "prestige" status in radiological meetings, journals or books. This is regrettable because the radiologist is frequently able to make a specific and very valuable contribution to the handling and management of trauma patients admitted to the emergency departments of our hospitals. Indeed, the radiologist, by virtue of his specific expertise, is able to provide excellent advice to clinicians concerning the choice and the sequence of examinations. He can thereby provide qualified support for rapid decisions that may be either vital for the patient's outcome or decisive for an early recovery without disability or long-lasting sequelae.

This book is unrivalled in its complete and meticulous coverage of the diagnostic imaging methods used in trauma patients. It is written by outstanding European experts and provides comprehensive coverage of all anatomical areas that may be involved in patients with skeletal or visceral traumatic lesions.

Professor M. Heller, Dr. A. Fink, and their team in Kiel have long-standing experience and a solid international reputation in the field of radiological imaging and management of trauma. They have been assisted in their task by several other well-known specialists in this area.

This book will certainly be welcomed by all general radiologists and by radiologists in training since it will fully update their knowledge in trauma radiology, based on the progress achieved by the new imaging modalities.

Leuven   ALBERT L. BAERT

Preface

The care, diagnosis, and treatment of patients with multiple traumatic injuries are challenging tasks. When dealing with acutely and severely injured patients, many decisions have to be made under severe time constraints. Nurses, technicians, and physicians of different specialities have to cooperate and communicate very efficiently, and medical supplies, operating rooms, and technical equipment need to be available at short notice and at all times. A great deal of knowledge, experience, and teamwork is necessary to provide good emergency services.

The editors of and contributors to this book have acquired their experience mainly in large hospitals that serve as major trauma centers. The book is designed to assist the general radiologist and in particular those in training to prepare for the diagnosis of trauma victims, increasing their confidence and practical knowledge. However, those in other disciplines should also benefit from this book in that they will learn what radiology now has to offer. Communication and cooperation are much easier if one specialist knows what to expect from another, what question to ask, and which information to supply.

We have tried to provide an update of modern trauma diagnostics. Against the background of conventional radiology, the book points out the opportunities that modern equipment has to offer: the advantages of fast (spiral or helical) CT, the value of three-dimensional CT in assisting surgeons to plan operations, and the current status of ultrasonography and how it compares with CT and peritoneal lavage. MRI is covered, with discussion of when and how it can replace arthrography or stress examinations. Knowledge of pitfalls and regular follow-up are equally important in the achievement of good results in trauma patients.

It should, however, be pointed out that not only patients with life-threatening injuries are covered by this volume; much attention is given to sprained ankles, broken arms, etc. If not diagnosed and treated adequately, these injuries can cause lifelong sequelae.

We are indebted to those who taught us and to those whose books we read during our training. Our goal was to concentrate on significant and relevant issues while leaving out as much academic discussion as possible. We have tried to pass on our experience and opinions to others, and would welcome criticisms and suggestions as to how this book might be further improved.

We would like to thank the editors of *Medical Radiology*, and in particular Prof. A.L. Baert, for their encouragement and support, and U.N. Davis and R. Mills from Springer-Verlag for their help and patience.

Last but not least, we feel that a word on the ubiquitous subject of health care costs is warranted: In many hospitals, both large ones that serve as trauma centers and smaller ones, a great many people spend more time working at unsocial hours than in most other professions and work with great motivation. They work at Christmas and at weekends for not more than a regular wage because they accept the responsibility that comes with their job. A community has a right to expect good medical service and these people stand ready to do their best, but this service is not and never will be cheap.

Kiel, June 1996
MARTIN HELLER
ANDREAS FINK

Contents

1 General Aspects of Trauma Radiology

M. Heller and A. Fink

CONTENTS

1.1 Introduction

Trauma usually occurs unexpectedly and anyone at any age may be affected. The severity of traumatizing forces resulting from travel accidents, accidents at home, sport activities, or crime and the situation when and where the accident happens influence the medical management. Efficient diagnosis and treatment require knowledge about the accident or – if that is not available – a good theory of what happened and how it happened.

An efficient emergency ambulance system, including the availability of helicopters, increases dramatically the number of severely injured patients who reach the hospital alive and the severity of their injuries. In addition, the expectations of the public over recent decades have risen to the point where not only survival of the patients is expected but also the maximum possible restitution that modern medicine has to offer. To achieve this requires a very high degree of cooperation between the individual medical specialties. This point cannot be stressed enough: the best possible outcome for the patient can only be achieved if the best knowledge of the individual medical specialties is put to work in a coordinated manner.

First one should, of course, differentiate between minor and potentially life-threatening injuries. However, while the requirement to do so is obvious, the decision, unfortunately, sometimes is not. Fortu-

M. Heller, MD, PhD, Professor and Direktor der Klinik für Radiologische Diagnostik, Klinikum der Christian-Albrechts-Universität zu Kiel, Arnold-Heller-Straße 9, 24105 Kiel, Germany
A. Fink, MD, Klinik für Radiologische Diagnostik, Klinikum der Christian-Albrechts-Universität zu Kiel, Arnold-Heller-Straße 9, 24105 Kiel, Germany

nately, the vast majority of trauma patients are not suffering from life-threatening injuries. So, stabilizing the injured organ or extremity in order to prevent worsening has a high priority and the pain should be treated adequately. While time is not as crucial as with life-threatening injuries, a decision as to whether or not to operate within the 6-h limit obviously has to be made fairly quickly.

After the trauma victim's breathing and circulation have been stabilized, a brief but careful examination by an experienced surgeon will determine the necessary further examinations. As a first step life-threatening injuries have to be excluded or diagnosed. Thus, an anteroposterior chest radiograph and sonography of the abdomen and chest (pleural effusion!) are probably the minimum steps required to evaluate a polytraumatized patient. To these procedures a lateral view of the spine should be added if such an injury is suspected. The frequently requested and performed three views the skull (anteroposterior, lateral and Towne's), for example, are time consuming and often yield only insignificant information. If an intracranial injury is suspected, computed tomography (CT) should be performed immediately. Very soon a decision has to be made as to whether additional examinations are warranted and whether the patient's vital status permits them. Also, if found necessary, additional specialists, e.g., a neurosurgeon or an ophthalmologist, will then have to become involved. At this stage the patient's well-being is dependent to a large extent on efficient medical management; good intentions and sound medical knowledge are essential but by no means sufficient. Good communication and cooperation between the physicians and the medical staff involved are mandatory.

While usually one of the surgeons or the anesthesiologist takes the lead, the radiologist should assume responsibility for managing the diagnostic imaging. She or he should be able to estimate whether angiography, CT-angiography or urography is necessary or whether CT can be planned in such a way as to allow the assessment of the kidneys and the urinary tract equally well.

1.2 Computed Tomography

Over the past 10–15 years CT has become the single most important tool for the diagnosis of trauma. It has, however, also become very complex. Spiral (or helical) CT, for example, is a powerful method to examine a patient very quickly but it is quite possible to miss the bolus of contrast medium completely, making the diagnosis of an aortic dissection difficult. This is particularly true if the circulation is impaired. A second attempt is often not possible due to time constraints or because the maximum amount of contrast medium has already been administered. Therefore, a radiologist with sufficient knowledge about trauma and the required equipment needs to plan the examination carefully.

After the vital functions have been secured and artificial respiration established, the patient should be taken to the CT room. This room needs to be equipped with an adequate respirator and all necessary supplies – oxygen, infusions, and drugs – to meet the anesthesiologist's needs. Blankets (possibly including electrical blankets) to prevent the body from cooling down too much are a good idea. Since it is difficult and possibly dangerous for the patient to be moved, an efficient examination strategy has to be devised first. If a head or cervical spine injury is likely, one should start by scanning the brain, then the cervical spine, then the mid face. For scanning the brain a standard procedure is usually established. When searching for fractures, thin sections with gaps are advisable. After a fracture has been found, and if three-dimensional reconstructions are desired, the gaps should be scanned. Without sacrificing much accuracy, this saves a lot of time compared to continuous scanning with thin slices, and it is much more sensible for fractures than, for example, continuous 5-mm slices.

One should then proceed by fastening the patient's arms above the head, and continue with a topogram (scout view) of the chest. A trial run is usually advisable in order to assure that all lines and hoses are loose enough to allow for the 20 to 50 or more cm of table movement. Patients *have* been extubated as a result of failure to take this precaution!

The topogram is often insufficiently appreciated. It offers an excellent overview of the chest and in particular of the abdomen, mainly because it is acquired with almost no scattered radiation (Figs. 1.1, 1.2). It not only should be used for selecting the scan areas but should be scrutinized for such "minor details" as, for example, the proper position of respiratory and stomach tubes. Next, three or four slices of the chest should be performed as a standard procedure – whether a chest CT is requested or not. Three slices do not take much time but offer a much better look at the lung than the chest radiograph. Pleural and cardiac effusions, lung contusions, and a minor pneumothorax can be demonstrated or excluded easily. To a lesser extent, this also holds true for spleen, liver, and kidney injuries and free intra-abdominal fluid.

The pelvis and spine are prime examples for the ability of modern CT not only to aid in diagnosing fractures but also to assist greatly in treatment planning. If significant fracture dislocations are found, the scanning should be planned so as to allow for adequate three-dimensional reconstructions. The surgeons should be asked which views they need for planning their operation, and the processing done after the patient has left the CT room.

All this requires that the responsible radiologist is present during the scanning and closely watches the examination on the CT monitors. On the other hand, sufficient clinical information must be provided by the surgeons to allow for adequate planning of the examination by the radiologist, and, of course, all images previously taken must accompany the patient.

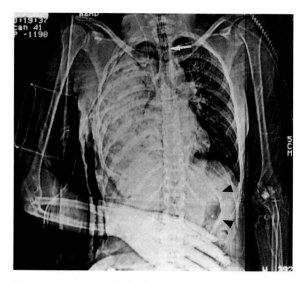

Fig. 1.1. Topogram clearly Illustrating a major injury to the right lung, which in the transverse sections (not shown) can be identified as an intrapulmonary hematoma resulting from a lung laceration. Also-note the proper positions of the respiratory (*arrow*) and gastric (*arrowhead*) tubes

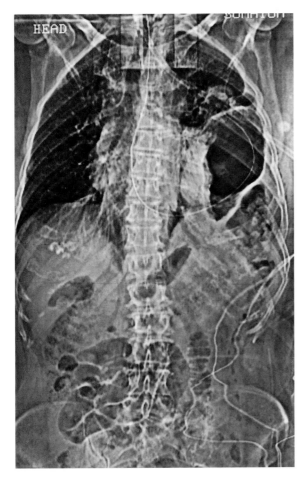

Fig. 1.2. Rupture of the left diaphragm. Parts of the stomach. Including the gastric tube, have been dislocated into the left lung. Also note the compression atelectasis of the left lower lobe. This topogram offers a much better overview than the transverse images and should be documented on the CT film *in addition* to a topogram indicating the slice positions with lines

1.3 Magnetic Resonance Imaging

There seem to be very few indications for magnetic resonance imaging (MRI) during acute emergency diagnostics. Up to now, examination times of 3–8 min per sequence, problems with metal and magnetic equipment, and the spatial restrictions of the magnet itself have prevented the standard use of MRI in severely traumatized patients. The only exception is the so-called spinal emergency: neurological deficits occurring without apparent trauma that are suspected to have their origin in a spinal cord disorder. With the advent of ultra fast sequences, so-called breath-hold sequences of 20 s or less, the availability of antimagnetic equipment, and the introduction of

"open" MRI systems, this might change. For the detection of intracerebral bleeding in the acute stage, CT still outperforms MRI.

For an increasing number of joints, MRI is evolving as a primary diagnostic tool. As well as patients with knee and shoulder problems, those with ankle and wrist injuries are increasingly often referred to MRI immediately after the initial x-rays are taken – and this not only because of the oft-heralded superb diagnostic capabilities of MRI in soft tissues, but also because of its ability to detect or exclude bone abnormalities. High-resolution STIR imaging (short tau inversion recovery) with its additive T1 and T2 weighting and its fat suppression characteristics is a very sensitive tool to diagnose even minor injuries such as radiologically otherwise invisible stress fractures or beginning inflammation. In this respect it competes with the sensitivity of scintigraphy. MRI is also beginning to replace stress examinations and arthrography of the ankle.

1.4 Technical Assistants

A very important aspect is the support offered by well-trained x-ray technicians. The increasing complexity of CT scanners, MRI, digital subtraction and digital x-ray equipment requires constant job rotation and training of technicians (and physicians, of course) in order to be able to adequately operate these machines. With the high cost involved in providing optimal medical care and the ongoing attempts to reduce medical expenditure, we find it increasingly difficult to staff our facilities with technical assistants and to have them on call around the clock. There is, unfortunately, very little time during an emergency to consult the manuals. Therefore, the ability to handle emergencies requires a lot of foresight and planning.

1.5 Coping with Shortcomings

Logistics can be complicated by spatial shortcomings. While an emergency department is usually equipped with at least the basic x-ray equipment and a movable sonography machine, CT scanners and much more so MR scanners have often been installed later and may not be located adjacent to the emergency rooms. Transportation of the patient, blood samples, medical supplies, and important images, e.g., CT images, to the neurosurgeon is then of utmost importance and must be available around the clock. Unfortunately, there is very little one can do about this in the short run; again, planning and thinking ahead are required.

Finally, we have found it extremely helpful to discuss the images with the different specialists involved while the patient is still in the CT or x-ray rooms. Then, additional images can be acquired without losing much time. Immediately after the patient has left the radiology department, the findings should be documented briefly and then sent on to accompany the patient. Otherwise, the risk of information getting lost – which is in any case a major risk – will be increased tremendously.

2 Skull, Brain, and Face

F.E. Zanella and U. Dietrich

CONTENTS

2.1 General Considerations

Traumatic brain injury represents a major health problem in all countries of the world. Trauma is the leading cause of death for individuals younger than 40 years, with more than half of these deaths related to severe head injury. Two-thirds of head trauma victims are men; preexisting brain lesions are very seldom. Alcohol intoxication, however, is implicated in a large number of head injuries. The primary goal in treating craniofacial trauma is to preserve the patient's life and neurological functions. Neuroimaging plays a vital role in early and correct diagnosis. The secondary goal is to identify those lesions that may determine the outcome of patients following head injury.

Injuries of the skull, brain, or face often present an emergency situation that requires immediate medical or surgical treatment following stabilization of respiratory and cardiopulmonary functions. In some cases severe thoracic or abdominal trauma takes priority over head injuries. On the other hand, possible fractures and instability of the spine must be detected. The radiological methods include plain film radiography, computed tomography (CT), angiography, ultrasonography, and magnetic resonance imaging (MRI). Investigations in the emergency room should be limited to chest x-rays, abdominal ultrasonography, and radiography of the spine and pelvis. For evaluation of head injuries CT is the method of choice, because of its ability to demonstrate cerebral parenchymal injuries as well as craniofacial fractures and injuries of the craniocervical junction. In cases of solitary head injury CT is the first-choice diagnostic tool, enabling immediate surgical evacuation of intracranial hematomas. Injuries not related to vital functions may be evaluated postoperatively. Even in cases of vascular injury, cranial CT should precede angiography to detect cerebral parenchymal injuries. Radiography of the skull has assumed a lesser role in emergency situations except for evaluating skull fractures which elude CT detection. MRI has gained increasing interest in the assessment of patients with symptoms which do not accord with CT findings.

Severely traumatized patients require fast and accurate evaluation through a skilled and experienced team combining the possibilities of surgical and intensive care treatment. Severely injured patients often have difficulty in cooperating during examinations, and examinations are some-

F.E. ZANELLA, MD, Professor, Direktor des Instituts für Neuroradiologie am Klinikum der J.W. Goethe-Universität, Schleusenweg 7-10, 60528 Frankfurt, Germany
U. DIETRICH, MD, Klinik für Neuroradiologie, Universitätsklinikum Essen, Hufelandstr. 55, 45122 Essen, Germany

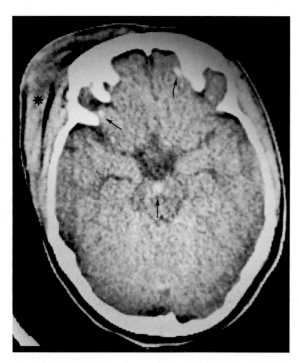

Fig. 2.1. Subgaleal hematoma. Axial CT scan demonstrates soft-tissue swelling (*asterisk*) located beneath the gelea aponeurotica and above the temporalis muscle. Small intracerebral parenchymal hemorrhages (*arrows*) suggest diffuse axonal injury

2.2 Skull

2.2.1 Scalp Injuries

The skull bones and the soft tissues of the scalp have an important role in distributing and decreasing an impact force to the head. Scalp injuries are common with head trauma varying from minor scalp wounds to severe laceration of the scalp. Hemorrhage in the soft tissues of the scalp can occur at three levels resulting in (1) subcutaneous, (2) subgaleal (subaponeurotic), and (3) subperiosteal hematoma. Subcutaneous hematoma results in caput succedaneum. This occurs in pediatric patients and represents an edematous swelling beneath the skin and above the galea aponeurotica. A subgaleal hematoma is a collection of blood beneath the galea aponeurotica and above the periosteum of the skull (Fig. 2.1). CT or MRI reveals a soft tissue swelling or hematoma extending over a large area of the skull beneath the subcutaneous layer and above the temporalis muscle. Subperiosteal bleeding results in cephalhematoma and again occurs in pediatric patients. It is situated beneath the temporalis muscle and does not cross suture margins.

2.2.2 Fractures

The evidence and type of a fracture often allow an indication as to the character and the quantitative force of the factors having produced the head injury. Linear fractures, comminuted fractures, and sutural diastasis usually result from broad-based traumatic violence, while depressed fractures are more often the product of circumscribed trauma to the head. Fractures may be induced in locations removed from the place of the primary traumatic event through transmission of forces within the skull bones, e.g., fractures of the skull base. Severe brain injuries correspond with skull fractures in about two-thirds of the patients. The absence of a fracture, however, does not exclude the possibility of brain injury. Fatal brain injury without associated fracture can be found in a significant number of cases.

Skull fractures may involve the cranial vault or the skull base. They are divided into linear, depressed, diastatic, and comminuted fractures. Linear fractures can also extend into sutures and give rise to sutural diastasis. A sutural diastasis can even occur without an accompanying fracture. It can be recognized when the width of the suture is more than 3 mm. Because the lambdoid suture closes latest, it is

times disrupted by an unforeseen need to manage vital functions. Time often permits only examinations that ascertain gross details of the primary injury. The role of the radiologist during emergencies is to determine within the immediate situation an effective balance between detailed, complex radiological procedures and the need for quick and coarse evaluation of injuries that may lead to irreversible brain damage.

On the other hand, however, it is equally important to remember that a single CT examination upon hospital admission will in many cases fail to identify threatening mass lesions that will only evolve later. This is particularly relevant if the first CT scans have been performed within a few hours after trauma. Early detection and early evacuation of an extracerebral hematoma, for example, should not divert attention from recognizing later developing mass lesions that remain inapparent for a time. Renewed CT scans should be performed at the first signs of new or worsening neurological deficit, when there are increases in measured intracranial pressure, in cases where surgery has been performed, and routinely within 12–24h in stable cases.

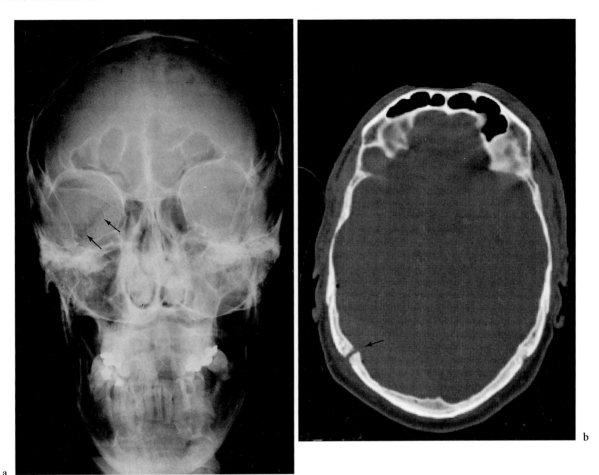

Fig. 2.2a,b. Diastatic fracture. The right lambdoid suture (*arrows*) is widened on posteroanterior plain film (**a**) and on CT scan (**b**)

more commonly involved than the coronal suture in adult patients (Fig. 2.2). Often there is a combination of several fractures having multiple divergent or convergent fracture lines, or with multiple small and large bone fragments. This is the case in so-called comminuted fractures, burst fractures, or complex fractures (Fig. 2.3). Fractures that communicate with the outside are classified as external compound fractures if they communicate with the scalp, and as internal compound fractures if there is communication with the paranasal sinuses.

Fractures of the cranial vault are visible on high-quality x-ray film, including anteroposterior (a.p.), lateral, and Towne's views. CT is the procedure of first choice for patients with suspected brain injury; radiography of the skull is usually performed later. CT scans should be displayed in soft tissue as well as in bone target modes to demonstrate skull fractures in one examination. High-resolution CT is optimal for the demonstration of fractures. CT evaluation of

the skull base and of the temporal bone requires sections of 2 mm or thinner. The ability to detect vault fractures depends on the plane chosen for the sections in relation to the direction in which the fractures run. Fractures parallel to or within the section plane may not always be visible on CT scans. Fractures oblique to the section plane are seen more readily. Additional coronal CT sections may also prove necessary.

The presence of a linear skull fracture increases the likelihood of an epidural or subdural hematoma, whereas depressed fractures are more often associated with localized parenchymal injury. Minor head injuries are almost always present without skull fractures, whereby, however, intracranial complications cannot be ruled out. For patients with minor head injury, skull radiography proves of little significance. Clinical guidelines for the correct indication to utilize plain skull radiography are clearly necessary. Plain film skull radiography should follow CT scan

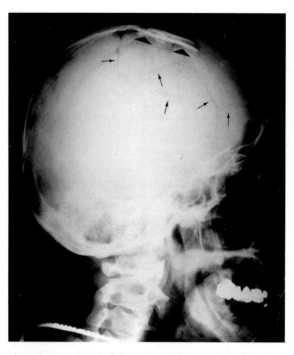

Fig. 2.3. Complex skull fractures. A depressed skull fracture (*arrowheads*) is combined with multiple divergent fracture lines (*arrows*)

fractures are wider in their midportion and narrow at their ends. The width usually does not exceed 3 mm. Fractures in thin portions of bone, e.g., the temporal squama, as well as fractures in young children may not always be visible. Calvarium fractures with an oblique course through the inner and outer tabulae and fractures of the skull base may also evade radiographic detection. A linear fracture is often only identifiable in one single plane of the standard radiographic projections, remaining invisible in the others (Fig. 2.4c). An area of soft tissue swelling becomes visible when the skull films are examined under a bright light. This may indicate the location of the trauma and can give a hint as to the side on which a fracture may be located. Displacement of the calcified pineal may be an indicator of space-occupying intracranial lesions such as hematoma or unilateral edema.

A skull fracture may take from several months to several years to heal completely. In some cases the fracture margin never completely obliterates. During healing the margins in time become less distinct and the fracture is often difficult to distinguish from a vascular impression. Repeat examination should demonstrate evidence of healing in a true fracture.

for patients with depressed fractures, for patients with suspicion of foreign bodies intra- or extracranially, and sometimes for comatose patients with an unknown history. Some authors recommend skull radiography for patients with loss of consciousness, amnesia, neurological deficits, injuries of the face or scalp, oto- or rhinorrhea, hemorrhage from the ear, periorbital hematoma, or a history of previous craniotomy. The identification of a skull fracture on plain film radiography may give a hint as to the severity of trauma, but does not play a role in the current management of head-injured patients.

2.2.2.1 Linear Fractures

A linear fracture appears in skull radiography as a translucent line having a well-defined margin. Such fractures may be confused with vascular channels, whereby the fractures, however, do not branch and fail to show corticated margins. Indeed, they often cross vascular markings (Fig. 2.4a). A fracture is more radiolucent than a vascular marking; it is generally straight or changes direction at sharp angles (Fig. 2.4b). The fracture line is thin and appears more detailed when the side of the skull containing the fracture is placed nearest the film. Skull

2.2.2.2 Depressed Fractures

Depression of bone fragments under the intact calvarial margins is called a depressed fracture. It may have a round and stellate or spoked-wheel appearance if multiple fracture lines radiate from the central point. There is frequently a zone of increased density at the fracture site due to overlapping of fragments beneath the adjacent calvarium (Fig. 2.5). Linear fractures may surround the depressed fracture. Tangential views are necessary to determine the amount of depression, whereby, however, CT scanning remains the more sensitive method for this evaluation.

Depressed fractures increase the risk of dural tear and may damage the underlying brain, thereby increasing the incidence of underlying cerebral contusions. Compound depressed fractures carry the risk of intracranial infection. The depressed fracture is considered to be of surgical significance if the fragments are depressed below and through the adjacent inner table or if they lie over a major dural sinus or over an eloquent cortical region of the brain. CT has the advantage of demonstrating in a single examination both the amount of bony depression and concomitant cerebral injury (Fig. 2.6).

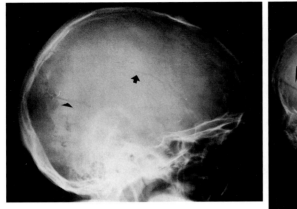

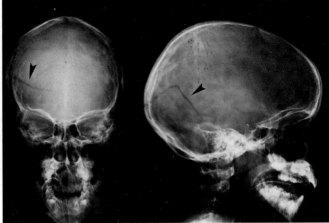

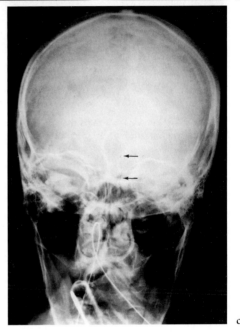

Fig. 2.4a–c. Linear skull fractures. **a** Occipital (*arrowhead*) and temporal (*arrow*) skull fractures; the latter crosses the groove of the anterior branch of the middle meningeal artery. **b** Temporo-occipital skull fracture (*arrowhead*) with a sharp angle. **c** Anteroposterior view of an occipital paramedian skull fracture (*arrows*) which is only visible on the anteroposterior view; extension into the foramen magnum, however, would have been better demonstrated on Towne's view

2.2.2.3 Fractures of the Skull Base

Skull base fractures are difficult to depict on plain film radiography and the basal view projection is seldom of benefit. Fractures of the cranial vault may extend downwards toward the skull base, and fractures of the skull base may extend upwards toward the cranial vault. Until the advent of high-resolution thin-section CT these fractures were more often diagnosed clinically than radiographically. Clinical features are bleeding from the middle ear, oto- or rhinorrhea, ecchymosis surrounding the orbit, subcutaneous hematoma around the mastoid process, and damage to cranial nerves. Plain films may reveal an air-fluid level in the sphenoid sinus, in the frontal sinus, or in the ethmoidal cells because of accumulation of blood or cerebrospinal fluid (CSF) in the sinuses. It is therefore recommended that skull films be obtained with the patient in the upright position, or that cross-table lateral films be acquired with the patient in supine position. Sometimes complete opacification of the paranasal sinuses or the mastoid cells is the only clue to a fracture. Fractures of the skull base are often associated with disruption of the dura mater. They become compound fractures when a communication exists between the intracranial and extracranial spaces. Presence of intracranial air indicates both a fracture and a dural tear with an extension to the paranasal sinuses or to the mastoid cells, whereby the risk of intracranial infection arises. Basilar fractures may extend across the foramina of the skull base and cause cranial nerve damage, lac-

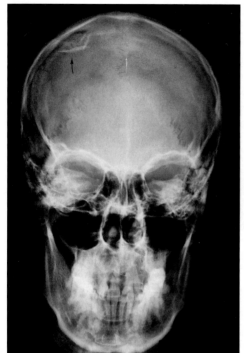

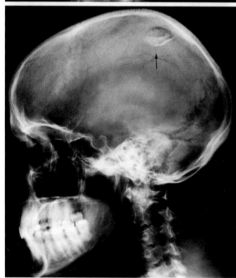

tures of the optic canal or the orbital apex as well as injury to the optic nerve. Fractures of the sphenoid bone can cause injury to the pituitary gland, to the carotid or ophthalmic arteries, to the cavernous sinus, and to the cranial nerves passing through the sinus. CT does not allow direct demonstration of cranial nerve injuries, but it is capable of showing fracture lines crossing the internal auditory canal, the jugular foramen, or the hypoglossal canal. Conventional pluridirectional tomography increases the likelihood of detecting skull base fractures in comparison with plain film radiography. CT scanning, however, has become the most effective method for diagnosis of these fractures and provides a more directed indication for surgical or conservative procedures. In cases with CSF fluid leak, or sometimes for

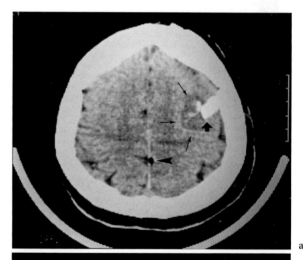

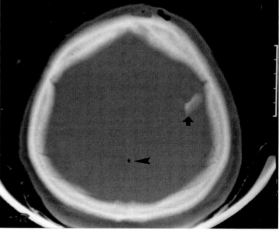

Fig. 2.5a,b. Right parietal depressed skull fracture (*arrow*). Anteroposterior (**a**) and lateral (**b**) skull films show areas of hyperlucency and hypolucency due to displacement of bone fragments beneath the level of the inner table of the skull

eration of great vessels, disturbance of pituitary gland function, or ossicular dislocation within the middle ear.

High-resolution thin-section CT scanning is the method of choice in the evaluation of basilar skull fractures. Fractures of the anterior and middle cranial fossae can extend into the frontal ethmoidal or sphenoidal sinuses. CT is able to demonstrate frac-

Fig. 2.6a,b. Compound depressed skull fracture (*large arrow*) with intracranial air bubble (*arrowhead*), underlying cerebral contusion (*small arrows*), soft tissue swelling, and subcutaneous air collection. CT scan with soft tissue (**a**) and bony (**b**) windows

evaluation of neural or vascular injury, it is necessary to perform CT scans in direct coronal sections. These have the advantage of being perpendicular to the skull base and can show fractures of the sinus roofs and of the temporal bone with better resolution than conventional a.p. view x-ray tomography, which becomes superfluous in almost all cases.

Fractures of the skull base are divided into (1) fractures of the anterior cranial fossa (frontobasal),

(2) fractures of the middle cranial fossa, i.e., of the sphenoid bone (sphenobasal) or of the temporal bone (laterobasal), and (3) fractures of the planum occipitale (Fig. 2.7). The fractures of the temporal bone are subdivided into longitudinal fractures, transverse fractures, and complex fractures. Longitudinal fractures are the most common type. They run parallel to or in the long axis of the petrous pyramid and are more often associated with the following

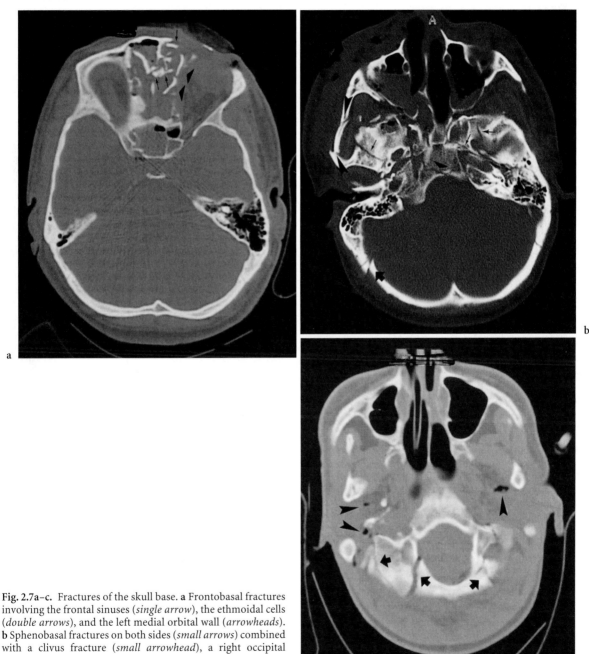

Fig. 2.7a–c. Fractures of the skull base. a Frontobasal fractures involving the frontal sinuses (*single arrow*), the ethmoidal cells (*double arrows*), and the left medial orbital wall (*arrowheads*). b Sphenobasal fractures on both sides (*small arrows*) combined with a clivus fracture (*small arrowhead*), a right occipital fracture (*large arrow*), and right zygomatic fractures (*large arrowheads*). c Multiple occipital fractures (*arrows*) and emphysema of the soft tissues (*arrowheads*)

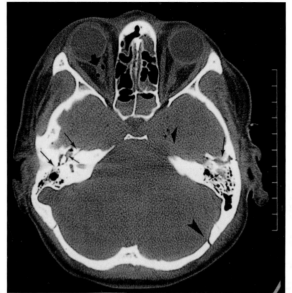

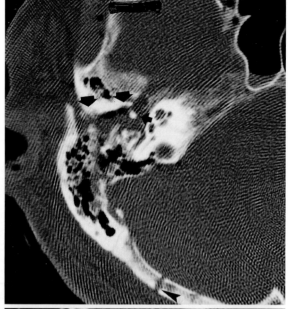

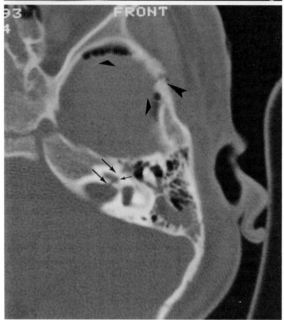

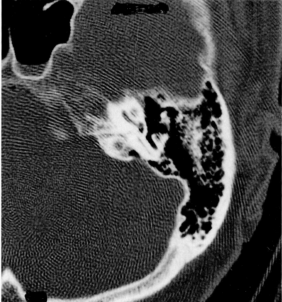

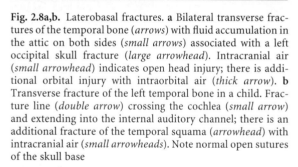

Fig. 2.8a,b. Laterobasal fractures. **a** Bilateral transverse fractures of the temporal bone (*arrows*) with fluid accumulation in the attic on both sides (*small arrows*) associated with a left occipital skull fracture (*large arrowhead*). Intracranial air (*small arrowhead*) indicates open head injury; there is additional orbital injury with intraorbital air (*thick arrow*). **b** Transverse fracture of the left temporal bone in a child. Fracture line (*double arrow*) crossing the cochlea (*small arrow*) and extending into the internal auditory channel; there is an additional fracture of the temporal squama (*arrowhead*) with intracranial air (*small arrowheads*). Note normal open sutures of the skull base

Fig. 2.9. a Ossicular (incudomalleal) dislocation. There is a longitudinal fracture of the right temporal bone (*large arrows*) with hemorrhage into the middle ear and the mastoid cells. The isolated head of the malleolus (*small arrow*) is not in conjunction with the long process of the incus. An additional fracture of the occipital bone is present (*arrowhead*). Compare the normal "ice cream cone" on the left side (**b**)

complications: rupture of the tympanic membrane, hemotympanum, and ossicular disruption (Fig. 2.8a). Transverse fractures run perpendicular or oblique to the long axis of the pyramid and are fre-

quently complicated by vestibular dysfunction, hearing loss, or facial nerve palsy (Fig. 2.8b). Complex fractures usually show multiple fragments with either otorrhea through the disrupted tympanic membrane or rhinorrhea via the eustachian tube. Suspected ossicular disruption within the middle ear should always be evaluated using CT. The axial view is preferred for diagnosis of an incudomalleal dislocation. Incudomalleal separation appears as vacant or increased space between the head of the malleus and the body of the incus. The normal "ice cream cone" appearance is altered (Fig. 2.9a). Coronal sections are preferred in the evaluation of an incudostapedial separation. The long process of the incus points away from the oval window, causing loss of the normal "V form" between this structure and the stapes. In all cases it is important to obtain sections of the contralateral uninvolved temporal bone in order to allow comparison with the normal positions of the ossicles in the attic (Fig. 2.9b).

2.2.3 Complications of Fractures

The presence of a skull fracture does not imply that there is also intracranial injury. The fracture itself does not need any specific treatment. Complications, however, that may accompany skull fractures often require therapeutic measures. In some cases vascular injuries are treated surgically, in other cases medically. Damage involving a cranial nerve may require surgical decompression if there are fragments narrowing the neural foramen or canal. Depressed fractures may cause leptomeningeal scarring or gliosis and can give rise to epileptic seizures. Compound fractures carry the risk of infection. Fractures of the paranasal sinuses with CSF leakage tend to be persistent and must be treated surgically, whereas spontaneous closure is more probable in cases of laterobasal fracture with otorrhea. The most serious complication of a skull fracture is epidural hematoma leading to secondary compression of the brain, sometimes very quickly. This will be discussed in Sect. 2.3.1. Ossicular dislocation has been discussed in Sect. 2.2.1.

2.2.3.1 Growing Fracture (Leptomeningeal Cyst)

If the skull fracture has resulted in a tear in the dura mater, the arachnoid membrane may protrude through the dural fissure and become incarcerated between the bone fragments. Over months to years in such cases the continued transmission of CSF pulsation leads to a smoothing and widening of the fracture line, resulting in what is termed a "growing fracture." Failing closure of such a fracture may give rise to a palpable cystic mass, a leptomeningeal cyst, protruding outside the bony calvaria. The cyst may be porencephalic, i.e., in communication with the cerebral ventricles. Leptomeningeal cysts occur most

often in infants and children under 2 years of age and are most frequently found in the frontal and parietal regions. Radiographically a growing fracture is characterized by sclerotic or scalloped margins. For children with skull fractures clinical follow-up is sufficient to rule out this complication.

2.2.3.2 Cerebrospinal Fluid Leak

Fractures of the floor of the anterior and middle cranial fossae can extend into the frontal, ethmoidal, or sphenoidal sinuses. If the dura mater is torn, the result is leakage of CSF into the nasal cavities with rhinorrhea and the risk of intracranial infection. In a similar fashion air may enter the intracranial space and lead to pneumocephalus with or without evidence of CSF leakage. Pneumocephalus means the presence of intracranial air which can be found within the subarachnoid space, the ventricular system, the subdural space, the epidural space, or the cerebral parenchyma. The latter is called pneumatocele. Pneumocephalus does not always appear immediately after trauma and in most cases resolves spontaneously within days. Occasionally the air expands, causing tension pneumocephalus with signs like headache, neck stiffness, stupor, and papilledema. In most cases, however, pneumocephalus is an incidental finding on CT scans. Intracranial air is identified as foci of very low attenuation values on CT scans and as areas of absent signal on MR studies. Epidural air collection under a skull fracture is often found on CT scans. Epidural air tends to remain localized and does not change with alteration in head position. In this condition the dura mater is intact and no open head injury exists, so no CSF leakage should be expected. Subdural air often forms an air-fluid level and changes with head position. Subarachnoid air is multifocal and droplet shaped and often located within the cerebral sulci (Fig. 2.10). Intraventricular air is only seen with severe head trauma and is usually the result of extended skull base fractures.

Sometimes recurrent meningitis following head injury is the first sign of a compound skull base fracture. CSF leakage may be minimal and hardly evident in such cases. The incidence of CSF leakage is high after fractures of the paranasal sinuses, the leak usually developing after the brain swelling decreases and the blood in the paranasal sinuses regresses. CSF leakage may also occur following fractures of the temporal bone if communication develops between the subarachnoid space and the middle ear or the mastoid cells. Otorrhea indicates rupture of the tym-

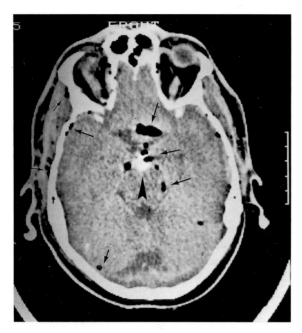

Fig. 2.10. Multiple subarachnoid air collections (*arrows*) indicate open head injury. Note subarachnoidal hemorrhage (*arrowhead*) and additional subcutaneous air collections (*small arrows*)

panic membrane whereas with an intact membrane the fluid will leak through the eustachian tube to the nasopharynx. CSF leakage following fractures of the paranasal sinuses is not likely to heal spontaneously if the rhinorrhea is persistent or recurrent. Fractures of the temporal bone with a CSF leak have a greater tendency to spontaneous closure and a period of initial waiting is justified.

The most difficult problem accompanying CSF leakage is identifying the site of the leak. The site of the fistula in traumatic rhinorrhea may be the frontal sinus, the ethmoidal sinuses, the cribriform plate, the sphenoidal sinus, or the petrous bone. The site of the leakage together with the possibility of bilateral occurrence is important for determining the surgical approach. Plain film radiography of the skull may reveal fracture lines through the paranasal sinuses in a small number of these cases. Demonstration of intracranial air is pathognomonic for a dural tear, but does not correlate with its location. The opacification of the paranasal sinuses or of the middle ear, and especially an air-fluid level, may give a hint as to the site of the leakage. Conventional tomography also often fails to disclose a convincing bone defect. Therefore it has been replaced by CT to demonstrate the site and extension of skull base fractures. CT is also superior for demonstrating opacification of paranasal sinuses and accumulation of intracranial

air. Axial slices are necessary to reveal defects of the posterior wall of the frontal sinus and of the lateral walls of the sphenoidal sinus, whereas coronal slices are better for delineation of defects of the roofs of the ethmoidal and sphenoidal sinuses and the cribriform plate.

In cases with extended fractures of the anterior and middle cranial fossae or in cases with rhinorrhea when no fracture is visible, a more precise localization of the leak is necessary. CT examination after intrathecal application of contrast agent can prove helpful. After lumbar puncture, 5–10 ml of a myelographic contrast agent is instilled and the patient is kept in a head-down position to allow entry of the contrast agent into the cerebral subarachnoid cisterns. The patient tries to provoke CSF leakage by coughing or pressing. Then CT cisternography can be performed with coronal sections of the paranasal sinuses. The site of the CSF leak is localized by (1) passage of contrast medium into the sinuses, (2) pooling of contrast medium in the sinuses, (3) bony or dural defect of the skull base, (4) soft tissue protrusion into the sinuses, or (5) deformity of the basal sulci (Fig. 2.11). CT cisternography is the most successful method for the examination of CSF

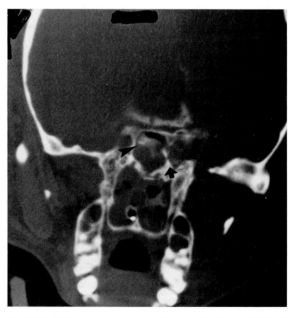

Fig. 2.11. Rhinorrhea. Coronal CT scan after intrathecal administration of contrast agent. A fracture of the lateral wall of the sphenoidal sinus (*arrow*) is demonstrated with air-fluid level within the sphenoidal sinus and pooling of contrast of the fluid collection (*arrowhead*). A small amount of contrast is seen in the left nose. Normal findings are a nasotracheal tube in the right nose and normal subarachnoid distribution of the contrast agent

liquorrhea and has replaced radionuclide cisternography. Adverse effects are seldom and consist of headaches, nausea, vomiting, and perceptual aberrations, depending on the amount and kind of contrast agent. A problem may arise in patients with intermittent liquorrhea examined in the so-called non-drop period. At that time there may be insufficient leakage of contrast agent into the paranasal sinuses, and only indirect signs such as bony defect, soft tissue prolapse or opacification of a sinus may indicate the site of the leak.

2.2.3.3 Posttraumatic Encephalocele

If the bony and meningeal disruption at the site of the basal skull fracture is sufficiently large, herniation of brain parenchyma into the defect can occur. These acquired cephaloceles can occur at any location but are most common in the basifrontal area. Such an encephalocele increases greatly the predisposition to intracranial infection. Detection with CT is easily accomplished and administration of intrathecal contrast agent is unnecessary. In some cases MRI may be preferred in order to demonstrate the herniated brain in pluridirectional sections. Often herniation or brain prolapse occurs into surgical trepanation defects of the calvaria after decompression of intracranial hematomas. CT will show not only the extent of prolapse but also adjacent parenchymal defects or porencephalic cysts.

2.2.3.4 Infection

Nowadays posttraumatic infection is not frequent. The risk is higher with penetrating head injuries and with fractures of the skull base and liquorrhea. Posttraumatic osteitis and osteomyelitis of the skull are uncommon diseases more likely to follow craniotomy than external compound fractures. Possible infections of the intracranial spaces are epidural empyema, subdural empyema, meningitis, and brain abscess. An epidural empyema usually arises after osteomyelitis, craniotomy, or infection of an epidural hematoma. A posttraumatic subdural empyema results from penetrating wounds, surgical procedures, or infection of subdural fluid collections. Meningitis and brain abscess are complications following open head injuries or neurosurgical procedures. Recurrent meningitis is a characteristic feature of CSF leakage, whereas posttraumatic brain abscess is more likely to be a consequence of an open head injury with intracranial organic material or foreign bodies or with broad open wounds. Posttraumatic ventriculitis may result from penetrating injuries, from retrograde extension of meningitis, from rupture of a cerebral abscess, or from surgical procedures, e.g., ventricular shunting. Radiological features in these cases do not differ from those of nontraumatic intracranial infection.

2.2.4 Vascular Injury

Trauma to the skull may cause damage to adjacent vascular structures. Direct damage to the great vessels is relatively rare following head trauma even for open penetrating injuries. Vascular trauma may present as transection or occlusion of arterial or venous vessels with disturbance of intracranial perfusion. Occasionally traumatic aneuryms or arteriovenous fistulae may develop following open or closed head injuries. Intracranial or cervical arterial dissection can lead to vessel occlusion either directly through narrowing of the lumen or by way of secondary emboli. Vascular damage may sometimes be clinically apparent, but often it is only detected after suspicions are aroused through CT scans, or when ischemic symptoms have presented. Angiography is required for a complete evaluation of these lesions in most cases and to determine the appropriate form of treatment.

2.2.4.1 Carotid Cavernous Sinus Fistula

A carotid cavernous sinus fistula represents an acquired intracranial arteriovenous shunt between the carotid artery and the cavernous sinus. Clinical findings are pulsating exophthalmos, pulse-synchronous intracranial bruit, palsy of cranial nerves III, IV, and VI, and chemosis of the eye. These fistulas are usually caused by major facial or craniocerebral trauma. The trauma may be blunt, with or without skull base fractures, or it may be penetrating from the orbita to the intracranial space.

Computed tomography provides a clue to this diagnosis when a fracture is seen traversing the sphenoid bone adjacent to the cavernous sinus. When the fistulous shunt has developed, CT shows bulging of the cavernous sinus, exophthalmos, and a dilated superior ophthalmic vein. MRI is superior to CT for visualization of the increased flow into the cavernous sinus, the distention of draining veins, and the

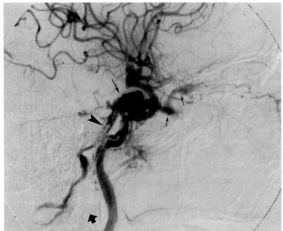

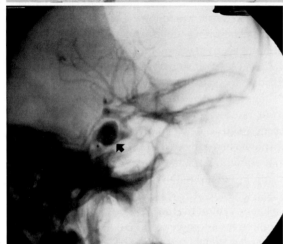

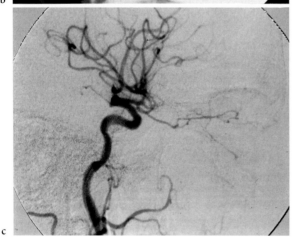

Fig. 2.12a–c. Carotid-cavernous fistula. **a** Angiography of the internal carotid artery shows simultaneously filling of the cavernous sinus (*large arrow*), the superior ophthalmic vein (*small arrows*), and the inferior petrosal sinus (*arrowhead*). **b** A detachable balloon (*arrow*) is placed and inflated within the cavernous sinus **c** Control angiography shows closure of the fistula and preservation of the carotid lumen

venous hypertension of the involved cerebral parenchyma. Angiographic evidence consists of early and dense opacification of the cavernous sinus, early filling of its draining veins (especially the superior ophthalmic vein), and poor opacification of cerebral vessels (Fig. 2.12a). It is important to perform angiography of both left and right carotid arteries and of the vertebrobasilar system. The pulsating exophthalmos may develop unilaterally (ipsilaterally or contralaterally), or bilaterally depending upon the venous outflow of the cavernous sinus. Bilateral carotid cavernous sinus fistulae may also occur. The fistula is usually supplied through a tear in the internal carotid artery; however, it may occasionally receive blood from branches of the internal or external carotid arteries or from the vertebrobasilar system via the posterior communicating artery. The venous drainage is primarily into the superior ophthalmic vein but also may extend into various venous outflows, including the contralateral cavernous sinus, the inferior ophthalmic vein, the pterygoid plexus, the sylvian veins, and the petrosal sinuses.

Nonsurgical, intravascular treatment is the method of first choice in these conditions. Closure of the fistula can be provided by means of detachable balloons or by coils delivered into the cavernous sinus (Fig. 2.12b). Preservation of the parent internal carotid artery can be achieved in most cases (Fig. 2.12c). If this is not feasible, the carotid artery may be occluded nonsurgically above and below the fistula using detachable balloons.

2.2.4.2 Dissection of Great Vessels

Rapid acceleration or deceleration of the skull can cause tears to the intima of major vascular structures. The most likely mechanism of injury is a sudden hyperextension or rotation of the head which leads to stretching of the internal carotid or vertebral arteries. It may be associated with fracture, dislocation, or subluxation of the cervical spine. Development of a subintimal or intramural hematoma results in vascular dissection. Besides trauma other factors such as hypertension, vascular diseases, drug abuse, or infection may play a role. Most commonly traumatic dissections involve the carotid artery beginning 2 cm distal to the carotid bifurcation and extending up to the skull base and the vertebral artery between the second cervical vertebra and the skull base. Arterial dissection can also occur with

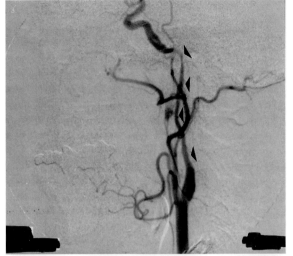

a

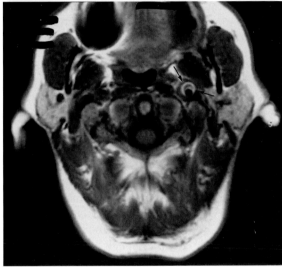

b

Fig. 2.13a,b. Dissection of the cervical internal carotid artery. **a** Angiography demonstrates long-distance narrowing of the lumen of the internal carotid artery (*arrowheads*). **b** MRI shows hematoma in the wall of the left internal carotid artery (*arrows*) with a peripherally high and centrally low signal intensity ring

minor trauma or no trauma at all. The dissection can resolve spontaneously, but may lead to peripheral embolization or total vascular occlusion. Clinical signs of vascular dissections are cerebral infarction with delayed onset, Horner's syndrome, and neck pain.

Angiographically the intimal flap is seen as a thin-lined negative structure within the contrast-filled lumen. Subsequent examinations often reveal narrowing and irregularity of the vascular lumen extending from the neck into the skull base and possibly further into the cranial vault (Fig. 2.13a).

Sometimes complete occlusion of the vessel will be present. CT or, preferably, MRI shows on the axial scans a narrowed vascular lumen with a surrounding ring-shaped thrombus, appearing hypodense on CT scans or hyperintense on MR images (Fig. 2.13b). MRI studies superior to the luminal injury will reveal an absent or asymmetric flow void of the involved artery. Intracranial scans may reveal areas of ischemia following embolization due to fragmentation of a thrombus. Fractures of the skull base or the cervical spine adjacent to the carotid canal or the foraminae transversariae of the cervical spine should be taken as a clue to vascular injury. Fat-suppressed axial T1-weighted images are highly sensitive for dissection. If MR findings confirm the clinically suggested dissection, angiography is not necessary in all cases.

2.2.4.3 Traumatic Pseudoaneurysms

Disruption of the vessel wall can also lead to traumatic aneurysm formation. A periarterial hematoma forms and is contained only by adjacent soft tissues and subsequent encapsulation. Traumatic aneurysms of the internal carotid artery occur in the petrous, cavernous, or supraclinoid segment of the vessel. The major clinical sign is severe recurrent epistaxis following nonpenetrating or penetrating head injury, often combined with monocular blindness and damage to the cranial nerves supplying the orbit. The bleeding may have a delayed onset and occurs through the sphenoidal sinus or the fractured skull base into the nasopharynx. Traumatic aneurysms of the petrous segment of the internal carotid artery may bleed via the eustachian tube into the nasopharynx and may be combined with auditory dysfunction and otorrhea. Traumatic aneurysms of the vertebral artery usually result from penetrating injuries but may also be caused by fractures of the cervical spine. In general, penetrating injuries, such as gunshot injury or injury through foreign bodies, may lead to laceration of a vessel, which in turn may cause occlusion, false aneurysms, or arteriovenous fistulae (Fig. 2.14a).

Although CT scans can suggest the presence of such damage, angiographic studies are mandatory to evaluate these lesions. On angiography, a traumatic pseudoaneurysm has an irregular contour and no or a broad-based aneurysmal neck (Fig. 2.14b). The pseudoaneurysm can thrombose spontaneously. The mass that is seen on CT or MRI will be considerably

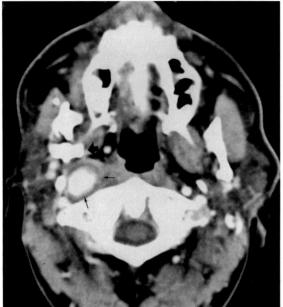

a

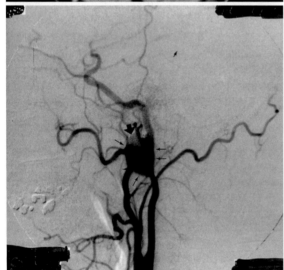

b

Fig. 2.14a,b. Traumatic aneurysm of the internal carotid artery as a sequela of a gunshot injury. **a** Aneurysmatic dilatation (*small arrows*) of the cervical carotid artery just behind the bullet (*thick arrow*) is demonstrated on axial contrast-enhanced CT scans. **b** Angiography of the common carotid artery, lateral view, confirms traumatic pseudoaneurysm of the cervical internal carotid artery

greater than the opacified lumen on angiography. The lesion is contiguous with the patent arterial lumen but projects outside the vessel wall. MRI is the best method for analyzing the size of the aneurysm, the degree of patency, the extent of the thrombus, and the relationship to the surrounding hematoma. Angiography, however, is still mandatory to plan surgical or endovascular procedures.

2.2.5 Traumatic Lesions of the Craniocervical Junction

2.2.5.1 Fractures

When evaluating trauma to the skull base the possibility that the craniocervical junction has also been injured must be considered. Linear fractures of the occipital bone are demonstrated adequately using conventional skull radiography; Towne's view, in particular, enables detection of occipital bone fractures extending to the foramen magnum. Fractures of the occipital condyle, however, should be evaluated using high-resolution CT with thin sections. CT has supplanted pluridirectional conventional tomography in detecting fractures of the occipital and temporal regions. CT has proven to be indispensable for evaluating fractures of the internal auditory canal, the jugular foramen, and the hypoglossal canal.

2.2.5.2 Atlanto-occipital Dislocation

Transverse CT scans may fail to show axial atlanto-occipital dislocation, whereby the empty articulation space between the occipital condyles and the lateral masses of the atlas is the only radiographic evidence of this dislocation. The separation between the skull and the cervical spine is seen to better advantage on lateral plain films or on the lateral scout view of the CT scan (Fig. 2.15). Although MRI demonstrates better the ligamentous disruption, the stretching of the vertebral arteries, and damage to the medulla oblongata or the cervical spinal cord, it cannot always be utilized. This injury has a very high mortality and patients are deeply comatose at the time of examination.

2.3 Brain

Head injury is categorized firstly clinically according to severity into three groups comprising mild, moderate, and severe head trauma. There is, however, a lack of clear and consistent definition. Mild head injury is a clinical syndrome exhibiting various single or combined symptoms such as transient alteration of consciousness, amnesia, and disturbances of vision, mobility, or sensation for a short period after the trauma. Severe head injury is defined as coma lasting 6 hours or longer, whereas moderate head trauma is used to describe conditions between

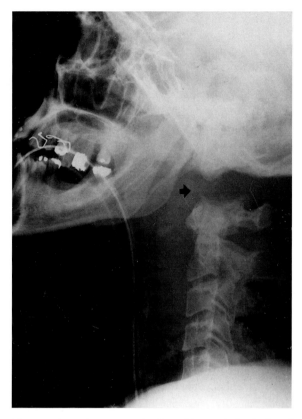

Fig. 2.15. Lateral x-ray examination of the cervical spinal cord with evident atlanto-occipital dislocation (*arrow*)

these two forms. Radiological findings do not, however, influence the clinical classification. Secondly, head injuries are classified into closed and open injuries depending upon the presence of a communication between the subarachnoid space and the outside. Thirdly, primary head injuries such as hematoma, contusion, and shearing injury are differentiated from secondary lesions such as infarction, swelling, thrombosis, and infection.

2.3.1 Extra-axial Lesions

Extra-axial fluid collections develop either from injuries of the brain parenchyma or from injuries of the surrounding bones, meninges, and vessels. Common to both epidural and subdural hematoma is an extra-axial collection of fluid which displaces the gray matter of the cortex inwards. If the space-occupying lesion is sufficiently large, secondary damage to the brain with midline shift, herniation, and ischemic brain damage may occur. Subarachnoid hemorrhage is a frequent extra-axial finding concomitant with cerebral contusions, which has, however, no space-

occupying effect. Intraventricular hemorrhage is also classified as extra-axial but is confined to the ventricular system.

2.3.1.1 Epidural Hematoma

Because of the firm attachment of the dura mater to the inner table of the skull, an epidural space does not exist under normal conditions. The vascular supply to the dura mater lies on the surface of the dura adjacent to the inner table of the skull. Fractures of the calvaria may lead to laceration of these vessels with arterial bleeding of sufficient pressure to strip the dura from the skull. Usually rapidly enlarging hematoma is the result but delayed onset of epidural hematomas is not uncommon. Arterial thrombosis and a tamponading effect through resistance of the underlying brain may limit this enlargement. The most common site of epidural hematoma is the temporoparietal region, the hematoma arising from laceration of the trunk of the middle meningeal artery or of its anterior or posterior branch. Skull fractures are found in almost all patients exhibiting epidural hematoma. In young children, however, the periosteum can separate from the inner table and blood may collect in the epidural space without the necessity of a fracture. Epidural hematomas are found less commonly at the frontal pole, in the parieto-occipital region, high convex in the midline, or in the posterior fossa. Epidural hematomas in these locations are most often of venous origin, deriving from fractures which disrupt the superior sagittal sinus, the torcular Herophili, or the lateral sinuses (Fig. 2.16). Whereas in the supratentorial region subdural hematoma is much more common than epidural hematoma, in the posterior fossa epidural hematoma predominates.

Epidural hematoma occurs in approximately 10% of all patients with severe head trauma. It is less common in infants and elderly persons. Clinical features are loss of consciousness or worsening of coma grade due to secondary compression of the brain. Frequently there is no evidence of brain injury. After a minor head trauma these patients are awake – the so-called lucid interval. If the epidural hematoma remains undiagnosed and untreated they may deteriorate with headache and rapid loss of consciousness. Ipsilateral oculomotor nerve palsy and contralateral hemiparesis or extension spasms indicate tentorial herniation with compression of the midbrain. The mortality of surgically treated

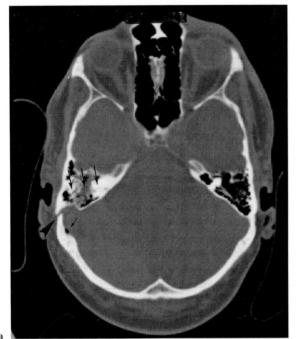

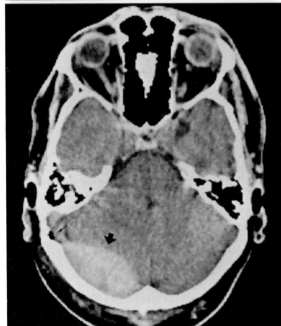

Fig. 2.16a,b. Venous epidural hematoma of the posterior fossa. a CT scan with a bony window demonstrates fracture through the sulcus sigmoideus (*arrowhead*), additional fracture of the petrous bone (*large arrows*), and a small epidural air accumulation (*small arrow*). b The soft tissue window shows adjacent epidural hematoma (*arrow*)

epidural hematomas has dropped from 30% to 5%–10% since the advent of CT. This emphasizes the need for an early diagnosis and for early surgical treatment.

Epidural hematoma presents on CT scans as a high-density lenticular-shaped collection of blood beneath the inner table of the calvaria (Fig. 2.17). Since the dura is still attached at the margins, the hematoma does not freely communicate over the cerebral hemisphere. An exception is epidural hematomas in the sagittal region, which can cross the midline and may have ill-defined margins. It is not, however, always possible to localize extra-axial hematomas as belonging to the epi- or subdural space (Fig. 2.18). Furthermore the coincidence of epidural and subdural hematoma is not uncommon, either unilaterally or contralaterally. There may be lucent areas within the acute hematoma representing unclotted blood (Fig. 2.19). Radiolucent areas or encased air bubbles within an epidural hematoma are considered a sign of instability and a warning that the hematoma may enlarge. After the peracute phase the entire hematoma will appear as a homogeneous hyperdense collection. In cases of chronic epidural hematoma the density of the collection decreases according to organization and resorption of blood elements. The displaced dura will demonstrate contrast enhancement similar to the rim enhancement of the capsule in subdural hematomas. Distinguishing chronic epidural from chronic subdural hematomas can therefore be difficult. The fracture itself may be visible in the bony

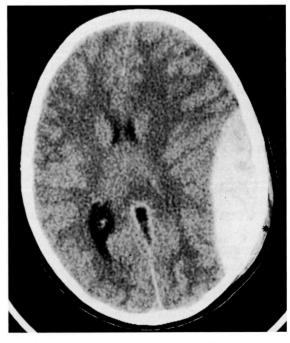

Fig. 2.17. Epidural hematoma with typical lenticular shape and midline shift. There is an overlying scalp injury (*asterisk*)

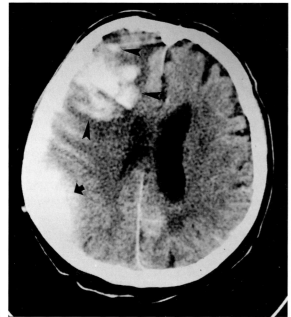

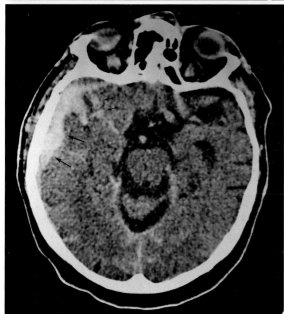

Fig. 2.18. Combination of epidural hematoma (*thick arrow*) with contusions (*arrowheads*) (**a**), subdural hematoma (*thin large arrows*), and subarachnoid hemorrhage (*thin small arrows*) (**b**)

window of the CT scans. Skull radiography which demonstrates a skull fracture crossing the vascular groove of the middle meningeal artery points to the possibility of an epidural hematoma. A more or less prominent displacement of the adjacent brain tissue is another sign of extracerebral hematomas on CT. Hemorrhagic contusions and cerebral swelling may contribute substantially to the mass effects of the hematoma. If an acute epidural hematoma has been the only traumatic lesion, CT most often shows return of the ventricle system to the midline following evacuation of the hematoma. However, in cases with associated subdural hematoma, cerebral contusions, or cerebral swelling, the midline shift may still remain postoperatively evident and parenchymal lesions will become more apparent. The advent of CT scanning has shown that not all epidural hematomas are of clinical significance. Frequently a small biconvex-shaped blood collection is visible under the course of a skull fracture. These fracture hematomas require clinical and CT follow-up but usually undergo resorption without surgical treatment (Fig. 2.20). CT is the most effective diagnostic method in demonstrating epidural hematomas. If MRI is nevertheless performed, epidural hematoma usually shows an increased signal intensity on both T1- and T2-weighted images, with the dura appearing as a low signal intensity rim outlining the periphery of the hematoma.

2.3.1.2 Subdural Hematoma

Subdural hematoma is the most common posttraumatic intracranial hematoma. The subdural space is

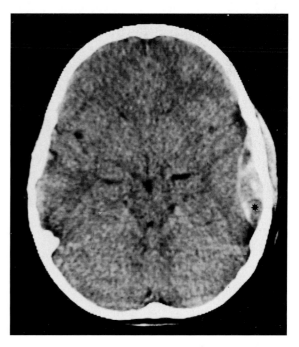

Fig. 2.19. Hyperacute epidural hematoma with hypodense areas (*asterisk*) representing unclotted blood or active bleeding

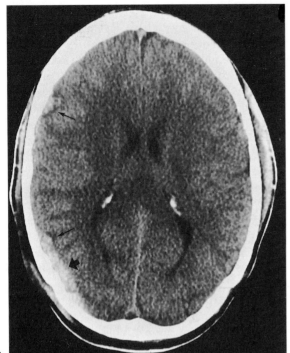

a

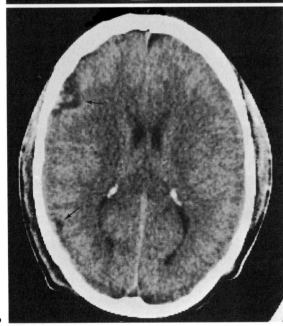

b

Fig. 2.20. a Small epidural ("fracture") hematoma (*arrow*) with two contusions (*small arrows*). **b** Follow-up CT shows resorption of the epidural hematoma and more clearly visible contusions

the room between the dura mater and the leptomeninges. Subdural hematoma may be classified as either acute, subacute, or chronic according to clinical, pathological, radiological, and traditional criteria. Unfortunately, no precise nomenclature exists and classification solely on the basis of the attenuation values of CT scanning allows only a rough correlation. Some authors divide subdural hematomas only into acute and chronic categories, which are easier to differentiate according to clinical and radiographic features. In addition, subdural hematomas can be classified as complicated or simple according to the presence or absence of accompanying parenchymal injury. Complicated subdural hematomas are those arising from cerebral injury. Acute subdural bleeding may be combined with other intracranial hematomas, such as epidural, intracerebral, or chronic subdural hematomas.

2.3.1.3 Acute Subdural Hematoma

Acute subdural hematoma follows severe head trauma in up to 20% of cases and usually presents within hours after injury. Rarely, delayed manifestation of up to 1 week can occur. Acute subdural hematoma is nearly always associated with underlying brain injury. The blood most commonly derives from damage to cortical or subcortical vessels, not only from bridging veins but also from arterial feeders. Occasionally, however, an expanding intracerebral hematoma may rupture into the subdural space and thereby become a subdural hematoma, often in the coup or contrecoup location. Patients with acute subdural hematoma are usually comatose and may show hemiparesis or decerebrate signs. Morbidity and mortality are higher than with other posttraumatic lesions. The mortality ranges from 50% to 90% correlating with the patient's preoperative neurological status. In children acute subdural hematoma may occur following ventricular shunting for hydrocephalus or other congenital brain anomalies. This is a consequence of sudden collapse of the brain with rupture of bridging veins, though clinical symptoms may be only minimal or absent.

Acute subdural hematoma appears on CT as a peripheral collection of blood lying between the inner table of the skull and the cerebral hemisphere. The majority of subdural hematomas are located over the cerebral convexity. These accumulations vary from small to very large amounts of blood. Because there is free communication within the subdural space, the hemispheres may be surrounded with hematoma from front to back and from top to bottom. Frequently blood extends into the interhemispheric fissure and above or beneath the tentorium. Sometimes subdural hematomas arise in

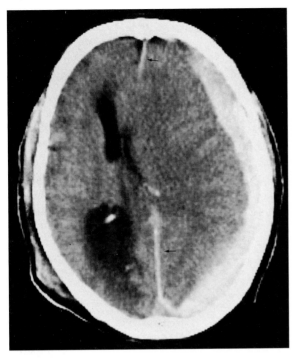

Fig. 2.21. Acute subdural hematoma with typical crescent shape, midline shift, and dilatation of the contralateral ventricle, and subarachnoid hemorrhage in the interhemispheric fissure (*small arrows*)

atypical locations such as subfrontal, subtemporal, or infratentorial. Subdural hematoma presents as a hyperdense fluid collection with a crescent shape (Fig. 2.21). Sometimes, however, the extracerebral accumulation of blood is so small that it is barely visible on CT scans. In these cases a substantial mass effect with sulcal effacement, cerebral swelling, and ventricular shift may nonetheless be evident. Midline displacement may appear with ipsilateral ventricular compression and contralateral dilatation. The mass effect, however, is due not only to the hematoma itself but also to associated cerebral contusion and swelling. If an expected corresponding midline shift is not identified, one should suspect a contralateral mass lesion the mass effect of which blocks the midline structures from shifting. Frequently parenchymal injuries become visible following surgical evacuation of the hematoma (Fig. 2.22). These injuries often demonstrate an increasing mass effect resulting in herniation of brain tissue through the postoperative bony defect. On CT scans acute subdural hematomas may appear iso- or hypointense due to several possible factors: presence of active bleeding, low blood hemoglobin, coagulopathy, mixing of subdural blood with cerebrospinal fluid, or serum extrusion during

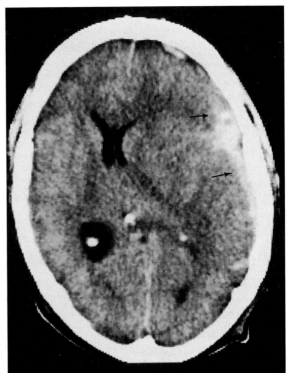

a

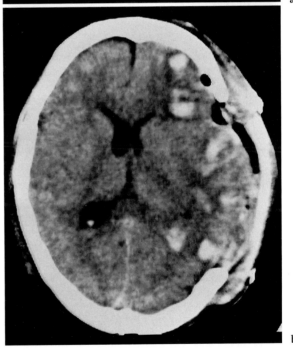

b

Fig. 2.22. a Smaller acute subdural hematoma (*arrows*) with midline shift. b Postoperative control demonstrates multiple contusions, intracerebral hematomas of the left hemisphere, intraventricular hemorrhage, and herniation through the postoperative bony defect

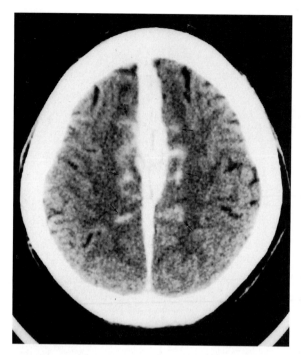

Fig. 2.23. Acute interhemispheric subdural hematoma in an elderly person. Adjacent subarachnoid hemorrhage (*small arrows*)

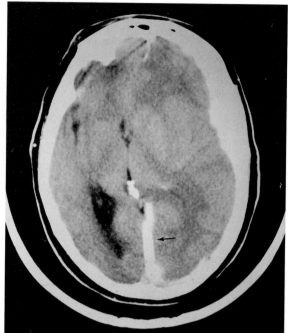

a

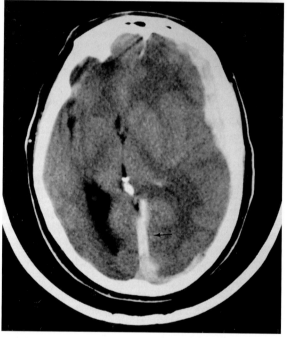

b

Fig. 2.24. a Acute subdural hematoma with extension into the posterior interhemispheric fissure (*arrow*) **b** Image with increased window width and level, better delineating hematoma from the skull

the early phase of clot retraction. Additionally there may appear horizontal fluid phenomena (hematocrit level) due to sedimentation of blood components if the patient has remained supine for a prolonged period. Sometimes an acute subdural hematoma is found to be located predominantly within the interhemispheric fissure. Blood derives in these cases from rupture of bridging veins (Fig. 2.23).

Plain film radiography may or may not reveal a skull fracture. A shift of the calcified pineal gland can sometimes be detected. This sign, however, is absent if bilateral subdural accumulations or contralateral edema exist, or when hematoma develops in the posterior fossa. CT scanning should be performed using varying window widths and levels, not only to show skull fractures, but also to better delineate the hyperdense hematoma between the cerebral cortex and the inner table of the skull (Fig. 2.24).

2.3.1.4 Subacute Subdural Hematoma

The subacute stage of a subdural hematoma lies 1–3 weeks following trauma. Larger acute subdural hematomas are usually evacuated surgically. Smaller

subdural hematomas demonstrate an evolution towards spontaneous volume decrease or disappearance. Development from an acute subdural hematoma into a chronic subdural hematoma is therefore unusual. In the first week following injury a gradual density decrease occurs within the hematoma. The subdural accumulation will be less crescentic and more lentiform, mimicking the shape of an epidural hematoma. A hematocrit effect may be seen.

2.3.1.5 Chronic Subdural Hematoma

Chronic subdural hematomas are thought to arise through a slow effusion of venous blood into the subdural space over a period of weeks to months. They are not usually a result of focal cerebral parenchymal injury. A history of trauma may be completely lacking or the injury may have been quite minor. Membranes develop differently on the dural and the arachnoid sides of the hematoma. The dural membrane is vascular with fragile vessels giving rise to multiple episodes of rebleeding at minor injuries. The exact pathogenesis of a chronic subdural hematoma is unclear because small acute subdural hematomas are resorbed completely and do not evolve to the chronic stage. Chronic subdural hematomas are common in the elderly and in patients with cerebral atrophy, chronic alcoholism, or coagulopathy. The clinical signs are headaches, gradual onset of neurological deficits, epilepsy, disorientation, or gradual loss of consciousness.

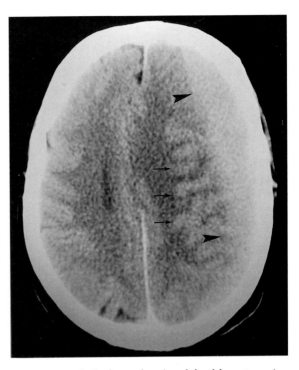

Fig. 2.26. Nearly isodense chronic subdural hematoma (*arrowheads*) recognized by inward shift of the corticomedullary junction (*arrows*)

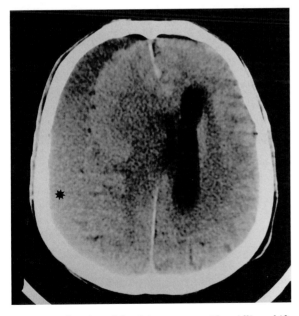

Fig. 2.25. Chronic subdural hematoma with midline shift. Note sedimentation of hyperdense blood products (*asterisk*) in the posterior portion

A chronic subdural hematoma can present with low density, high density, or isodensity on CT scans depending upon the interval since the last episode of bleeding. The fluid usually appears hypodense relative to the brain parenchyma, and only slightly denser than CSF. Fresh blood elements are hyperdense and gravitate to the more dependent portion of the hematoma (Fig. 2.25). A fluid level with increased density in the dependent portion and low density in the upper portion may therefore develop. Formation of compartments with fibrous septa is possible with differing densities in the various compartments. The hematoma tends to conform to the convexity of the brain, but a biconvex lenticular configuration is also possible. Isodense hematomas can be recognized indirectly through midline shift, displacement of the ventricles, inward displacement of the gray-white matter interface, compression of the sulci, or inward displacement of cortical veins (Fig. 2.26). Chronic subdural hematomas are found bilaterally in 25% of all cases (Fig. 2.27). If they are isodense, this can be difficult to detect on CT scans. A characteristic feature is, however, the symmetrical compression of the anterior horns of the lateral ventricles, resembling "rabbit ears." Contrast media enhancement of hematoma

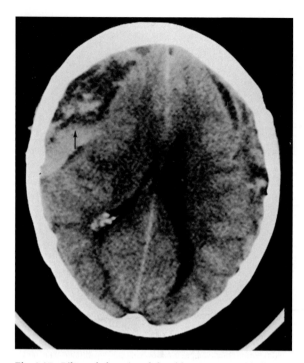

Fig. 2.27. Bilateral chronic subdural hematomas with "hematocrit" level on the right side (*arrow*) and multiple septations of both hematomas

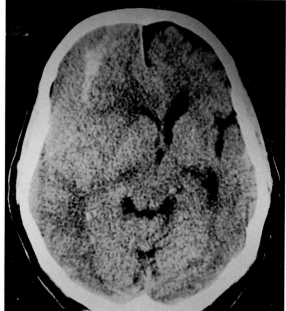

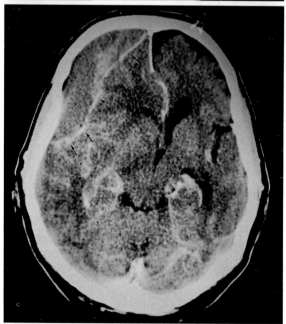

Fig. 2.28a,b. Chronic subdural hematoma. **a** Unenhanced CT scan and **b** enhancing membrane (*small arrows*) following contrast administration

membranes and of shifted cortical blood vessels also allows delimitation of the hematoma (Fig. 2.28). Chronic subdural hematomas may occasionally show calcification, particularly following shunting of hydrocephalus.

Under certain circumstances MRI images are very helpful to identify the exact location of blood accumulation because hematomas present with high signal intensity on T1-weighted images. MRI is particularly successful in showing smaller collections of blood below the tentorium, over the convexity, and under the temporal or occipital lobes (Fig. 2.29). The decrease in high signal intensity on T1-weighted images occurs more rapidly, however, with chronic subdural hematomas than with intracerebral hematomas. This is a consequence of dilution, absorption, and degrading of hemoglobin. The remaining signal intensity of the subdural fluid collection depends upon its protein content. Consequently, 30% of chronic subdural hematomas are iso- or hypointense compared to CSF on T1-weighted MRI studies. On T2-weighted images most chronic subdural hematomas are hyperintense and are without hemosiderin deposition. MRI can also show layering effects of the hematoma which are best demonstrated on T2-weighted images. When repeated hemorrhage has occurred, the MRI scans reveal multiple compartments composed of acute, subacute, and chronic hemorrhage.

Following evacuation of chronic subdural hematomas, the subdural space remains enlarged and the brain remains displaced. There is only a gradual return of the brain to its normal contour, leaving sufficient subdural space for possible repeated accumulation of fluid.

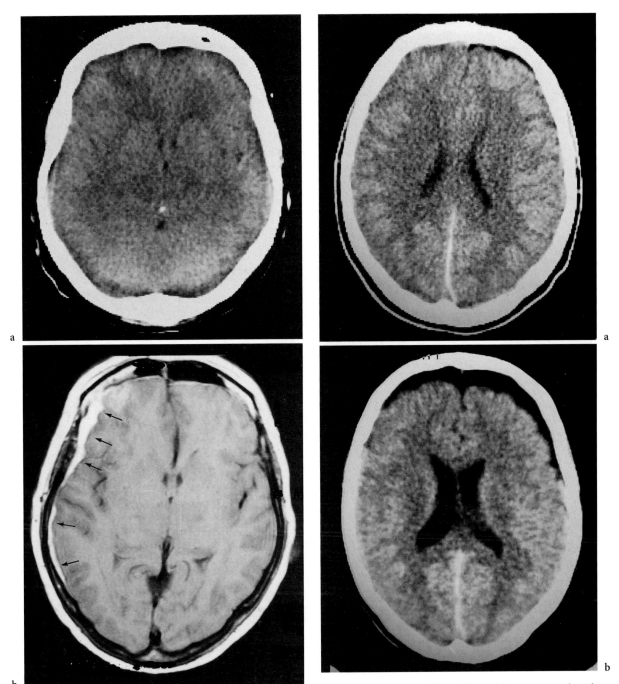

Fig. 2.29. Subacute subdural hematoma not visible on nonenhanced CT scan (a) but clearly visible on the T1-weighted MR image (*arrows*) (b)

Fig. 2.30. Evolution of bilateral frontal hygromas on the 5th (a) and 15th days (b) after head injury. Note concomitant widening of the ventricular system

2.3.1.6 Subdural Effusion (Hygroma)

Subdural effusions (hygromas) occur frequently following head injuries. The mechanism is not well understood. Apparently, a tear occurs in the arachnoid membrane with a valve mechanism allowing CSF to enter the subdural space, resulting in extracerebral accumulation. Subdural hygromas usually present when the cerebral contusion and the swelling are resolving, most commonly at the end of the first week (Fig. 2.30). The clinical signs of subdural hygromas may be the same as those for subacute subdural

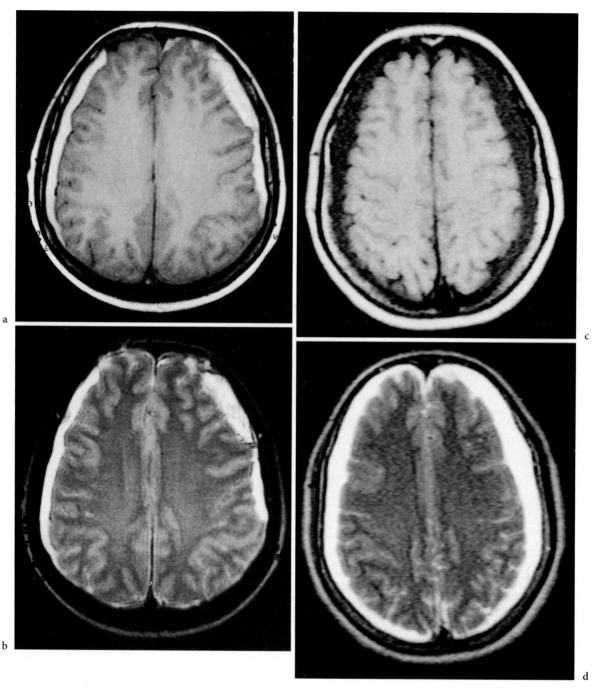

Fig. 2.31a–d. Bilateral subdural hygroma and hematoma. Compare the high signal of the hematoma on the T1-weighted MR image (a) and the discrete less bright signal intensity on the T2-weighted image (b), with CSF-like signal intensity of the hygromas on both T1- (c) and T2-weighted images (d)

hematomas. In most cases, however, the symptoms will be masked by those resulting from the primary brain injury. Therefore these effusions often appear clinically silent. The extracerebral fluid collections usually reabsorb spontaneously and can be managed conservatively. In patients with symptomatic hygromas, however, improvement is achieved through drainage of the hygroma.

Hygromas present on CT scans as crescentic extracerebral fluid collections over one or both hemispheres and may extend into the interhemispheric fissure. Major cortical sulci are usually preserved and there is only a mild mass effect. Subdural hygromas show low attenuation values and may be indistinguishable from chronic subdural hematomas. The attenuation values of hygroma fluid are very similar to those of ventricular CSF, whereas chronic hematomas present slightly higher density on CT scans. MRI often permits better differentiation between these two lesions. The signal intensity of a subdural hygroma resembles the signal intensity of cerebrospinal fluid, whereas a chronic subdural hematoma appears brighter than CSF on all pulse sequences (Fig. 2.31).

2.3.1.7 Subarachnoid Hemorrhage

Subarachnoid hemorrhage (SAH) is a frequent finding following brain injuries. In most cases, however, it can be considered clinically insignificant. SAH derives from injury to small cortical veins passing through the subarachnoid space. It is found in closed head injuries, with or without skull fracture. In addition it often occurs in conjunction with cerebral contusions, hematomas, penetrating brain injuries, and intraventricular hemorrhage. The most common complication of SAH is communicating hydrocephalus due to obliteration of the pacchionian granulations and decreased resorption of CSF.

On CT scans SAH appears as serpentine linear areas of high attenuation filling out the sulci and cisterns, e.g., within the interpeduncular cistern or the sylvian fissure. Traumatic SAH within the basal cisterns and the sylvian fissure may resemble hemorrhage following rupture of an aneurysm. Traumatic SAH, however, is more often focal and found adjacent to the site of contusion as well as collecting in the interhemispheric fissure and along the tentorium (Fig. 2.32). The normal falx or calcification of the falx may be mistaken for SAH. Increased density due to SAH adjacent to the falx or to the tentorium disappears, however, within a week following injury. The subarachnoid blood becomes progressively less visible over time through decrease in attenuation. The cisterns, fissures, and sulci will appear to be obliterated, mimicking brain edema, during that time interval when the SAH attenuation is isodense to brain. In addition SAH into a preexisting arachnoid cyst can be confused with an epidural hematoma or hemorrhagic intracerebral neoplasm. Finally, posterior interhemispheric SAH can mimic the "empty delta sign" and should not be mistaken for dural sinus thrombosis.

Acute SAH cannot be reliably imaged using MRI; rather, CT is the method of choice. In subacute and chronic stages, however, MRI has been shown to be superior. Increased signal intensity can be noted within the cisternal spaces on T1-weighted images during the subacute stage of an SAH. During the chronic stage superficial hemosiderosis appears as a thin layer of signal loss surrounding the subarachnoid spaces and is best demonstrated on T2-weighted images.

2.3.1.8 Intraventricular Hemorrhage

Intraventricular hemorrhage may arise through rupture of an intracerebral hematoma into the ventricular system, shearing injury of subependymal veins, reflux of subarachnoidal blood, or penetrating head injury. Traumatic intraventricular hemorrhage is relatively uncommon and usually indicates severe head injury. CT may show a varying amount of blood in the ventricles; in mild cases there is only a faintly hyperdense blood level in the occipital horns (Fig. 2.33). Sometimes rounded blood clots can be seen in the lateral ventricle, which disappear subsequently

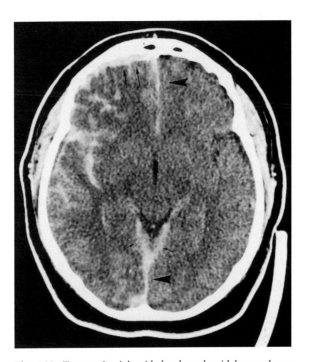

Fig. 2.32. Traumatic right-sided subarachnoid hemorrhage. There is also subarachnoid hemorrhage in the interhemispheric fissure (*arrowheads*) and along the tentorium (*small arrows*), as well as a small frontal subdural hematoma (*large arrows*)

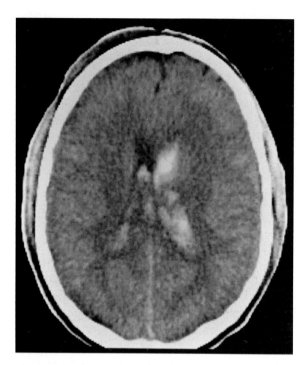

Fig. 2.33. Traumatic intraventricular hemorrhage in both lateral ventricles, which is more extended on the left side

on follow-up examinations. Occasionally a focal hemorrhage into the choroid plexus can be identified. MRI demonstrates fluid levels within the ventricle or complete filling of the ventricle with material differing in signal intensity from that of CSF. Intraventricular hemorrhage may cause ependymal proliferation with subsequent stenosis or occlusion of the cerebral aqueduct leading to occlusive hydrocephalus.

2.3.2 Intra-axial Lesions

2.3.2.1 Cerebral Contusions

Contusions are traumatic lesions of the cerebral cortex and underlying white matter characterized by hemorrhages and mechanical damage. With increased severity of the injury, hemorrhages coalesce into a focal rounded hematoma. Therefore, a contusion and a hematoma are often not distinct entities. Some authors distinguish between lacerations (cut or torn tissue) and contusions (bruised tissue). Contusions occur when the cerebral parenchyma strikes the skull or when the skull is pushed inward and strikes the brain. Contusions are the most frequent traumatic parenchymal lesions seen on CT and are found in about half of all patients with severe head trauma. They are often multiple and they are often

associated with other intracranial hematomas, especially subdural hematoma, but sometimes also with diffuse axonal injury or with brain stem trauma. Hemorrhagic contusions and intracerebral hematomas show a delayed evolution in severe head trauma, either increasing in size or appearing as new lesions within the first 12 h. Coup contusions result at the site of the direct trauma. They are found in the temporal, frontal, parasagittal, or occipital regions. Such contusions develop when, for example, the brain scrapes across the orbital roof, the cribriform plate, the sphenoid wings, or locations with a relatively fixed dura, e.g., the arachnoid granulations. Typical locations are the temporal tip, the inferior temporal and frontal surfaces, the frontal poles, and the cortex around the sylvian fissure. Contrecoup contusions occur at a site remote from the point of impact, e.g., contralateral temporal contusions or frontal contusions after occipital trauma (Fig. 2.34). Fracture contusions occur beneath skull fractures, especially beneath depressed fractures (Fig. 2.6a). Cerebellar contusions are relatively rare, despite the frequency of occipital fractures. Clinically, contusions may present with confusion, unconsciousness, focal cerebral dysfunction, or seizures. They may, however, also present without neurological deficits.

Computed tomography is the modality with which cerebral contusions are most often first detected. Contusions can be superficial within the cerebral cortex but often also extend into the white matter. On CT scans they are most frequently hemorrhagic with ill-defined areas of increased and decreased density (Fig. 2.35). CT is limited in its ability to reveal all contusions. They may be too small or too superficially situated to be visible or they may present with only a minimal hemorrhage. Sometimes they are obscured by artifacts or through value averaging of the adjacent bone. MRI is able to reveal contusions that CT does not detect; this, however, usually has little clinical significance.

Contusions develop through a series of phases. In the acute phase CT shows a hemorrhagic mass of increased density mixed with areas of decreased density representing necrosis or edema. There is only a mild mass effect in the first 3 days. In the second phase, edema develops between the fourth and the seventh day. The contusion may present a decreased density on CT examination, but swelling and edema produce an increasing mass effect (Fig. 2.36). Some contusions that escaped prior CT detection may now become visible. The third phase is characterized by disturbance of the blood-brain barrier. CT shows the contusion as an isodense area with decreasing mass

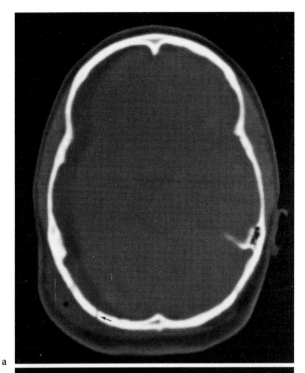

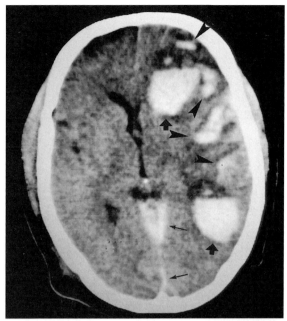

Fig. 2.35. Multiple cerebral contusions (*arrowheads*) of the left hemisphere concomitant with two larger intracerebral hematomas (*thick arrows*) showing fluid levels and subarachnoid hemorrhage (*small arrows*)

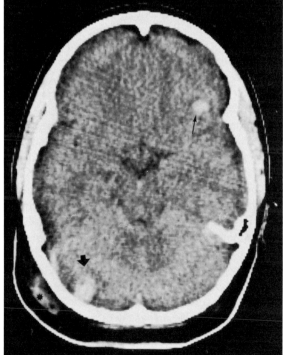

a

b

Fig. 2.34. Right occipital skull fracture (*arrow*) (**a**) with overlying soft tissue swelling (*asterisk*) and underlying coup contusion (*thick arrow*) and left frontal contrecoup contusion (*small arrow*) (**b**)

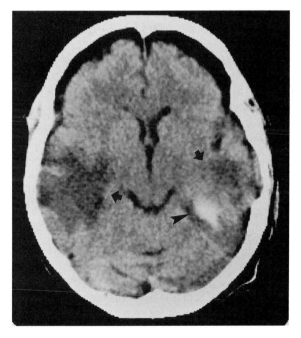

Fig. 2.36. Edematous phase of bilateral temporal contusions (*arrows*). The blood on the left side is a remnant of a subdural hematoma (*arrowhead*); bifrontal hygromas are present

effect. Intravenous administration of contrast agents reveals enhancement at the site of contusion similar to that observed with cerebral infarcts. The history of previous injury with resolving contusions prevents

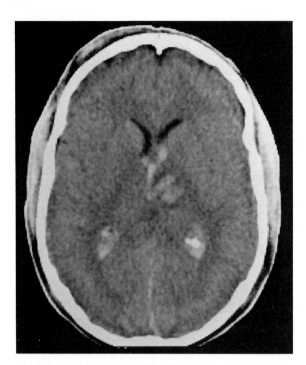

Fig. 2.37. Traumatic intracerebral hematoma of the left thalamus and intraventricular hemorrhage

the possibility of mistaking these areas of enhancement for infection, cerebral infarct, or tumor. Contrast-enhanced CT studies, however, are only important to rule out infection of the brain for patients with open head injuries or with fractures of the skull base. Apart from this, contrast enhancement is usually not necessary for evaluation of acute head injuries. In the final stage of cerebral contusions, cystic cavities are formed within the brain parenchyma, presenting with CSF density and often leading to enlargement of cortical gyri and adjacent ventricular structures. T2-weighted MRI studies may show cystic cavities with surrounding gliosis and deposition of hemosiderin.

2.3.2.2 Intracerebral Hematoma

Intracerebral hematoma is due to blood vessel rupture and bleeding into the white matter of the brain. The frontal and temporal lobes are predominantly involved. The hematoma may rupture into the ventricular system or the subarachnoid space. Intracerebral hematomas occur significantly less frequently than contusions. Like contusions, they may be associated with other traumatic lesions and may occur bilaterally. A solitary traumatic intracerebral

hematoma is indistinguishable from spontaneous hemorrhage and angiography may be required to exclude a primary vascular lesion (Fig. 2.37). A traumatic intracerebral hematoma generally develops within 4–24h following trauma; however, some intracerebral hematomas present after a delay of up to 7 days following head injury. They occur at sites of contusion or of parenchymal ischemia and sometimes after removal of an extracerebral hematoma. Delayed intracerebral hematoma is an important cause of secondary deterioration in conjunction with head injury.

On CT examination intracerebral hematomas appear as well-defined, rounded areas of increased density from 50 to 80 Hounsfield units. A fluid level can occasionally be identified within the hematoma, analogous to the hematocrit effect within an extracerebral hematoma (Fig. 2.35). A rim of decreased density may represent extravasation of serum or small edema. In the first week the edema and the mass effect tend to increase. In the following weeks the hematoma decreases in size and mass effect. The density values change progressively from hyper- to iso- and subsequently to hypodense. The resorption of the hematoma occurs slowly over a prolonged period. Contrast enhancement of a peripheral rim around the resolving hematoma can usually be demonstrated on CT. Without an accurate history it may not be possible to differentiate a ring-enhancing hematoma from a neoplasm, abscess, or infarction. Late follow-up CT studies in cases of intracerebral hematoma may show a cavity with CSF density and with dilatation of the adjacent ventricular system and overlying cortical sulci.

The role of MRI in the management of acute head injuries remains secondary. Limited availability of MRI, long scanning times, and difficulties in utilizing life support systems under MR field strengths are only part of the problem. Experience with MRI to date suggests that acute extra- or intracerebral collections of blood following trauma are only difficult to visualize on early MR scans. Because of its sensitivity for the presence of blood, either intra- or extracerebrally, CT remains the imaging technique of choice. MRI, on the other hand, is more sensitive than any other diagnostic method in demonstrating subacute and chronic hemorrhagic lesions as well as all nonhemorrhagic lesions which may follow head injury. This advantage should find increased utilization in patients in whom CT provides unremarkable findings after head injury.

In the very acute stage (1–2h following trauma) the MR signal intensity is similar to edema. In the acute stage (2–12h) the hematoma is isointense or slightly hypointense on T1-weighted images and markedly hypointense on T2-weighted images. In the subacute stage (3 days to 1 month) the outer portion of the hematoma appears with high signal intensity on the T1-weighted images. The hyperintensity extends gradually over time inwardly to involve the entire hematoma. Finally it shows high signal intensity on both T1- and T2-weighted images. The chronic stage (1 month and onwards) is characterized by CSF-filled cavities surrounded by a ring of low intensity on T2-weighted images and of isointensity or low intensity on T1-weighted images (Fig. 2.47b). Although subdural and epidural hematomas behave similarly, their appearance may be modified throughout the above stages by a decreased resorption and varying degrees of liquefaction. Acute subarachnoid hemorrhage may not be discernible from CSF on MR scans.

2.3.2.3 Brain Swelling

Increased intracranial pressure is considered to be the most important factor causing secondary brain injury. Cerebral swelling is characterized by an increase in brain volume due to cerebral hyperemia and consequent cerebral edema. Brain injury may lead to disturbance of the blood-brain barrier, of cerebral blood flow and autoregulation, and of cerebral metabolism. The result is cerebral hyperemia and edema. Cerebral edema accompanies all forms of acute cerebral injuries. Focal brain swelling appears on CT as ill-defined zones of low attenuation with an associated mass effect. Unilateral brain swelling is often seen with subdural hematomas, intracerebral hematomas, or multiple contusions.

Bilateral generalized cerebral swelling can occur by itself following trauma without other forms of brain injury. This results in stiffening of the brain and diminution of the CSF spaces. All types of edema can occur following head trauma, vasogenic edema being the most common. Traumatic hyperemic brain swelling is seen in 10%–20% of severe brain injuries. It usually develops within the first 2 days and is more common in children than in adults. Clinical findings are impairment of consciousness, coma, or decerebrate status with a mortality of up to 50%.

Acute bilateral cerebral swelling is best demonstrated on CT scans. It manifests as compression or obliteration of the lateral and third ventricles and the perimesencephalic cisterns; cortical sulci, cerebral fissures, and basilar cisterns are effaced (Fig. 2.38).

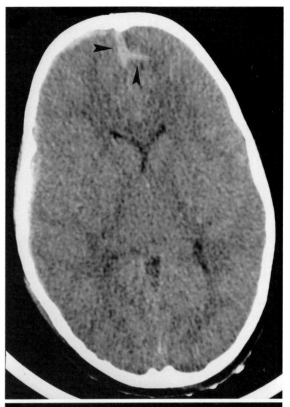

a

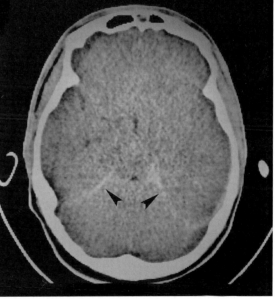

b

Fig. 2.38. a Bilateral brain swelling demonstrated by diffuse hypodensity of the hemispheres and compression of the ventricular system. Additional subarachnoid hemorrhage is present (*arrowheads*). **b** A different case with bilateral brain swelling shows narrowing of the basal cisterns and subarachnoid hemorrhage (*arrowheads*)

The cerebral surface appears to be flattened and discrimination between gray and white matter is poor. The dural sinuses may appear slightly hyperdense on noncontrast scans. The cerebral hemispheres typically exhibit homogeneous decreased attenuation values. Changes due to minor swelling, however, may be difficult to assess, especially in children. Diagnosis of brain swelling therefore can only be considered after taking into account the range of normal variance, the slice thickness and volume averaging, and the clinical manifestations. Often diagnosis becomes sure only after follow-up studies have shown that ventricles and cisterns have returned to normal size. Following resorption of cerebral edema, transient enlargement of the subarachnoid space and collection of extracerebral fluid may also occur.

2.3.2.4 Diffuse Axonal Injury (Shearing Injury)

Rapid acceleration or deceleration of the brain can give rise to shearing stress along the white matter axons within the cerebral parenchyma. Disruption of axons may occur through which small blood vessels are lacerated. Multiple and usually minor hemorrhages result at typical sites along gray/white matter junction zones centrally and peripherally. Such hemorrhages may be delayed, occurring hours or even days after injury. These patients are typically unconscious from the moment of traumatic impact, whereby, however, CT scans reveal only minor lesions, if any. Diffuse axonal injury is believed to be present in about half the cases with severe closed head injury. Clinical findings are coma with minimally or nonreacting pupils, hemiparesis, tetraparesis, or decerebrate posturing. When patients survive, they often suffer from neurological and mental deficits.

Subtle changes may be present on CT scans, such as blood in the subarachnoid space, blood in the lateral ventricles, rounded or oval areas of hemorrhage at the gray/white matter junction zones, and small lateral ventricles produced by edema (Fig. 2.39). Most characteristic of diffuse axonal injury are small hemorrhages that occur at the gray-white matter interface of the hemispheres, in the corpus callosum, the upper brain stem, the cerebellar peduncles, and the internal capsule. Three areas of the brain are known as the "shearing injury triad": the lobar white matter, the corpus callosum, and the upper brain stem. Lobar white matter injury appears as multiple small focal ovoid lesions with long axes parallel to

the direction of the affected axons within the subcortical white matter. Shearing injury to the corpus callosum most often occurs at the splenium, presenting as a focal midline hemorrhagic lesion. Brain stem axonal injury is almost always associated with multiple hemorrhages within the lobar white matter and corpus callosum. It has a predilection for the dorsolateral quadrant of the mesencephalon.

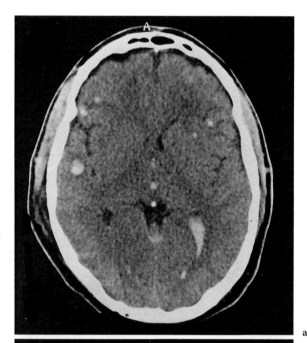

a

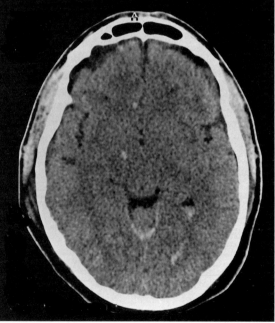

b

Fig. 2.39a,b. Diffuse axonal injury suggested by multiple subcortical and deep hemorrhages as well as intraventricular and subarachnoid hemorrhage

Magnetic resonance imaging is more sensitive for detecting these changes, including in cases where CT scan is normal. Small areas of increased signal intensity on the T1-weighted MR images at the above-mentioned locations represent hemorrhagic lesions, whereas areas of increased signal intensity only on T2-weighted images represent nonhemorrhagic lesions. Diffuse axonal injury may appear more extended on gradient-echo images because of their enhanced sensitivity to the presence of blood products. These lesions become more conspicuous when the imaging study is performed several days after the initial injury. Very late changes are enlargement of the ventricles and cortical sulci and sometimes encephalomalacic or porencephalic cystic lesions.

2.3.2.5 Brain Stem Injury

Brain stem injuries are either primary, occurring directly from trauma, or secondary, resulting from transtentorial herniation. Diffuse axonal injury is the most common type of traumatic primary brain stem injury. Torsion or impingement of the brain stem may produce hemorrhage and edema. Injury to the brain stem is assumed for unconsciousness trauma victims who do not otherwise demonstrate a mass lesion. Mortality in this patient group is high. Primary brain stem injuries are typically located in the dorsolateral region. Not all brain stem lesions, however, can be recognized on CT scans and due to minimal hemorrhage they may not appear hyperdense. Indirect evidence of brain stem injury is provided by swelling of the brain stem and obliteration of the surrounding cisterns. Diagnostic caution, however, is necessary because subarachnoid hemorrhage as well as swelling of the cerebellum or of the medial temporal lobes also may obliterate the same cisterns. Evidence of supratentorial shearing injury often implies primary brain stem injury as well.

Secondary injury to the brain stem results most frequently from transtentorial herniation following development of a supratentorial mass lesion (Fig. 2.40). Vascular damage results from shearing-off or compression of small perforating pontine and mesencephalic vessels. Demonstration of secondary brain stem injury using CT is not always possible, but minor hypodense or hyperdense areas centrally located within the brain stem favor this diagnosis. Obliteration of the perimesencephalic cisterns and widening of the lateral ventricles may be associated

findings. Brain stem injury can be better demonstrated on MR images without artifacts and with a higher sensitivity to edema or hemorrhage. Single or multiple secondary hemorrhages in the central tegmentum are called Duret hemorrhages. Kernohan's notch is an edema, ischemia, or hemorrhage of the contralateral cerebral peduncle resulting from compression against the tentorial edge following transtentorial herniation. Late findings on CT scans are focal defects within the brain stem or wallerian degeneration of the corticospinal tracts.

2.3.3 Open Head Injury

The term "open head injury" implies that there is a communication between the outside environment and the brain. Clinical signs are penetration of brain substance or CSF through the wound, rhinorrhea or otorrhea, or posttraumatic intracranial infection. A *first type* of open head injury is a compound depressed fracture with laceration of the dura (Sect. 2.2.2). A *second type* comprises fractures of the skull base or laterobasal fractures with a dural tear communicating with the paranasal sinuses, the middle ear, or the mastoid cells (Sect. 2.2.3).

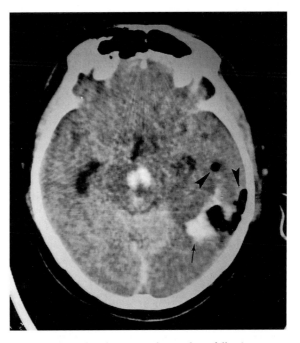

Fig. 2.40. Secondary brain stem hemorrhage following evacuation of a left-sided subdural hematoma. Some blood (*arrow*) and air (*arrowheads*) collections are still visible on the left side and the ventricular system is slightly enlarged

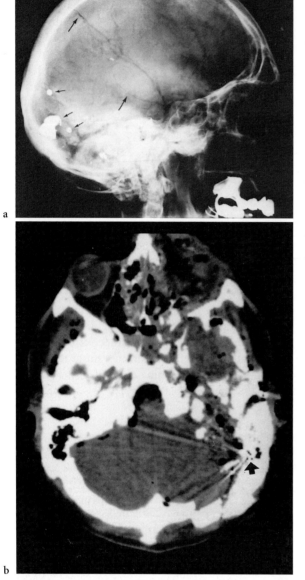

Fig. 2.41a,b. Penetrating gunshot injury. a Several skull fractures (*long arrows*) and fragments of the bullet (*short arrows*) are visible on lateral x-ray films of the skull. b CT demonstrates the gunshot canal with destruction of the left orbit and the comminuted fractures of the temporal fossa extending into the posterior fossa on the left side where the metallic fragment (*arrow*) is still intracranial. Air collections are present intracranially and soft tissue emphysema extracranially

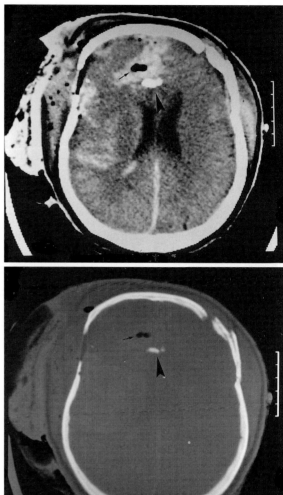

Fig. 2.42. a Perforating gunshot injury with entrance injury on the right side, hemorrhagic wound canal with contusion, subarachnoid hemorrhage, inclusion of air (*arrow*) and bone fragments (*arrowhead*), and exit injury on the left side with outward displacement of bone. b Bone window confirms the inward driven bone fragments; no metallic bullet fragments are present

A *third type* of open head injury is the *penetrating head injury*. Most gunshot wounds penetrate the scalp and skull. Other such injuries are stab wounds and occupational accidents. Surgical management is not always indicated in these patients. The canal of a penetrating injury is usually small and is closed by

hematoma, edematous tissue, or later by granulation tissue. Infection occurs more often from fragments of bone, scalp, or organic material driven into the brain than from inorganic metallic material. Missile injuries are classified into superficial, depressed, penetrating, and perforating types depending on their extent. Patients with nonballistic injuries often present in the emergency room with the penetrating agent still in place. The location of the penetrating injury determines its severity, whereby brain stem injury is usually fatal.

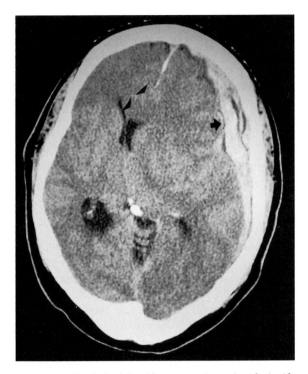

Fig. 2.43. Left-sided subdural hematoma (*arrow*) with significant midline shift and subfalcial herniation (*arrowheads*)

Plain radiography and CT are usually performed to estimate the depth and location of the injury and of possible foreign bodies (Fig. 2.41). The inner table of the skull is often more fractured than the outer table. Brain laceration is characteristically canalicular and hemorrhagic, but contusive injury at a distance from the laceration may also be found (Fig. 2.42). The diameter of the wound canal increases with the size and with increasing velocity of the penetrating agent. Radiography and CT show whether the missile is situated intracranially or extracranially or has perforated out of the skull. MRI should not be performed in these patients because the penetrating material may have a metallic content bearing smaller or larger amounts of ferromagnetic substances.

2.3.4 Brain Herniation

"Brain herniation" means displacement of brain tissue from one compartment to another. Several types of brain herniation are recognized: subfalcial, transtentorial, tonsillar, and external. Transtentorial herniation includes medial (uncal), descending, and ascending herniation.

Subfalcial herniation results in displacement of the cingulate gyrus beneath the falx cerebri and above the corpus callosum. MR or CT scans reveal displacement of the cingulate gyrus, tilting of the corpus callosum, and corresponding midline shift (Fig. 2.43). The ipsilateral lateral ventricle is compressed and the contralateral ventricle enlarges due to obstruction of the foramen of Monro. Anterior mass lesions lead to displacement of the anterior cerebral or pericallosal artery, while posterior mass lesions to displacement of the internal cerebral veins, whereby posttraumatic infarction is uncommon (Fig. 2.44).

Unilateral uncal herniation results from a temporal lobe mass lesion. Bilateral uncal herniation is usually due to large bilateral supratentorial lesions (hematoma, edema, hydrocephalus). The first radiological sign is effacement of the ambient cistern by the herniating medial temporal lobe (Fig. 2.45). The ipsilateral cerebral peduncle is compressed by the adjacent uncus and the contralateral cerebral peduncle is compressed against the free edge of the tentorium. Bilateral compression of the mesencephalon causes flattening of its transverse diameter. Finally uncal herniation can lead to compression of the posterior cerebral artery or of the veins of Rosenthal and Galen, whereby infarction of the posterior cerebral artery is more common (Fig. 2.46). In cases with severe transtentorial

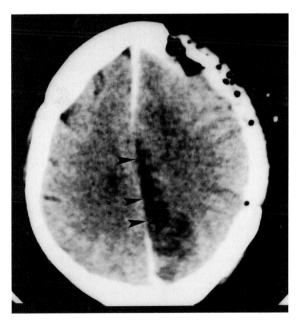

Fig. 2.44. Infarction in the vascular territory of the left anterior cerebral artery (*arrowheads*) following evacuation of an ipsilateral subdural hematoma

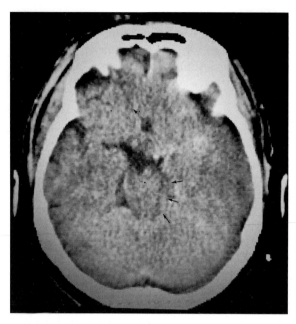

Fig. 2.45. Unilateral uncal herniation indicated by compression of the left ambient cistern (*arrows*) in a case with left-sided cerebral contusions

herniation CT scans show obliteration of all basal cisterns.

Descending transtentorial herniation is caused by supratentorial masses which cause downward displacement of the diencephalon, the basal ganglia, and the mesencephalon through the tentorial incisura. Under these circumstances secondary brain stem hemorrhage may occur. On CT scans caudal displacement of the diencephalon and the brain stem may be difficult to recognize. Radiological signs are obliteration of the basal cisterns, compression of the diencephalon, and inferior herniation of the gyri recti. Usually descending and medial transtentorial herniation occur together.

Ascending transtentorial herniation occurs when a mass lesion within the posterior fossa causes displacement of the cerebellum superiorly through the tentorial opening. It is often also associated with tonsillar herniation. CT features are compression of the fourth ventricle and of the mesencephalon with consequent hydrocephalus.

Tonsillar herniation comprises herniation of cerebellar tissue inferiorly with compressed cerebellar tonsils extending through the foramen magnum. This can be a consequence of a traumatic posterior fossa mass lesion, but also occurs when bilateral supratentorial mass lesions (e.g., brain swelling) cause downward displacement through the tentorium and compression of the cerebellum. CT scans show effacement of the cisterna magna and herniation of the cerebral tonsils through the foramen magnum. Infarction of the posterior inferior cerebellar artery may occur.

External herniation is not uncommon following surgical evacuation of posttraumatic intra- or extracerebral hematoma. Brain swelling causes herniation of brain parenchyma through the bone defect. The degree of the herniation is also dependent upon whether the dura is intact or not.

2.4 Special Features of Trauma in Children

Trauma is the leading cause of death in infancy and childhood. The major causes of pediatric head injury are falls and motor vehicle and bicycle accidents. Additional and unique groups of head trauma in this population are birth trauma and child abuse. In infancy, ultrasonography is often the first desirable method for diagnosing head injury sequelae. In other cases CT is generally sufficient, with MRI remaining for special questions.

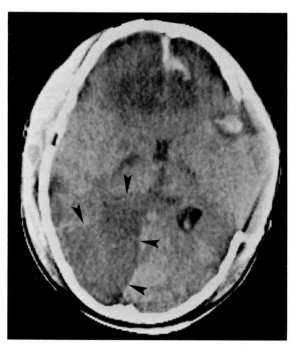

Fig. 2.46. Infarction in the territory of the right posterior cerebral artery (*arrowheads*) following decompression of a contralateral subdural hematoma. Frontal and temporal contusions with edema are still present

2.4.1 Birth Trauma

Head trauma occurring during delivery may result in intracranial hemorrhages. Intraventricular hemorrhage is the most common form within the neonatal age group. Intracerebral hematoma, solitary or multiple, may be found in peripheral locations of the cerebral hemispheres. Nontraumatic hemorrhages, however, resulting from Rhincompatibility, disseminated intravascular coagulopathy, or sepsis, may also be multifocal and peripherally located. Ultrasonography has proven to be effective in the evaluation of most forms of perinatal intracranial hemorrhage. CT is sometimes required if subarachnoid hemorrhage or subdural hematoma is suspected. Sequelae such as hydrocephalus, cerebral atrophy, or porencephaly may result from peri- and postnatal intracranial hemorrhage.

2.4.2 Skull Injury

Development of growing fractures by impingement of leptomeningeal tissue in the fracture line has been discussed in Sect. 2.2.3.1. Because the skull bone of children is thin, overlapping skull fractures and depressed fractures can occur readily. A special kind of depressed fracture is the so-called celluloid fracture whereby a localized depression of the bone, resembling an impressed ping pong ball, occurs without fracture lines.

2.4.3 Extra-axial Lesions

Epidural hematomas are less common in children than in adults, and they are rare in infancy. In children and infants, epidural hematomas more often have a venous than an arterial origin and may occur without skull fracture. When they do occur in childhood, subdural hematomas are more extensive than those in the adult population, more often bilateral, and more often interhemispheric. Chronic subdural hematoma in children only occurs following ventricular shunting for hydrocephalus. Posttraumatic subdural hygroma is more common than in adults.

2.4.4 Intra-axial Lesions

Children tend to have contusions rather than intracerebral hematoma, whereby the incidence of both is much lower than in adults. On the other hand, trau-matic cerebellar hemorrhage is more common in children. In general, children have a higher incidence of diffuse and shearing injuries and have fewer focal mass lesions than adults. Cerebral swelling represents a frequent form of response to head trauma in young patients. It is the most common manifestation of intra-axial pediatric head injury. Hypoxia and ischemia are important secondary factors causing intra-axial injury in children and can be found in many cases without head trauma. They result most commonly from asphyxia following cardiorespiratoy arrest, aspiration, smothering, strangulation, pneumothorax, or chest compression.

2.4.5 Child Abuse

The true incidence of child abuse is unclear. Many cases remain unknown, either unreported altogether or not recognized properly by evaluating physicians who lack specific knowledge regarding the manifestations of child abuse. The great majority of victims are young children, usually younger than 2 years. Child abuse or battered child syndrome has a mechanism of injury different from that associated with accidental head trauma. Beside direct impact to the head there may be indirect impact in the form of shaking, asphyxia, and nutritional deprivation. Neurologically, the battered child syndrome presents with seizures, lethargy, or coma. Many such children show external injuries or retinal hemorrhages. Subdural hematomas are the most common intracranial injuries presenting on CT scans in abused children with or without signs of external head trauma. Interhemispheric subdural hematoma is described as a classic finding in the shaken baby syndrome. Other common intracranial findings in the battered child are subarachnoid hemorrhage and brain edema. Small contusions, focal areas of edema, and small extra-axial collections may be demonstrated whereby the sensitivity of MRI is much greater for these lesions than that of CT (Fig. 2.47). Intracranial hemorrhages showing different stages of evolution are an important clue in recognizing recurrent trauma and child abuse. Identification of skull fractures by plain radiography is important as well. Fractures, as a whole, are the most common radiographically evaluated injuries in such children. The demonstration of multiple injuries in different stages of healing is in general the most compelling evidence for repeated abuse, a fact which must be borne in mind by the evaluating radiologist.

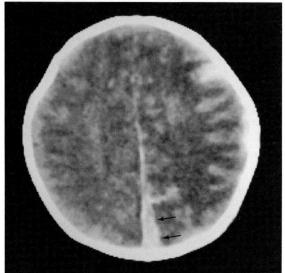

a

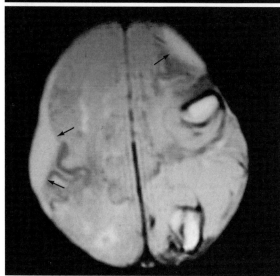

b

Fig. 2.47. Child abuse was suggested by the discrepancy between fresh subarachnoid hemorrhage over the left hemisphere and small interhemispheric subdural hematoma (*arrows*) on CT scans (**a**) and chronic intracerebral hematomas and bilateral subdural hematomas (*arrows*) on MR scans (**b**)

2.5 Sequelae of Head Injury

2.5.1 Encephalomalacia and Atrophy

Two to six months following injury, atrophy or encephalomalacia may be observed. Focal tissue loss is referred to as posttraumatic encephalomalacia and diffuse tissue loss as posttraumatic atrophy, whereby, however, they are often concomitant. Encephalomalacia presents on CT scans as a hypodense parenchymal defect with a similar density to

CSF. The adjacent cortical sulci and ventricular system are widened. MRI may show a central area of macrocystic gliosis isointense to CSF and a peripheral zone of microcystic gliosis with increased signal intensity on proton-weighted sequences. If there is deposition of hemosiderin products, MRI may show these areas with a characteristic dark ring allowing diagnosis of a previous hemorrhagic lesion.

Posttraumatic atrophy means widening of the entire ventricular system and of all sulci and fissures. It may occur after diffuse brain injuries such as diffuse axonal injury, brain swelling, increased intracranial pressure, or hypoxic damage. The etiology is often multifactorial. Posttraumatic atrophy may be focal and asymmetrical, particularly in cases with preexisting focal lesions. Discrimination of posttraumatic hydrocephalus has to be taken into consideration. Wallerian degeneration of the corticospinal tract is a tissue involution along the tract distal to the site of injury and can best be seen on axial slices through the midbrain on CT or MRI scans.

2.5.2 Hydrocephalus

Posttraumatic subarachnoid bleeding can lead to the development of a communicating hydrocephalus. Fibroblastic proliferation may obliterate the cortical sulci, preventing reabsorption of CSF. Intraventricular bleeding can lead to a proliferative aseptic ependymitis with subsequent ventricular obstruction and noncommunicating hydrocephalus. Following head injury, however, both forms of hydrocephalus often occur concomitantly. Clinical findings accompanying posttraumatic hydrocephalus may be stagnating recovery or worsening of consciousness. The dilatation of the temporal and frontal horns, the effacement of the cortical sulci, and the periventricular lucency caused by posttraumatic hydrocephalus often help to distinguish hydrocephalus from ventriculomegaly. The latter arises from diffuse parenchymal atrophy with enlargement not only of internal but also of external CSF spaces and without any increase in intraventricular pressure.

2.5.3 Infarction

The most common posttraumatic infarction occurs in the supply area of the posterior cerebral artery as a consequence of transtentorial herniation with impingement of the artery against the tentorium.

Infarction due to herniation with impingement of the anterior cerebral or the posterior inferior cerebellar arteries is much less common. In addition infarction may occur through hypotension resulting in border zone infarcts, through congestive venous infarction, and through embolic infarction, e.g., fat embolism. Posttraumatic thrombosis of dural sinuses is a rare condition which sometimes occurs in conjunction with skull fractures. In the acute stage vascular infarcts are masked by brain swelling and space-occupying lesions and thereby often escape early diagnosis. Only those patients who survive later present the typical hypodense lesions corresponding to the regions of the involved vessels.

2.6 Face

2.6.1 General Considerations

Injury to the facial bones, orbits, and adjacent soft tissue structures may occur as a component of multiple injuries or alone. Severe trauma to the face is always a strong indication for radiological investigation, whereby diagnostic imaging for facial trauma should only be done after the patient's vital functions and possible cervical fractures have been stabilized.

The radiological imaging modalities for facial trauma are conventional plain films, CT, and MRI. The *routine plain film facial series* includes Waters, Caldwell, Towne's, and lateral views, which are sometimes supplemented by special projections such as zygomatic arch views or base projections. If possible, all plain films should be obtained with the patient in an upright position. This enables the radiologist to identify air-fluid levels and prevents the orbital floor from being obscured by diffuse density caused by fluid within the maxillary sinus.

The viscerocranium consists of a complex bony anatomy in all three axes, and the possibilities of evaluation on plain films are limited. CT is therefore often necessary in facial trauma to visualize relevant anatomical structures and changes. CT is performed using a high-resolution bone algorithm technique with 2- to 4-mm contiguous scans in the axial and coronal planes through the whole bony orbits and all facial bones. In severe trauma, however, direct coronal CT imaging should only be performed after demonstrating that the cervical spine is normal. If a complementary soft tissue window is necessary, it is obtained from the bone algorithm data. If secondary reconstruction of the coronal and oblique sagittal planes following acquisition of thin axial slices is able to demonstrate intraorbital structures and the orbital floor satisfactorily enough for the evaluation of trauma, direct coronal imaging may become unnecessary.

Magnetic resonance imaging may be extremely helpful for assessment of injuries of the eyeball itself and in cases with suspicion of orbital hematoma or optic nerve damage. Bone fractures and their sequelae, e.g., displaced fragments and structures, vessel and neural dissection, and disruption of neurocranial integrity, are, however, the most important aspects in maxillofacial trauma. Because of its inferior demonstration of bony details, MRI visualizes fractures poorly when compared with CT. Furthermore, MRI is strictly contraindicated in the presence of ferromagnetic foreign bodies. If there is a history of exposure to such foreign bodies, e.g., industrial accidents, metallic components have to be ruled out before MRI by means of preliminary plain films.

2.6.2 Paranasal Sinuses and Facial Bones

2.6.2.1 Emphysema

Emphysema, encased air in tissues, following facial trauma is found particularly if bony injury creates a passage for air from a paranasal sinus to non-pneumatized spaces or structures. Orbital floor and/ or orbital wall fractures may be complicated by orbital emphysema caused by air entering the orbit from the ethmoid sinuses or maxillary antrum (Fig. 2.48a,b). The extent of the emphysema of the orbit and/or face depends on the severity of trauma. Logically, it is observed regularly and obviously in the Le Fort III fracture type and the nasoethmoidal complex fracture (see Sects. 2.6.2.5.3 and 2.6.2.5.4).

2.6.2.2 Hemorrhage

Inferior orbital rim fractures may be nondisplaced or there may be a step-off between the medial and lateral fragments. Frequently, there is associated edema or hematoma with mucosal thickening in the adjacent maxillary antrum or even an antral fluid level (Fig. 2.48a,c). Mostly in cases of severe injuries there may be bleeding into the orbit, sinuses, and nasal cavity, either diffusely into the soft tissues or more circumscribed with hematoma formation.

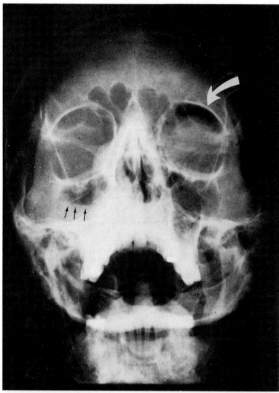

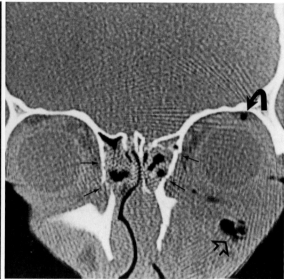

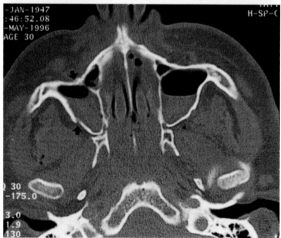

Fig. 2.48a–c. Sequelae of trauma to the face. a Waters view demonstrates an air-fluid level within the right maxillary sinus (*small black arrows*) and a large orbital emphysema (*curved white arrow*). b Direct coronal CT scan better demonstrates smaller amounts of emphysema within the soft tissues (*open arrow*) and the orbit (*curved arrow*). Note the bilateral fractures of the medial orbital wall (*straight arrows*). c Axial CT scan in the bone window setting with bilateral fluid levels within the maxillary sinuses, better seen than on plain films. Note the fractures of the anterior and posterolateral wall of the right maxillary sinus (*arrows*)

Ruptured branches of the maxillary artery may cause severe nosebleeding, sometimes necessitating surgical or – as is more often today – endovascular closure of the bleeding vessel. Rarely, a pseudoaneurysm may develop. A further bleeding complication of facial trauma may be a septal hematoma, resulting from separation of the perichondrium from the septal cartilage. In the event of septal hematoma there is a high risk of necrosis or inflammation of the septum, which may cause severe deformity of the nose.

2.6.2.3 Nasal Fractures

The nasal bones are in an exposed, unprotected, and centrally located position. This frequently leads to fractures if a force is exerted on the midface. Logically the paired nasal bones are the most frequently fractured bones of the facial skeleton. Most nasal fractures take a course perpendicular to the long axis of the nasal bones. They vary from nondisplaced linear fractures to severe comminution with multiple fragments. Fractures of the nasal bones are often as-

Skull, Brain, and Face

sociated with injury of the osseous and/or cartilaginous portion of the anterior nasal septum. While the osseous septum is often fractured, the cartilaginous portion is usually only deflected. A feared complication is septal hematoma, which can cause diminished blood supply to the cartilage and result in rapid necrosis of the septum, leading to the so-called saddle-nose deformity. Bacterial infection of the hematoma can occur because of its exposure to outside air and may lead to subsequent septal abscess.

Nasal fractures are not always obvious during the first clinical examination because of associated edema. However, it is important to recognize nasal fractures because they can later cause an uncorrectable deformity. Plain film series demonstrate the nasal bones best on an underpenetrated lateral view (Fig. 2.49a). CT is necessary only in very few cases (Fig. 2.49b), especially if there is comminution or complication.

2.6.2.4 Zygomaticomaxillary Complex Fractures

The separation of the zygoma from the remainder of the facial skeleton is defined as zygomaticomaxillary complex (ZMC) fracture. Other terms for this fracture type are tripod or trimalar fracture. The body of the zygoma is typically displaced inward and rotated slightly because the classical history is an impact force against the anterolateral face. The typical course of the fracture lines is the inferior orbital rim, the zygomaticofrontal suture with widening, the (postero)lateral wall of the maxillary sinus, and the zygomatic arch with a variable degree of depression. Compared with the later described "inferior blowout" fracture, the associated floor fracture in the ZMC fracture is usually not significant, probably because of the more lateral involvement of the orbital floor. If the ZMC fracture has resulted from application of a particularly severe traumatic force, however, marked displacement or comminution of fragments may occur, requiring special treatment of a significant inferior displacement of the orbital floor and other displaced components of the fracture.

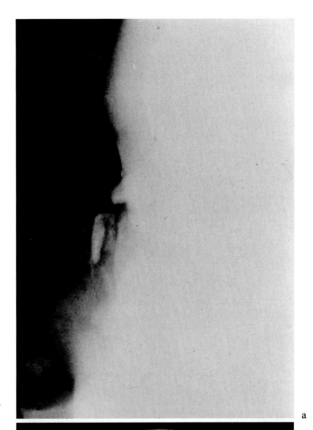

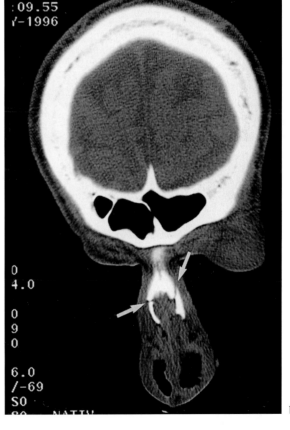

Fig. 2.49a,b. Nasal fractures. a Underpenetrated lateral view of the nose demonstrates a severely dislocated fracture of the nasal bone. b Direct coronal CT scan demonstrates a linear lucency (*arrows*), characteristic of a nondisplaced nasal fracture

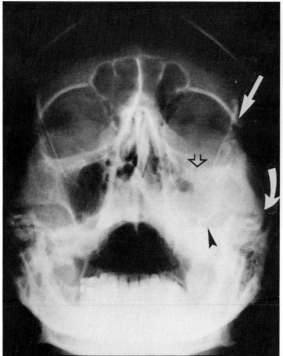

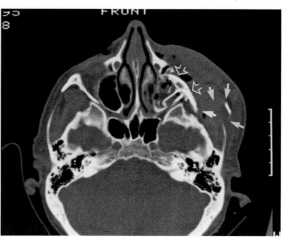

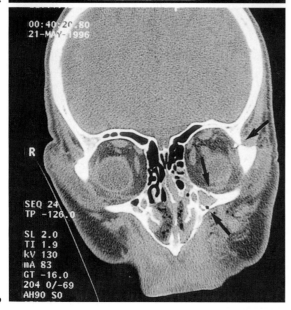

Fig. 2.50a–c. Zygomaticomaxillary complex fracture. **a** Waters view demonstrates the fracture lines and the dislocation well. Note the disruption of the four articulation sites of the zygoma [zygomaticofrontal suture (*large arrow*), inferior orbital rim (*open arrow*), posterolateral wall of the maxillary sinus (*arrowhead*), and zygomatic arch (*curved arrow*)]. **b** Direct coronal CT scan also demonstrates a nondisplaced tripod fracture with fracture lines of the zygomaticofrontal suture, orbital rim, and lateral wall of the maxillary sinus (*arrows*). Note the small fragment and the fluid within the left maxillary sinus. **c** Axial CT scan demonstrates marked depression of the left malar eminence (*open arrows*). Note the fracture of the orbital floor, the posterolateral wall of the maxillary sinus, and especially the displacement of the zygomatic arch (*straight arrows*). There is marked emphysema of the adjacent soft tissue

Comminution of the zygoma body is very rare and nearly always caused by a gunshot injury.

The aforementioned components of ZMC fractures can usually be identified on conventional plain films (Fig. 2.50a). CT scans are mandatory, however, in all cases where severe force to the face has resulted in considerable displacement and/or clinical symptoms such as periorbital edema/hematoma, crepitus, limitation of mouth opening, trismus, or displace-

ment of the globe. CT optimally demonstrates the course of the fracture lines and of the rotation and displacement of the various fragments (Fig. 2.50b,c). Furthermore, in the case of severe trauma, CT best visualizes the fractured infraorbital rim, providing an answer to the important question of whether depression and defects in the floor have developed as a consequence of the frature. As described later for "blow-out" fractures ZMC fractures are often ac-

Fig. 2.51. Fracture lines of the different Le Fort fractures

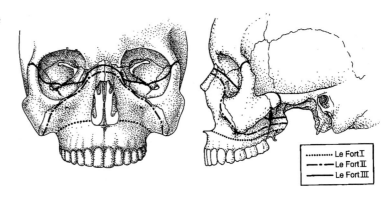

··········· Le Fort I
— · — Le Fort II
——— Le Fort III

companied by increased density in the maxillary antrum with or without a fluid level, edema in the nasal cavity, and increased density in the adjacent ethmoidal sinus. Possible soft tissue injuries within the orbit with involvement of the globe and the canthal ligaments are also optimally evaluated with CT. Because severe forces applied to the anterolateral orbital wall are not infrequently transmitted to the middle cranial fossa, CT is also considered important to rule out concomitant intracranial injuries of the basal parts of the brain. Although both of the latter complications may also be well demonstrated on MRI, MRI has no important role in the overall assessment of ZMC fractures.

2.6.2.5 Medial Fractures

The typical Le Fort fractures (Fig. 2.51) are uncommon today, because owing to safety belts the incidence of crushing facial injuries in high-speed motor vehicle accidents (Le Fort's original experiments) has been reduced. Among the Le Fort fractures the Le Fort type II is the most common, followed by type I. Today the medial fractures are often associated with ZMC fractures, frontal sinus fractures, and mandibular fractures.

2.6.2.5.1 Le Fort I Fracture (Transverse). The Le Fort I fracture corresponds to a transverse fracture through the maxilla, above the alveolar portion (Fig. 2.51). The course of the fracture lines extends through the inferior nasal cavity above the hard palate, the floor of the maxillary antrum (Fig. 2.52a), and the lower pterygoid plates bilaterally. Clinically there is a horizontal separation of the caudal maxilla. On physical examination there is a freely movable alveolar portion of the maxilla against the upper viscerocranium, and malocclusion of the teeth.

Coronal CT evaluates the Le Fort I type optimally, because in this plane the facial fractures are oriented perpendicular to the plane of section (Fig. 2.52b,c). This type of fracture is often missed by plain film radiographs and on axial CT scans because of the horizontal course of the bony interruption, which only rarely exhibits displacement.

2.6.2.5.2 Le Fort II Fracture (Pyramidal). The typical Le Fort II fracture separates the complete midface from the cranium and lateral aspect of the face, because here the nasal bones are involved (unlike in the type I fracture), usually fracturing near the nasofrontal suture and the frontal process of the maxilla (Fig. 2.51). The fracture lines extend laterally on both sides with involvement of the inferior orbital rim and floor, and posteriorly through the zygomatic and/or maxillary bones and pterygoid plates. Because of their typical shape, these fractures are also defined as pyramidal fractures. If they extend more inferiorly and cause fractures in the maxillary sinuses, increased density and/or a fluid level within the maxillary sinus may be seen. However, the medial walls of the maxillary sinus are typically spared, which differentiates these fractures from the Le Fort I type. There is often severe swelling of the face, including the soft tissue structures of both orbits, especially the lids.

As in type I fractures, conventional plain film views are of only limited value for evaluating Le Fort II fractures. CT scanning in the axial and coronal planes alone allows a detailed assessment of this fracture type (Fig. 2.53), particularly if surgery is planned. Varying intensities of impact force and direction are responsible for the significant morphological variability within this fracture form as well as for the varying degrees of displacement and comminution. The fracture may also extend into the frontal and anterior ethmoids, leading to the possible com-

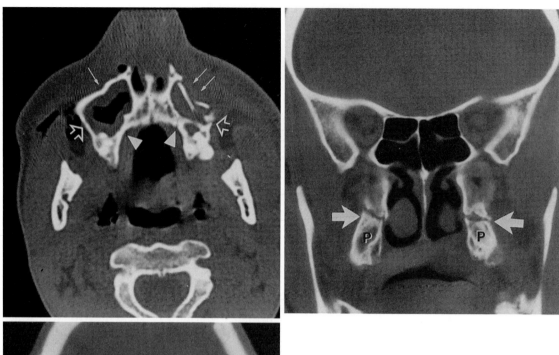

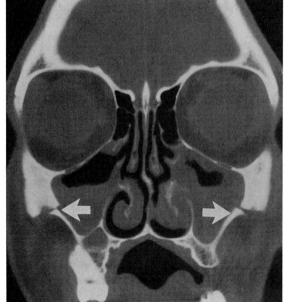

Fig. 2.52a–c. Le Fort I fracture. **a** Axial CT scan demonstrates bilateral fractures of the anterior (*straight arrows*), medial (*arrowheads*), and posterolateral (*open arrows*) walls of the maxillary sinus, which are more clearly seen on the left side than on the right. The Le Fort I fracture is the only Le Fort fracture to disrupt all walls of the maxillary sinus (and the pterygoid plate). **b,c** Direct coronal CT scans demonstrate the transverse nature of the Le Fort I fracture best. Note the fracture of the pterygoid plates (*P*), and of the walls of the maxillary sinus (*arrows*)

plication of a CSF leak. MRI again plays no important role in evaluating fractures of this kind.

2.6.2.5.3 Le Fort III Fracture (Craniofacial Dysjunction).
The Le Fort III fracture is also named craniofacial dysjunction, because this worst Le Fort fracture type detaches the middle third of the facial skeleton completely from the base of the skull. The typical clinical finding is movement of the whole face in relation to the skull. To achieve this kind of movement, there

usually must be a severe trauma to the face and – in addition to the Le Fort II fracture – a disconnection of the lateral walls of both orbits (Fig. 2.51). The fracture lines extend additionally through the nasal bones, medial walls of both orbits, ethmoidal sinuses, and cribriform plates with frequent extension into the sphenoidal sinus and occasional extension into the optic canals. Because of this extension, all paranasal sinuses normally demonstrate increased density with fluid levels, including the sphenoidal

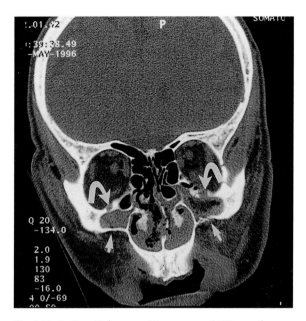

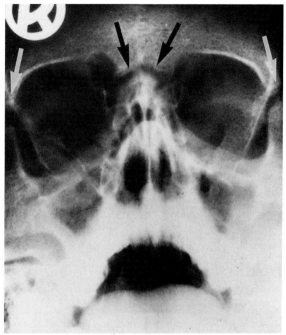

Fig. 2.53. Le Fort II fracture. Direct coronal CT scan demonstrates the pyramidal character of this fracture type best. Note the bilateral fractures of the orbital rim (*curved arrows*) and the lateral walls of the maxillary sinus (*straight arrows*). Uncharacteristic of a typical Le Fort II fracture is the questionable disruption of the left zygomaticofrontal suture (mediolateral fracture type)

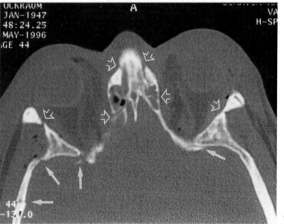

sinus. The necessary force to create such a fracture always causes marked soft tissue swelling of the whole face, and often severe orbital soft tissue injuries (see Sect. 2.6.3.2).

In addition to the often obvious severe emphysema of the face and/or orbit, a pneumocephalus with air in the subarachnoid space and/or ventricles may develop if a communication through the frontal, ethmoidal, and sphenoidal sinuses and cribriform plate has been produced by the fracture. Such a communication, on the other hand, can frequently lead to rhinorrhea, occurring immediately or developing later, with an accompanying risk of intracranial infection.

The degree of severity of this facial injury can already be preliminarily assessed on conventional plain films (Fig. 2.54a). Even more so, however, than for Le Fort types I and II, CT is the modality of choice to provide a detailed demonstration of the sites and extensions of multiple fracture lines (Fig. 2.54b). Only CT is able to show the amount of comminution and the frequently associated intracranial findings. CT scanning should be done with a bone window setting in the axial and coronal projections. The severity of injury often prohibits early direct coronal

Fig. 2.54a,b. Le Fort III fracture. a Conventional plain film demonstrates the fracture lines additionally through the nasal bones and the lateral orbital walls (*arrows*), leading to a complete detachment of the facial skeleton from the base of the skull. b Axial CT scan in the bone window setting demonstrates the multiple fracture lines (*open arrows*) optimally. Uncharacteristic of a typical Le Fort III fracture are the fractures of the temporal bone and the posterior orbital wall (*arrows*)

plane scanning and coronal reconstructions should be made from axial scan data if necessary. MRI is again only of limited value in early posttraumatic assessment; it better demonstrates associated globe and optic nerve injuries and can be utilized later according to clinical suspicion and the patient's general condition.

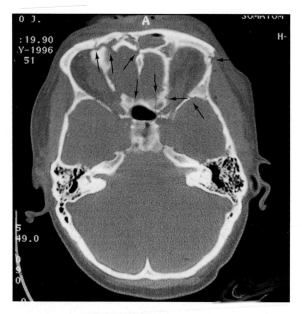

Fig. 2.55. Nasoethmoidal complex fracture (smash injury). Axial CT scan demonstrates significant posterior displacement and comminution of the nasofrontal region. Note the fractures of the frontal skull base, the lateral orbital walls, and the anterior and posterior walls of the frontal sinus (*arrows*)

2.6.2.5.4 Nasoethmoidal Complex Fracture (Facial Comminution). Some authors mention the nasoethmoidal complex fracture or "smash injury" as a worse form of the Le Fort III type fracture with destruction and posterior displacement of the whole nasofrontal region and ethmoid labyrinth (Fig. 2.55). This type of injury is caused by a very severe force, often leading to marked comminution of the nasal bones, along with multiple fractures in the cribriform plate area and adjacent frontal and ethmoidal sinuses, including the lamina papyracea. Due to bone shattering in the frontobasal region, such complications as have already been discussed for Le Fort type III, involving the orbit and CSF rhinorrhea, are more severe and more frequent. In severe trauma, pseudohypertelorism may be noted on physical examination, often associated with horizontal gaze limitation and diplopia.

This type of fracture is also frequently associated with epistaxis, septal hematoma, and injury to the nasolacrimal drainage system, either unilaterally or bilaterally. The most frequent finding is obstruction of the nasolacrimal duct near its junction with the nasolacrimal sac, which can be demonstrated by dacryocystography. The contrast column then reveals marked narrowing or complete occlusion of the upper nasolacrimal duct leading to a dilatation of the lacrimal sac.

2.6.3 Orbit

2.6.3.1 Foreign Bodies

The exposed position of the eye and orbit explains the frequency of traumatic eye injuries with or without foreign bodies. Many different substances such as metal, glass, plastic, stones, and wood may penetrate into the globe and/or orbital cavity, and cause different diagnostic problems. Not only the material of the foreign body but also the differentiation between its location inside or outside the eyeball is important from the clinical point of view because surgical extraction is not necessary in many cases of nonreactive foreign bodies in the orbital cavity.

Conventional films reveal metallic foreign bodies larger than 1.2 mm, including glass with a high lead content. However, there may be problems concerning its exact site inside or outside the globe. This differentiation is especially important if there is blood within the globe, making detailed clinical evaluation impossible. There are many reasons to designate CT the modality of choice for demonstrating orbital foreign bodies. Firstly, CT scans performed in contiguous 2-mm axial plane sections and supplemented by secondary reconstructions of the coronal and sagittal planes are sufficient to precisely localize a foreign body within the globe in nearly all cases (Fig. 2.56a,b). Secondly, the damage caused by the penetrating foreign body may be more clinically relevant than the foreign body itself; CT can best demonstrate such damage in most cases. Thirdly, CT is also able to visualize optimally less dense substances such as glass and plastic material. Demonstration of foreign bodies by MRI makes sense only in certain special cases. It is superior in the detection of wooden foreign bodies (Fig. 2.56c), as these are usually not detected on early posttraumatic CT scans. Wooden splinters are visualized by CT when they are dry and filled with air, or if inflammation develops around them. One of the most important limitations of MRI, however, is its absolute contraindication when there is suspicion of ferromagnetic foreign bodies.

2.6.3.2 Soft Tissue Injury

Foreign bodies and/or orbital fractures may be associated with different soft tissue injuries. Potential ocular injuries are a ruptured globe (Fig. 2.57a), hyphema, a dislocated lens, choroidal hematoma,

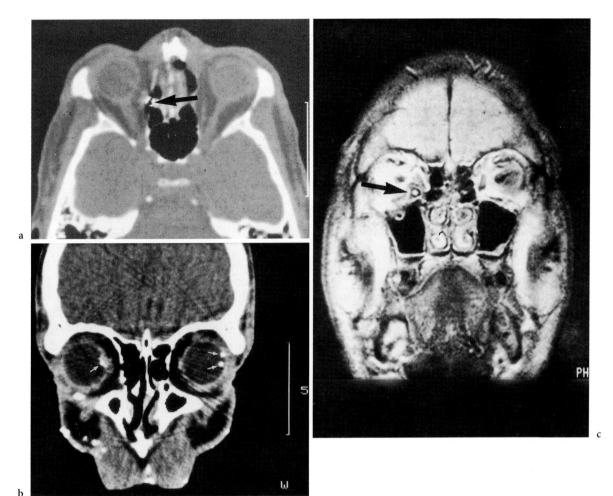

Fig. 2.56a–c. Foreign bodies within the orbit. a Axial CT scan and b direct coronal CT scan best demonstrate the number and location of intraorbital foreign bodies. a Axial scan demonstrates a single metallic foreign body (*arrow*) in the extraconal compartment medial to the right medial rectus muscle. b Direct coronal CT scan demonstrates multiple foreign bodies (pellets of a gun shot) (*arrows*) in both globes. c T2-weighted MRI demonstrates a wooden foreign body in the extraconal compartment of the right orbit (*arrow*). There is high signal intensity because of the wet wood

and a detached retina with subretinal fluid collection. Severe injury to the globe may give rise to phthisis bulbi, which is characterized by a shrunken, irregular globe with increased density and scattered calcifications on CT (Fig. 2.57b).

Intraorbital soft tissue structures such as the extraocular muscles, the retro-orbital fat, the optic nerve, and the superior ophthalmic vein are easily identified on high-resolution CT studies. Extraconal soft tissue structures are the lacrimal drainage system, the canthal ligaments, and the soft tissue of the eyelids. There may be diffuse orbital cellulitis following penetrating orbital wounds with or without a retained foreign body. Soft tissue swelling caused by inflammation can be optimally demonstrated by axial CT (Fig. 2.57c).

2.6.3.3 Orbital Wall Fractures

2.6.3.3.1 Orbital Floor Fractures (Inferior Blow-out Fractures). This fracture typically involves the middle (and anterior) third of the orbital floor in the region of the infraorbital canal. The classical "blow-out fracture" occurs in isolation, showing no association with other fractures in the facial bones or another rim fracture. Although only the floor of the orbit is fractured, there is a wide spectrum of lesion variations ranging from short linear to slightly comminuted fractures up to fractures accompanied by marked depression whose inferiorly displaced fragments leave a variable degree of dehiscence in the floor.

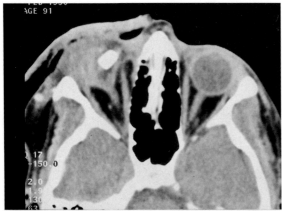

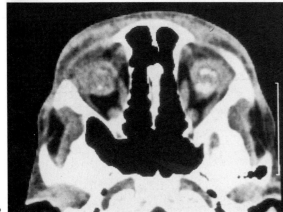

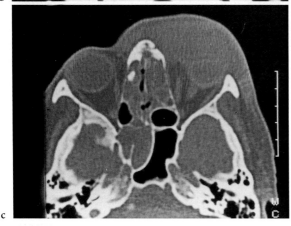

Fig. 2.57a–c. Soft tissue changes of the orbit. **a** Axial CT scan demonstrates an intraocular lead-bearing glass foreign body with a ruptured right globe. **b** Shrunken, irregular globe bilaterally with increased density and scattered calcifications as a typical finding of a phthisis bulbi. **c** Axial CT scan demonstrates extensive orbital cellulitis following penetrating orbital wound

Linear and only slightly comminuted orbital floor fractures may be difficult to recognize on conventional films. Clinically significant orbital floor fractures are, however, nearly always seen and therefore best evaluated first with conventional orbital films.

Nevertheless, CT should be performed for detailed assessment and always in cases with clinical ophthalmological findings. This need not be done in the acute stage of the trauma, but within a few days and prior to surgery. Because small bone fragments may impinge on the inferior rectus muscle and cause diplopia, CT is mandatory in all cases where clinical ophthalmological examination shows corresponding limitation of eye movement arousing suspicion of orbital muscle entrapment. CT should be performed in the coronal and axial planes (Fig. 2.58a), whereby in many cases 2-mm axial sections with coronal and lateral reconstructions are sufficient. In cases of severe orbital floor fractures and planned surgery, CT measurement techniques should be utilized to quantitatively determine the coordinates and dimensions of fracture extension.

The adjacent soft tissue structures are also usually well demonstrated on CT scans. This is especially important in cases with displacement or entrapment of the inferior rectus muscle or with possible enophthalmos caused by marked depression of the orbital floor into the maxillary antrum. MRI does not play an important role in the acute-phase evaluation of orbital floor fractures. It may be particularly useful, however, in the assessment of herniating soft tissue displacement of the inferior rectus muscle or adjacent fat tissue through a defect into the maxillary sinus (Fig. 2.58b).

2.6.3.3.2 Medial and Lateral Orbital Wall Fractures. Medial wall fractures occur less commonly than orbital floor fractures even though the lamina papyracea is significantly thinner than the floor of the orbit. Their associated occurrence, frequently bilaterally, with orbital floor fractures is found in up to 30% of cases. They are frequently not detected because they often present no clinical symptoms. However, in cases where ophthalmological examination following trauma has demonstrated horizontal gaze limitation, suspicion of bony entrapment of the medial rectus muscle in a medial orbital wall fracture may be entertained. This is comparable to entrapment sequelae following orbital floor fractures with downward displacement of the inferior rectus muscle.

Because the lamina papyracea is extremely thin, nondisplaced fractures usually remain undetected on plain films. They may be suspected in cases with increased density within the neighboring ethmoidal cells due to bleeding and/or associated orbital emphysema. CT axial plane scans in the bone window setting are the method of choice for detailed assess-

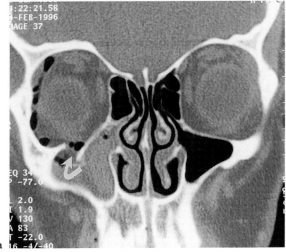

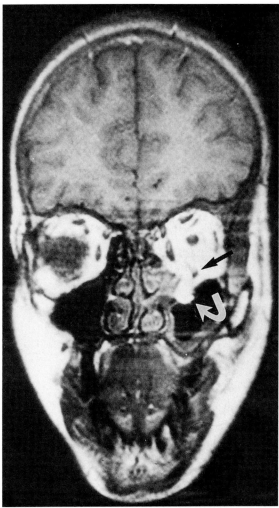

Fig. 2.58a,b. Orbital floor fracture. **a** Direct coronal CT scan demonstrates the characteristic trapdoor appearance (*curved arrow*) of an inferior blow-out fracture on the right side. The inferior rectus muscle is not identified clearly. Note the fluid filling the right maxillary sinus, and the emphysema within the right orbit caused by the connection to the maxillary sinus. **b** T1-weighted MRI demonstrates herniation of intraorbital fat tissue through the bony defect into the maxillary sinus (*curved arrow*). Note the inferior rectus muscle (*straight arrow*), which is not involved by the displacement

ment of medial wall fractures (Fig. 2.59a). CT scanning in a plane chosen orthogonal to a structure's anatomical extension and parallel to the usual direction of fragment displacement best demonstrates bony displacement from the structure. For fracture identification, axial plane CT scans optimally visualize the lamina papyracea with its anterior-posterior extension, clearly demonstrating typical fracture interruptions with a variable degree of medial fragment displacement. Similar to inferior rectus muscle entrapment in orbital floor fractures, entrapment of the medial rectus muscle may be recognized in the CT soft tissue window by displacement of the muscle into the medial wall fracture site (Fig. 2.59b), sometimes in association with edema and swelling of the muscle. MRI may also reveal medial displacement of the muscle, but CT is usually sufficient for assessment.

Lateral orbital wall fractures frequently present as isolated fractures. In most cases there will be dehis-

cence of the zygomaticofrontal suture, but fractures may also present above or below the suture. Although these fractures often show little or no displacement, significant comminution with displacement can sometimes be found, occurring particularly in cases caused by severe direct traumatic forces.

Conventional plain film series including lateral, Waters, and Caldwell projections normally allow a clear definition of lateral orbital wall fractures (see Sect. 2.6.2.4). Should detailed assessment prove necessary, however, e.g., for surgical reconstruction procedures, CT scanning in the axial and coronal planes becomes mandatory (Fig. 2.60).

2.6.3.4 Orbital Roof Fractures

Depending on the direction of the force to the orbit, there may be "blow-out" fractures of the orbital roof

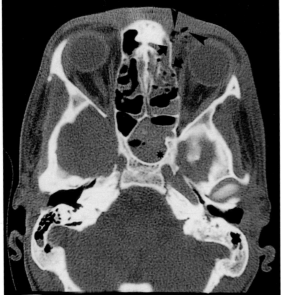

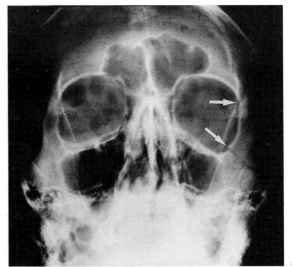

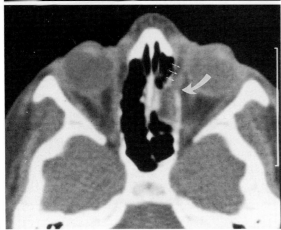

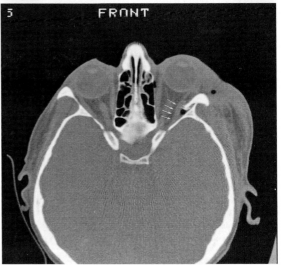

Fig. 2.59a,b. Medial orbital wall fracture. **a** Axial CT scan demonstrates a minimally displaced fracture of the left medial orbital wall. Note the fracture lines (*arrows*), not optimally seen because of the thin lamina papyracea. Note the fluid levels within the adjacent paranasal sinus (***), and the emphysema of the soft tissues in the extraconal compartment (*arrowheads*). **b** Axial CT scan demonstrates displacement of the left medial rectus muscle (*arrowheads*) through the bony defect into the adjacent ethmoid air cells (*curved arrow*)

Fig. 2.60a,b. Lateral orbital wall fracture. Waters projection demonstrates two fracture lines (*arrows*) of the lateral wall of the left orbit. The fractures and the small amount of fragment-dislocation are well recognized on conventional plain film (**a**). **b** Axial CT scan in the bone window setting (different patient) demonstrates severe displacement of the anterior fragment with dislocation of the lateral rectus muscle (*arrows*). Note the emphysema inside and outside the bony orbit

characterized by cranial displacement of parts of the orbital roof, or "blow-in" fractures with caudal displacement. Both fracture types frequently involve the frontal sinus, and additional intracranial injuries such as contusion, pneumocephalus, and dural tear may occur. Comminution of these fractures may lead to associated orbital emphysema with air from the frontal sinus. Inferior displacement of fragments is often injurious to the superior rectus or levator palpebrae muscles, and/or to the superior division

of the oculomotor nerve. On rare occasions an orbital roof fracture may create a defect through which meninges and brain are able to herniate into the orbital cavity (orbital menigocele, orbital meningo-encephalocele).

Orbital roof fractures may cause various complications due to bleeding. Diffuse bleeding into the orbital fat can produce proptosis with stretching of the optic nerve. This normally happens immediately after the injury. Subperiosteal hematoma can develop beneath the orbital roof for anatomical reasons. This

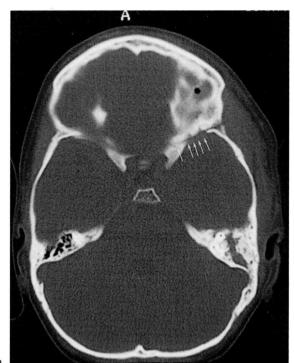

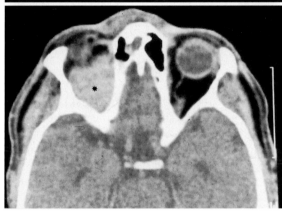

Fig. 2.61a,b. Orbital roof fracture. **a** Axial CT scan demonstrates a linear fracture (*arrowheads*) running through the left orbital roof. Note the emphysema within the left orbit. **b** Nonenhanced axial CT demonstrates a subperiosteal hematoma as a relatively well-defined high-attenuation mass located within the posterosuperior aspect of the right orbit

posttraumatic lesion, also known as orbital hematocyst or epidural hematoma, corresponds to a focal hemorrhage caused by a tear in the subperiosteal vessels. Hematomas in the orbit may also occur without a visible fracture, probably due to rapid movement of the intraorbital soft tissues caused by direct force. The space-occupying character of intraorbital hematomas may persist long after trauma and remain obvious when using imaging procedures.

Orbital roof (and orbital floor) fractures can be easily missed on axial plane CT scans because of their horizontal course (Fig. 2.61a). Scanning in the coronal plane is therefore helpful, and indeed often necessary to diagnose this type of fracture. In cases of diffuse retrobulbar bleeding CT may not reveal increased densities of blood at the early stage. As soon as clot formation is initiated, the typical findings of hematoma are demonstrated by diffuse increased densities secondary to the high attenuation values of hematoma formation on the CT scan (Fig. 2.61b). MRI in the coronal and/or sagittal plane best reveals meningoceles, encephaloceles, and subperiosteal hematoma because of the readily identifiable characteristic signal intensities. MRI also shows various abnormal signal intensities specific to the different ages of hemorrhage from deoxyhemoglobin to methemoglobin and hemosiderin formation.

2.6.3.5 Fractures of the Orbital Apex (Optic Foramen)

Fractures of the optic foramen are uncommon. They are usually caused by a severe force to the face and skull. Although they may occur as an isolated fracture, they are more often found in association with other fractures of the viscero- or neurocranium such as the Le Fort III fracture or an extensive orbital floor fracture. They tend to extend into the sphenoid sinus and in these cases cause an increased density and an associated fluid level within the sinus. The optic nerve is nearly always involved in cases of a fracture of the optic foramen because of its close relationship to the bony canal. The degree of injury varies significantly, however, depending on the extension and comminution of the fracture. Stretching forces to the optic nerve may cause its swelling or surrounding bleeding because the intracanalicular portion of the optic nerve is fixed. In these cases temporary loss of vision may occur. If bony fragments of a comminuted fracture injure the nerve itself, however, there will be partial interruption of the optic nerve fibers or even complete disconnection of the nerve, leading to persistent loss of vision.

For fractures of the orbital apex, conventional plain films make no sense because the hidden site of the optic foramen cannot be demonstrated sufficiently. Again, CT with a bone window setting optimally demonstrates these fractures and especially their relationship to the optic canal. The bony margins of the orbital apex are well seen in the axial plane. Therefore CT should be done primarily in the

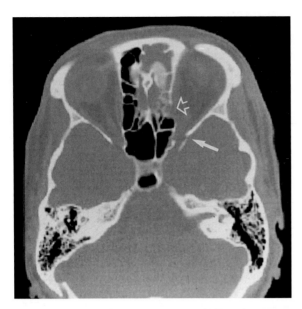

Fig. 2.62. Fracture of the orbital apex. Axial CT scan in the bone window setting demonstrates a displaced fracture of the left orbital apex (*arrow*). Note also the fracture of the medial wall of the left orbit (*open arrow*)

axial plane using thin-section high-resolution scanning (Fig. 2.62). If changes within the adjacent soft tissues have to be demonstrated or ruled out, MRI must be considered the best radiological modality. The investigation should be done with 2- to 3-mm thin T1-weighted images in the axial, coronal, and sagittal planes along the longitudinal axis of the optic nerve without administration of contrast medium. T2-weighted images are very helpful in the identification of fluid, e.g., edema of the optic nerve, fluid around the optic nerve, and fluid within the adjacent paranasal sinuses. Injuries to the optic nerve in its retrobulbar part, in the canal, and in the intracranial cavity also can be best demonstrated using MRI. In cases of severe trauma to the apex of the orbit, a carotid-cavernous sinus fistula may develop rapidly or slowly after a fracture. As already mentioned in Sect. 2.2.4, concerning trauma to the base of the skull, angiography is the diagnostic method of choice in detecting such fistulae, and can often be combined with immediate endovascular treatment (Fig. 2.63).

2.6.4 Mandible

2.6.4.1 General Considerations

The architectural structure of the mandible is strongly influenced by the pattern of stress to which

it is subjected. Like other stress-bearing bones, it has a characteristic tubular structure best configured for resisting lateral forces. In profile the mandible is L-shaped, with a vertical ascending ramus and a horizontal body on each side. The typical horseshoe shape is seen if the mandible is observed from above or below. The horizontal body and the ascending ramus join at the angle of the mandible, which carries the main muscles of mastication. The coronoid process is the superior projection of the anterior aspect of the ascending ramus. The narrow condylar neck with the surmounted condyle is the superior projection of the posterior margin of the ascending ramus. The mandibular canal contains the major portion of the third division of the trigeminal nerve and extends from the medial part of the ascending ramus through the cancellous bone of the body to the mental foramen, which perforates the lateral cortex adjacent to the bicuspid roots. These structural characteristics create several sites which are predisposed to fracturing when subjected to abnormal forces. These sites include the mental foramina, tooth sockets, crypts of impacted teeth, and condylar neck.

2.6.4.2 Fractures of the Mandible

The prominent site of the mandible makes this bone vulnerable to injury, similarly to the nasal bones and the orbit. About 40% of patients with severe maxillofacial injury have one or more fractures of the mandible. There are different kinds of fractures. There may be only a single line of fracture (simple fracture) or more fracture segments (complex or comminuted fracture). Especially in children greenstick-type fractures or incomplete fractures are found.

Malocclusion, trismus, tenderness, swelling, pain, limitation of mandibular motion, and intraoral bleeding are common clinical findings with mandibular trauma. Because the majority of mandibular fractures communicate either directly with the outside environment via a laceration or indirectly via the periodontal space, they are prone to secondary infectious complications.

2.6.4.2.1 Fractures of the Temporomandibular Joint. The temporomandibular joint (TMJ) is divided into two separate joint spaces by an intervening meniscus where the upper joint space is the larger one. The TMJ is a combined hinge-sliding articulation with great individual variations in the shape of the mandibular condyle, capped by articular cartilage. The

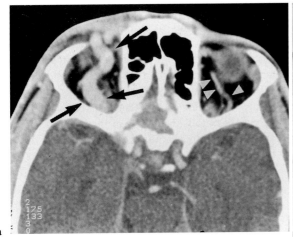

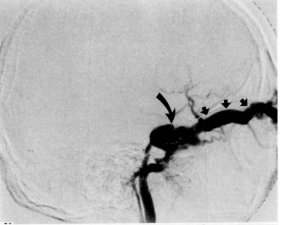

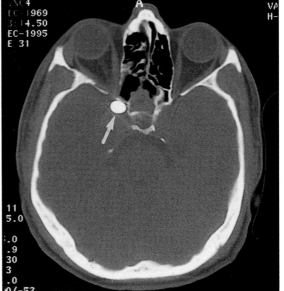

Fig. 2.63a–c. Traumatic carotid-cavernous sinus fistula. **a** Axial CT scan after administration of contrast medium demonstrates the widened superior ophthalmic vein (*arrows*) within the right orbit. Note the normal vein on the opposite site (*arrowheads*). Subsequently, digital subtraction angiography (**b**) demonstrates in the lateral view a large fistula between the internal carotid artery and the cavernous sinus (*curved arrow*) draining into the extremely widened superior ophthalmic vein (*arrows*). **c** Axial CT scan after an interventional procedure demonstrates the inflated balloon (*arrow*) within the fistula

meniscus has a roughly oval shape; it is posteriorly attached to the temporal bone and anteriorly to the superior head of the lateral pterygoid muscle. The majority of fractures in this region involve the condyle. They may be divided into three types: first, fractures with involvement of the intracapsular portion of the condylar head; second, fractures of the extracapsular portion of the condylar neck; and third, the more caudal subcondylar fractures (Fig. 2.64a). Fracture treatment with overly late mobilization may lead to ankylosis (Fig. 2.64b) of the TMJ with growth arrest in children.

The most frequently utilized plain film radiographs for evaluating TMJ fractures are the lateral, base, and Towne's projections. The TMJ is located in direct projection to the petrous bone and the mastoid air cells. Therefore lateral views should be done with craniocaudal angulation of the beam to avoid overlapping with the neighboring structures. Some authors also recommend "corrected" images, because the condyles are inclined approximately 10° posteromedially. CT has great value for the detection of lesions of the TMJ. Beside the routinely obtained axial plane scans, supplementary reconstructed sagittal plane thin slices are helpful for evaluation. Reconstructions are utilized because direct sagittal scanning is complex. Two-component arthrography under fluoroscopy or videofluoroscopy is a highly reliable and established diagnostic procedure, but this method is an invasive procedure. Arthrography is superior to CT and MRI for diagnosis of capsular adhesions and the detection of small ruptures involving the meniscus attachments or demonstration of meniscus derangements following joint

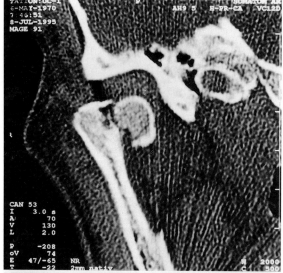

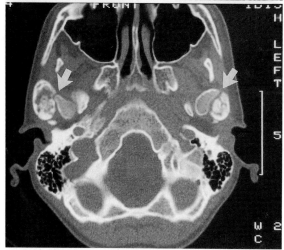

Fig. 2.64a,b. Fracture of the temporomandibular joint. **a** Direct coronal CT scan demonstrates fracture of the mandibular condyle. Note the typical medial displacement of the condyle. **b** Axial CT scan in the bone window setting demonstrates bilateral ankylosis of the temporomandibular joint (*arrows*)

2.6.4.2.2 Fractures of the Mandibular Ramus and Angle. This group of fractures includes the subcondylar fracture, the coronoid fracture, the ramus fracture, and the angle fracture. The most common among these sites of fracture is the subcondylar neck. When this fracture occurs, the condyle is characteristically angulated or pulled medially by the lateral pterygoid muscle. Fractures of the coronoid process and the ascending ramus are rare because of the protecting influence of the overlying zygomatic arch and muscles of mastication. In the event of a direct force to the chin, there are often bilateral condylar neck fractures with or without a concomitant fracture in the parasymphyseal region. Condylar neck fractures may be diagnosed as a solitary fracture, but they frequently occur in combination with a fracture of the contralateral body or angle (so-called contrecoup injury).

Fractures of the ramus and the angle of the mandible are usually adequately demonstrated on plain films. The routine mandible series consists of a posteroanterior view, of bilateral oblique posteroanterior views of the mandible, the of a Towne's view. The horizontal Panorex (zonarc) study is especially helpful in detecting fractures of the posterior third of the mandible (Fig. 2.65a,b). CT can be helpful in evaluating severely comminuted or displaced fractures as well as postoperative complications. Direct coronal CT scan reveals dislocated subcondylar fractures best, demonstrating the angulated and medially displaced condyles (Fig. 2.65c). On axial CT scans, the so-called empty TMJ is a reliable sign of displacement of the mandibular condyle.

Mandibular fractures differ from other facial fractures because of the distracting influence of the attached muscles. The physiological attachment of the muscles must be familiar to the evaluating radiologist in order to be able to estimate correctly possible amounts of bone fragment displacement, which depends not only upon the extent of the fracture but also upon the muscle traction. Muscle pull may keep the fracture elements together or distract them depending on the course of the fracture line. Muscle pull is responsible for some dangerous types of mandible fractures through which obstruction of the upper airway can occur. The flail mandible consists of a fracture of the parasymphyseal region in conjunction with bilateral subcondylar, ramus, or angle fractures presenting the danger of posterior displacement of the fragments due to the above-mentioned pull of the attached muscles.

injuries, but it has no indication in the detection of fractures in acute trauma. Surface coil MRI has changed the diagnosis of TMJ derangements fundamentally; it is the procedure of choice because of its multiplanar imaging capabilities, noninvasive character, and superior soft tissue contrast resolution. But once again, MRI does not serve well for the assessment of bone damage in acute trauma. The vast majority of cases of acute maxillofacial trauma are therefore imaged with CT, allowing superior demonstration of bony injury while usually providing adequate soft tissue information for initial patient management.

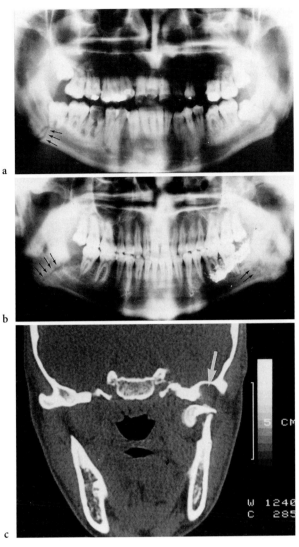

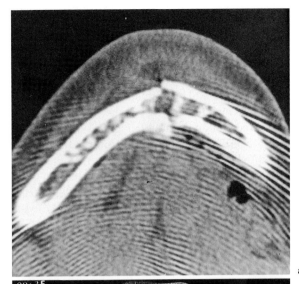

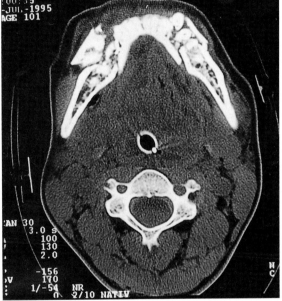

Fig. 2.65a–c. Fractures of the mandibular ramus and angle. **a** The horizontal Panorex study demonstrates a fracture without significant dislocation of the right mandibular angle (*arrows*). Note the connection to the tooth-bearing portion of the mandible, leading to an "open" fracture with a high risk of infection. **b** Another horizontal Panorex study demonstrates nonunion of a bilateral fracture of the mandibular angle (*arrows*) following infection. **c** Direct coronal CT scan best demonstrates the dislocation of a fracture of the neck of the condyle. Note the typical medial displacement of the fragment and the "empty" left temporomandibular joint (*arrow*)

Fig. 2.66a,b. Fractures of the mandibular body. **a** Axial CT scan in the bone window setting clearly demonstrates a simple fracture of the mandibular body. However, the axial CT scan is more helpful in the case of severe comminuted or compound fractures (**b**), demonstrating the amount of displacement best, particularly preoperatively

Posttraumatic mandibular complications include ankylosis of the TMJ, permanent anesthesia of V_3, malunion of the fracture (nonapproximation), and nonunion of the fracture due to infection or mobility during healing. Especially ankylosis of the TMJ joint is well seen on CT scans in the bone window setting with thin sections in the coronal plane. Nonunion can be recognized on both plain films and CT scans, although healing of a mandibular fracture is defined clinically by the extent of mobility and pain at the fracture site. Radiographically it may be impossible to define the evidence of healing because a lucency in the region of the fracture may present for several months.

2.6.4.2.3 Fractures of the Mandibular Body and Dentoalveolar Fractures. This group includes the body fracture, the symphyseal fracture, and the dentoalveolar fracture. The tooth-bearing alveolar process is surmounted on the basal cortical bone of the body. All fractures traversing the tooth-bearing portion of the mandible are presumed to be compound injuries because of the communication with the oral cavity. This explains the high risk of infections in compound mandibular fractures, sometimes leading to malunion or chronic osteomyelitis.

The edentulous mandible requires special attention because of the missing structural stability of the mandibular alveolus and dentition. In this context another type of dangerous displacement of fragments due to the pull of the adjacent muscles must be mentioned. The bilateral edentulous mandibular fracture may be associated with significant displacement of the anterior fragment by the suprahyoid musculature, leading to the possibility of rapid obstruction of the upper airway. Additionally it is in general important to examine the chest film when a fracture involves the alveolar process of the mandible in order to rule out the presence of aspirated teeth.

From the radiological point of view, fractures of the body of the mandible including the parasymphyseal region are normally seen adequately on plain films. The most helpful projections are the occlusal view, the Panorex, the posteroanterior mandible view, and the right and left oblique mandible views. CT may be very helpful in cases of comminuted or compound fractures, particularly in the symphyseal or parasymphyseal regions (Fig. 2.66). Often there will be extensive soft tissue swelling, better seen on CT scans than on plain films. Fractures of the mandibular body can be demonstrated by CT in the axial as well as in the direct coronal view. MRI has no role in the detection of fractures in these localizations. With regard to lesions of the teeth or rootnerves, there are certain special plain films used mainly by dentists which will not be discussed here.

References

Aldrich EF, Eisenberg HM, Saydjari C et al. (1992) Diffuse brain swelling in severely head-injured children. J Neurosurg 76:450–454

Baker SR, Gaylord G, Lantos G, Tabbador K, Gallagher J (1984) The use of restrictive criteria for emergency skull radiography (abstract). Radiology 153(P):20
Davis JM, Zimmerman RA (1983) Injury of the carotid and vertebral arteries. Neuroradiology 25:55–69
Drayer BP, Wilkins RH, Boehnke M, Horton JA, Rosenbaum AE (1977) Cerebrospinal fluid rhinorrhea demonstrated by metrizamide CT cisternography. AJR 129:149–151
Fobben ES, Grossman RI, Atlas SW, Hackney DB, Goldberg HI, Zimmerman RA, Bilaniuk LT (1989) MR characteristics of subdural hematomas and hygromas at 1.5 T. AJNR 10:687–693
Gean AD (1994) Imaging of head trauma. Raven, New York
Gentry LR, Godersky JC, Thompson B (1988) MR imaging of head trauma: review of the distribution and radiopathologic features of traumatic lesions. AJNR 9:101–110
Gomori JM, Grossman RI, Goldberg HI, Zimmerman A, Bilaniuk LT (1985) Intracranial hematomas: imaging by high field MR. Radiology 157:87–93
Hackney DB (1991) Skull radiography in the evaluation of acute head trauma: a survey of current practice. Radiology 181:711–714
Hamilton M, Wallace C (1992) Nonoperative management of acute epidural hematoma diagnosed by CT: the neuroradiologist's role. AJNR 13:853–859
Isherwood I (1992) Radiology of head injuries. In: Harwood-Nash DC, Petterson H (eds) Neuroradiology. NICER Series on Diagnostic Imaging. Merit Communications, London
Kelly AB, Zimmerman RD, Snow RB, Gandy SE, Heier LA, Deck MDF (1988) Head trauma: comparison of MR and CT – experience in 100 patients. AJNR 9:699–708
Manelfe C, Cellerier P, Sobeel D, Prevost C, Bonafe A (1982) Cerebrospinal fluid rhinorrhea: evaluation with metrizamide cisternography. AJR 138:471–476
Mirvis SE, Wolf AL, Numaguchi Y, Corradino G, Joslyn JN (1990) Posttraumatic cerebral infarction diagnosed by CT: prevalence, origin, and outcome. AJNR 11:355–360
Newton TH, Hasso AN, Dillon WP (1988) Computed tomography of the head and neck. Raven, New York
Osborn AG (1994) Diagnostic neuroradiology. Mosby, St. Louis
Samii M, Brihaye J (1983) Traumatology of the skull base. Springer, Berlin Heidelberg New York
Sato Y, Yuh WTC, Smith WL, Alexander RC, Kao SCS, Ellerbroek CJ (1989) Head injury in child abuse: evaluation with MR imaging. Radiology 173:653–657
Servadei F, Nanni A, Nasi MT, Zappi D, Vergoni G, Giuliani G, Arista A (1995) Evolving brain lesions in the first 12 hours after head injury: analysis of 37 comatose patients. Neurosurgery 37:899–907
Som PM (1985) CT of the paranasal sinuses. Neuroradiology 27:189–201
Taveras JM, Ferrucci JT (1992) Radiology. Diagnosis, imaging, intervention, vol 3. Neuroradiology and radiology of the head and neck. J.B. Lippincott, Philadelphia

3 Spine

C.H. Buitrago-Téllez, F.J. Ferstl, and M. Langer

CONTENTS

3.1 General Considerations

Spinal injuries represent a major source of disability in modern society, especially when they occur in conjunction with longstanding neurological deficits. The overall rate of neurologic damage following spinal injuries ranges from 10% to 23%.

A bimodal age percentage distribution of patients with vertebral injuries has been reported, showing that young adult males are most commonly affected, followed by elderly females (Riggins and Krauss 1977). A common aspect of spinal trauma is therefore its disabling effect on young productive patients with a high economic, psychological, and occupational impact.

Depending on the series, motor vehicle (Dorr et al. 1982) or occupational accidents (Wimmer 1989) are the largest single external cause of spinal trauma, followed by falls, home accidents, sports and recreational activities, and suicide attempts.

Fractures associated with spinal cord injury most often occur in the cervical spine, especially C1/C2 or C4/C7, and in the thoracolumbar junction. Recently, upper thoracic spinal fractures have been associated with neurological injury in up to 63% of the cases (Meyer 1989; El-Khoury and Whitten 1993).

Another important aspect to be taken into account is the high incidence of multilevel spinal injuries, which occur in 17%–30.4% of cases. Common sites for second noncontiguous fractures of the thoracic spine are the upper cervical spine and the thoracolumbar junction. It is therefore mandatory to search for other spine fractures once a fracture is detected, especially in polytraumatized patients.

3.2 Anatomy and Biomechanics

3.2.1 Anatomy

3.2.1.1 General Characteristics

The spinal column includes 7 cervical, 12 thoracic, 5 lumbar and 5 fused sacral vertebrae. Except for C1, C2, and the sacrum, each vertebra has similar osseous morphologic characteristics. Diskoligamentous structures differ slightly according to the spinal level (Yu et al. 1991).

The typical osseous structures of a vertebra include the body and the neural arch. The neural arch or osseous posterior element consists of both pedicles, articular pillars with their superior and inferior processes, posterolateral laminae, and transverse and spinous processes.

C.H. Buitrago-Téllez, MD, Abteilung Röntgendiagnostik, Radiologische Universitätsklinik, Klinikum der Albert-Ludwigs-Universität Freiburg, Hugstetterstraße 55, 79106 Freiburg, Germany
F.J. Ferstl, MD, Abteilung Röntgendiagnostik, Radiologische Universitätsklinik, Klinikum der Albert-Ludwigs-Universität Freiburg, Hugstetterstraße 55, 79106 Freiburg, Germany
M. Langer, MD, FICA, Professor and Director, Abteilung Röntgendiagnostik, Radiologische Universitätsklinik, Klinikum der Albert-Ludwigs-Universität Freiburg, Hugstetterstraße 55, 79106 Freiburg, Germany

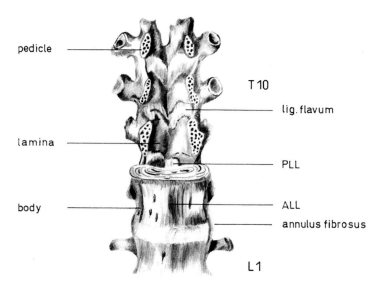

pedicle

T 10

lig. flavum

lamina

PLL

body

ALL

annulus fibrosus

L 1

Fig. 3.1. Ligamentous structures of the thoracic and lumbar spine. *PLL,* Posterior longitudinal ligament; *ALL,* anterior longitudinal ligament. (Modified from Moore 1982)

The spinal canal, formed by the adjacent vertebral foramina, contains the posterior longitudinal and flava ligaments, an organized venous plexus, the dural sac, spinal cord, cerebrospinal fluid, and nerve roots.

The neural or intervertebral foramina are bound by the vertebral bodies and intervertebral disks anteriorly, the incisurae of the adjacent pedicles superiorly and inferiorly, and the facet joints posteriorly. Each foramen contains the spinal nerve, blood vessels, and fat.

The spinal ligaments throughout the entire spine include the anterior and posterior longitudinal, interspinous, supraspinous, flaval and capsular ligaments (Fig. 3.1). The anterior longitudinal ligament attaches at the anterior and lateral surfaces of the vertebral bodies, extending from the occipital bone down to the sacrum. The posterior longitudinal ligament is a thin and narrow band of dense fibrous tissue consisting of a superficial layer without contact to the vertebral bodies and a deep layer along the posterior margin of vertebral bodies attached to the posterior disk surface (PRESTAR and PUTZ 1982).

3.2.1.2 Cervical Spine and Craniocervical Region

The osseous structures in the craniocervical region are unique and include the occipital condyles and the foramen magnum (anterior border: basion; posterior: opisthion), as well as the atlas and axis. The atlas, consisting of a ring structure formed by the anterior and posterior arches, is located in the neighborhood of lateral masses and transverse processes.

The axis is characterized by the presence of the dens, and also contains a vertebral body, pedicles, lateral masses and transverse and spinous processes. Odontoid dimensions, especially at the neck level of the dens, are particularly important for surgical planning in cases of unstable fractures (NUCCI et al. 1995). The minimum dens transverse width at this level ranges from 6 to 10mm (XU et al. 1995).

Ligaments connecting the occiput and the axis include the tectorial membrane, the cruciate ligament, the apical ligament, and the paired alar or occipitodental ligaments (Fig. 3.2). The transverse portion of the cruciate ligament or transverse ligament extends between both osseous tubercles at the inner surface of the lateral masses of the atlas dorsal to the dens.

The characteristic structures of the cervical vertebrae are the transverse foramina from C3 to C7, which contain, with the exception of C7, the vertebral artery. The facet joints are oriented in an oblique plane and angled 45° with respect to the coronal plane when it parallels the vertical axis of the cervical spine. The facet joints are also 45° to the axial plane when the axial plane is perpendicular to the vertical axis. These facts are important for the 2D computed tomographic (CT) reconstructions and the biomechanics of the cervical spine.

3.2.1.3 Thoracic and Lumbar Spine

The upper thoracic spine has some peculiarities relevant to spinal trauma. Firstly, the ovoid or rounded lumen of the spinal canal has its narrowest segment

Fig. 3.2. Ligamentous structures at the craniocervical junction. *ant.,* Anterior; *lig.,* ligament; *trans.,* transverse; *inf.,* inferior; *sup.,* superior; *post.,* posterior. (Modified from BULAS et al. 1993)

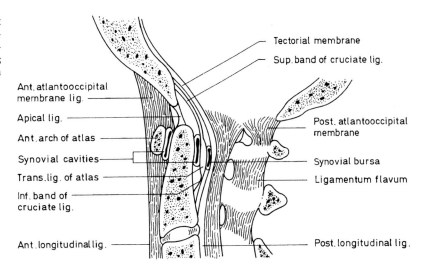

Ant. atlantooccipital membrane lig.

Apical lig.

Ant. arch of atlas

Synovial cavities

Trans. lig. of atlas

Inf. band of cruciate lig.

Ant. longitudinal lig.

Tectorial membrane

Sup. band of cruciate lig.

Post. atlantooccipital membrane

Synovial bursa

Ligamentum flavum

Post. longitudinal lig.

at the thoracic spine. Thus, even minimal narrowing of the spinal canal may be accompanied by neurologic lesions. Secondly, the presence of the costovertebral and costotransverse joints is characteristic of the thoracic spine, increasing resistance against trauma. Throughout T1 to T10 the facets are in the coronal plane, with the articulating facets being situated on the posterior surface of the superior articular process and ventral surface of the inferior process. Thus, they actively limit sagittal translation.

The lower dorsal vertebrae (T11/T12) differ from the typical dorsal morphology, having only a single vertebral facet to articulate with the corresponding 11th and 12th ribs. Moreover, facets begin to change their orientation to simulate the lumbar pattern (oblique sagittal).

The lumbar spine is characterized by the greater dimension of the vertebral bodies and spinal canal in comparison to their cervical and thoracic counterparts. The oblique sagittal orientation pattern of the facet joints limits rotation.

3.2.2 Biomechanics

3.2.2.1 General Aspects

The analysis of biomechanics in the setting of spinal trauma requires knowledge of the normal function of the spine, the injury mechanism, and the mechanics of therapeutic approaches. In the following, a succinct survey of the mechanics of the normal spinal column will be presented. The injury mechanisms will be discussed in Sect. 3.3.

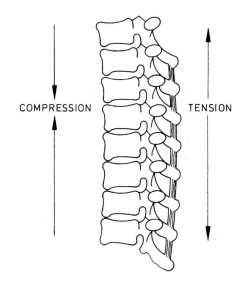

COMPRESSION   TENSION

Fig. 3.3. Biomechanical model of Whitesides: an anterior weight-bearing column of vertebral bodies/intervertebral disks and a posterior column of neural arches/ligaments resisting tension (modified from WHITESIDES 1977)

According to the biomechanic model of WHITESIDES (1977), the basic function of the spine is to maintain the erect position and to protect the neural elements that pass through it. In order to maintain this erect position, and considering the localization of the center of gravity anterior to the cervical spine, he proposed a two-column structure of the spine: an anterior weight-bearing column of vertebral bodies/intervertebral disks and a posterior column of neural arches/ligaments resisting tension (Fig. 3.3).

According to Whitesides' model, rotatory stability of the spine is provided by the facet alignment and all the ligamentous complexes. Experimental studies on the characteristics of vertebral structures seem to support this model. Vertebral bodies are essential to withstand axial forces. Mechanical stress within a vertebra during axial compression is directly proportional to the load applied, and inversely proportional to the cross-sectional area of the bone. Thus, smaller vertebrae, as in the case of females, may diminish axial load tolerance (GILSANZ et al. 1994).

Among the posterior elements responsible for withstanding tension, the strong supraspinous ligament and the flaval ligament deserve special mention. The posterior longitudinal ligament, although not part of the posterior ligamentous complex, is essential to withstand tension posteriorly under hyperflexion/distraction, having a tolerance of up to 180 N.

As regards the motion of contiguous spinal segments, the most accepted model of biomechanics of spinal movement is based on a motion segment consisting of two adjacent vertebrae together with the connected ligamentous structures. In accordance with this concept, WHITE and PANJABI (1990) presupposed six degrees of freedom of spinal motion: flexion, extension and left and lateral translation through a horizontal laterolateral x-axis, axial compression, axial distraction and clockwise and counterclockwise rotation through a craniocaudal vertical y-axis and lateral flexion to either side and anterior or posterior translation through a dorsoventral horizontal z-axis. This model allows an individual analysis of any motion component in a specific spinal injury.

3.2.2.2 Regional Aspects

Functional stability of the occipito-atlanto-axial joints depends on the surrounding ligaments that connect the occiput to the axis and atlas. The tectorial membrane and paired alar ligaments are primary stabilizers of the cranium (BULAS et al. 1993). The transverse ligament is essential for stability of the atlantoaxial unit.

In the cervical region the articular facets are small, flat, and angled 45° from the horizontal plane. This orientation explains the great degree of motion allowed, as well as the relative ease with which cervical facets subluxate, dislocate, and lock.

Throughout the upper thoracic spine, the coronal oriented facets provide significant resistance to anterior translation. Biomechanically, the rib cage provides additional strength and energy-absorbing

capacity, especially with respect to rotational and compressional forces.

The thoracolumbar and lumbar pattern of facet orientation – oblique sagittal – limits rotation but has less effect on anterior translation, thus making facet dislocation more frequent than in the upper thoracic spine.

3.3 Classification

3.3.1 Stability

One of the major purposes of diagnostic imaging in the setting of spinal trauma is to assess whether a fracture is stable or unstable. This apparently simple differentiation has significant therapeutic implications. Unfortunately, there is no agreement concerning the definition of stability. Some researchers such as WHITE and PANJABI (1990) and WHITESIDES (1977) have tried to include in their definitions general aspects applicable to the entire spine.

WHITE and PANJABI (1990) defined clinical instability as "the loss of the ability of the spine under physiological loads to maintain relationships between vertebrae in such a way that there is neither initial damage nor subsequent irritation to the spinal cord or nerve roots and, in addition, there is no development or incapacitating deformity or pain due to structural changes."

WHITESIDES (1977) also introduced into his definition biomechanical aspects concerning physiological loads. He considered a stable spine as one "that can withstand axial compressive forces anteriorly through the vertebral bodies, tension forces posteriorly, and rotational stresses, thus being able to function to hold the body erect without progressive kyphosis and to protect the spinal contents from further injury."

These definitions are conceptually important in understanding the meaning of an unstable spine. However, concrete signs or facts are necessary to define instability in the acute clinical setting. In this respect, the decisive initial proposal was made by Sir Frank HOLDSWORTH (1970), who considered instability of a spinal injury below C2 to be present if the "posterior ligamentous complex" consisting of the interspinous and supraspinous ligaments, the capsules of the lateral joints, and the ligamentum flavum was damaged. WHITESIDES (1977) redefined the two-column concept of Holdsworth, differentiating an anterior weight-bearing column of vertebral bodies and a posterior column of osseous and ligamentous

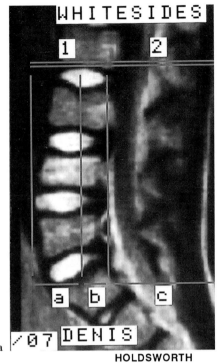

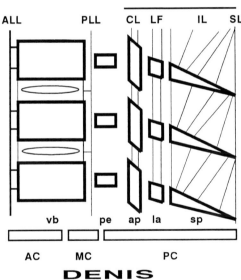

Fig. 3.4a,b. Two- versus three-column concept of the spine. **a** Sagittal T2-weighted image with a type A compression fracture of L4 demonstrating the structures of the anterior (*1*) and posterior (*2*) columns of Whitesides as well as the anterior (*a*), middle (*b*), and posterior (*c*) columns of Denis. **b** Schematic representation of the spine underlying the posterior ligamentous complex as defined by Holdsworth. *CL,* Capsular ligament; *LF,* ligamentum flavum; *IL,* interspinous ligament; *SL,* supraspinous ligament; *vb,* vertebral body; *pe,* pedicle; *ap,* articular pillar; *la,* lamina; *sp,* spinous process. Note the different attachments of the anterior longitudinal ligament (*ALL*) and posterior longitudinal ligament (*PLL*). The three colums of Denis are also marked (*AC,* anterior column; *MC,* middle column; *PC,* posterior column)

elements resisting tension. Based on experimental evidence revealing that isolated complete rupture of the posterior ligamentous complex was insufficient to create instability in flexion, extension, rotation, and shear, DENIS (1983) proposed the three-column concept, which added a middle column of great importance for the diagnosis of stability.

Supporting the three-column concept, MCAFEE et al. (1983) specified the limits of the three columns, the *anterior column* consisting of the anterior longitudinal ligament, the anterior two-thirds of the vertebral body, and the anterior part of the annulus fibrosus, the *middle column* comprising the posterior third of the vertebral body, the posterior part of the annulus fibrosus, and the posterior longitudinal ligament, and the *posterior column* including the facet joint capsules, the flaval ligaments, the osseous neural arch, the supraspinous and interspinous ligaments, and the articular processes. The different column concepts are represented in Fig. 3.4.

According to the three-column theory, the middle column is the key to instability: Lesions of the posterior column are unstable if one structure of the middle column is also affected, and lesions of the anterior and middle columns are unstable at least in flexion/compression. By contrast, isolated lesions of the anterior or posterior column are stable. Lesions of all three columns are unstable. Denis' system of classification into minor and major injuries was too extensive for practical use, and was consequently modified by MCAFEE et al. (1983) according to the type of failure of the middle osteoligamentous complex as visualized by CT (Table 3.1). MCAFEE et al. (1983) differentiated between stable and unstable burst fractures on the basis of whether or not the posterior column is involved, i.e., involvement of the posterior column is indicative of an unstable burst fracture. Wedge compression fractures are stable and the other groups show increasing instability, especially the translational injuries. Although primarily conceived for the thoracolumbar spine, the three-column concept may be applied to the middle and lower cervical spine. WOLTER (1985) proposed

Table 3.1. Classification of thoracolumbar fractures according to MCAFEE et al. (1983)

Wedge compression fracture
Stable burst fracture
Unstable burst fracture
Chance fracture
Flexion-distraction injury
Translation injury

Table 3.2. Radiographic criteria for instability of the spine below C2 according to DAFFNER et al. (1990)

Displaced vertebrae
Widened interlaminar or interspinous distance
Perched or dislocated facet joints
Increased interpediculate distance
Disrupted posterior vertebral line

Table 3.3. Radiographic signs of instability with reference to the involved column (according to JEND and HELLER 1989)

Anterior column
Teardrop: rupture of the anterior longitudinal ligament
Compression of more than 50%
Tilting of vertebral bodies by more than 11° in comparison to adjacent vertebrae

Middle column
Irregularity of the posterior vertebral line
Translation of the posterior vertebral margin >3.5 mm
Diminished posterior vertebral height
Increased interpediculate distance

Posterior column
Widened interspinous distance
Fracture of posterior elements
Lateral dislocation of the articular processes
Facet dislocation >5 mm
Facet articulation <50%
Facet luxation

Table 3.4. Signs suggesting instability in the occipito-atlanto-axial region (modified from JEND and HELLER 1989)

Dens–basion distance
    Adults >4–5 mm
    Children >12 mm
Difference on flexion/extension >1 mm
Atlantodental distance >3 mm
Displacement of the lateral masses of the atlas >7 mm
Soft tissue swelling at C2 >7 mm
Ratio of basion-posterior arch of C1/opisthion-anterior arch of C1 >1
Widening of atlanto-occipital joint >5 mm

quantification of the narrowing of the spinal canal as a further criterion for classification, distinguishing between four degrees of narrowing: 0 (no narrowing), 1 (33%), 2 (66%), and 3 (complete obstruction). Unfortunately, there is clinical evidence of a lack of correlation between spinal canal narrowing and neurological deficit (RIGGINS and KRAUSS 1977; WIMMER 1989).

Some researchers (MAIMAN and PINTAR 1992) have questioned the three-column concept for the upper thoracic spine. Furthermore, DAFFNER et al. (1990) proposed a model based on radiographic criteria for instability that would apply to the entire

spine below C2: if one or more of the proposed radiographic signs is present, the injury is to be considered unstable (Table 3.2).

In this context, JEND and HELLER (1989) undertook a complete review of the radiographic signs of instability based upon the analysis of the three columns of Denis (Table 3.3) or topographic features of the occipito-atlanto-axial region (Table 3.4), the middle and lower cervical spine (Table 3.5), and the thoracolumbar spine (Table 3.6). These signs are helpful, especially in the careful analysis of conventional radiographs. However, the fact that up to 16% of spinal fractures observed to be unstable on CT are primarily misdiagnosed as stable on plain films (WIMMER 1989) underlines the need for knowledge of the type of injuries associated with instability and a further diagnostic step if uncertainty persists.

In this setting, there are two classifications in respect of the upper cervical spine which have been widely accepted because of their relevance in indicating stability. These are the classifications of ANDERSON and D'ALONZO, 1974 for odontoid frac-

Table 3.5. Signs suggesting instability of the middle/lower cervical spine (from JEND and HELLER 1989)

Widening of the interspinous distance
Decreased intervertebral space anteriorly
Dislocation >3.5 mm
Tilting >11°
Widening of zygapophyseal joints
Facet articulation <50%
Facet subluxation >5 mm
Prevertebral soft tissue swelling at C6 >22 mm
Bilateral facet dislocation
Anterior-basal teardrop fragment

Table 3.6. Signs suggesting instability of the thoracolumbar spine (modified from JEND and HELLER 1989)

Lateral view
Compression of posterior vertebral margin
Anterior compression of vertebral body with signs of rupture of the posterior longitudinal ligament
Dislocation of the vertebral bodies >2–3 mm
Tilting of more than 5° (thoracic) or 11° (lumbar) in comparison to adjacent vertebrae
Fracture of posterior elements
Translation >16% on flexion views, and >12% on extension views (lumbar spine)

Anteroposterior view
Lateral vertebral body compression with signs of rupture of the posterior longitudinal ligament
Widening of the vertebral body
Increased interpediculate distance
Translation of spinous processes

TYPE I   TYPE II   TYPE III

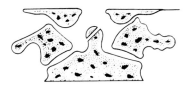 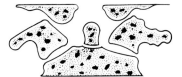 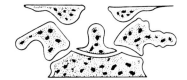

Fig. 3.5. Anderson and D'Alonzo's classification for odontoid fractures: type I, oblique fracture through the upper part of the odontoid process; type II, fracture line at the junction of the odontoid process with the vertebral body of C2; type III, fracture through the body of the atlas (modified from ANDERSON and D'ALONZO 1974)

TYPE I   TYPE II   TYPE III

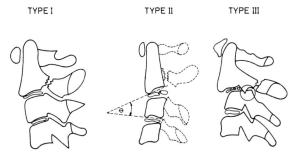

Fig. 3.6. Effendi's classification for traumatic spondylolisthesis of the axis (hangman's fractures/ring fractures of the axis: type I, nondisplaced, C2/C3 disk intact; type II, significant angulation (>15°) and/or translation (>3 mm) of C2 over C3 and disrupted C2/C3 disk; type III, same as type II with C2/C3 locked facets (modified from LEVINE and EDWARDS 1985)

tures (Fig. 3.5, Table 3.7) and of EFFENDI et al. (1981) for traumatic spondylolisthesis of the axis (hangman's fractures: Fig. 3.6, Table 3.8).

3.3.2 Injury Mechanism

Spinal injuries may be classified on the basis not only of their stability but also the presumed mechanism of injury. A combination of both is desirable, but there are some classifications that emphasize the injury pattern.

According to the mechanistic classification of ALLEN et al. (1982), the pattern of injury may allow one to infer the mechanism of injury. They proposed six categories depending on the injury mechanism: compressive flexion, distractive flexion, lateral flexion, translational, torsional flexion, vertical compression, and distractive extension.

Recently, MAGERL et al. (1994) simplified these concepts and presented a system for the classification of thoracic and lumbar injuries according to the main mechanism of injury, pathomorphological uniformity, and prognostic aspects (Table 3.9). These

authors considered just three types of spinal injury taking into account the main injury mechanisms acting on the spine: compression (type A), distraction (type B) and axial torque (type C) (Fig. 3.7).

This classification, based upon the review of 1445 spinal injuries, uses the widely accepted AO fracture classification system identifying three types of fracture (A/B/C) which are divided into three groups (A1–A3, B1–B3, C1–C3), each of which contains three subgroups with specifications. Also noteworthy is its relationship to the biomechanical model of WHITESIDES (1977), in which the spine is divided into two columns, as previously explained.

Table 3.7. Anderson and D'Alonzo's classification of odontoid fractures

Type	Definition	Stability
I	Oblique fracture through the upper part	Stable
II	Neck fracture at the junction with the body	Unstable
III	Fracture extending through the body of the axis	Stable

Table 3.8. Effendi's classification of traumatic spondylolisthesis of the axis (hangman's fractures)

Type	Definition	Stability
I	Fracture involving posterior part of the body of C2 or any part of the ring (Non-displaced) C2/C3 disk intact	Stable
II	Fracture as I Anterior displacement >3 mm Angulation >15° of C2 over C3 C2/C3 disk disrupted	Unstable
III	Features as II Uni- or bilateral C2/C3 locked facet	Unstable

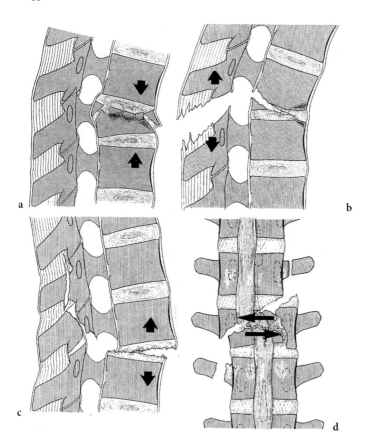

Fig. 3.7a–d. Magerl's AO classification system for spinal fractures: (**a**) type A compression fractures; (**b**) type B distraction injuries with posterior disruption; (**c**) type B distraction injuries with anterior disruption; (**d**) type C rotation injuries (from MAGERL et al. 1994)

Table 3.9. Comprehensive classification of thoracic and lumbar fractures according to MAGERL et al. (1994)

Type	Group
A. Vertebral body *compression*	A1 Impaction A2 Split A3 Burst
B. Anterior and posterior element injury with *distraction*	B1 Flexion-distraction injuries, predominantly ligamentous (posterior disruption) B2 Flexion-distraction injuries, predominantly osseous (posterior disruption) B3 Hyperextension shear injury (anterior disruption through the disk)
C. Anterior and posterior element in injury with *rotation*	C1 Type A with rotation C2 Type B with rotation C3 Rotational shear injuries

According to Magerl et al.'s classification, *type A* injuries result from failure to withstand unphysiologic axial compression forces and are therefore focused on the vertebral body. However, posterior osseous elements may be compromised in burst fractures (A3) without evidence of ligamental

rupture. *Type B* injuries result from failure to withstand pathologic tensional forces posteriorly with the subsequent transverse disruption of anterior and posterior elements with distraction (B1/B2) or anteriorly with anterior disruption of both columns (B3). Finally, *type C* injuries result from the impossibility of resisting rotational forces and therefore may be superimposed on type A (C1) or B (C2) fractures or represent the most unstable spinal injuries (rotational/shear injuries: C3).

This classification has, however, been subjected to criticism because of some overlap in the order of severity and stability of spinal injuries. GERTZBEIN (1994) therefore proposed modification of the system, especially with respect to type B and C fractures. According to this proposal, type C fractures are redefined as multidirectional with translation and further divided into three groups: C1 corresponding to anteroposterior dislocation, C2 to lateral shear injuries, and C3 to rotational shear or burst injuries. The basic difference consists in the definition of rotational injuries as a group (C3) and not as a type (i.e., type C). Additionally, sagittal dislocations, which may be classified among B1 or B2 fractures according to MAGERL et al. (1994), are considered as a single

Table 3.10. Classification of cervical spinal injuries according to injury mechanism and stability (modified from GREENSPAN 1993)

Injury mechanism	Stability
Flexion:	
Subluxation	Stable
Facet dislocation	
Unilateral	Stable
Bilateral	Unstable
Clay shoveler's fracture	Stable
Wedge fracture	Stable
Flexion-teardrop fracture	Unstable
Burst fracture	Stable/unstable
Odontoid fractures	
I/III	Stable
II	Unstable
Extension:	
Isolated posterior arch fracture of the atlas	Stable
Hangman's fracture	
I	Stable
II/III	Unstable
Hyperextension-teardrop fracture	Stable
Hyperextension fracture	Unstable
Dislocation	
Compression:	
Jefferson fracture	Unstable
Burst fracture	Stable/unstable
Compression	Stable
Shear:	
Lateral compression fracture	Stable
Lateral dislocation	Unstable
Avulsion of transverse processes	Stable
Isolated fracture of the lateral mass	Stable
Rotation:	
Fracture dislocation	Unstable
Fracture of the articular pillar and facet	Stable/unstable
Fracture of transverse process	Stable
Distraction:	
Hangman's fracture	
I	Stable
II/III	Unstable
Atlantoaxial subluxation	Stable/unstable

group (C1). This approach tries to combine severity concepts with the systematic analysis of MAGERL et al. (1994), but is not based on significant new data. Therefore, the AO classification system of Magerl et al. (Table 3.9) may be considered as a basis for the standardization of documentation of spinal injuries and for a rational therapeutic approach. For the assessment of stability, a detailed analysis should be made of the features of the specific fracture, taking into account the three-column concept of DENIS (1983).

It has been suggested that Magerl et al.'s system might also serve for the classification of injuries occurring in the lower cervical spine (C3–C7). How-

ever, considering the injury mechanism and stability of clinically common fractures, GREENSPAN (1993) proposed a classification system for the cervical spine (Table 3.10) which may be clinically useful if the typical features of the listed fractures can be identified.

3.4 Examination Methods

Safe and accurate radiographic diagnosis is essential for the evaluation and treatment of spinal trauma. The general purposes of spinal imaging are to detect and assess the extent of osseous, ligamentous, neural, and other soft tissue injuries and to help evaluate instability. The introduction of CT and MRI has yielded important additional diagnostic information, thereby facilitating the achievement of these objectives. In the following, a general survey of the relevant examination methods and their potential and limitations is presented.

3.4.1 Plain Film Radiography

Conventional radiography has retained its importance in the diagnosis of spinal trauma, although some of its inherent limitations must be taken into account. In all acutely injured patients with clinical signs of spine or spinal cord injury, and in all noncommunicating patients in whom a spinal injury is suspected based on the severity of the trauma, a radiographic survey of the entire spine should be performed.

Plain film radiographs may be generated using the analog or the digital storage technique. Although of lower spatial resolution, digital luminescence radiographs offer some advantages in the setting of traumatized patients since they avoid exposure difficulties, especially on lateral radiographs. The major application of radiographs lies in the evaluation of the osseous elements of the spine. As previously noted, several signs of instability may be identified on plain radiographs, especially concerning bony malalignment and extent of fractures. Other advantages include the short exposure and examination times, and the potential to provide a general survey of the entire structure of the spinal column. The main limitation is the poor visualization of soft tissues because of the inherently limited contrast resolution. Moreover, bony structures at the craniocervical and cervicothoracic junctions may be obscured by superimposition.

The reported sensitivity of plain film radiographs in detecting fractures ranges between 58% (WOODRING and LEE 1992) and 93% (STREITWIESER et al. 1983), while specificity values lie between 60% and 71%.

There is not universal agreement on the number of radiographic views that may be considered sufficient in the acute situation. The standard screening views of the cervical spine should at least include lateral, anteroposterior, and open mouth views (EL-KHOURY et al. 1995). Optional views include the right and left oblique views, the pillar view, and the swimmer's view. For the pillar view, a slight cervical hyperextension and a 30°–35° tilting of the x-ray tube in the craniocaudal direction are necessary. On this view fractures of the articular processes or the pillars are readily detected. For the swimmer's view, the patient must be able to lie prone with 180° abduction of the left arm and adduction of the right arm with the x-ray tube centered on the cervicothoracic junction. This view is indicated in a collaborating patient with inadequate visualization of the cervicothoracic junction on the lateral view.

Anteroposterior and lateral radiographs represent the mainstay of diagnostic imaging of the thoracolumbar spine. Anteroposterior radiographs are suitable for the evaluation of the vertebral bodies, while lateral radiographs are helpful in assessing vertebral body height, disk height, endplate irregularities, erosions, and alignment.

3.4.2 Conventional Tomography

It is known that conventional tomography is more sensitive than plain radiographs for detecting fractures, especially in the cervical spine (BINET et al. 1973; ACHESON et al. 1987). Conventional tomograms also may be indicated in the follow-up of the healing process of spinal fractures, particularly of the dens. However, despite its attributes, conventional complex motion tomography has been replaced by CT in the evaluation of the acute phase of spinal trauma, subsequent to the use of plain radiography. While it is widely accepted that conventional tomography may have advantages in detecting undisplaced dens and facet fractures (EHARA et al. 1992; WOODRING and LEE 1992), advocates of CT (KEENE et al. 1982; BRANT-ZAWADZKI et al. 1981) have reported that CT combined with standard radiography may be equal or superior to conventional tomography in assessing overall spinal trauma. Moreover, CT offers some relevant advantages in comparison to conventional tomography: less mobi-

lization, diagnosis of soft tissue or associated injuries in the trauma setting, the possibility of two- and three-dimensional reconstructions, and a lower radiation dose to the patient.

3.4.3 Functional Examinations

The purpose of functional examinations is to detect segmental instability in patients having no signs of osseous or ligamentous injuries on initial plain film evaluation but clinical symptoms suggesting diskoligamentous injuries in the cervical or lumbar spine such as localized pain and tenderness. They are seldom indicated in the acute phase and may be postponed several days until cooperation from the patient may be adequate. It must be emphasized that flexion/extension views of the cervical spine should be obtained only in an alert patient who is able to limit these maneuvers himself, if necessary. Lateral flexion and rotational views may be important in certain cases depending on clinical signs.

Functional examinations are especially relevant in the diagnosis of soft tissue instabilities, which have a potential for poor healing and may be progressive, especially in children (LOUIS 1977).

The most frequent indication for functional examinations is the so-called whiplash syndrome consisting in a wide range of symptoms after forcible hyperextension secondary to rear-end collisions. If the findings are initially negative, follow-up 1–4 weeks later is necessary to rule out a subacute late instability.

Functional imaging also may be performed in conjunction with MR imaging and CT. According to WEIDENMAIER (1994), MR imaging, performed at different degrees of flexion/extension in patients with negative radiographic functional images, may reveal up to 81% of unsuspected pathology. However, a rather selected group of patients were included in his series.

Three-dimensional CT functional images have also been suggested for the study of rotational instabilities but there is still no evidence of their accuracy in large series, and the radiation dose to the adjacent thyroid gland may be a limiting factor (BRAUNSCHWEIG and BILOW 1994).

3.4.4 Computed Tomography

The introduction of CT made possible the acquisition of important additional diagnostic information

Table 3.11. CT protocol for evaluation of spinal trauma

Standard
1–2 mm (cervical) and 3 mm (thoracolumbar) slice
  thicknesses
High-resolution algorithm in bone window (data storage)
Standard algorithm in soft tissue window
2D reconstructions (hemisagittal: Figs. 3.11b, 3.15b;
  parasagittal/oblique, coronal: Fig. 3.9a)

Optional
3D reconstructions (frontal, lateral, dorsal, oblique, and
  hemisection)

in the setting of spinal trauma because of its better soft tissue contrast and lack of superimposition in comparison with plain radiographs.

Computed tomography is particularly useful for the assessment of structures of the middle and posterior columns of Denis, thus being essential for diagnosing instability. It also allows the detection of an impingement of the thecal sac and spinal cord from extradural sources, such as retropulsed bone fragments, herniated disks, and epidural hematomas. Current indications for CT include inadequate radiographic visualization of the craniocervical (C0/C2) and cervicothoracic junction (C6/T1) in polytraumatized patients, preoperative evaluation of radiographically evident unstable fractures, neurological deficits in an apparently stable injury and uncertainty concerning instability after thorough review of plain films of good quality. Minor wedge compression fractures are usually not indications for a CT examination. However, if there is more than a 50% collapse of the vertebral body as assessed by plain radiographs, CT is necessary to exclude middle as well as posterior column disruption. Multiple adjacent wedge compression fractures are also an indication for CT due to the risk of late instability secondary to middle column involvement and neural deficit secondary to progressive kyphosis (McAfee et al. 1983).

To obtain the maximum diagnostic information from CT a standardized protocol should be followed (Table 3.11). It is important to scan at least one vertebral level above and below the injured vertebra to allow therapy planning and rule out the frequent contiguous vertebral fractures. The main disadvantage of axial CT is the difficulty in visualizing horizontally oriented fractures, such as bicolumn transverse fractures of the thoracolumbar spine ("Chance fractures", Fig. 3.26). Therefore, 2D reformations in the sagittal and coronal planes are mandatory. Sagittal 2D reconstructions are especially important for the evaluation of indirect signs of disruption of the posterior elements as in type B1 and

B2 distraction injuries. They also facilitate the differentiation between fracture, subluxation, and complete facet dislocation. Oblique reconstructions are necessary in the cervical spine according to the orientation pattern of facets.

Some controversy exists with respect to the value of 3D CT reconstructions. Initially (Zinreich et al. 1990; Vogel et al. 1990), 3D reformations were considered to yield additional diagnostic information concerning vertebral body fractures, spinal malalignment, and foraminal narrowing following spinal fractures. However, Saeed et al. (1994) concluded that 3D CT was no better than axial CT with 2D reformations, especially in the diagnosis of nondisplaced fractures and posterior element injuries. Nonetheless, they agreed with literature reports (Zinreich et al. 1990) concerning the ability of 3D images to detect a rotational component. The fact that signs of rotation represent the ultimate criterion for distinguishing a type A or B from a type C1 fracture according to Magerl's classification underlines the increasing importance of 3D reconstructions. The overall sensitivity of CT for fracture detection lies between 90% and 99% (Woodring and Lee 1992; Acheson et al. 1987).

3.4.5 Magnetic Resonance Imaging

Magnetic resonance imaging has expanded the imaging evaluation of spinal trauma by supplying unique diagnostic information concerning soft tissue and cord injuries. Currently, MR imaging may be considered the method of choice after initial plain radiography for patients with neurological deficits without evidence of bony injuries. In the past, spinal cord lesions were solely assessed by clinical evaluation, as proposed by Frankel et al. (1969) (Table 3.12). Now, MR imaging allows distinction between edema, hemorrhage, and transection of the spinal cord. A classification of spinal cord lesions on MR images using a similar scheme to that of Frankel et al. is proposed in Table 3.13. Two patterns of spinal cord hemorrhage have been described by Kulkarni et al. (1987): the intraparenchymal, which has the worst

Table 3.12. Assessment of neural level of function after spinal trauma according to Frankel et al. (1969)

A: Complete spinal cord deficit
B: Sensation present but no motor function
C: Motor function present but useless
D: Motor function useful
E: Neurally intact

Table 3.13. Assessment of the severity of spinal cord injuries using MRI

A: Complete spinal cord transection
B: Spinal central hematoma
   B1: Intraparenchymal, increasing with time
   B2: Petechial, resolving with time
C: Cord edema
D: Cord compression and impingement
E: Intact spinal cord

Table 3.14. Signal characteristics of acute spinal injuries on MR imaging

Ligament rupture
Anterior/posterior longitudinal ligament:
   Abrupt discontinuity of the low-intensity stripe on sagittal
     images (T1/T2)
Interspinous ligament:
   Focal increase in signal intensity on T2-weighted images
     and widening of interspinous distance
Capsular ligaments: subluxation >3 mm

Intraspinal lesions
Cord transection
   Complete discontinuity of cord accompanied by
     hemorrhage and edema
Cord hematoma
   Iso-/hypointense on T1-weighted images
   Hypointense on T2-weighted images
Cord edema
   Hypointense on T1-weighted images
   Hyperintense on T2-weighted images

Extradural lesions
Epidural hematomas
   Hyperintense on T1-weighted images
   Iso-/hyperintense on T2-weighted images
Disk herniation/rupture: extruded disk material
Retropulsed bone fragments: elevated posterior longitudinal
   ligament if not ruptured

prognosis, and the petechial, which may resolve. Cord edema also has a better prognosis than hematoma. The optimum time for prognostic imaging is 24–72h after injury since better evaluation of the extension of the cord involvement can be achieved at this time.

Acute spinal ligament disruption is also best assessed by MR imaging, the overall sensitivity being 79% according to cadaveric studies (KLIEWER et al. 1993). Lesions of the anterior and/or posterior longitudinal ligaments are better depicted than those of the capsular, interspinous, or flaval ligaments. A summary of the signal characteristics of ligament injuries is given in Table 3.14. MR imaging is also accurate in the diagnosis of injuries of the intervertebral disk. Moreover, flexion/extension views, as previously noted, may be obtained to search for the causes of segmental instabilities or neurological symptoms

after whiplash injury. MR imaging is further indicated in the follow-up of late sequelae after spinal cord injuries, such as atrophy, myelomalacia, and syringohydromyelia.

T1- and T2-weighted sagittal images are the minimum requirement for adequate evaluation of the presence of a spinal injury and ligamental disruption. Fat-suppressed sequences may facilitate the diagnosis of epidural hematoma.

3.4.6 Myelography

The inherent disadvantage of myelography in the acute setting of spinal trauma results from the mobilization of the patient and intrathecal contrast medium administration. As previously noted, it may be performed in combination with CT (myelo-CT) to study radiculopathies secondary to traumatic avulsion of nerve roots or dural tears. If MR imaging is not available or is inconclusive in cases of suspected dural tears, nerve root avulsions, or soft tissue stenosis, CT with metrizamide myelography may be performed.

3.5 Trauma Patterns and Pathomorphology of Spinal Injuries

3.5.1 Cervical Spine

Spinal injuries of the occipito-atlanto-axial region are so unique in their trauma pattern that they will be considered separately in a topographic approach.

The middle and lower cervical spine, although differing from the thoracolumbar spine by virtue of its greater range of motion, may be included in the AO classification system of MAGERL et al. (1994). In the following, the most frequent injuries are listed under the basic types A, B, and C. Furthermore, a fourth type of injury consisting of isolated injuries of posterior elements, not considered by MAGERL et al. (1994) but often present in the cervical spine, will be briefly discussed.

Traumatic rotatory atlantoaxial dislocation has to be distinguished from reversible rotatory atlantoaxial subluxation after acute infection of the upper respiratory tract with a painful rotational block of the neck or a minor trauma, particularly in children. The true dislocation is the result of a forced rotational movement leading to rupture of the joint capsules. It may be unilateral or bilateral depending on the location of the center of rotation (WIMMER et

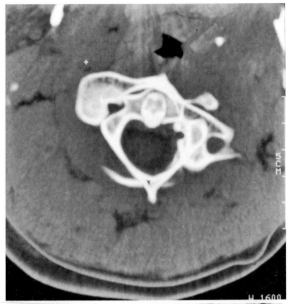

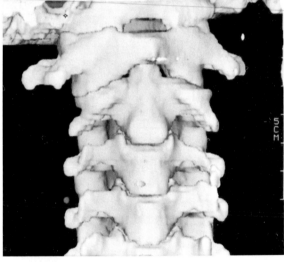

Fig. 3.8a,b. Bilateral rotational atlantoaxial dislocation. a Computerized addition of two transverse cuts demonstrating bilateral dislocation of the lateral masses of the atlas in the opposite direction. The image represents the simultaneous display of two adjacent axial slices to demonstrate the dislocation. **b** 3D CT underlines the anterior dislocation of the right lateral mass and, less clearly, the posterior dislocation of the left lateral mass

al. 1990). If the rotational axis passes through the dens, the dislocation will be bilateral (Fig. 3.8), whereas if it lies in the atlantoaxial joint it will be unilateral. Plain film radiography may be suggestive of this condition, especially in the AP projection, demonstrating a narrowing of the atlantodental distance on the side of the dislocation. CT is, however, the method of choice because of its ability to demonstrate the axial relationship of the atlas and axis. The

addition of two adjacent axial CT images as well as 3D-CT reformations may be helpful for diagnosis (Fig. 3.8).

Atlas fractures may appear isolated or, as in half of the cases, simultaneously with axis fractures. Five types of fracture have been described (WIMMER et al. 1990): burst fractures (Jefferson's fractures), injuries of the posterior arch, horizontal fractures of the anterior arch and fractures of the lateral mass of the atlas and of the transverse process.

Jefferson's fractures consist of burst fractures of the anterior and posterior arches resulting from axial compression by a blow on the vertex of the head. They may be unilateral (Fig. 3.9) or bilateral and stability depends on the associated disruption of the transverse ligament. Plain films may show indirect signs of transverse ligament rupture consisting in displacement of the lateral masses exceeding 6.9 mm on the open mouth view (SPENCE et al. 1970) or widening of the predental space to more than 3 mm on the lateral flexion view (ODA et al. 1991). However, lateral mass offset is not specific for atlas fractures (it is also seen in anterior-posterior clefts, partial aplasia, and children under 4 years), and there may be Jefferson's fractures without lateral displacement.

3.5.1.1 Occipito-atlanto-axial Region

Fractures of the occipital condyles must be considered in the differential diagnosis of localized pain and tenderness in the upper part of the cervical spine. They have been classified by ANDERSON and MONTESANO (1988) according to their pattern and stability. Type I fractures are impacted fractures of the condyle resulting from axial loading of the skull. Type II fractures occur at the base of the skull, extend into the occipital condyles, and are produced by direct trauma. Both type I and II fractures are stable. Type III fractures consist of avulsions of the occipital condyles by the alar ligaments because of excessive rotation or lateral bending and are consequently unstable. Plain film radiographs are frequently normal and diagnosis relies on axial CT, showing the displacement and extension (EL-KHOURY et al. 1995).

Traumatic *atlanto-occipital dislocation* should be considered in patients involved in motor vehicle accidents, especially if rapid deceleration with either hyperextension and distraction or hyperflexion can be inferred. This injury is more frequent in children and neurology may range from immediate death to initially normal findings. Therefore, an accurate radiographic diagnosis is essential. Plain film radiography is the cornerstone of diagnosis. The trauma pattern typically consists in anterior displacement of the basion from its normal position superior to the odontoid, with a distance from the basion to the tip of the dens exceeding 12 mm in children (BULAS et al. 1993) or 5 mm in adults (JEND and HELLER 1989). A malalignment between the spinolaminar line of C1 and the posterior margin of the foramen magnum and a failure of the clival line to intersect the odontoid are further specific signs (see Table 3.4). CT may be helpful in equivocal cases provided 2D sagittal reconstructions and soft tissue window settings demonstrate hemorrhage along the tectorial membrane and alar ligaments as an indirect sign of this injury. CT is also the method of choice to confirm Jefferson's fractures, allowing the accurate detection of associated osseous avulsion of the transverse ligaments and lateral subluxation of the atlantoaxial joint (Fig. 3.9).

Isolated fractures of the posterior arch of C1 occur from axial compression and hyperextension and may be clearly detected on lateral views with occasional tilting if the fractures are bilateral. Oblique or sagittal nondisplaced fractures are stable injuries that can be exactly evaluated by CT (Fig. 3.10). The other types of atlas fractures are also stable and can be well detected by CT. It is important to emphasize that the gantry needs to be aligned precisely parallel to the plane of the atlas to avoid missing nondisplaced fractures (LEVINE and EDWARDS 1991).

Fractures of the odontoid process most frequently result from motor vehicle accidents with forced extension and ventral and lateral flexion. As previously noted, the classification of ANDERSON and D'ALONZO (1974) is the basis for diagnosing stability

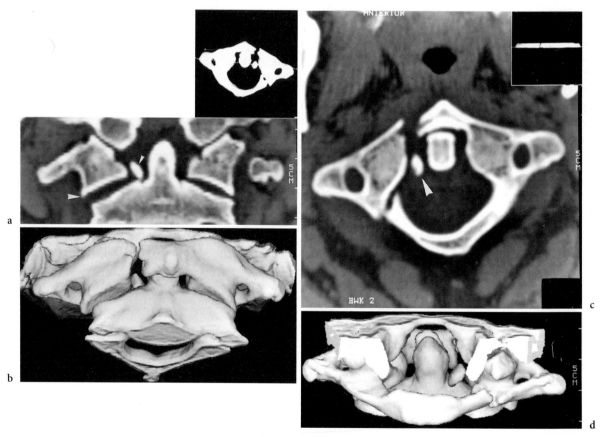

Fig. 3.9a–d. Unilateral Jefferson's fracture. **a** Coronal 2D reconstruction showing a lateral displacement of the lateral mass of the atlas (*large arrowhead*) and an avulsed bone fragment medially (*small arrowhead*). **b** Frontal 3D view demonstrating the anterior arch fracture and the subluxation of the lateral atlantoaxial joint. **c** Axial image revealing the unilateral fractures of the anterior and posterior arch of C1 with an avulsed bone fragment (*arrowhead*) as an indirect sign of transverse ligament disruption. **d** A dorsal 3D view underlines the discrete caudal dislocation of the fractured right fragment of the atlas

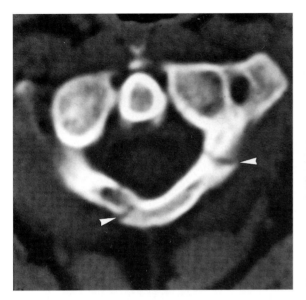

Fig. 3.10. Isolated posterior arch fracture of C1: an axial CT slice reveals nondisplaced oblique fractures (*arrowheads*)

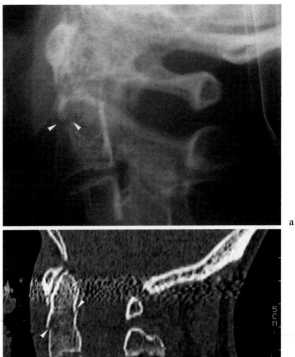

a

b

Fig. 3.11a,b. Undisplaced odontoid process fracture type II. **a** Lateral view revealing a fracture line through the neck (*arrowheads*). **b** 2D CT sagittal reconstruction showing a minimal interruption of the anterior and posterior cortical lines at the neck level (*arrowheads*)

(Fig. 3.5, Table 3.7). *Type I* fractures are oblique fractures through the tip of the dens secondary to alar ligament avulsion and are considered stable. *Type II* fractures occur at the junction of the dens with the body of the axis (Fig. 3.11), are unstable, and are associated with a higher risk of nonunion and neurologic damage. In *type III* fractures the fracture line extends downward into the cancellous portion of the body as a fracture through the body of the axis (Fig. 3.12). Each type may be displaced (Fig. 3.12) or undisplaced (Fig. 3.11). Plain film radiography and particularly the open mouth view are best to demonstrate odontoid fractures, especially type I and type III fractures. Type II fractures are best detected on lateral views. Indirect signs, such as widening of the prevertebral soft tissue by more than 7mm at the level of the axis, require CT.

If CT with sagittal reconstructions (Fig. 3.11) does not demonstrate a horizontal nondisplaced fracture and plain films are suggestive, lateral tomograms are indicated (PATHRIA and PETERSILGE 1991). Displaced and nondisplaced oblique fractures are well detected by CT.

Traumatic spondylolisthesis of the axis consists in bilateral avulsion of the neural arches from the vertebral body. EFFENDI et al. (1981) (Fig. 3.6, Table 3.8) classified *hangman's fractures* into three types: Type I fractures involve the posterior part of the body of C2 or any part of the ring without evident angulation or displacement. In type II fractures there is additional anterior displacement of C2 over 3mm or an

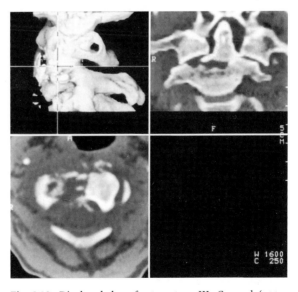

Fig. 3.12. Displaced dens fracture type III. Coronal (*upper right*) and axial (*lower left*) 2D reconstruction based on a lateral 3D image (*upper left*), demonstrating a typical fracture line through the body of the axis with signs of lateral atlantoaxial subluxation (coronal reconstruction)

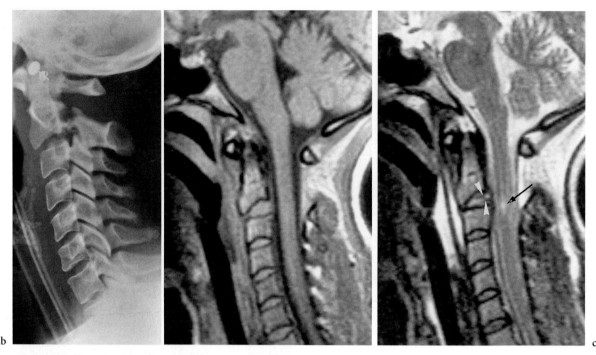

Fig. 3.13a–c. Unstable hangman's fracture type II. **a** Bilateral avulsion of the neural arches from the vertebral body with an angulation of more than 15° of C2 over C3. **b** MR imaging underlines the dislocation of C2 over C3 on a sagittal T1- weighted image. **c** A T2-weighted images confirms the fragmentation of the intervertebral disk C2/C3 (*arrowheads*) and increased signal intensity in the spinal cord at the same level as a sign of cord edema (*arrow*)

angulation of more than 15° (Fig. 3.13). Type III fractures are type II injuries accompanied by unilateral or bilateral C2–3 locked facet. Type I and II fractures result from hyperextension and axial compression while type III fractures are caused by flexion followed by rebound extension.

The key to stability is the integrity of the C2–3 disk. As it is disrupted in type II and III lesions, these are unstable. Plain lateral radiographs demonstrate these fractures accurately in up to 90% of cases. CT may be an adjunct to detect nondisplaced type I fractures as they are well suited to axial CT because of its vertical direction. MR imaging may be necessary for further evaluation of type II and III fractures before surgical stabilization to rule out spinal cord damage and to exclude protruded disk material (Fig. 3.13b,c).

3.5.1.2 Middle and Lower Cervical Spine

The simple *wedge compression fracture* consists of comminution of the anterosuperior end plate of the vertebra without concomitant injury to the posterior aspect of the vertebral body, posterior longitudinal ligament, or posterior bony elements. These injuries are stable. Plain film radiographs are sufficient to diagnose such injuries.

Burst fractures of the cervical spine are clinically important because of the high risk of neurologic injury. They result from axial compression with comminution of the vertebral body and are similar in the thoracic and lumbar region.

Retropulsed fragments causing an extradural compression of the cord are frequently found. The anterior and posterior longitudinal ligaments are usually intact. A vertical split through the arch may be present, but the posterior ligament complex is intact.

Diagnosis is based on initial plain radiographs showing interpediculate widening on the AP view, greater than 50% or 20° of compression of the vertebral body on the lateral view, loss of posterior vertebral body height, and an apparent posterior vertebral cortex fracture or canal fragment.

CT is indicated to evaluate the extent of the injury as regards the presence of retropulsed fragments with narrowing of the spinal canal, the detection of associated fractures of the posterior elements and the assessment of the adjacent vertebrae for therapy planning. MR imaging is often indicated to assess the extent of spinal cord damage. These injuries are un-

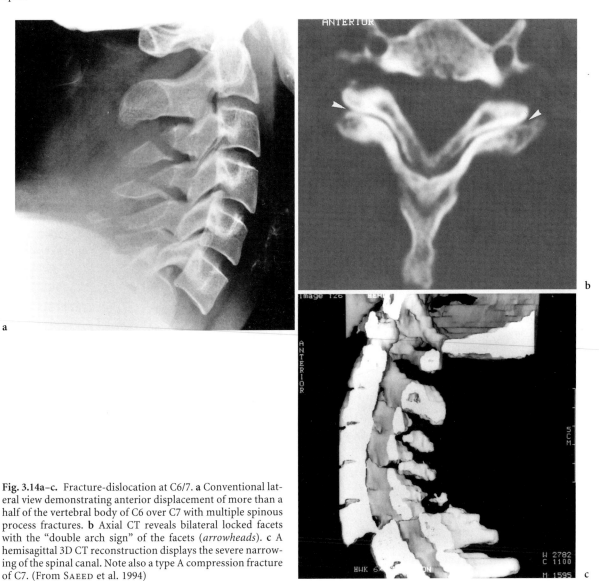

Fig. 3.14a–c. Fracture-dislocation at C6/7. **a** Conventional lateral view demonstrating anterior displacement of more than a half of the vertebral body of C6 over C7 with multiple spinous process fractures. **b** Axial CT reveals bilateral locked facets with the "double arch sign" of the facets (*arrowheads*). **c** A hemisagittal 3D CT reconstruction displays the severe narrowing of the spinal canal. Note also a type A compression fracture of C7. (From SAEED et al. 1994)

stable, at least in flexion/compression (MAGERL et al. 1994). Further aspects regarding stability will be discussed in Sect. 3.5.2.

The highly unstable *bilateral facet dislocation* occurs secondary to severe flexion-distraction forces that cause complete ligamentous disruption of the posterior and middle columns. It rarely occurs in isolation; rather it is usually associated with anterior or posterior bony lesions (Fig. 3.14). This ligamentous injury is readily detected on lateral radiographs showing anterior displacement of the superior vertebrae of more than half the width of the vertebral body. CT may be indicated to document the degree of narrowing of the spinal canal and associated fractures of the posterior elements usually

obscured at the cervicothoracic level (Fig. 3.14). MR imaging is emerging as an adjunct in the assessment of these injuries, not only to evaluate possible spinal cord damage but also to rule out occlusion of a vertebral artery, which may be associated with this injury.

The unstable bilateral facet dislocation may be included in the group of flexion-distraction injuries characterized by a posteroanterior dislocation with bilateral facet dislocations or fractures of the articular processes. A type A fracture of the vertebra above may be associated. Anteroposterior fracture-dislocations are less common and are the result of hyperextension/shear injuries with frequent disruption through the disk. As all three columns of Denis

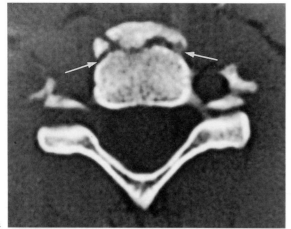

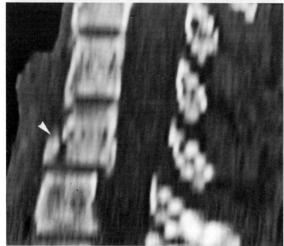

Fig. 3.15a,b. Teardrop fracture of C6. **a** Axial CT demonstrating the coronal split fracture (*arrows*) in the anterior third of the vertebral body with smaller anterior fragments. **b** A hemisagittal (sagittal plane through the middle of the vertebral body) 2D reconstruction underlines the typical appearance: a smaller, triangular fragment anteroinferiorly aligned with the vertebral below (*arrowhead*) and interruption of the posterior vertebral line by retropulsion of the larger fragment, narrowing the spinal canal

are involved, these injuries are highly unstable. Diagnosis is evident on plain radiographs demonstrating the sagittal dislocation of the vertebral body and associated fractures of the anterior or posterior elements. CT is especially useful when there is inadequate visualization of the cervicothoracic junction.

Flexion-teardrop fractures, which occur more often in the lower cervical spine (C5–C7), are the result of a combination of flexion and compression forces. Moreover, a distraction component must be considered because of the associated disruption of the posterior ligamentous complex with widened interspinous and interlaminar distances and facet

subluxation as an indirect sign of capsular ligament injury.

A *distraction-flexion-teardrop fracture* may be diagnosed in the presence of anterior displacement of the cervical spine above the fractured vertebra. By contrast, the classical *flexion-teardrop fracture* is characterized by posterior displacement of the vertebrae above, which are aligned with the posterior fractured fragment. Furthermore, typically the flexion-teardrop fracture consists of a coronal split through the vertebral body (Fig. 3.15) dividing it into two principal fragments, a smaller anterior triangular "teardrop" fragment frequently associated with a rupture of the anterior longitudinal ligament and a larger posterior fragment that is retropulsed into the

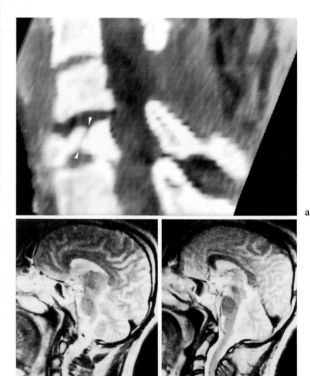

Fig. 3.16a,b. Teardrop fracture at C6/C7 with spinal cord damage. **a** Parasagittal 2D CT reconstruction revealing the typical coronal fracture (*arrowheads*) with a discrete displacement of the posterior vertebral fragment. **b** MR imaging (proton-weighted sagittal image) 4 months later demonstrates a cystic spinal cord lesion (*black arrows*) corresponding to syringohydromyelia. Note also the loss of height of the fractured vertebral body (*white arrowhead*)

spinal canal. The lateral radiographic view reveals the typical anteroinferior "teardrop" fragment, which may be aligned with the anterior margin of the vertebra below, and the interruption of the posterior vertebral line by the retropulsion of the larger fragment.

CT is the next diagnostic step, often revealing an associated sagittal fracture component as well as injuries of the posterior elements, such as lamina fractures or facet subluxation. Due to the complete disruption of the annular and ligamentous structures, the flexion-teardrop fracture is a highly unstable injury often complicated by spinal cord damage. In this context, MR imaging may be indicated in the acute or late phase (Fig. 3.16).

Hyperextension injuries are more common in the cervical than in the thoracolumbar spine and may range from a pure diskoligamentous injury to a hyperextension fracture-dislocation. Hyperextension injuries may be divided into two groups: those with fractures and those with no evidence of bony injury. Among the former group the *hyperextension-teardrop fractures* must be emphasized because of the possibility of misdiagnosing them as flexion-teardrop fractures. In these injuries, a small osseous fragment typically undergoes avulsion from the anteroinferior corner of the vertebral body, frequently in association with injury of the anterior longitudinal ligament. Unlike in the case of flexion-teardrop fractures, the posterior vertebral line is not interrupted and no lesions of the posterior elements are described. Thus, these injuries may be considered stable. They occur more frequently at the C2–C3 level and CT may be necessary to rule out

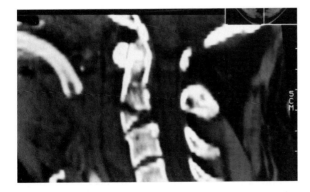

Fig. 3.17. Hyperextension teardrop fracture. Although demonstrated at C2, this case shows the typical appearance of these injuries in the middle and lower cervical spine: widening of the disk space, prevertebral soft tissue swelling, and an anterior teardrop fragment without interruption of the posterior vertebral line

involvement of the posterior elements or misalignment of the posterior "instability" vertebral line (Fig. 3.17).

In the group of hyperextension injuries without bony lesions, the most common trauma is the so-called *whiplash injury*, a soft tissue lesion usually seen after rear-end collisions with forced hyperextension. A wide range of symptoms may follow, including neck and craniofacial tenderness. Radiological documentation of this diffuse injury may be difficult. Plain film radiography may just reveal indirect signs suggesting soft tissue damage such as loss of the cervical lordosis or actual kyphosis, scoliotic curvature, widening of the anterior part of the intervertebral disk or even narrowing of one or more intervertebral foramina (EL-KHOURY et al. 1995; WIMMER et al. 1990). Functional flexion/extension views may be necessary to rule out segmental instabilities. Persisting symptoms or progressive neurological deficit may demand an MR imaging examination, which may be performed with different degrees of flexion/extension according to clinical findings. Functional imaging must not be done in unconscious patients or where neurological deficits suggest a spinal cord injury. Moreover, fractures must be ruled out before functional imaging.

Unilateral facet dislocation is usually caused by flexion combined with a rotational component. This lesion may or may not be associated with fractures. Solely ligamentous injuries have an increased prevalence of spinal cord damage or radiculopathy. As the posterior longitudinal ligament and the disk are usually intact, the injury is stable, except against further rotation because of the torn capsular ligaments. Plain radiographs reveal a discrete anterior translation of the vertebral bodies (3–4 mm), a "butterfly" appearance of the facet with a change from a strict lateral view below the damaged segment to an oblique view above on the plain lateral film, and a deviation of spinous processes on the AP view. CT may be indicated to rule out associated facet fractures as well as narrowing of the intervertebral foramina in the presence of neuropathy. MR imaging may be necessary to define spinal cord damage or vertebral artery occlusion if clinical signs are present.

Fractures of the *articular pillars and processes or the lamina* result from a combination of extension and rotation and are not associated with vertebral body fractures. The pillar fractures may be of two types: the fracture-separation and the avulsion fracture (WIMMER et al. 1990). In the fracture-separation type the fracture line runs through the pillar and then

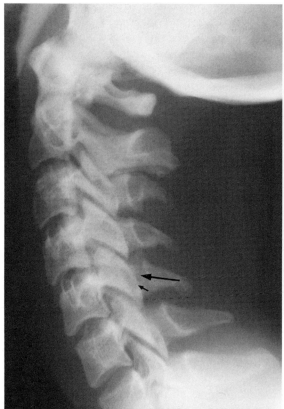

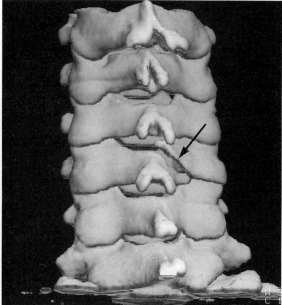

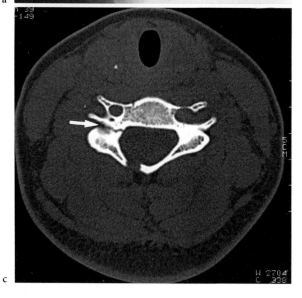

Fig. 3.18a–c. Fracture-separation of the articular pillar of C5. **a** Lateral view showing an oblique fracture through the lamina of C5 (*arrowheads*). **b** Dorsal 3D CT view underlining the extent of the arch fracture (*arrow*). **c** Axial CT delineates the horizontal fracture through the pillar (*arrow*) with disruption of the lamina and discrete widening of the spinal canal secondary to the outer rotation at the pillar

sagittally through the arch (Fig. 3.18). This injury may be difficult to visualize on plain radiographs unless there is an evident rotation with abnormal joint interspace on the AP view or a fracture line through the arch on the lateral view. Usually, CT is indicated to assess the extent of rotation and involvement of the arch as well as narrowing of the intervertebral foramina.

Isolated fractures of the articular processes with involvement of the facet joints result from lateral flexion with or without rotation. They may not be detected on plain films, especially if they are non-displaced. CT or conventional tomography may be the next diagnostic step if the clinical findings demand further investigation. Parasagittal or oblique reconstructions facilitate the diagnosis.

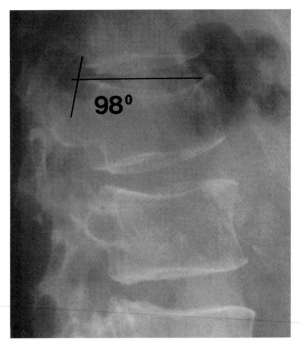

Fig. 3.19. L1 wedge compression fracture (A1) demonstrated on a lateral view. Note the superior posterior vertebral body angle of less than 100° and the compression of less than 50% of the vertebral body

The *clay shoveler's fracture* involves the spinous processes of C6 or C7, resulting from avulsion of the supraspinous ligament. These lesions are stable and readily detected on plain film radiographs.

3.5.2 Thoracic and Lumbar Spine

In the following section, the AO classification system proposed by Magerl et al. (1994) for the thoracic and lumbar spine serves as the basis for the description of the different trauma patterns (Table 3.9).

3.5.2.1 Type A: Compression Fractures

Type A compression fractures result from axial loading with or without flexion (Fig. 3.7a) and range from stable wedge fractures to the unstable burst fractures described by McAfee.

The impaction fracture injury group includes *endplate impaction* with wedging of up to 5°, *wedge impaction fractures* with angulation of more than 5°, and *vertebral body collapse* of the endplates, as often seen in osteoporotic spines. On the basis of the involvement of the anterior column of Denis, these injuries can be considered stable. Plain film radio-

graphy is sufficient to diagnose them accurately. However, detailed analysis is necessary to differentiate wedge fractures from potentially unstable burst fractures requiring CT examination.

According to Ballock et al. (1992) 20% of all patients with a burst fracture would be misdiagnosed as having a wedge compression fracture if plain films alone were used to evaluate these injuries. Classic signs of burst fractures, such as widening of the interpediculate distance or loss of posterior vertebral body height, may not be present in up to 45% of cases. Therefore, other signs, such as compression of more than 50% of the vertebral height or increased (>100°: burst fractures) superior or inferior posterior vertebral angles (Fig. 3.19) may suggest the need for CT to distinguish impaction from burst fractures (McGrory et al. 1993).

In the group of compression fractures, split fractures are characterized by a sagittally or coronally oriented split fracture through the vertebral body (Roy-Camille et al. 1979). The risk of nonunion exists especially if the gap between fragments is filled by disk material (Fig. 3.20). Plain film radiographs reveal the fracture lines but CT is indicated to rule out extension to the posterior vertebral margin and extrusion of disk material. The fractures are usually stable, unless the posterior column of Denis is involved or fragments are displaced anteriorly, reducing stability in flexion/compression.

Burst fractures have been defined by Holdsworth (1970) as those resulting from axial compression forces with fracture of one or the other vertebral end plates and "explosion" of the vertebral body secondary to the forcing of nucleus pulposus into the body. The posterior ligament complex is intact and retropulsed bone fragments may narrow the spinal canal with risk of spinal cord compression.

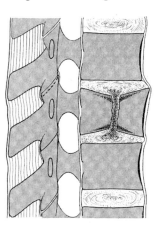

Fig. 3.20. Schematic coronal split fracture (from Magerl et al. 1994)

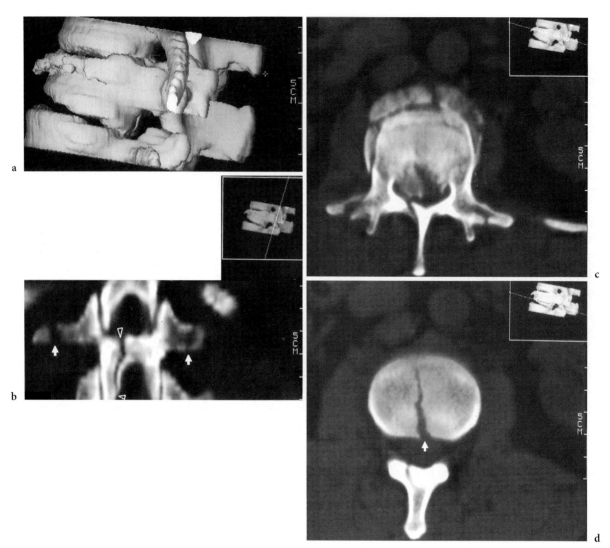

Fig. 3.21a–d. Typical unstable superior burst-split fracture of L1 (A3). **a** Lateral 3D CT reconstruction showing the wedge-shaped comminution of the superior part of the vertebral body. **b** Oblique coronal reconstruction revealing a vertical split fracture of the right lamina (*arrowheads*) as well as associated transverse process fractures (*arrows*). **c** An axial recon-struction at the superior half of the vertebral body reveals the severe narrowing of the spinal canal with retropulsed bone fragments, as well as the comminution of the vertebral body. **d** An axial reconstruction at the lower half of the vertebral body reveals the characteristic sagittal split fracture (*arrow*)

McAFEE et al. (1983) proposed a differentiation between *stable* and *unstable* burst fractures depending on the involvement of the posterior osseous elements of the neural arch. Unstable ones are those in which the neural arch or the facet articulations are also fractured (Figs. 3.21–3.23). Other authors, such as MAGERL et al. (1994), underline the fact that even in *incomplete burst fractures* (half of the body burst, half intact) stability is reduced in flexion/compression with the risk of further retropulsion of fragments and increasing kyphosis.

In *burst-split fractures* one-half of the vertebral body has burst, whereas the other is split sagittally. The laminae or spinous processes are split sagittally (Fig. 3.21). The *complete burst fractures* (entire body burst) may be divided into pincer, complete flexion (Fig. 3.22), and complete axial (Fig. 3.23) fractures. They are usually accompanied by a split fracture of the neural arch and are unstable in flexion-compression.

Plain film radiography, as previously discussed, has its limitations in distinguishing between a wedge compression and a burst fracture. A careful analysis of plain films is necessary to select the cases with a higher likelihood of being burst fractures. In these cases, CT is indicated to confirm the diagnosis, to evaluate further injuries of the posterior elements, to quantify the degree of narrowing of the spinal canal,

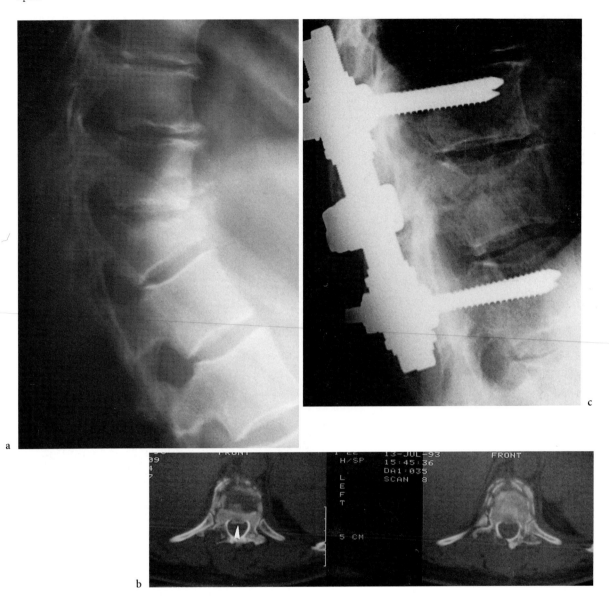

Fig. 3.22a–c. Complete flexion burst fracture of T12 (A3). **a** Lateral view revealing a wedge compression greater than 50% of the vertebral body. **b** Axial CT demonstrates involvement of the middle column with discrete narrowing of the spinal canal (*arrowhead*) and avulsion injuries of the transverse process and the right lamina. **c** Postoperative control after stabilization with a fixateur interne showing adequate repositioning, especially of the anterior vertebral height

and for therapy planning (anatomic survey of morphology of adjacent vertebral bodies and pedicles before screw placement). MR imaging is usually unnecessary, unless a neurologic deficit is not adequately explained by CT or progression is clinically evident.

3.5.2.2 Type B: Distraction Injuries

Predominantly ligamentous flexion-distraction injuries (Fig. 3.7b: B1) are characterized by a posterior disruption through the supraspinous, interspinous, and flaval ligaments. This disruption of the posterior ligamentous complex is associated with bilateral subluxation, dislocation, or facet fracture. The lesion of the anterior column may be through the disk or occur in association with a type A fracture (Fig. 3.24). The most severe injuries of this group are those associated with a *posteroanterior fracture-dislocation* (Fig. 3.25).

As all three columns are involved, these injuries are unstable in flexion but less so in rotation. They are stable against axial loading unless they are accompanied by a type A fracture.

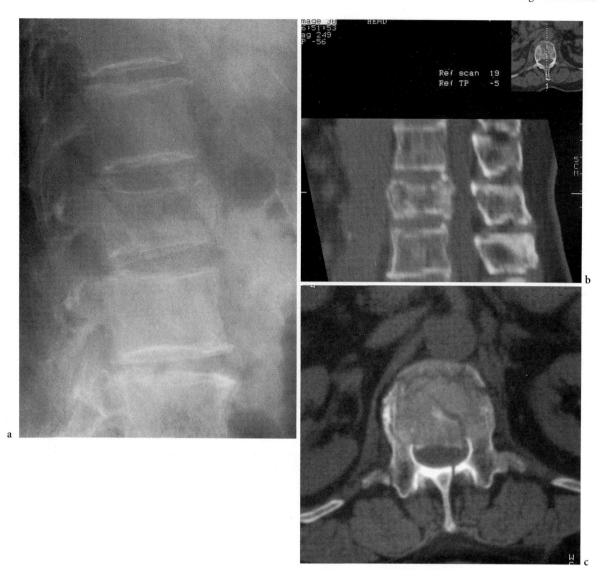

Fig. 3.23a–c. Unstable complete axial burst fracture of T12 (A3). In contrast to flexion burst fractures, the height of the comminuted vertebral body is evenly reduced, as seen on the lateral view (a) and sagittal 2D CT reconstruction (b). Note also the accompanying split fracture of the lamina and the retropulsed fragment on an axial image (c)

Plain film radiography may be suggestive of this type of distraction injury. The main features are found on the lateral view and consist of widening of the interspinous distance and evidence of rupture of the supraspinous and interspinous ligaments. A widening of the dorsal aspect of the disk also may be present.

CT may be useful to define the pattern of facet dislocation. The "naked facet sign", consisting of an exposed facet on several transverse scans without articulation with the adjacent facets, represents an indirect sign of rupture of the joint capsule. Additionally, CT allows exact definition of the injury if there is an associated type A fracture (Fig. 3.24).

With predominantly osseous flexion-distraction injuries (B2), the main fracture line runs horizontally through the lamina and pedicles or the isthmi and may continue through the vertebral body, as in cases of transverse bicolumn fractures (Chance fractures: Fig. 3.26). It may also run anteriorly through the disk or occur in conjunction with an associated type A fracture of the vertebral body. These fractures were often referred as seat belt injuries or pure distraction injuries.

Plain film radiographs are characteristic in the case of bicolumn fractures, demonstrating the fracture edges through the spinous processes, the neural arch, and the vertebral body. The horizontal cleft in

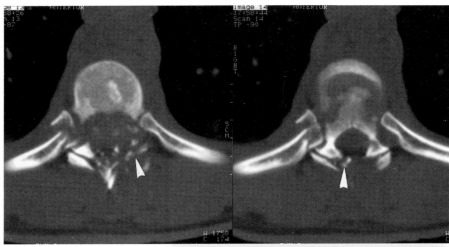

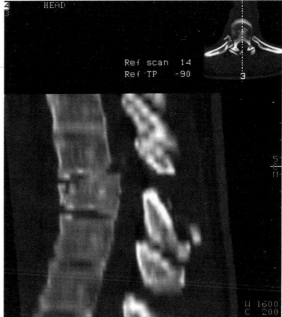

Fig. 3.24a,b. Flexion-distraction injury with posterior disruption that is predominantly ligamentous (B1). **a** Axial CT shows bilateral facet fractures (*arrowheads*) as well as multiple bone fragments within the spinal canal. **b** A 2D hemisagittal reconstruction reveals widening of the interspinous distance as evidence of rupture of the posterior ligamentous complex, anterior displacement of T10 over T11 with narrowing of the spinal canal, and a wedge compression (A1) fracture of T11. The findings are typical of a posteroanterior dislocation with fractures of the articular processes and a type A fracture of T11

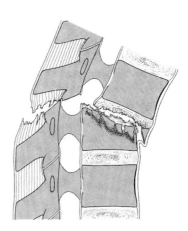

Fig. 3.25. Posteroanterior fracture-dislocation with bilateral facet dislocation corresponding to a B1 fracture associated with a type A fracture and sagittal translation (B1 subgroup) (from MAGERL et al. 1994)

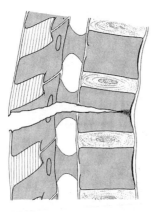

Fig. 3.26. Transverse bicolumn fracture ("Chance" fracture; B2 subgroup) (from MAGERL et al. 1994)

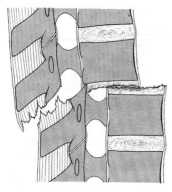

Fig. 3.27. Anteroposterior dislocation secondary to hyperextension-shear forces (B3 subgroup) (from MAGERL et al. 1994)

the vertebral body is also evident in the AP view. CT is inherently limited in the detection of horizontally oriented fractures, especially if they are less distracted and a slice thickness of more than 5 mm is used. Nevertheless, fractures are often oblique and 2D reconstructions, especially coronal, may be helpful in detecting the fracture line. On the other hand, CT is very accurate when a fracture is associated with flexion-distraction injuries because of its ability to depict vertebral body comminution, narrowing of the spinal canal, and associated dislocated or fractured facets (Fig. 3.24).

Conventional tomography remains the alternative to CT when a transverse bicolumn fracture is still suspected and not evidenced by CT. The considerations that apply to MR imaging of B1 fractures also apply to B2 injuries.

Hyperextension-shear injuries (Fig. 3.7c: B3) are characterized by a transverse anterior disruption of the disk that may extend to the posterior column.

Pure diskoligamentous injuries are rare in comparison to such injuries of the cervical region. An associated fracture of the isthmus may cause a *hyperextension-spondylolysis*. The most severe subgroup of these injuries comprises *anteroposterior dislocations and fracture-dislocations* with sagittal translation and severe neurologic damage, generally associated with paraplegia (Fig. 3.27). These lesions are unstable and may display poor healing because of their soft tissue nature. In accordance with the high proportion of diskoligamentous lesions among this group of injuries, MR imaging is emerging as the next diagnostic step after plain film radiography in all types of hyperextension injuries, particularly in the absence of bony injuries.

3.5.2.3 Type C: Rotation Injuries

Type A injuries may be complicated by a rotational component, thus leading to increased rotational instability. This is especially important for burst fractures. A rotational component may be difficult to visualize on plain radiographs or axial CT with 2D reformations, as demonstrated by SAEED et al. (1994). Therefore, 3D CT may be an important adjunct when a rotational component is suspected (Fig. 3.28). Rotation may be through the dorsoventral z-axis (lateral bending to either side) or through the craniocaudal vertical axis (clockwise and counterclockwise rotation).

Distraction injuries with rotation represent severely unstable lesions resulting from strong forces. This group includes the *lateral distraction injuries* described by DENIS and BURKUS (1991) and other variants of fracture-subluxation, especially those associated with unilateral or bilateral facet dislocation or fracture. Plain film radiographs readily delineate the unstable features of these injuries with frequent sagittal or lateral translations. CT remains the cornerstone for the diagnosis of narrowing of the spinal canal and pattern of facet involvement (MANASTER and OSBORN 1987). 3D CT reconstructions may facilitate the distinction between B and C2 fractures (Fig. 3.29).

Rotational shear injuries (C3) include the most unstable spinal injuries. Instability results from the potential for multidirectional translations in any plane. The *slice fracture of Holdsworth* consists of a rotational fracture-dislocation characterized by lateral rotation, unilateral or bilateral articular process fractures, and a slice disruption of the upper border of the adjacent lower vertebra (Fig. 3.30). The *oblique*

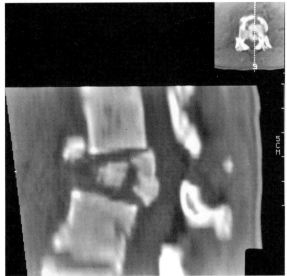

a

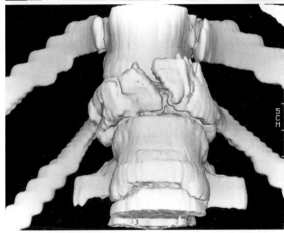

b

Fig. 3.28a,b. Rotational burst fracture (C1). **a** Hemisagittal 2D reconstruction revealing the typical features of burst fractures, consisting in retropulsed fragments with narrowing of the spinal canal. **b** A frontal 3D view documents clearly the lateral rotation to the right of the fractured L1 with evident translation of the vertebra above in comparison to the vertebra below

fracture with craniocaudal and lateral translation is also included in this group (Fig. 3.31). Radiographic diagnosis of these evidently unstable injuries starts with plain radiographs, which allow an accurate assessment of stability. CT may be performed as an adjunct if operative stabilization is planned.

In an unconscious patient, MR imaging may play an important role in the evaluation since findings on plain radiographs may equivocally suggest transection of the spinal cord. As reported by some authors (EL-KHOURY and WHITTEN 1993; SIMPSON et al. 1990), there may be evident fracture-dislocations without spinal cord damage. A "floating

laminae" or "floating arches" protective mechanism has been postulated. Therefore, there should be careful handling of the unstable spine and consideration of an early MR examination under these circumstances.

3.6 Special Features of Spinal Trauma in Children and Adolescents

Fractures of the vertebral column in children are uncommon in comparison to fractures of other regions. The distribution of spinal injuries reveals a predisposition toward lesions of the cervical and thoracic spine.

With regard to the occipito-atlanto-axial region, two aspects deserve special mention. Firstly, *traumatic atlanto-occipital dislocation* must be considered in all children involved in motor vehicle accidents. Children are especially vulnerable to this injury because of the larger size of the head relative to the body, increased laxity of ligaments, horizontally oriented occipito-atlanto-axial joints, and hypoplastic occipital condyles (BULAS et al. 1993). Secondly, *odontoid fractures* in children under the age of 7 are actually lesions of the cartilaginous plate (synchondrosis) separating the odontoid process from the body of the axis. Such lesions are usually not accompanied by neurological deficits, but closed or open reduction is necessary to avoid late instability.

As regards the middle and lower cervical spine, a preponderant distribution of injuries at the C2–C4 level has been described, supporting the theory (CATTEL and FILTZER 1965) that the fulcrum of cervical movement in children is located at a higher level. Realization of this fact is important if one is to avoid interpreting the frequent wedging of the ossification center of C3 and C4 in infants and children as a compression fracture (SWISCHUK et al. 1993). Compression fractures are extremely rare but if doubt exists, MR imaging (Fig. 3.32) may be performed in order to confirm the fracture, which is demonstrated by an increased signal intensity on T2-weighted images in up to 83% of cases (ALLGAYER et al. 1990). CT is only indicated if an involvement of the posterior vertebral margin is suspected.

Thoracic spinal injuries in children are usually stable and associated with a multilevel injury. Fracture-dislocations are more common in the thoracolumbar spine and injuries at the lumbar level are uncommon.

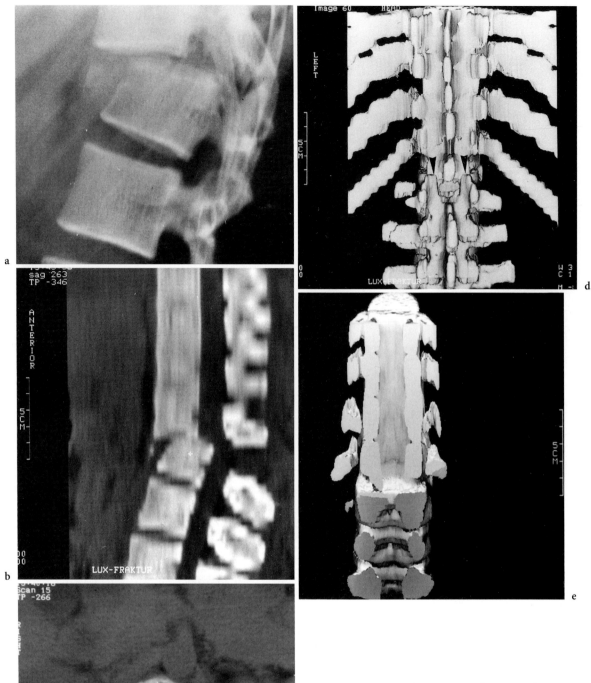

Fig. 3.29a–e. Type C2 injury. **a** Lateral view revealing anterior displacement of T12 over L1 with a type A compression fracture of L1. **b** Hemisagittal 2D CT reconstruction underlining the severe narrowing of the spinal canal as well as widening of the interspinous distance at T12/L1 as a sign of rupture of the posterior longitudinal complex (B1 distraction injury). **c** Axial CT demonstrating the naked facets (*arrowheads*) of the superior articular processes of L1 because of the bilateral facet dislocation. **d** A posterior 3D CT view underlines the bilateral facet dislocation of T12/L1 by the posterior location of the superior articular process of L1 (*black arrowheads*). **e** Finally, a 3D-CT dorsal view using a "cut function" to remove the neural arches reveals a clockwise rotation above L1 not previously suspected (C2 injury)

Fig. 3.30. Holdsworth's slice fracture (from MAGERL et al. 1994)

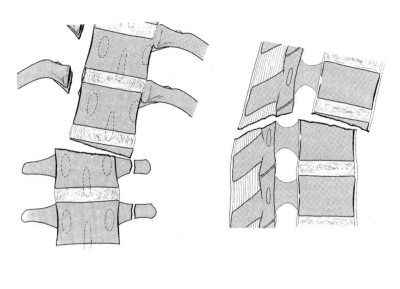

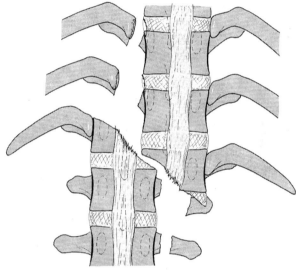

Fig. 3.31. Oblique translational fracture (from MAGERL et al. 1994)

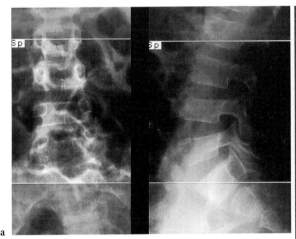

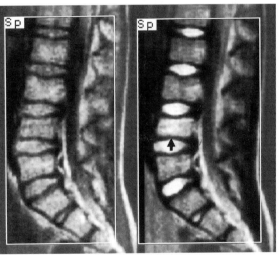

Fig. 3.32a,b. Type A compression fracture in a 7-year-old child after falling from a tree. **a** AP and lateral plain film views reveal a discrete wedging of L4. **b** Proton-weighted (*left*) and T2-weighted (*right*) images. Diffusely increased signal intensity is seen on the T2-weighted image (*arrow*), reflecting bone edema after fracture

In evaluating children with spinal trauma some peculiarities must be considered. In particular, one must take account of (a) the potential for further progression of untreated unstable injuries, and (b) the ability of the immature spine to remodel the vertebral body, especially after wedge compression fractures. Another important feature is the frequent presentation of posttraumatic spinal cord lesions in children in the absense of skeletal injury (GOVERNDER et al. 1990). These lesions may be related to hyperflexion or hyperextension mechanisms in the cervical spine with cord damage (McPHEE 1981). In this setting, MR imaging should be performed after plain film evaluation. Conventional radiographs must be carefully evaluated, as only slight changes, such as a widening of greater than 10 mm between the spinous processes of C1–C2 on the lateral view may be the only sign of associated spinal cord damage (ALLINGTON et al. 1990).

A further special aspect is the possibility of child abuse presenting as spinal trauma. Spinal injuries associated with abuse may be stable or unstable and are often associated with vertebral notching at the anterior margin of the superior endplate. According to histopathological studies the most common pattern is characterized by compression fractures affecting the anterior aspect of the vertebral endplates (KLEINMAN and MARKS 1992). Fractures of the spinous processes appear also to occur in the shaken infant syndrome. Radiological skeletal survey in cases of suspected abuse should include a minimum of two views. A high degree of suspicion in the presence of compression fractures without adequate trauma should alert the radiologist to search for other signs of child abuse.

3.7 Follow-up, Sequelae, and Complications

Spinal injuries may be considered in an acute phase within 3 weeks after trauma, as during this period most fractures behave like fresh fractures and surgical reduction is still possible (QUENCER 1988). An *immediate postoperative follow-up* is imperative to evaluate therapy results.

Plain film radiography allows the assessment of the adequacy of implantation of osteosynthetic material (Fig. 3.22), particularly in relation to adjacent critical structures such as the spinal canal or the neural foramina (HÄBERLE et al. 1994). Moreover, it allows an assessment of repositioning or dislocation of fractured bone fragments. Unfortunately, it is not

as accurate as CT in evaluating residual stenosis of the spinal canal. Furthermore, CT allows one to rule out immediate postoperative complications, such as extraspinal hematomas or extruded or sequestered disk material. It identifies accurately the location of intracorporeal bone grafts (Fig. 3.33).

In the *subacute (>3 weeks) and long-term follow-up* after conservative or surgical treatment, imaging studies are necessary to evaluate the fracture healing process, the development of late instabilities, the changes in osteosynthetic material, and the presence of complications such as pseudarthrosis, infection, or late neurological sequelae.

Intraosseous fracture healing is difficult to assess radiologically and conventional tomograms are often indicated, especially in cases of dens fractures. Periosteal consolidation reveals a progressive smoothing of the fractured cortical surface. Follow-up films should be obtained at intervals of 3–4 weeks until complete consolidation occurs (around 3 months after trauma). Plain radiographs may also detect pathological changes in the healing process such as nonunion, intervertebral spontaneous fusion, posttraumatic osteoarthrotic changes, vertebral body deformities, and scoliotic deformities.

CT is widely used to assess the remodelling of the spinal canal after reposition of burst fractures with retropulsed fragments (Fig. 3.33). As KUNER et al. (1992) have demonstrated, a near-normal reduction of the spinal canal is achieved through ligamentotaxis for fractures between T12 and L2, whereas for fractures between L3 and L5 an incomplete reduction is observed. Ligamentotaxis is the surgical term for the indirect reduction mechanism of retropulsed bone fragments after fixateur-interne osteosynthesis of burst fractures.

MR imaging is an alternative modality to evaluate the relevance of the remaining spinal canal stenosis (Fig. 3.33h,i) or to rule out neurologic sequelae of spinal trauma such as spinal cord atrophy, tethering, myelomalacia, and syringohydromyelia (Fig. 3.34b,c). The latter may be localized at the injury site or extend into neighboring regions of the cord (KERSLAKE et al. 1991).

Functional images are necessary to evaluate late instability, segmental hypomotility, or ankylosis of the affected segments. WEBER and WIMMER (1991) correlated the degree of segmental posttraumatic lesions with the loss of income capacity for medicolegal reasons. They proposed individual analysis of involved segments according to their con-

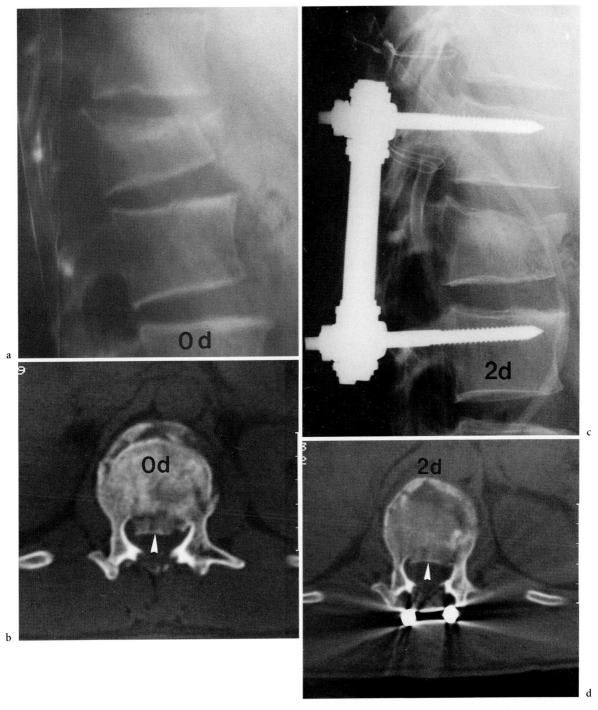

Fig. 3.33a–i. Type A3 burst fracture. **a** Lateral view showing compression of around 50% of the anterior vertebral height. **b** Axial CT demonstrating a narrowing of 50% of the lumen of the spinal canal (*arrowhead*). **c** Lateral view 2 days after osteosynthetic reduction and trabecular bone graft. A wedged vertebra is still present. **d** Axial CT at the same level as preoperatively underlines a partial reduction of the retropulsed bone fragment (*arrowheads*). **e** Normal appearance (*arrows*) of correctly positioned trabecular bone graft through the left pedicle. **f** Axial CT 1 year after trauma and after removal of the fixateur interne in the vertebra above, showing adequate location of transpedicular screws not beyond the anterior cortical line. **g** An axial slice at the same level as 1 year before shows the complete remodelling of the spinal canal. **h** T1- and **i** T2-weighted MR images reveal discrete bulging of the disks at L1/L2 and L2/L3 without relevant narrowing of the spinal canal. Note also residual kyphotic deformity of the fractured L1 (*arrows*)

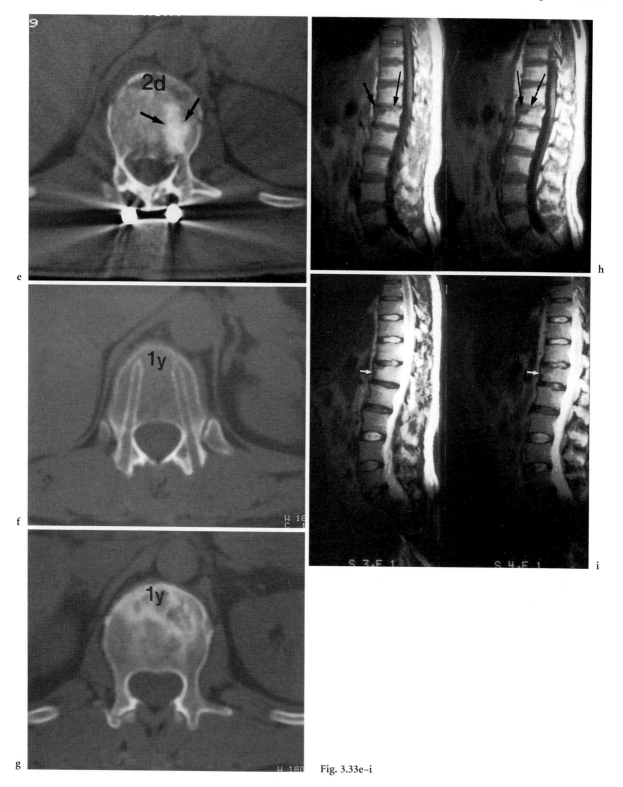

Fig. 3.33e–i

tribution to movement and a final addition to obtain the reduction of working capacity.

Finally, bone scintigraphy may be performed to follow the posttraumatic healing process, especially in the presence of complications such as pseudarthrosis or infection. It also helps to differentiate fresh from old fractures (ALLGAYER et al. 1990).

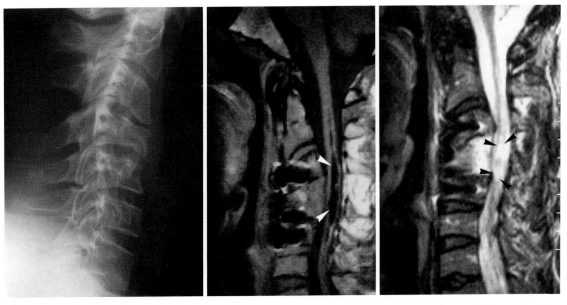

a,b   c

Fig. 3.34a–c. Posttraumatic syringomyelia. **a** Plain radiograph 1 year after C3 fracture with anterior fusion. Note narrowing of the disk space C2/C3 with osteoarthrotic changes. **b** T1-weighted MR image revealing a rounded syringohydromyelia from C2 to C4 (*arrowheads*), characterized by intraspinal low signal intensity. **c** T2-weighted image showing bone edema of the posterior aspect of the vertebral body of C3 and the high signal intensity of the syrinx (*black arrowheads*)

3.8 Diagnostic Algorithm and Important Facts

The purpose of diagnostic imaging in the setting of spinal trauma is to obtain the maximum information with the minimum of risk to guarantee the most adequate treatment according to the severity of the spinal injury. A proposal for the sequence of imaging modalities is presented in Fig. 3.35.

It is important to remember the following points when imaging the injured spine:

– Due to the high incidence of multilevel spinal injuries, it is mandatory to search for other spinal fractures when a fracture is detected, especially in polytraumatized patients.
– An exact knowledge of anatomic characteristics of the spine is the basis for the objective analysis of any type of injury.
– The posterior ligamentous complex of HOLDSWORTH (1970), the two-column theory of WHITESIDES (1977) and the three-column concept of DENIS (1983) form the basis for assessment of stability in conjunction with imaging modalities.
– The AO classification system of MAGERL et al. (1994) for thoracic and lumbar spine injuries is based upon the main mechanism of injury and may be applied to the cervical spine below C2.
– Plain film radiography remains the best screening examination for acute injuries of the spine. The three-view (AP, lateral, and open mouth views) examination of the cervical spine together with the two-view (AP and lateral views) approach to the thoracic and lumbar spine are the basis for further imaging studies.
– CT has replaced conventional tomography as the second step in the evaluation of unstable or potentially unstable spinal injuries. Its major advantage lies in the assessment of the craniocervical and thoracolumbar junctions while its major limitation lies in the detection of nondisplaced horizontally oriented fractures.
– 2D CT reconstructions are mandatory while 3D CT is optional in the acute phase. 3D CT may be obtained to confirm or display a rotational component of unstable fractures.
– Conventional tomography remains a standard alternative for the detection of axially oriented fracture lines in cases of dens, facet, or Chance fractures.
– MR imaging has emerged as the method of choice to evaluate patients with progressive or incomplete neurological damage because of its unique ability to display spinal cord damage, ligamental disruption, and intervertebral disk pathology.
– The most unstable fracture of the cervical spine is the flexion-teardrop fracture; the latter must be distinguished from the hyperextension-teardrop fracture, which is stable.

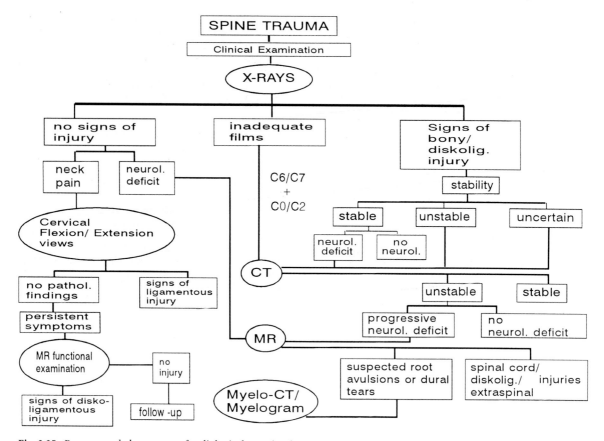

Fig. 3.35. Recommended sequence of radiological examinations

- Type A1 and A2 compression fractures are stable while type A3 fractures (burst fractures) are unstable at least in flexion/compression.
- Type B distraction fractures may be associated with sagittal translation and are thus highly unstable.
- Type C rotation fractures are characterized by instability with the potential for multidirectional translation; this is especially true for group C3.
- Instability in children may progress if adequate treatment is not performed.
- An atlanto-occipital dislocation must be ruled out on plain films in any child after a motor vehicle accident.
- Compression fractures or multiple vertebral notches at the superior endplates of vertebral bodies in children with inadequate trauma should alert one to the possibility of child abuse.
- MR imaging is an invaluable tool for follow-up of neurological sequelae after spinal trauma, such as atrophy, syringomyelia, and myelomalacia.
- Finally, the Socratic principle of "primum non nocera" (first don't damage) applies to the diagnostic algorithm for the assessment of spinal injuries. Imaging studies should avoid further injury, as may potentially occur in the case of functional imaging in the acute phase of trauma, and must be terminated as soon as diagnostic information allows the most adequate therapeutic approach to be adopted.

References

Acheson MB, Livingston RR, Richardson ML, Stimac GK (1987) High-resolution CT scanning in the evaluation of cervical spine fracture: comparison with plain film examinations. AJR 148:1179–1185

Allen BL, Ferguson RL, Lehmann TR, O'Brian RP (1982) A mechanistic classification of closed indirect fractures and dislocations of the lower cervical spine. Spine 7:1–27

Allgayer B, Flierdt E, Gumppenberg SV, Heuck A, Matzner M, Lukas P, Luttke G (1990) Die Kernspintomographie im Vergleich zur Skelettszintigraphie nach traumatischen Wirbelkörperfrakturen. Fortschr Röntgenstr 152:677–681

Allington NJ, Zembo M, Nadell J, Bowen JR (1990) C1-C2 posterior soft tissue injuries with neurologic impairment in children. J Pediatr Orthop 10:596–601

Anderson LD, D'Alonzo RT (1974) Fractures of the odontoid process of the axis. J Bone Joint Surg [Am] 56:1663–1674

Anderson PA, Montesano PX (1988) Morphology and treatment of occipital condyle fractures. Spine 13:731–736

Ballock RT, Mackerse R, Abitbol J, Cervilla V, Resnick D, Garfin SR (1992) Can burst fractures be predicted from plain radiographs? J Bone Joint Surg [Br] 74:147–150

Binet EF, Moro JJ, Maramgola JP, Hodge CJ (1973) Cervical spine tomography in trauma. Spine; 2:163–172

Brant-Zawadzki M, Miller EM, Federle MP (1981) CT in the evaluation of spine trauma. AJR 136:369–375

Braunschweig R, Bilow H (1994) Radiologische Funktionsdiagnostik der Wirbelsäule – Erstdiagnose und Verlaufskontrolle. In: Bargon G (ed) Radiologie der Wirbelsäulenerkrankungen. Schnetztor-Verlag, Konstanz, pp 47–55

Bulas DI, Fitz CR, Johnson DL (1993) Traumatic atlanto-occipital dislocation in children. Radiology 188:155–158

Cattel HS, Filtzer DL (1965) Pseudoluxation and other normal variations in the cervical spine in children. J Bone Joint Surg [Am] 47:1296–1309

Daffner RH, Deeb ZL, Goldberg AL, Kandabarow, Rothfus WE (1990) The radiologic assessment of post-traumatic vertebral stability. Skeletal Radiol 19:103–108

Denis F (1983) The three column spine and its significance in the classification of acute thoracolumbar spinal injuries. Spine 8:817–831

Denis F, Burkus JK (1991) Lateral distraction injuries to the thoracic and lumbar spine. A report of three cases. J Bone Joint Surg [Am] 73:1049–1053

Dorr LD, Harvey JP, Nickel VL (1982) Clinical review of early stability of spine injuries. Spine 7:545–550

Effendi B, Roy D, Cornish B, Dussault RG, Laurin CA (1981) Fractures of the ring of the axis. J Bone Joint Surg [Br] 63:319–327

Ehara S, El-Khoury GY, Clark CR (1992) Radiologic evaluation of dens fracture: role of plain radiography and tomography. Spine 17:475–479

El-Khoury GY, Whitten CG (1993) Trauma to the upper thoracic spine: anatomy, biomechanics, and unique imaging features. AJR 160:95–102

El-Khoury GY, Kathol MH, Daniel WW (1995) Imaging of acute injuries of the cervical spine: value of plain radiography, CT, and MR imaging. AJR 164:43–50

Frankel HL, Hancock DO, Hyslop G (1969) The value of postural reduction in initial management of closed injuries of the spine with paraplegia and tetraplegia. Paraplegia 7:179–192

Gertzbein SD (1994) Spine update: classification of thoracic and lumbar fractures. Spine 19:626–628

Gilsanz V, Boechat MI, Gilsanz R, Loro ML, Roe TF, Goodman WG (1994) Gender differences in vertebral sizes in adults: biomechanical implications. Radiology 190:678–682

Govender S, Charles RW, Rasool MN (1990) Spinal injuries in children. Injury 21:403–406

Greenspan A (1993) Skelettradiologie: Orthopädie, Traumatologie, Rheumatologie, Onkologie. 2. ed. VCH Verlagsgesellschaft, Weinheim, Basel, Cambridge, New York

Häberle HJ, Rilinger N, Tomczak R, Arand M (1994) Osteosynthetische Versorgung von Wirbelsäulenverletzungen im Röntgenbild. In: Bargon G (ed) Radiologie der Wirbelsäulenerkrankungen. Schnetztor-Verlag, Konstanz, pp 46–55

Holdsworth F (1970) Fracture, dislocations, and fracture-dislocations of the spine. J Bone Joint Surg [Am] 52:1534–1551

Jend HH, Heller M (1989) Stabilitätsbeurteilung bei Wirbelsäulenfrakturen. Fortschr Röntgenstr 151:63–68

Keene JS, Goletz TH, Lilleas F, Alter AJ, Sackett JF (1982) Diagnosis of vertebral fractures. J Bone Joint Surg [Am] 64:586–595

Kerslake RW, Jaspan T, Worthington BS (1991) Magnetic resonance imaging of spinal trauma. Br J Radiol 64:386–402

Kleinman PK, Marks SC (1992) Vertebral body fractures in child abuse. Radiologic histopathologic correlates. Invest Radiology 27:715–722

Kliewer MA, Gray L, Paver J, Richardson WD, Vogler JB, McElhaney JH, Myers BS (1993) Acute spinal ligament disruption: MR imaging with anatomic correlation. Magn Reson Imag 3:855–861

Kulkarni MV, McArdle CB, Kopanicky D, Miner M, Cotler HB, Lee KF, Harris JH (1987) Acute spinal cord injury: MR imaging at 1.5 T. Radiology 164:837–843

Kuner EH, Kuner A, Schlickewei W, Wimmer B (1992) Die Bedeutung der Ligamentotaxis für die Fixateur-interne-Osteosynthese bei Frakturen der Brust- und Lendenwirbelsäule. Chirurg 63:50–55

Levine AM, Edwards CC (1991) Fractures of the atlas. J Bone Joint Surg [Am] 73:680–691

Levine AM, Edwards CC (1985) The management of traumatic spondylolisthesis of the axis. J Bone Joint Surg [Am] 67:217–225

Louis R (1977) Les théories de l'instabilité. Rev Chir Orthop 63:423–425

Magerl F, Aebi M, Gertzbein SD, Harms J, Nazarian S (1994) A comprehensive classification of thoracic and lumbar injuries. Eur Spine J 3:184–201

Maiman DJ, Pintar FA (1992) Anatomy and clinical biomechanics of the thoracic spine. Clin Neurosurg 38:296–324

Manaster BJ, Osborn AG (1987) CT patterns of facet fracture dislocations in the thoracolumbar region. AJR 148:335–340

McAfee PC, Yuan HA, Fredrickson BE, Lubicky JP (1983) The value of computed tomography in thoracolumbar fractures. J Bone Joint Surg [Am] 65:461–479

McGrory BJ, Vanderwilde RS, Currier BL, Eismont FJ (1993) Diagnosis of subtle thoracolumbar burst fractures. A new radiographic sign. Spine 18:2282–2285

McPhee IB (1981) Spinal fractures and dislocations in children and adolescents. Spine 6:533–537

Meyer PR (1989) Vascular anatomy of the spinal cord: T1 to T10. In: Meyer PR (ed) Surgery of spine trauma. Churchill Livingstone, New York, pp 85–106

Moore KL (1982) Anatomía: orientación clínica. Editorial Médica Panamericana, Buenos Aires

Nucci RC, Seigal S, Merola AA, et al. (1995) Computed tomography evaluation of the normal adult odontoid: implications for internal fixation. Spine 20:264–270

Oda T, Panjabi MM, Crisco JJ III, Oxland TR, Katz L, Nolte L-P (1991) Experimental study of atlas injuries. II. Relevance to clinical diagnosis and treatment. Spine 16:466–473

Oxland TR, Panjabi MM, Lin RM (1994) Axes of motion of thoracolumbar burst fractures. J Spinal Disord 7:130–138

Panjabi MM, Krag MH, Goel VK (1981) A technique for measurement and description of three-dimensional six degree-of-freedom motion of a body joint with an application to the human spine. J Biomech 14:447–460

Pathria MN, Petersilge CA (1991) Spinal trauma. Radiol Clin North Am 29:847–865

Prestar FJ, Putz R (1982) Das ligamentum longitudinale posterius. Morphologie und funktion. Morphol Med 2:118–181

Quencer RM (1988) The injured spinal cord. Evaluation with magnetic resonance and intraoperative ultrasonography. Radiol Clin North Am 26:1025–1046

Riggins RS, Krauss JF (1977) The risk of neurologic damage with fractures of the vertebrae. J Trauma 17:126–133

Roy-Camille R, Saillant G, Berteaux D, Mary-Anne S (1979) Early management of spinal injuries. In: McKibbin B (ed) Recent advances in orthopedics. 3. Churchill Livingstone, Edinburgh, pp 57–87

Saeed M, Buitrago-Téllez CH, Ferstl FJ, Boos S, Wimmer B, Langer M (1994) Three-dimensional CT in the diagnosis of spinal trauma: comparison with plain film and two-dimensional CT examinations. Eur Radiol 4:161–166

Simpson AHRW, Williamson DM, Golding SJ, Houghton GR (1990) Thoracic spine translocation without cord injury. J Bone Joint Surg [Br] 72:80–83

Spence KF, Decker S, Sell KW (1970) Bursting atlantal fracture associated with rupture of the transverse ligament. J Bone Joint Surg [Am] 52:543–549

Streitwieser DR, Knopp R, Wales LR, Williams JL, Tonnemacher K (1983) Accuracy of standard radiographic views in detecting cervical spine fractures. Ann Emerg Med 12:538–542

Swischuk LE, Swischuk PN, John SD (1993) Wedging of C-3 in infants and children: usually a normal finding and not a fracture. Radiology 188:523–526

Vogel W, Dingler WH, Schütz M, Deininger HK (1990) Preliminary results for CT examinations of spinal fractures with a Somatom Plus 3-D software program. In: Felix R, Langer M (eds) Advances in CT. Springer, Berlin Heidelberg New York, pp 144–153

Weber M, Wimmer B (1991) Die klinische und radiologische Begutachtung von Wirbelsäulenverletzungen nach dem Segmentprinzip. Unfallchirurgie 17:200–207

Weidenmaier W (1994) MRT-Funktionsdiagnostik der Halswirbelsäule nach Schleudertrauma. In: Bargon G (ed) Radiologie der Wirbelsäulenerkrankungen. Schnetztor-Verlag, Konstanz, pp 56–62

White AA III, Panjabi M (1990) Clinical biomechanics of the spine. Lippincott, Philadelphia

Whitesides TE JR (1977) Traumatic kyphosis of the thoracolumbar spine. Clin Orthop 128:78–92

Wimmer B (1989) Computertomographie beim Wirbelsäulentrauma. Radiologe 29:441–446

Wimmer B, Hoffmann E, Jacob A (1990) Trauma of the spine. Springer, Berlin Heidelberg New York

Wolter D (1985) Vorschlag für eine Einteilung von Wirbelsäulenverletzungen. Unfallchirurg 88:481–484

Woodring JH, Lee C (1992) The role and limitations of computed tomographic scanning in the evaluation of cervical trauma. J Trauma 33:698–708

Xu R, Nadaud MC, Ebraheim NA, Yeasting RA (1995) Morphology of the second cervical vertebra and the posterior projection of the C2 pedicle axis. Spine 20:259–263

Yu S, Haughton VM, Rosenbaum AE (1991) Magnetic resonance imaging and anatomy of the spine. Radiol Clin North Am 29:691–710

Zinreich SJ, Wang H, Abdo F, Bryan N (1990) 3-D CT improves accuracy of spinal trauma studies. Diagn Imaging Int 4:24–29

4 Neck

C.H. Buitrago-Téllez, F.J. Ferstl, and M. Langer

CONTENTS

4.1 General Considerations

Injuries to the neck represent one of the major challenges for adequate diagnosis and therapy in the setting of acute trauma. These lesions may be fatal or associated with life-long morbidity.

Establishing an adequate airway is one of the priorities in the care of the trauma patient. Thus, airway compression secondary to a soft tissue cervical injury must be recognized early and treated.

Neck trauma may be classified into blunt or penetrating injuries. Blunt neck trauma includes the fre-

C.H. Buitrago-Téllez, MD, Abteilung Röntgendiagnostik, Radiologische Universitätsklinik, Klinikum der Albert-Ludwigs-Universität Freiburg, Hugstetterstraße 55, 79106 Freiburg, Germany
F.J. Ferstl, MD, Abteilung Röntgendiagnostik, Radiologische Universitätsklinik, Klinikum der Albert-Ludwigs-Universität Freiburg, Hugstetterstraße 55, 79106 Freiburg, Germany
M. Langer, MD, FICA, Professor and Director, Abteilung Röntgendiagnostik, Radiologische Universitätsklinik, Klinikum der Albert-Ludwigs-Universität Freiburg, Hugstetterstraße 55, 79106 Freiburg, Germany

quent cervical spine injuries discussed in Chap. 3. Penetrating injuries extend beyond the platysma muscle and often require an immediate surgical approach, especially in cases of severe vascular injuries. Furthermore, a topographic analysis of the organs involved in the trauma may be helpful in defining the most adequate imaging and therapeutic approach.

Laryngeal injuries result most commonly from motor vehicle accidents, followed by sports and recreational activities (Peppard 1984). On the other hand, cervical vascular injuries are more frequently seen after penetrating wounds related to violence. These facts account for the higher incidence of such injuries among young adults.

Another important aspect to keep in mind is the possible association between cervical spinal trauma, laryngeal fracture, and blunt carotid artery injuries secondary to hyperextension injuries.

4.2 Anatomy and Mechanisms of Injury

4.2.1 Anatomy

Detailed knowledge of the complex anatomy of the neck containing the different viscera, blood vessels, and nerves is a prerequisite for evaluation of the different injuries.

Spatial anatomy of cervical structures is based upon the superficial and deep cervical fascias (Figs. 4.1, 4.2).

The *superficial fascia* is a thin layer that encloses the platysma muscle. The deep cervical fascia is divided into three layers. These three layers cleave the neck into two functional spaces converging on the hyoid bone: the suprahyoid and the infrahyoid part of the neck (Harnsberger and Osborn 1991; Smoker and Harnsberger 1991). The superficial or investing layer of deep cervical fascia encircles the neck, splitting to enclose the sternomastoid and trapezius muscles. The space external to the superficial layer of deep cervical fascia is the *superficial space*. It contributes to the formation of the carotid sheath.

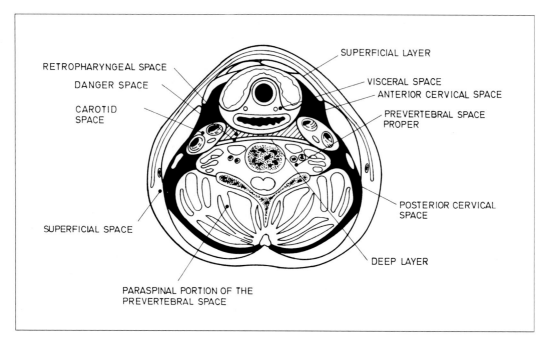

Fig. 4.1. Axial scheme through the infrahyoid neck at the level of the thyroid gland, showing the superficial, middle (surrounding the thyroid gland), and deep layers. Note also the superficial, visceral, carotid, retropharyngeal, danger, anterior, and posterior cervical spaces. (Modified from Parker and Harnsberger 1991)

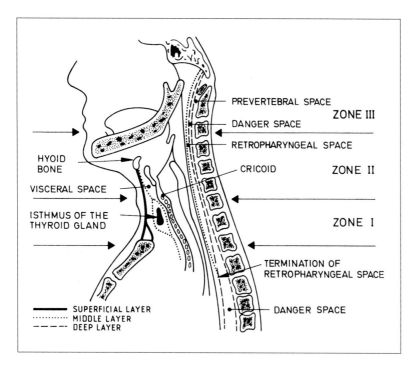

Fig. 4.2. Midsagittal section demonstrating the different fascial layers and spaces of the infrahyoid portion of the neck. Note also the three anatomic areas considered in the setting of penetrating trauma (zones I, II, and III). (Modified from Smoker and Harnsberger 1991)

The pretracheal or *middle layer* attaches above to the thyroid and cricoid cartilages and extends into the chest, where it blends into the pericardium. The main portion of the middle layer forms a fascial sheath encompassing the *visceral space*. A capsule for the thyroid gland is formed by a splitting of the middle layer. The posterior aspect of the middle layer forms the anterior wall of the *retropharyngeal space*.

Finally, the prevertebral or *deep layer of deep cervical fascia* covers the prevertebral muscles attaching to transverse processes and thus subdividing the *prevertebral space* into the anterior prevertebral space proper and the posterior paraspinal portion of the prevertebral space. The anterior aspect of the deep layer splits into the alar (anterior) and prevertebral (posterior) portions, forming the "*danger space,*" so called because it may facilitate the spread of hematoma or abscess of the retropharyngeal space to the mediastinum. The alar portion forms the posterior and lateral walls of the retropharyngeal space.

The *retropharyngeal space* is important in the setting of trauma, because of the frequent location of hematomas in this space, causing life-threatening airway obstruction (DAVIS et al. 1990; O'NEILL 1977). Furthermore, it is a frequent location of air secondary to laryngeal fractures.

Also of importance is the division into three anatomic areas with respect to surgical accessibility in cases of penetrating cervical injuries (ROON and CHRISTENSEN 1979). *Zone I injuries* are considered to be at the base or root of the neck and extend from above the clavicle to the cricoid. *Zone II* is the midneck and comprises that region from the cricoid cartilage to the angle of the mandible. *Zone III injuries* involve the area above the angle of the mandible (NOLPH and RICHARDSON 1987). These zones are correlated with the midsagittal diagram of the neck in Fig. 4.2.

Zone I includes the proximal carotid arteries, the subclavian vessels, and major vessels in the chest, lung, upper mediastinum, esophagus, trachea, and thoracic duct. Zone II includes the most important cervical vascular structures and is the easiest to evaluate and explore surgically. Both zone III and zone I are difficult to explore surgically, because of their proximity to the thoracic inlet and skull base, respectively.

4.2.2 Mechanisms of Injury

Penetrating injuries result from stab wounds, gunshot wounds, and wounds caused by other sharp objects. Paradoxically, a partial section of a cervical artery is more life-threatening than a complete section, because of the protecting retraction of both ends of the sectional vessels with reflex vasoconstriction (LEDGERWOOD and LUCAS 1984).

Gunshot wounds have a wide spectrum of injury patterns. These lesions range from localized bleeding into the surrounding soft tissues to massive bleeding, when the injury is adjacent to a cavity, such as a hemithorax, esophagus, hypopharynx, or trachea. Additionally, the energy transmitted by a bullet leads to destruction of soft tissues far distant from the actual missile path. This may affect the cartilaginous structures of the larynx and its mucosa. The mucosal involvement and edema may compress the airway and must therefore be evaluated in the acute phase of penetrating injuries.

Blunt injuries are related to either acceleration-deceleration forces or direct blows to cervical structures. During acceleration and rapid deceleration, anterior neck structures are forced against the cervical spine, causing compressional and shear injuries to soft tissues. An acute angulation at a carotid artery may result in an intimal tear, causing a localized occlusion, a dissection, or an embolus. Additional laryngeal injuries may result from the same mechanism. Moreover, an anatomic weak area at the hypopharyngeal-esophageal junction may predispose this area to perforation with blunt trauma (THAL 1988).

Direct blows to the neck, especially to the laryngeal structures, may result from altercations, sports or a hyperextension injury, in which the head is thrown backward while the larynx may directly strike the dashboard.

4.3 Classification of Cervical Soft Tissue Injuries

As previously emphasized, in the classification of cervical soft tissue injuries, a *penetrating trauma* is considered present when the injury extends beyond the platysma muscle. Furthermore, penetrating injuries may be classified according to the level of injury (zones I, II, and III).

Blunt neck trauma usually results from motor vehicle accidents and frequently occurs in conjunction with cervical spine injuries. Furthermore, blunt injuries may be present with impairment of the airway secondary to outer compression by hematoma or edema or fracture of the laryngeal skeleton.

Laryngeal injuries may be classified as *internal* or *external*. Internal injuries are either iatrogenic after intubation or endoscopy or secondary to burns. External injuries, which refer to the typical blunt or penetrating trauma, may be classified according to the direction of the forces or the anatomic areas involved. Laryngeal fractures resulting from anteroposterior forces are usually associated with a midline vertical fracture line as well as injuries of the internal laryngeal structures such as the vocal cords, articulations, and muscles. Lateral forces typically cause multiple fragment fractures with unilateral luxations of the cricoarythenoid or cricothyroid articulations (RICHTER 1992). A further classification of laryngeal injuries is based upon anatomic location and considers *supraglottic*, *transglottic*, *cricoid*, and *cricotracheal* injuries.

4.4 Examination Methods

4.4.1 Conventional Radiography

The evaluation of the stabilized patient with blunt neck trauma starts with a three-view series of the cervical spine (AP, lateral, and open mouth views).

Plain films allow an accurate evaluation of bony structures (Fig. 4.3) as well as the extent of airway narrowing, retropharyngeal hematoma or fracture-dislocation of the laryngeal skeleton. Subcutaneous emphysema, soft tissue swelling, and displacement of the trachea are also indirect signs of soft tissue damage (SWEENEY and MARX 1993).

A chest radiograph is also indicated in the acute setting of neck trauma, especially when evaluating

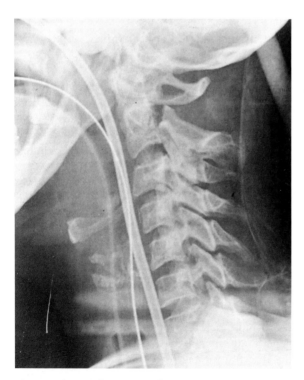

Fig. 4.3. Blunt neck trauma with traumatic spondylolisthesis of the axis ("hangman's fracture"). Note the bilateral avulsion of the neural arch at its junction with the body of C2, clearly delineated on the lateral cervical view

zone I penetrating injuries with increased risk of hemothorax or pneumothorax.

Conventional tomography may reveal laryngeal fractures in the acute phase. However, it has been replaced by computed tomography (CT), with its better soft tissue contrast for such injuries. Nevertheless, conventional tomography may also be helpful in the follw-up after laryngeal trauma.

4.4.2 Oral Contrast Studies

An oral contrast study with water-soluble contrast media is indicated in the patient with clinical or radiological signs of esophageal rupture who is in a stable condition. It is also included in the diagnostic workup of penetrating injuries. Unfortunately, water-soluble contrast studies have a significant rate of false-negative results (CHEADLE and RICHARDSON 1982), so that barium is frequently used to disclose mucosal tears. Nevertheless, the risk of barium-induced mediastinitis must be kept in mind.

4.4.3 Duplex Ultrasonography

Duplex ultrasonography is a noninvasive alternative for the evaluation of stable patients after blunt neck trauma with potential cervical vascular injuries. According to BYNOE et al. (1991), the sensitivity of duplex ultrasonography in characterizing vascular injuries of the cervical and extremity vessels such as arterial disruptions, intimal flaps, acute pseudoaneurysms, and arteriovenous fistulas may be as high as 95%. A disadvantage of this method is the high user-dependence. However, it should be considered as a screening method available for cases with clinical signs suggesting vascular injury (MARTIN et al. 1991).

4.4.4 Angiography

Arteriography, if available promptly, is useful in stable patients with suspected cervical vascular injury.

Biplane arteriography, usually done by the transfemoral route, is a highly sensitive examination with the capability to detect accurately vascular injury patterns such as completely or partially transected vessels with extravasation of contrast medium (Fig. 4.4), pseudoaneurysms, intimal flaps

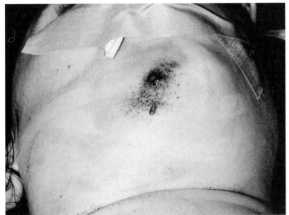

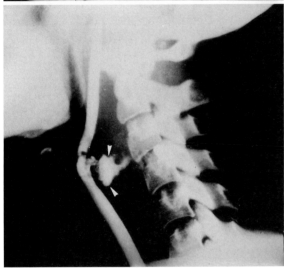

Fig. 4.4a,b. Penetrating neck trauma secondary to gunshot injury. **a** Note massive cervical hematoma and the missile entrance lesion at zone II (midneck). **b** Conventional angiography reveals an injury of the right common carotid artery with extravasation of contrast medium (*arrowheads*)

posure, the delay in therapy with the risk of development of neurologic deficit, and the high sensitivity of clinical findings in this region in predicting vascular injury (BEITSCH et al. 1994), others suggest that angiography be used to evaluate zone II lesions in stable patients with a significant cervical hematoma (MENAWAT et al. 1992; SCLAFANI et al. 1991; see Fig. 4.4).

If a diagnostic evaluation with selective exploration is preferred, arteriograms are routinely performed to rule out a relevant vascular injury.

4.4.5 Computed Tomography

Computed tomography has emerged as the second step in the imaging evaluation of blunt cervical trauma. It is especially accurate in ruling out cervical spine fractures, soft tissue hematomas (Fig. 4.6) or swelling, and fractures of the laryngeal structures (MANCUSO and HANAFEE 1979; see Fig. 4.7) and of the hyoid bone (SZEREMETA and MOROVATI 1991). It is also an adequate method for excluding associated pathology such as thoracic vascular disorders extending into the neck, mimicking an increasing hematoma (e.g., increasing thoracic aneurysm: Fig. 4.8). Moreover, CT has the potential to localize occlusions of the cervical vessels as well as extravasal contrast medium collections.

or dissections (Fig. 4.5), traumatic arteriovenous fistulas, and major venous injuries (SCHENK 1992).

High-quality conventional angiography (Fig. 4.4b) or intra-arterial digital subtraction angiography (Fig. 4.5) both may be adequate techniques. Intravenous digital subtraction angiography may be useful in single cases (PRINGLE and CHARIG 1994), but cannot be recommended as the standard technique. Indications for angiography depend to a great extent upon the treatment approach followed by surgeons (SCHENK 1992).

If mandatory exploration of any penetrating injury is considered, angiography is indicated in stable patients with zone I and III injuries. However, there is still controversy with respect to zone II injuries: While the majority of authors reject angiography in zone II injuries because of the adequate surgical ex-

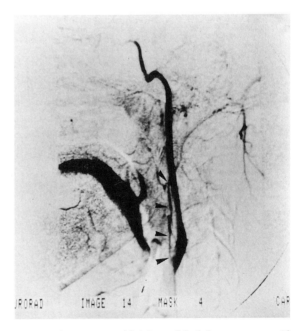

Fig. 4.5. Blunt trauma with injury of the left common carotid artery: intra-arterial digital subtraction angiography reveals an intimal tear with spontaneous dissection (*arrowheads*). Clinically, a right-sided hemiparesis was evident

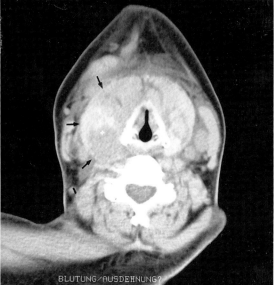

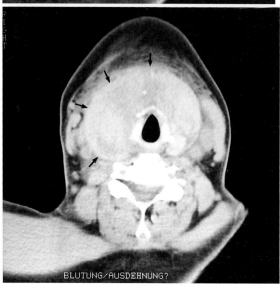

Fig. 4.6a,b. Thyroid hematoma: **a** and **b** demonstrate contiguous axial slices revealing high-density (47 HU) structures within the thyroid capsule (*arrows*) in the visceral space

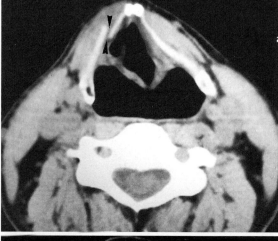

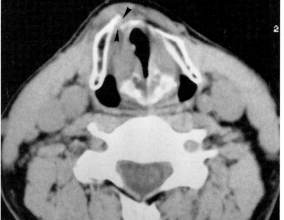

Fig. 4.7a,b. Laryngeal fracture. **a** Axial CT demonstrates a displaced vertical fracture (*arrowheads*) of the right ala of the thyroid cartilage. **b** An axial slice caudally shows the continuity of the vertical thyroid alar fracture through the lamina of the crycoid cartilage (*arrowheads*). (Images courtesy of Prof. M. Heller, Kiel)

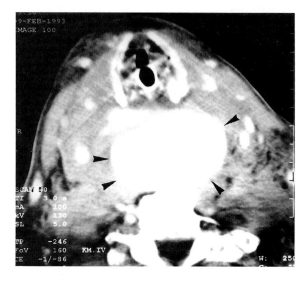

Fig. 4.8. Unconscious patient with an increasing mass in the neck. Axial CT scan demonstrated a large enhanced mass (*arrowheads*) in front of the cervical spine, displacing the carotid arteries. Angiography (not shown) confirmed a posttraumatic aortic arch aneurysm with extension up to the suprahyoid region

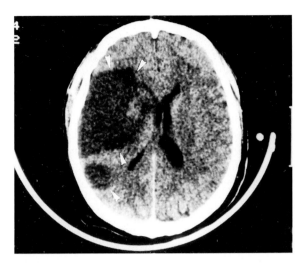

Fig. 4.9. Blunt carotid artery trauma. Follow-up CT of the head reveals an ischemic insult in the supply area of the right medial cerebral artery (*arrowheads*). Such infarctions result from intimal tears of the carotid arteries, causing an embolus

In patients with progressive neurological deterioration, a head CT may reveal infarct zones secondary to blunt carotid or vertebral artery trauma.

4.5 Trauma Pattern and Pathomorphology of Cervical Soft Tissue Injuries

4.5.1 Vascular Injuries

An arterial injury may result from a directly penetrating wound or from a blunt trauma, causing either major hemorrhage with hypovolemia and shock or ischemia in the supply area of the damaged vessel (Fig. 4.9).

Zone I injuries require aortic arch arteriography with selective studies depending on the case. Multiple views are necessary and the search for vascular injuries must include visualization of the venous system (PHILLIPS 1992). Zone II injuries are studied with selective imaging of the cervical course of the appropriate carotid or vertebral arteries or both, including the visualization of the venous system. The same procedure is recommended for zone III injuries.

Blunt injuries to the carotid artery may initially be missed. The intimal tear may progress to complete occlusion of the involved vessel, dissection (Fig. 4.5), or embolization to a more distal location within the brain (Fig. 4.9). Other lesions described include dissection, pseudoaneurysm, and local contusion (PRETRE et al. 1994). Blunt carotid artery injuries

must be ruled out in patients with neck hyperextension injuries or with cervical spine fractures as well as in patients with neurologic deficits not explained by intracranial trauma (MARTIN et al. 1991). Duplex scanning and magnetic resonance (MR) imaging may be useful noninvasive studies, which may decide the need for angiography.

Traumatic vertebral artery lesions are often associated with cervical spinal injuries, especially at the level C1–2 or with concomitant uni- or bilateral dislocation. MR imaging may be a noninvasive means of diagnosing this complication of cervical spine trauma (PRABHU et al. 1994), which may cause cerebellar infarctions in young patients (GARG et al. 1993). Angiography may confirm the diagnosis.

Posttraumatic aneurysms of cervical vessels not only may be diagnosed by angiography, but also may be treated by intravasal application of special coils, such as platinum coils (WEBER et al. 1993). Moreover, embolic occlusion of injured vessels has been successfully described for zone III injuries (RAO et al. 1993), and may be theoretically applied to injuries of other zones.

4.5.2 Laryngeal Injuries

Soft tissue injuries including mucosal lacerations, hematomas, edema, and cricoarytenoid dislocation may be well detected by CT.

Supraglottic injuries require the evaluation of the thyroid cartilage; this may be carried out by conventional radiographs (lateral view: conventional tomograms) but is better achieved by CT, which reveals transverse or vertical thyroid alar fractures (AVRAHAMI et al. 1994; MANCUSO and HANAFEE 1979; see Fig. 4.7). Ligamentous lesions are not well detected. Free air in the neck is an indirect sign of a fracture of the laryngeal skeleton. A distorsion as well as a narrowing of the airway may be present.

Transglottic injuries may combine a vertical fracture of the thyroid cartilage with an avulsion of the vocal cord. CT demonstrates the fracture as well as edema and hemorrhage of the avulsed vocal cord.

A *cricoid or subglottic injury* may be life-threatening because of the potential for severe airway narrowing secondary to dislocated fragments and edema as evidenced by CT.

A complete *separation of the trachea from the cricoid* also may be present, and diagnosis must be made as early as possible to avoid thoracic retraction of the trachea.

Although not belonging to the laryngeal skeleton, the hyoid bone is tightly attached to it and may also fracture in blunt neck injuries. Its fracture results more commonly from strangulation and may cause severe airway compromise (SZEREMETA and MOROVATI 1991). Diagnosis is sometimes difficult and CT readily reveals the posteriorly dislocated fragments.

4.5.3 Esophageal Injuries

Esophageal injuries may result either from penetrating neck injuries or from a sudden increase in intraluminal pressure after a thoracic trauma. A water-soluble contrast study may reveal the perforation site and, if negative, the study may be repeated with barium, although the risk of mediastinitis must be considered. Alternatively or complementarily, endoscopic examination should be performed.

4.5.4 Thyroid and Submandibular Gland Injuries

Blunt cervical trauma may be complicated by severe damage to glandular tissue. Thyroid injury may result in an important hematoma (Fig. 4.6) due to the high blood supply of this organ. These lesions may be initially asymptomatic but may progress. CT (RUPRECHT et al. 1994; see Fig. 4.6) or ultrasonography may reveal the extent of the hematoma. From the salivary glands at risk of blunt cervical trauma the submandibular gland may present as a slowly expanding posttraumatic neck mass. Both CT and sialographic evaluation may demonstrate the fracture of this gland, which is encapsulated in the superficial layer of the deep cervical fascia (ROEBKER et al. 1991).

4.6 Special Features of Cervical Soft Tissue Injuries in Children and Adolescents

Vertebral artery injuries result from cervical blunt trauma and may be associated with posttraumatic strokes affecting the cerebellar hemispheres. This complication is observed more frequently in children and adolescents (GARG et al. 1993; ROSMAN et al. 1992). Prognosis for neurologic recovery is good and early diagnosis should be made with the use of MR imaging in cases of neurologic deficits after any significant neck trauma, especially if it is associated with a cervical spine fracture or facet dislocation.

Blunt laryngotracheal injuries are rare in the pediatric group due to anatomic considerations. Firstly, the lowest margin of the larynx of children lies significantly higher (C4) than in adults (C7); thus in children the mandibula protects the larynx from direct trauma (RICHTER 1992). Secondly, the cartilaginous skeleton of the larynx of children is more flexible and the structures will rebound rather than undergo actual fracture and permanent deformation. Nevertheless, laryngeal injuries may be present in children suffering direct strong forces with secondary cartilaginous fractures. They are usually associated with severe impairment of the airway and therapy should not be delayed because of diagnostic studies (KADISH et al. 1994).

4.7 Follow-up, Sequelae, and Complications

Injuries to the neck may recover adequately without sequelae or lead to death secondary to cervical spine injury, airway impairment from massive bleeding and tracheal compression, or neurologic damage due to carotid artery injury.

The major complication of vascular injuries is cerebral ischemia due to carotid artery injury presenting usually as a unilateral neurological deficit which becomes apparent after the acute phase. In these patients CT documentation of cerebral injury may be important, not only in the acute setting but also in follow-up. Further complications related to cervical vascular trauma reflect more the hypovolemic shock rather than specific injuries to the cervical vessels and include adult respiratory distress syndrome, renal insufficiency, and infectious sequelae.

The most feared complication after laryngeal trauma is airway stenosis. According to OLSON (1984) there are certain findings that predispose to stenosis, including displaced cartilage fragment with edges exposed to the lumen of the larynx, collapse of the cricoid cartilage, and airway collapse requiring immediate or urgent tracheotomy. Furthermore, a vocal cord lesion may result in an impairment or loss of the voice.

Posttraumatic laryngeal stenosis may be recognized on the lateral cervical view, but often conventional tomograms or CT is necessary to evaluate the extent of stenosis and its location. Sequelae affecting vocal cord quality require laryngological functional studies (RICHTER 1992).

4.8 Diagnostic Algorithm and Important Facts

Diagnostic imaging procedures in the setting of acute trauma of the soft tissues of the neck, excluding the cervical spine, must be postponed until stabilization of the patient is achieved. A diagnostic algorithm taking into account the distinction between blunt and penetrating neck injuries is proposed in Fig. 4.10.

For further information on cervical spine fractures, the reader is referred to Chap. 3.

The following points should be kept in mind in imaging the injured neck:

– Clinical suspicion of a hyperextension mechanism of injury should alert the radiologist to the need to rule out combined injuries of the cervical spine and of the laryngeal skeleton and blunt injuries of the carotid arteries.

– Detailed analysis of the lateral view should allow recognition of a retropharyngeal hematoma, which may compromise the airway, as well as indirect signs of visceral injuries, such as free air in the cervical soft tissues.

– Knowledge of the spatial anatomy of the neck is especially useful for localizing specific lesions on axial imaging modalities, such as CT or MR imaging.

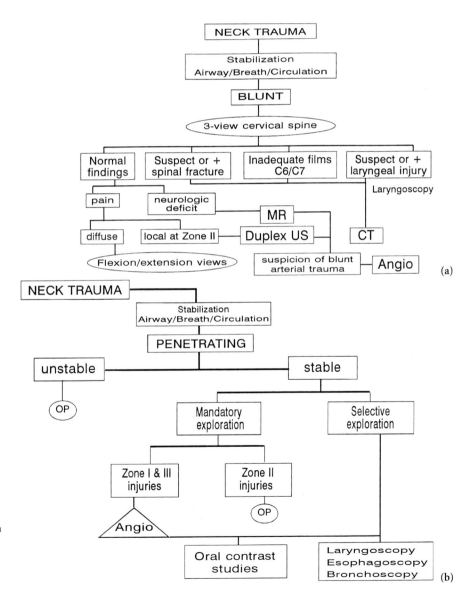

Fig. 4.10. Sequential algorithm for the evaluation of blunt (**a**) and penetrating (**b**) neck trauma (modified from SCHENK 1992)

– The division of the neck into zones I (base of the neck), II (midneck), and III (above the mandibular angle) has therapeutic and diagnostic implications for the management of penetrating neck injuries.

– Based upon the mandatory explorative approach, injuries of zones I and III constitute indications for angiography in the stable patient, while injuries of zone II are immediately operated on.

– The alternative diagnostic evaluation with selective exploration implies the study of all stable patients with penetrating injuries with angiography, oral contrast studies, and triple endoscopy (laryngoscopy, esophagoscopy, and bronchoscopy).

– CT has emerged as an adjunct to laryngoscopic evaluation of laryngeal fractures, allowing an exact evaluation of the extent of narrowing of the airway and the degree of comminution of the larynx.

Acknowledgement. Special thanks are due to Prof. G. Spillner, Department of Cardiovascular Surgery, University of Freiburg, for support in the documentation of clinical cases.

References

Avrahami E, Havel M, Englender M (1994) CT evaluation of displaced superior cornu of ossified thyroid cartilage. Clin Radiol 49:683–685

Beitsch P, Weigelt JA, Flynn E, Easley S (1994) Physical examination and arteriography in patients with penetrating zone II neck wounds. Arch Surg 129:577–581

Bynoe RP, Miles WS, Bell RM, Greenwold DR, Sessions G, Haynes JL, Rush DS (1991) Noninvasive diagnosis of vascular trauma by duplex ultrasonography. J Vasc Surg 14:346–352

Cheadle W, Richardson JD (1982) Options in management of trauma to the esophagus. Surg Gynecol Obstet 155:380–384

Davis WL, Harnsberger HR, Smoker WRK, Watanabe AS (1990) Retropharyngeal space: evaluation of normal anatomy and diseases with CT and MR imaging. Radiology 174:59–64

Garg BP, Ottinger CJ, Smith RR, Fishman MA (1993) Strokes in children due to vertebral artery trauma. Neurology 43:2555–2558

Harnsberger HR, Osborn AG (1991) Differential diagnosis of head and neck lesions based on their space of origin. 1. The suprahyoid part of the neck. AJR 157:147–154

Kadish H, Schunk J, Woodward GA (1994) Blunt pediatric laryngotracheal trauma: case reports and review of the literature. Am J Emerg Med 12:207–211

Ledgerwood AM, Lucas CE (1984) Cervical vascular injury. In: Mathog RH (ed) Maxillofacial trauma. Williams and Wilkins, Baltimore, pp 78–88

Mancuso AA, Hanafee WN (1979) Computed tomography of the injured larynx. Radiology 133:139–144

Martin RF, Eldrup-Jorgensen J, Clark DE, Bredenberg CE (1991) Blunt trauma to the carotid arteries. J Vasc Surg 14:789–793

Menawat SS, Dennis JW, Laneve LM, Frykberg ER (1992) Are arteriograms necessary in penetrating zone II neck injuries? J Vasc Surg 16:397–400

Nolph MB, Richardson JD (1987) Cervical injuries. In: Richardson JD, Polk HC, Flint LM (eds) Trauma: clinical care and pathophysiology. Yearbook Medical Publishers, Chicago, pp 433–450

O'Neill JV (1977) Retropharyngeal hematoma secondary to minor blunt trauma in the elderly patient. J Otolaryngol 6:43

Olson NA (1984) Laryngeal and tracheal stenosis. In: Mathog RH (ed) Maxillofacial trauma. Williams and Wilkins, Baltimore, pp 385–402

Parker GD, Harnsberger HR (1991) Radiologic evaluation of the normal and diseased posterior cervical space. AJR 157:161–165

Peppard SB (1984) Laryngeal trauma. In: Mathog RH (ed) Maxillofacial trauma. Wiliams and Wilkins, Baltimore, pp 374–384

Phillips CD (1992) Emergent radiologic evaluation of the gunshot wound victim. Radiol Clin North Am 30:307–324

Prabhu VC, Patil AA, Hellbusch LC, McConnell JR, Leibrock LG (1994) Magnetic resonance angiography in the diagnosis of traumatic vertebrobasilar complications: a report of two cases. Surg Neurol 42:245–248

Pretre R, Reverdin A, Kalonji T, Faidutti B (1994) Blunt carotid artery injury: difficult therapeutic approaches for an underrecognized entity. Surgery 115:375–381

Pringle MB, Charig MJ (1994) The use of digital subtraction angiography in penetrating neck injury – a very instructive case. J Laryngol Otol 108:522–524

Rao PM, Ivatury RR, Sharma P, Vinzons AJ, Nassoura Z, Stahl WM (1993) Cervical vascular injuries: a trauma center experience. Surgery 114:527–531

Richter WC (1992) Kopf- und Halsverletzungen: Klinik und Diagnostik. Thieme, Stuttgart

Roebker JJ, Hall LC, Lukin RR (1991) Fractured submandibular gland: CT findings. J Comput Assist Tomogr 15:1068–1069

Roon AT, Christensen N (1979) Evaluation and treatment of penetrating injuries to the neck. J Trauma 19:319–397

Rosman NP, Wu JK, Caplan LR (1992) Cerebellar infarction in the young. Stroke 23:763–766

Rupprecht H, Rumenapf G, Braig H, Flesch R (1994) Acute bleeding caused by rupture of the thyroid gland following blunt neck trauma: case report. J Trauma 36:408–409

Schenk WG III (1992) Neck injuries. In: Moylan JA (ed) Principles of trauma surgery. Gower Medical Publishing, London, pp 15.1–15.15

Sclafani SJ, Cavaliere G, Atweh N, Duncan AO, Scalea T (1991) The role of angiography in penetrating neck trauma. J Trauma 31:557–562

Smoker WRK, Harnsberger HR (1991) Differential diagnosis of head and neck lesions based on their space of origin. 2. The infrahyoid portion of the neck. AJR 157:155–159

Sweeney TA, Marx JA (1993) Blunt neck injury. Emerg Med Clin North Am 11:71–79

Szeremeta W, Morovati SS (1991) Isolated hyoid bone fracture: a case report and review of the literature. J Trauma 31:268–271

Thal ER (1988) Injury to the neck. In: Mattox KL, Moore EE, Feliciano DV (eds) Trauma. Appleton & Lange, Norwalk, Conn., pp 301–313

Weber R, Keerl R, Hendus J, Kahle G (1993) Der Notfall: das traumatische Aneurysma im Kopf-Hals-Bereich. Laryngorhinootologie 72:86–90

5 Chest

M. Galanski and A. Chavan

CONTENTS

5.1 General Considerations

5.1.1 Incidence and Distribution

Ten percent of all accident victims and 60% of patients with multiple traumatic injuries have associated thoracic trauma. The reported frequency of the various injuries to the chest wall, lungs, mediastinum, heart, and great vessels varies considerably and is dependent on the type of patients included in studies. Therefore the cited frequency of thoracic and associated injuries suffices only for orientation (Table 5.1).

M. Galanski, MD, Professor, Direktor der Abteilung Diagnostische Radiologie I der Medizinischen Hochschule Hannover, Konstanty-Gutschow-Straße 8, 30625 Hannover, Germany
A. Chavan, MD, Abteilung Diagnostische Radiologie I der Medizinischen Hochschule Hannover, Konstanty-Gutschow-Straße 8, 30625 Hannover, Germany

5.1.2 Mechanisms of Injury

Seventy-five percent of thoracic injuries occurring in daily life are attributable to traffic accidents; a further 18% result from a fall from a height and 7% are industrial accidents or injuries sustained at work. The number of stab and gunshot wounds is low and can vary regionally depending on social factors and criminality. Combat injuries include a higher percentage of gunshot and blast injuries. Differentiation between nonpenetrating blunt thoracic trauma and penetrating trauma is necessary.

The most common causes of blunt thoracic injury, which accounts for more than 90% of chest trauma in civil life, are direct or indirect forces, such as in the case of acceleration and deceleration injuries.

The severity of a penetrating injury is dependent not only on the localization (depth and involvement of the pulmonary hilum and mediastinum), but also on the kinetic energy. Hence, gunshot injuries, and especially those caused by high-velocity bullets (>500 m/s) are a more severe form of penetrating trauma than stab injuries irrespective of their localization unless vital organs such as the heart and great vessels are involved. Tissue cavitation caused by high-velocity projectiles produces lesions 20–30 times the size of the projectile.

Blast or shock wave injuries constitute a special form of trauma. Although they are rare in civil life, they require special mention on account of the magnitude of damage they may cause. They cause severe contusions and tears at air–tissue interfaces not only in the lungs but also in other air-containing organs such as the stomach and intestines. These may necessitate immediate artificial respiration, albeit at an increased risk of air embolism (Groskin 1992).

5.2 Imaging of Thoracic Trauma

5.2.1 Diagnostic Strategy

The ten important questions to be answered when confronted with chest trauma are listed in Table 5.2

Table 5.1. Frequency of various types of chest trauma and frequency of associated injuries (A = Swiss trauma study with 1500 patients; B = North American major trauma outcome study with 15000 patients). (Modified from LoCicero and Mattox 1989)

	Incidence A	Incidence B
Type of thoracic injury		
Chest wall	54%	45%
Pneumothorax	20%	20%
Hemothorax	21%	25%
Lung	21%	26%
Heart	7%	9%
Aorta and great vessels	4%	4%
Esophagus	7%	0.5%
Diaphragm	7%	7%
Miscellaneous	18%	21%
Associated injuries		
Head	51%	
Extremities	46%	
Spine	11%	
Abdomen	32%	

ultrasonography to assess the pleural and pericardial spaces as well as the heart and abdomen.

Computed tomography (CT) is being increasingly used in cases of thoracic trauma. It is more sensitive in the detection of pneumothorax and in the differentiation of unclear intrathoracic opacities. Suspected mediastinal, vascular, and diaphragmatic injuries are clear indications for CT (Goodman 1982; Heiberg et al. 1983; Kearns and Gay 1990; Smejkal et al. 1991).

Magnetic resonance imaging (MRI) at present plays only a limited role in the emergency management of acute chest trauma not only because it provides no additional information compared to other diagnostic measures, but also because of the practical difficulties in carrying out the examination.

Angiography may be necessary to prove or exclude vascular injury requiring immediate surgery when CT is unable to provide adequate information or is not possible due to shortage of time.

(Gens 1992; Glinz 1981, 1986). The first four points concern the respiratory and circulatory status (ABC = airway, breathing, and circulation). These questions are of vital importance and have to be answered immediately; urgent management without further investigation may be required if the patient's respiratory or circulatory status is critical. Only after taking care of these vital parameters should radiological diagnostic measures be undertaken as shown in the flow chart in Fig. 5.1. Even today the supine chest x-ray is the primary investigation and is indicated in virtually every patient with chest or multiple trauma. Nowadays it is usually supplemented by

Table 5.2. The ten most important questions in cases of blunt thoracic trauma (the main points are highlighted in italics)

1. *Circulatory status: hypovolemia?*
2. *Respiratory status?*
3. *Tension pneumothorax?*
4. *Pericardial tamponade?*
5. Flail chest?
6. Pneumothorax?
   Soft tissue/mediastinal emphysema?
7. Hemothorax?
8. Aortic rupture?
9. Diaphragmatic rupture?
10. Myocardial contusion?

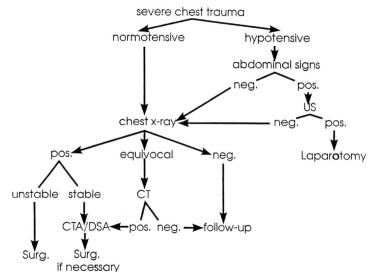

Fig. 5.1. Diagnostic strategy in severe chest trauma

Table 5.3. The most suitable modalities to answer specific clinical questions

Indication	Diagnostic modality
Basic examination	Chest x-ray
	US
Hemothorax	Chest x-ray/US
(therapy-refractory:	
vascular injury?)	DSA
Pneumothorax	Chest x-ray/CT/US
(therapy-refractory:	
tracheobronchial tear?)	Bronchoscopy/spiral-CT
Mediastinal emphysema	
(therapy-refractory:	
tracheobronchial tear?	Bronchoscopy
esophageal rupture?)	Endoscopy/contrast examination
Mediastinal widening	CT
Aortic rupture	CTA/DSA
Diaphragmatic rupture	US/CT/contrast examination

US, Ultrasonography; DSA, digital subtraction angiography; CT, computed tomography; CTA, computed tomography-angiography

Contrast examinations of the esophagus, stomach, and bowel are necessary only in selected cases, e.g., esophageal or diaphragmatic ruptures. Other radiological examinations such as conventional tomography, bronchography, and lymphangiography are not justified nowadays.

The most suited modalities for specific indications are listed in Table 5.3 and the diagnostic spectrum of the various modalities is shown in Table 5.4.

5.2.2 Image Analysis of the Primary Chest Radiograph

While analyzing an emergency chest radiograph, specific attention should be paid to the following points (DUNBAR 1984; MIRVIS and RODRIGUEZ 1992; MOORE et al. 1993):

1. Position of tubes and catheters
2. Pathological lucencies and opacities (see Table 5.5)
3. Widening or shifting of mediastinum
4. Diaphragmatic contour
5. Thoracic skeleton, including the spine
6. Soft tissues

The important findings on a chest radiograph and their possible causes are listed in Table 5.5.

Certain radiological findings reflect specific pathology, e.g., pneumothorax or a pleural effusion. Other features, especially the opacities, may

be less specific and may require further diagnostic workup.

Although the different organs and structures can be injured in a variety of combinations, a topographic classification of the injuries is helpful. Thus one can classify the injuries as those involving the pleural space, the lungs, the tracheobronchial system, the mediastinal organs (heart and great vessels), and the diaphragm.

5.3 Thoracic Wall Injury

5.3.1 Thoracic Skeleton

With respect to anatomy, only the first rib requires special mention. It is susceptible not only to direct trauma but also to indirect traction injury caused by the scalene muscles. Due to its relatively firm attachment to the thoracic spine posteriorly and to the

Table 5.4. Diagnostic spectrum of the various modalities

Diagnostic modality	Indication/utility
Chest x-ray	Basic examination
US	Basic examination
	Pleural effusion/hemothorax
	Heart injury
	Sternal fracture
	Diaphragmatic rupture
Spiral-CT	Clarification of doubtful pathology
	Suspicion of aortic rupture (CTA)
	Suspicion of tracheobronchial tear
DSA	Vascular injury
Esophagogram	Suspected esophageal rupture
	Suspected diaphragmatic rupture
MRI	Spine injury

MRI, Magnetic resonance imaging; other abbreviations as in Table 5.4

Table 5.5. Main radiological findings and their possible etiology

Radiological finding	Possible etiology
Pathological lucencies	Pneumothorax
	Mediastinal/soft tissue emphysema
	Pneumatocele
	Diaphragmatic rupture
Pathological opacities	Contusion, laceration
	Hematoma
	Hemothorax
	Atelectasis
	Diaphragmatic rupture
Mediastinal widening	Hematoma
	Aortic rupture

manubrium and clavicle anteriorly, this rib has limited mobility and a strong contraction of the scalene muscles can easily cause traction injury. The subclavian vein and artery run along the upper surface of the first rib in a bony sulcus anterior and posterior to the scalene tubercle respectively.

5.3.1.1 Rib Fractures

Rib fractures constitute the most common skeletal injury. They may result either from trivial or from severe thoracic trauma. The frequency of rib fractures in blunt thoracic trauma is as high as 50%. Osteoporosis and advanced age are predisposing factors as the ribs gradually lose elasticity beyond the age of 30 years.

Hemothorax, pneumothorax, and subcutaneous emphysema are especially common if multiple rib fractures or markedly dislocated fragments are present (frequency 5%).

The 4th–9th ribs are most frequently affected. The upper three ribs are protected by the shoulder girdle (clavicle, scapula, musculature) and fractures affecting these ribs generally indicate a severe trauma. For this reason, as well as because of the close proximity to the brachial vessels and plexus, fractures involving the thoracic inlet are often accompanied by vascular or plexus injuries. Fractures of the 10th–12th ribs are often associated with injury to the upper abdominal and retroperitoneal organs (liver, spleen, kidneys).

Although fractures can affect any part of the rib, the middle and dorsal third are most frequently affected. Multiple fractures generally occur in a row (Fig. 5.2a; see also Fig. 5.5). Depending on the number of fractures, one can differentiate between isolated fractures, serial fractures (fractures involving more than two ribs), and fragmented fractures.

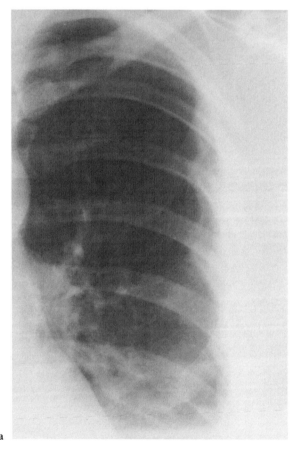

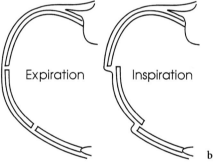

Fig. 5.2. a Multiple serial rib fractures. **b** Schematic diagram of paradoxical movement of a portion of the chest wall in flail chest

5.3.1.1.1 Radiological Projections. The standard roentgenograms include an anteroposterior (a.p.) and an oblique projection of the affected hemithorax, supplemented if necessary by an upper abdomen x-ray for the lower ribs. Additional projections increase the rate of detection of rib fractures. The chest x-ray is not optimally suited for the detection of all rib fractures. Due to the foreshortening and overlapping of the ribs along the lateral thoracic wall and the overlapping of the lower ribs by abdominal structures, fractures in these regions may be easily overlooked. As a rule not more than 70% of rib fractures are detected with standard chest roentgenograms.

As in many cases the detection of fractures has no therapeutic consequences, in patients with severe thoracic trauma the supine chest x-ray is adequate as the basic projection for detecting fractures and possible complications; for this reason an exhaustive roentgenological workup is not necessary.

5.3.1.1.2 Radiological Signs. In the presence of direct radiological fracture signs, detection of fractures poses no great difficulty (Fig. 5.2a). The signs are a break in cortical continuity which can be recognized best along the upper border of the rib, displacement of the fragments, and a fracture line which may be seen as a line of lucency or increased density (overlapping fragments) that often runs vertically or obliquely. Without dislocation, the detection of rib fractures may be difficult.

Indirect radiological signs of rib fractures are a spindle-shaped soft tissue density along the course of the rib (fracture hematoma), hemothorax or pneumothorax, and the presence of thoracic wall emphysema (which almost always suggests a rib fracture).

Apart from detection of the actual fracture, one can also encounter typical associated injuries which may be of grave clinical significance.

Fractures of the first three ribs may be associated with cardiac contusion, aortic rupture, and injury to the tracheobronchial system. Multiple rib fractures often cause complications such as hemothorax or pneumothorax. In up to 30% of patients with blunt thoracic injury, multiple rib fractures are bilateral. Respiratory insufficiency may result from paradoxical movement of a portion of the chest wall in patients with unstable fragmented fractures (flail chest), especially when the fractured fragment of the chest wall lies ventrally or laterally (Fig. 5.2b). Dorsal fragmented fractures are relatively stable due to the strong back musculature and hence do not necessarily denote an unstable chest. Serial rib fractures combined with invisible fractures at the costochondral or costosternal articulations also may cause a flail chest. Fractures of the lower ribs are often associated with injuries to the upper abdominal organs (spleen, liver) and kidneys. Fractures of the first rib associated with delayed development of an extrapleural hematoma should arouse suspicion of subclavian artery injury. This is caused by repeated irritation of the artery by the fracture fragments during respiration.

5.3.1.2 Sternal Fractures

Unlike rib fractures, sternal fractures are rare. They constitute less than 3% of fractures seen in the thoracic skeleton and not more than 0.5% of all fractures. They are almost always a consequence of direct trauma to the sternum, usually caused by direct impact of the steering wheel. The manubriosternal synchondrosis and the upper portion of the sternum are the most frequently injured sites.

The majority of sternal fractures are transverse fractures which, on conventional radiography, are normally recognizable only on the lateral projection. Since dislocation of the fragments does not occur often, a presternal soft tissue swelling or retrosternal opacity due to the fracture hematoma may be the only signs pointing towards the fracture. Especially in an emergency situation, in equivocal cases ultrasonography takes precedence over the time-consuming CT or conventional tomography for the diagnosis of sternal fractures (Fig. 5.3). Special attention should be paid to cardiac contusion in these patients. Sternal fractures associated with a widening of the mediastinum are strongly suggestive of injury to the aorta or the supra-aortic vessels (HARLEY and MENA 1986).

5.3.1.3 Injuries to the Sternoclavicular Joint

Injuries to the sternoclavicular joint are also rare. Ventral subluxation is the most common and does not cause any complications. Dorsal dislocations, in contrast, may cause compression of the trachea, esophagus, or supra-aortic vessels.

Conventional x-rays are inadequate for diagnosis. If such injuries are suspected clinically, one should proceed directly to ultrasonography or CT.

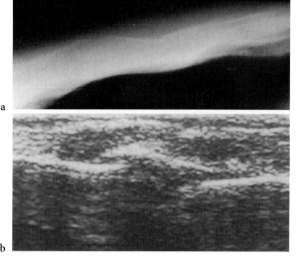

Fig. 5.3a,b. Sternal fracture. a Conventional roentgenogram. b Ultrasonography: note the break in continuity of the cortical echoes. The hypoechoic zone seen anterior to the fracture is a fracture hematoma

5.3.1.4 Thoracic Spine Injuries

Injuries to the thoracic spine may often go undiscovered on the routine preliminary chest x-ray (especially in unconscious patients) unless there is a significant dislocation or obvious neurological deficit. Radiological signs which may suggest a spinal injury include disalignment of the vertebral column, widening of the interpedicular distance, and displacement of the paravertebral line (Fig. 5.4). Caution should be exercised in diagnosing vertebral injury on the basis of displacement of the paravertebral line alone as atelectasis of the lower lobes or aortic rupture may give a similar appearance (WOODRING et al. 1988).

5.3.1.5 Soft Tissue Emphysema

Open injuries or injuries of both layers of the pleura with pneumothorax may be associated with soft tissue emphysema. As a rule, thoracic wall emphysema occurs in association with rib fractures. In most cases it is a trivial trauma. Only massive, rapidly progressive, therapy-resistant soft tissue emphysema requires special attention as a bronchopleural fistula may be the underlying cause. Soft tissue emphysema caused by a tracheostomy is usually seen in the cervical and supraclavicular region only.

5.3.2 Pleura and Pleural Space

Pleural injuries almost invariably occur in cases of perforating thoracic injuries, but they are also frequently associated with blunt thoracic trauma. Hemothorax, pneumothorax, and subcutaneous emphysema are particularly common in patients with multiple rib fractures, especially when fragments are dislocated.

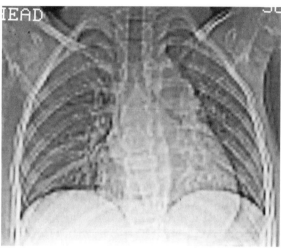

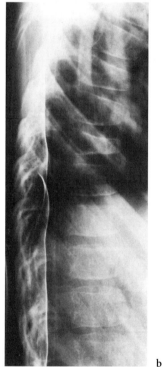

Fig. 5.4a,b. Fracture of the eighth thoracic vertebra with an associated hematoma causing displacement of the paravertebral line as seen on the digital CT scanogram (a). b The fractured vertebra as seen on the conventional lateral radiogram of the thoracic spine

5.3.2.1 Pneumothorax

Among patients requiring hospitalization, pneumothorax occurs in 15%–38% of those with blunt thoracic trauma and in less than 20% of those with
penetrating trauma (CONN et al. 1963; GROSKIN
1992). The reported incidence strongly depends on
the assessed patient population and the type of diagnostic modality used.

A small pneumothorax in a patient with pulmonary lesions compromising pulmonary function
may have greater importance than in an otherwise healthy lung (GROSKIN 1992). It is important
to bear in mind that a 1-cm-wide circular
pneumothorax reduces the lung volume by about
50%; a 5-cm-wide pneumothorax reduces it by about
80%–90%.

5.3.2.1.1 Radiological Examination. Whereas a large
pneumothorax can be detected on a chest x-ray without difficulty, small pneumothoraces may be easily
overlooked, especially on the supine chest film, due
to their ventral location. Such a location means that
the typical findings, such as the pleural line and the
loss of vascular markings, cannot be appreciated on
the aforementioned projection. Tangential oblique
projections of the injured side may be helpful and are
superior to lateral chest radiographs because the
overlapping of the contralateral side as well as of the
mediastinum can be avoided. Lateral decubitus films
are equally diagnostic but require positioning of
the patient with the risk of causing additional
injury.

Ultrasonography can aid in the detection of
pneumothorax as the movement of the parietal
versus visceral pleura is no longer visible and, hence,
the pleural interface is seen as a static line
(WERNECKE et al. 1987). Subcutaneous emphysema,
however, markedly reduces the diagnostic value of
ultrasonography.

Computed tomography is the best-suited modality for detecting small and ventrally or atypically
located pneumothoraces. Hence, the incidence of
pneumothorax detected by CT is higher. Thirty percent of the pneumothoraces detected by CT are not
seen on the supine chest radiograph (BROOKS and
OLSON 1989). However, the therapeutic relevance of
these small pneumothoraces is still controversial.

5.3.2.1.2 Radiological Findings. The following fea-
tures on a chest radiograph suggest a ventral
pneumothorax (Fig. 5.5) (GALANSKI et al. 1981;
MOSKOWITZ and GRISCOM 1976):

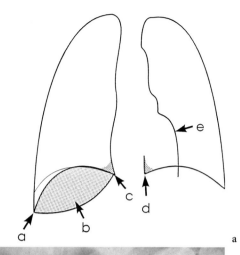

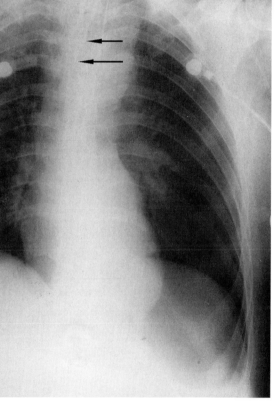

Fig. 5.5. **a** Ventrally located pneumothorax: radiological signs
on the supine chest x-ray. *a*, Deep lateral recess; *b*, increased
transparency of the diaphragmatic dome; *c*, sharply delineated
and accentuated angle between the diaphragmatic dome and
the cardiac border; *d*, sharply delineated diaphragmatic contour extending up to the vertebral column; *e*, unusually sharp
border of the mediastinum. **b** Ventrally located tension
pneumothorax. The pleural line is barely recognizable. Note
the increased transparency in the left lower zone, the sharp
border of the mediastinum and the left diaphragm, and the
unusually deep lateral recess. The tension component of the
pneumothorax is suggested by the displacement of the mediastinum, including the trachial tube, to the right. A ventrally
and medially located pneumothorax is present on the right
side, as is also recognizable from the sharply delineated diaphragmatic contour extending up to the vertebral column

1. Deep and sharply delineated costophrenic angle (deep sulcus sign)
2. Increased transparency of the upper abdominal region due to the overlapping air-filled pleural recess (basilar hyperlucency)
3. Unusually sharp definition of the cardiac and mediastinal borders, and in particular of the right cardiophrenic angle and the cardiac apex depending on the affected side
4. Sharp delineation of the diaphragm extending right up to the vertebral column

The clinically relevant pneumothorax is normally recognizable with the help of these signs on the supine chest radiograph.

Radiological signs of a tension pneumothorax are:

1. Shifting of the mediastinal organs to the contralateral side
2. Depression and flattening of the ipsilateral diaphragm
3. Compression atelectasis of the lung

Note that the last-mentioned sign may be completely absent if there is an accompanying lung contusion which prevents the collapse of the affected parts of

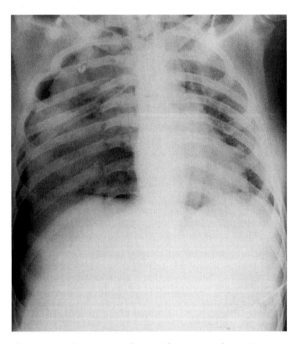

Fig. 5.6. Tension pneumothorax. The pneumothorax is recognizable from the lateral transparency associated with a deep lateral sulcus and increased translucency in the region of the right diaphragmatic dome. Only the shift of the mediastinum suggests the tension component. The normally associated collapse of the underlying lung is not seen due to the "stiff lung" resulting from intrapulmonary hemorrhage (lung contusion). Serial rib fractures are also seen

the lung (so-called stiff lung). In such cases one should not underestimate the magnitude of the tension pneumothorax despite the absence of lung collapse (Fig. 5.6).

One should, however, be aware of certain pitfalls. Lines caused by skin folds may mimic a pneumothorax on a supine film. Massive soft tissue emphysema may render the diagnosis of pneumothorax extremely difficult. Therapy-resistant pneumothorax should arouse suspicion of bronchial injury.

5.3.2.2 Hemothorax

Hemothorax may be observed in 25%–50% of patients with blunt chest injury and in 60%–80% of those with penetrating injury (Conn et al. 1963; Graham et al. 1979). The source of bleeding is generally the systemic vessels such as the intercostal vessels and vessels supplying the thoracic wall or diaphragm. Pulmonary vessels and the bronchial arteries are rarely injured.

5.3.2.2.1 Radiological Examination. Ultrasonography and CT are the best methods for detecting and quantifying small amounts of pleural fluid or blood. X-ray images are less sensitive. Pleural effusions are recognizable on the erect chest radiograph only when they exceed 200 ml. Reliable detection on the supine chest x-ray requires quantities of at least 500 ml (Mirvis and Rodriguez 1992).

5.3.2.2.2 Radiological Findings. On erect chest radiographs, pleural effusions are seen as haziness or obliteration of the pulmonary vascular markings in the posterior recess, as blunting of the costophrenic angle, as semilunar opacities ascending along the lateral chest wall, or (with increasing amounts) as opacification of the entire hemithorax associated with a broad opaque band around the compressed lung. Subpulmonary effusions may appear as pseudoelevation of the diaphragm.

Detection of a hemothorax on the supine chest radiograph is more difficult. Unless the hemothorax is massive, causing shifting of the mediastinum and compression of the lung, the only hints may be reduced transparency of the affected hemithorax with preservation of pulmonary vascular markings and/or ill-defined diaphragmatic contours.

It should be noted that in cases of massive therapy-resistant hemothorax, one must consider the possibility of arterial bleeding originating from the intercostal, internal mammary, or phrenic arter-

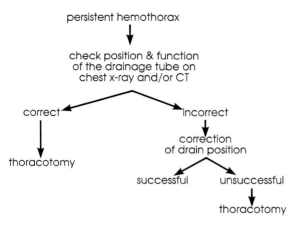

persistent hemothorax

check position & function
of the drainage tube on
chest x-ray and/or CT

correct   incorrect

thoracotomy

correction
of drain position

successful   unsuccessful

thoracotomy

Fig. 5.7. Diagnostic strategy in persistent hemothorax

ies, or even from aortic injury. A stepwise diagnostic strategy in cases of persistent hemothorax is suggested in the flow chart shown in Fig. 5.7.

5.3.2.3 Chylothorax

Chylothorax is an extremely rare complication of thoracic trauma. Apart from direct penetrating injury, hyperextension of the thoracolumbar spine may lead to tears of the thoracic duct with subsequent chylothorax.

If the thoracic duct is injured below the fifth thoracic vertebra, the chylothorax is encountered more frequently on the right side; rupture of the thoracic duct above this level is often associated with a chylothorax on the left. Chylothorax may also occur bilaterally. In hyperextension injuries, the thoracic duct is typically damaged at the level of the diaphragmatic hiatus (FRASER et al. 1991).

With imaging modalities, it is impossible to differentiate between chylothorax and other pleural effusions except bleeding. Chylothorax normally manifests 3–7 days after the thoracic trauma; thus, unexplained effusions developing a few days after trauma could represent chylothorax.

5.4 Parenchymal Lung Injuries

Radiologically visible parenchymal lesions are either a direct consequence of trauma or may be seen later due to secondary complications such as pneumonia, adult respiratory distress syndrome (ARDS), or atelectasis.

5.4.1 Pulmonary Contusion and Laceration

5.4.1.1 Patterns of Injury

Usually the radiologist and the surgeon (as opposed to the pathologist) differentiate between lung contusion and lung laceration (WAGNER et al. 1988). Lung contusion may be defined as multiple microscopic tears in the pulmonary tissue. The morphological equivalent is a serosanguineous exudation into the parenchyma, which in the majority of cases is of little clinical relevance (Table 5.6) and which rarely leads to complications.

Lung laceration can be regarded as a macroscopic tear in the lung parenchyma often associated with rupturing of the visceral pleura. Hematoma and pneumatocele caused by injury to small blood vessels or bronchioles represent special forms of lung laceration.

Blast injuries constitute a special form of lung contusion as they cause diffuse alveolar and capillary rupture with development of bronchovenous and alveolovenous fistulas often leading to air embolism. Due to the extensive and diffuse nature of the injury they rapidly progress to respiratory failure.

Lung contusions and lacerations are the most common traumatic lesions, occurring in 30%–60% of patients with blunt thoracic trauma. Traumatic lung herniation entails prolapse of the lung into a space lined by parietal pleura. Only rarely does it occur as a direct consequence of a trauma; more commonly it is iatrogenic, following a rib resection.

5.4.1.2 Radiological Features

Pulmonary contusions, lacerations, hematomas, and pneumatoceles all may have characteristic radiologi-

Table 5.6. Patterns of parenchymal pulmonary lesions and their clinical relevance

Type of injury	Clinical relevance
Lung contusion	Variable
Without respiratory depression	Generally not of relevance
With respiratory depression	Assisted ventilation (PEEP)
Lung laceration	Usually not of relevance except when centrally located
Pulmonary hematoma	Of no clinical relevance
Pneumatocele	Of no clinical relevance
Blast injury	Severe injury requiring assisted ventilation

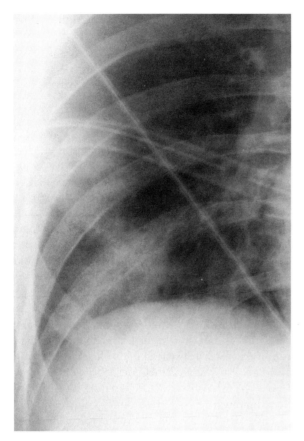

Fig. 5.8. Lung contusion: typical finding in lung contusion characterized by ill-defined scattered opacities located subpleurally

cal features. Often they are of little clinical relevance and it is important not to overestimate or misinterpret them, thus triggering unnecessary investigations.

Lung contusions manifest as ill-defined opacities which have a typical localization and pattern of progression and/or regression. The opacities are always close to the chest wall at the point where the trauma has occurred; they are generally clearly recognizable on the first radiograph as the development of such contusions takes just a few hours (Fig. 5.8). In uncomplicated cases complete regression may require 3–10 days depending on the extent of the lesion. Persistence or progression suggests more severe lung injury or complications such as aspiration or secondary infection.

Pulmonary lacerations are seen as dense and more extensive, often inhomogeneous opacities (Fig. 5.9). Spherical or oval shadows with relatively sharp boundaries represent hematomas and lucent areas with or without air–fluid levels represent pneumatoceles or so-called traumatic pseudocysts.

As with contusions, lacerations are usually located close to the chest wall in the region of maximum impact or near the opposing chest wall as a contrecoup effect (MANSON et al. 1993). Hematomas and pneumatoceles are initially often masked by surrounding contusions and may become clearly visible only after the latter regress. While the resolution of a hematoma may take weeks to months, traumatic pulmonary pseudocysts resolve within 1–3 weeks.

Unlike in blunt trauma, in *perforating injuries* hematomas and lacerations are small, well circumscribed, and restricted to the vicinity of the tract

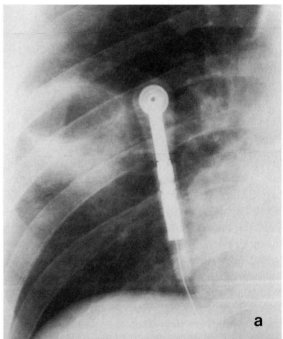

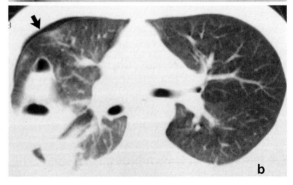

Fig. 5.9a,b. Lung lacerations often produce well-defined and dense shadows representing hematomas. Pneumatoceles are seen as well-defined circular or oval zones of transparency (**a**). Complex injuries are better evaluated with CT (**b**); note the small ventrally located pneumothorax in **b** which was not seen on the conventional chest radiograph (*arrow*)

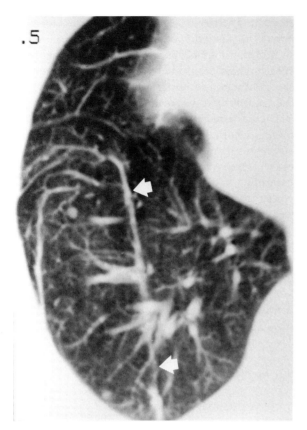

Fig. 5.10. Linear pulmonary scar resulting from an old gunshot injury (*arrows*)

caused by the penetrating object (Fig. 5.10). Whereas hemothorax is common, pneumothorax is often prevented by the blood tamponading the tear in the visceral pleura (GRAHAM et al. 1979).

Blast injuries may produce a radiological picture similar to that of pulmonary edema. As perforation of the gas-containing hollow viscera frequently occurs in association with blast injuries, appropriate radiological examination of the abdomen is always indicated (Fig. 5.11).

It is to be noted that pulmonary lesions resulting directly from trauma are almost always visible on the initial chest radiograph. Changes occurring later are therefore strongly suggestive of secondary complications. Clear-cut differentiation between a hematoma and a pneumatocele containing blood is not possible and also not necessary since they both result from a tear in the lung and have no great therapeutic consequences.

Computed tomography may be helpful in clarifying extensive but unclear findings seen on the chest radiograph (see, for example, Fig. 5.8). It is also more sensitive in the detection of discrete findings, but is

not indicated in such cases as the findings are not of great clinical significance. According to the literature, pulmonary lesions are detected thrice as often with CT as with standard supine chest radiography (FRASER et al. 1991; KEARNS and GAY 1990; SMEJKAL et al. 1991; WAGNER et al. 1988).

5.4.2 Pulmonary Complications Resulting from Trauma

If the initial posttraumatic changes do not regress as expected or if new radiological features develop that were not present initially, one should consider the possibility of secondary complications. These include pneumonia (including aspiration pneumonia), atelectasis, and ARDS.

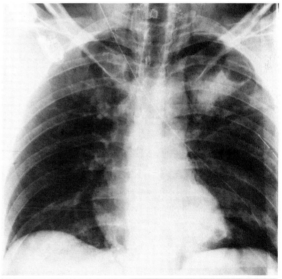

a

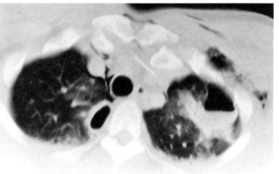

b

Fig. 5.11a,b. Blast injury. **a** Chest radiograph of a professional diver who suffered multiple pulmonary lacerations associated with intrapulmonary hematomas resulting from an underwater explosion. **b** The CT section shows the pneumatoceles on both sides as well as the presence of air in the mediastinum and the thoracic wall

Posttraumatic atelectasis generally results from luminal obstruction by mucous plugs or blood clots. A rare but important primary cause is tracheobronchial laceration. Inhomogeneous, sharply delineated opacities, loss of vascular markings, and signs of loss of volume (mediastinal shift to the ipsilateral side, raised dome of the diaphragm) are suggestive of atelectasis.

It should be noted that in patients with extensive basal opacities suggesting atelectasis or subpulmonary hematoma, thoracic drains are contraindicated prior to exclusion of diaphragmatic rupture. Therapy-resistant atelectasis should alert one to the possibility of bronchial injury.

Bronchopulmonary infections are difficult or even impossible to differentiate from traumatic lesions without appropriate clinical information and the availability of serial chest radiographs.

Other than direct parenchymal damage due to the trauma, aspiration, reexpansion edema, infection, and hypovolemic shock are all causes of ARDS. The basic pathology is an increase in capillary permeability leading first to interstitial edema followed by alveolar edema. Apart from clinical findings, the well-known leading features in the diagnosis of ARDS are the generalized bilateral opacities without associated effusions (Fig. 5.12).

A rare and difficult differential diagnosis in cases of secondary pulmonary lesions is fat embolism. Such embolisms may manifest radiologically as ill-defined disseminated nodular opacities 24–48 h after the embolic episode.

5.5 Mediastinal Injury

5.5.1 Mediastinal Emphysema

Mediastinal emphysema not infrequently follows chest trauma and most often results from pulmonary barotrauma. The air escapes from the alveoli into the interstitial space and from there via the pulmonary hilum into the mediastinum. This type of mediastinal emphysema often has no clinical relevance. Other possible causes include tracheobronchial injury, esophageal injury, retroperitoneal emphysema from duodenal or colonic perforation, cervical emphysema caused by tracheostomy, and perforating injuries including iatrogenic injuries.

The typical radiological findings on the a.p. film are the sharply demarcated mediastinal pleural lines, the sharp contour of the descending aorta up to the diaphragm, the sharp delineation of the aortopulmonary window, and visualization of the diaphragm in its entire course up to the vertebral column (continuous diaphragm sign). On the lateral radiograph, retrosternal air and linear lucencies in the middle mediastinum paralleling the trachea and esophagus suggest mediastinal emphysema. Subcutaneous emphysema is frequently an associated finding. Esophageal injury has to be ruled out in all patients with mediastinal emphysema or a penetrating injury to the posterior mediastinum.

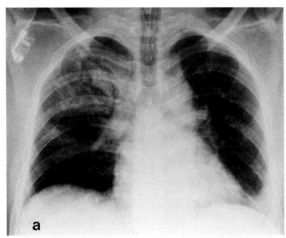

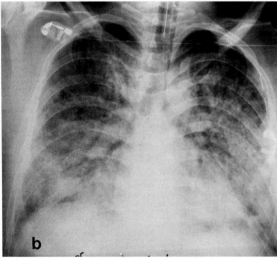

Fig. 5.12a,b. ARDS following chest trauma. **a** The initial chest radiograph shows irregular opacities in the right upper lobe caused by pulmonary contusion. **b** A repeat chest radiograph after a few days reveals extensive inhomogeneous opacities scattered over both lungs which are certainly not a primary consequence of the trauma, but suggest a seconary complication such as ARDS. Pulmonary contusions practically never progress and normally decrease rapidly with the passage of time, as seen in this case

5.5.2 Injuries of the Aorta and the Supra-aortic Vessels

About 1%–2% of patients with severe thoracic trauma suffer from an aortic injury. Only 10%–20% of these survive and in two-thirds of them the adventitia is not torn. It has been reported that in the absence of treatment, a further 50% of these patients die within the first 24 h and up to 75% within 3 weeks following trauma (PARMLEY et al. 1958b; STARK 1990); however, these figures are probably too high as they are based on autopsy material and do not take into consideration survivors with undetected lesions (FECZKO et al. 1992).

5.5.2.1 Mechanism of Injury

Perforating injuries most commonly affect the ascending aorta and the supra-aortic vessels and are generally fatal. Even perforations smaller than 1 cm are lethal. Severe compression trauma and accleration/deceleration injuries are the primary causes of aortic rupture in patients with blunt chest trauma. Horizontal acceleration forces may result in lesions of the descending aorta whereas vertical forces (fall from a height) may cause injury to the ascending aorta and the supra-aortic vessels.

5.5.2.2 Localization

Up to 90% of patients with aortic ruptures who survive the acute event have diagonal tears at the insertion of the ligamentum arteriosum. The incidence of rupture of the ascending aorta in clinical practice is very low since these lesions are almost invariably lethal and patients do not reach the hospital alive. As a result there is a discrepancy between the quoted incidence in clinical practice and in autopsy studies (FECZKO et al. 1992).

5.5.2.3 Clinical Features

Apart from hemodynamic shock, differences in the measured blood pressure between the two arms or hypertension in the upper extremities combined with hypotension in the lower extremities may be observed. Massive swelling of the lower neck or stridor may be present. Conscious patients may complain of pain which may be retrosternal or radiating to the back, hoarseness, dyspnea, and dysphagia. The indirect signs include a massive hemothorax, Horner's syndrome, oliguria, and paraplegia.

5.5.2.4 Radiological Features

The various radiological findings are listed in Table 5.7 in descending order of frequency and importance and are illustrated in Fig. 5.13.

The majority of the plain film findings are a consequence of the mediastinal hematoma (Figs. 5.14–5.16). Mediastinal hematoma is, however, non-specific because it is most often caused by rupture of

Table 5.7. Radiological findings in aortic rupture (STARK 1990) (findings shown in italics are those most suggestive of aortic rupture)

Radiological finding	Incidence
Widening of the mediastinum >8 cm	70%
Displacement of the tracheal/gastric tube to the right	63%/50%
Caudal displacement of the left main bronchus	40%
Obliteration of the aortic arch or descending aorta or opacity in the region of the aortopulmonary window	55%/67%
Obliteration of the left upper lobe margin (apical cap)	65%
Reduction of the carinal angle	65%
Widening of the right paratracheal stripe	53%
Displacement of the right or left paravertebral lines	33%/35%
A left-sided hemothorax	35%
Fracture of the first rib	16%

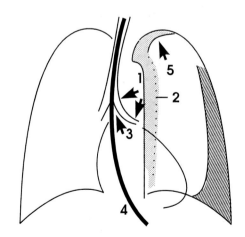

Fig. 5.13. Radiological signs in aortic rupture: *1*, displacement of the trachea to the right and of the left main bronchus caudally; *2*, blurring of the contour of the aortic knob and the descending aorta due to para-aortic hematoma (*dotted area*); *3*, displacement of the carina to the right with reduction of the carinal angle; *4*, displacement of the nasogastric tube to the right; *5*, apical cap; *hatched area*, hemothorax

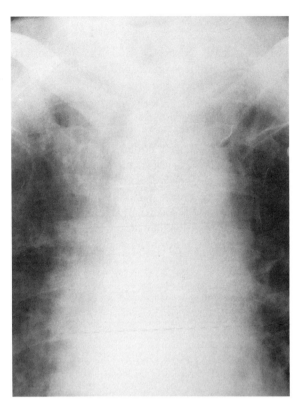

Fig. 5.14. Chest film in a patient with mediastinal hematoma. Note the widening of the superior mediastinum and tracheal displacement to the right, suggesting possible injury to the aorta or supra-aortic arteries

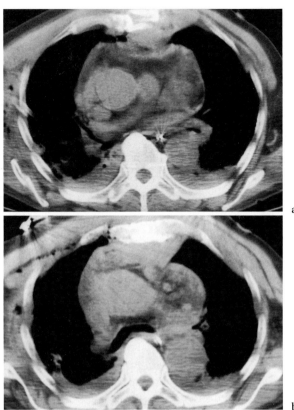

a

b

Fig. 5.15a,b. CT scans in a patient with mediastinal hematoma. Note the diffuse increase in density of the mediastinal fatty tissue. Hematomas are seen in the retrosternal (associated sternal fracture) and right para-aortic regions as well as in the region of the aortopulmonary window

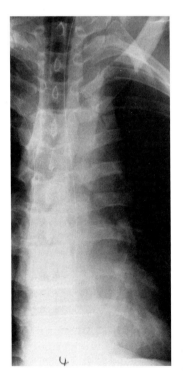

Fig. 5.16. A case of aortic rupture showing displacement of the paravertebral line continuing cranially as the so-called apical cap sign

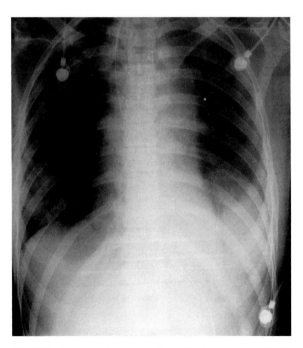

Fig. 5.17. Aortic rupture: note the widening of the mediastinum, displacement of the nasogastric tube to the right, blurring of the aortic contours, and the left hemothorax

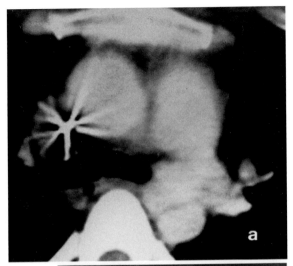

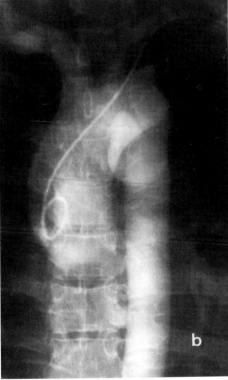

Fig. 5.18a,b. Traumatic aortic aneurysm in the typical location. **a** CT scan showing the aneurysm lateral to the left main bronchus with a flap of the aortic wall recognizable as a lucent line between the aneurysm and the aortic lumen. **b** Angiogram confirming the CT finding

small mediastinal vessels (MARNOCHA et al. 1984). Aortic rupture is often subadventitial and hematoma may result from seepage of blood through this tear into the mediastinum. Of the radiological features listed in Table 5.7, the features shown in italics are those most suggestive of aortic rupture since they

indicate massive hematoma under pressure (Fig. 5.17). Mediastinal widening, which is the most frequent finding, is not dependable for the diagnosis of aortic rupture as it may often be due to technical factors such as inadequate film focus distance or insufficient inspiration. It may also be a consequence of spine fractures (DENNIS and ROGERS 1989).

In centers with adequate experience with spiral CT, CT-angiography is the modality of choice for detecting aortic injury (Figs. 5.18, 5.19). Under these circumstances, angiography is necessary only in cases with equivocal CT findings or in highly unstable cases where the modality with the maximum probability of detecting the lesion has to be resorted to immediately (MORGAN et al. 1992; PAIS 1992; RAPTOPOULOS et al. 1992). Angiographically, however, a "ductus bump," a ductus diverticulum, or ulcerated plaques may all present differential diagnostic problems. If spiral CT is not available, angiography is still the modality of choice to clarify questions regarding aortic rupture.

Computed tomographic signs of aortic injury are a pseudoaneurysm, a periaortic or intramural hematoma, an intimal flap, a definitive dissection, or a localized irregularity of the aortic wall (RICHARDSON et al. 1991).

5.5.2.5 Diagnostic Strategy

Although the chest radiograph is not very specific, it is still the primary imaging modality. A negative chest radiograph practically excludes an aortic rupture as the quoted negative predictive value is about 0.98 (MIRVIS et al. 1987). In patients with suspected aortic rupture the diagnostic strategy illustrated in the flow chart in Fig. 5.20 may be useful.

5.5.3 Trauma to the Heart and Pericardium

The incidence of cardiac injuries in blunt chest trauma is about 5% (HEALEY et al. 1990). The spectrum of cardiac lesions is exceptionally wide. The most common mechanism of blunt injury to the heart is injury caused by the steering wheel. Less frequent are penetrating injuries, acceleration and deceleration trauma, and an acute intense increase in intrathoracic pressure.

Due to their anatomical location, the right ventricle, the left anterior descending coronary artery, and the left-sided cardiac valves are at maximum risk. One in 1000 patients with blunt thoracic injury

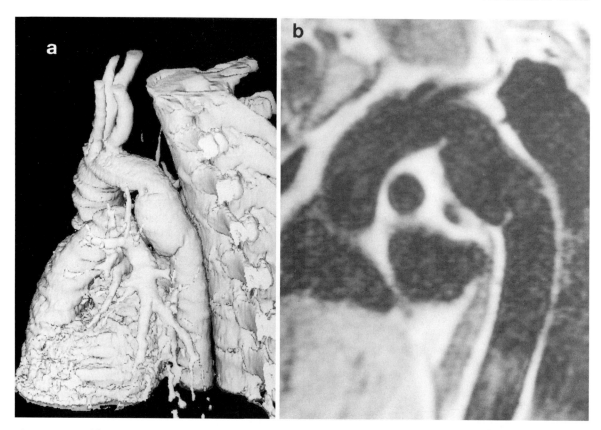

Fig. 5.19. Typical location of a traumatic aortic pseudoaneurysm demonstrated by 3D spiral-CT-angiography (**a**) and MRI (**b**)

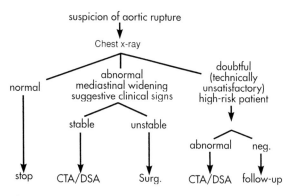

Fig. 5.20. Diagnostic strategy in suspected aortic rupture

has a pericardial rupture, which is typically located in the pleuropericardial region on the left (64%); other sites include diaphragmatic (18%), right pleuropericardial (9%), and the pericardial reflections in the superior mediastinum (9%) (PARMLEY et al. 1958a). Patients with penetrating injuries to the heart rarely survive unless the injury is very small or is followed by pericardial tamponade.

5.5.3.1 Clinical Features

Depending on the severity of trauma, chest pain, respiratory distress, cardiac arrhythmias, obstruction to venous return, hypotension, or cardiogenic shock may be the predominant feature.

5.5.3.2 Diagnosis

The primary diagnostic procedures in evaluating the cardiac status are echocardiography and electrocardiography (ECG). Hypokinesia or dyskinesia of the right ventricular wall on echocardiography suggests a cardiac contusion. ECG often shows arrhythmias, bundle block, and ST segment elevation with flattening of the T wave. Unlike with a cardiac infarct, the changes are seen after 24–48 h and start regressing after a few days (HAUF and LÖNNE 1989).

Laboratory tests have a low specificity because associated injuries to the liver and the musculoskeletal system often influence the enzyme levels.

5.5.3.3 Radiology

As the chest radiograph is often negative, it is of limited importance. Massive pericardial effusion or bleeding causes widening of the cardiac silhouette but smaller lesions cannot be detected on the chest radiograph. Sometimes, an elevation of the epicardial fat layer may suggest the presence of pericardial fluid. Pericardial hematomas and/or effusions can be detected equally well by CT and ultrasonography. The indirect signs of venous congestion are a widening of the inferior vena cava, the renal veins, and the hepatic veins, associated with periportal hypodensity in the liver.

A thin translucent line along the cardiac contour extending up to but not beyond the pericardial reflection at the root of the great vessels is suggestive of pneumopericardium. Unlike in cases of pneumomediastinum, in pneumopericardium the radiolucent line changes its location with alterations in patient position. In tension pneumopericardium, the so-called small heart sign is seen.

In patients with sternal fractures or parasternal rib fractures, one should always consider the possibility of a cardiac contusion. A pneumopericardium need not always be a direct consequence of the trauma; rather it may result from pulmonary barotrauma.

5.5.4 Tracheobronchial Rupture

Tracheobronchial injuries are rare (incidence 1.5% of all cases of blunt thoracic trauma). They generally occur as a consequence of sever direct or indirect thoracic trauma.

The exact mechanism of injury is still a matter of controversy. The postulated hypotheses include severe compression, e.g., due to steering wheel injuries or injuries sustained when driven over by vehicles, thoracic compression occurring in a phase of inspiration with a closed glottis (intraluminal rise in pressure), and strong shear forces resulting from acceleration or deceleration injuries.

The typical localization (80%–90%) is the first 2.5 cm of the main bronchus or the trachea in the vicinity of the carina. The rupture is generally unilateral, more frequently on the right.

5.5.4.1 Radiological Features

Radiological features are generally nonspecific (Fig. 5.21). The indirect signs are listed in Table 5.8. The most common but nonspecific signs are therapy-resistant pneumothorax and atelectasis. Specific signs such as bayonetting of the bronchial outlines or the "falling lung sign" requiring a nearly complete tear of the bronchus are extremely rare.

Tracheobronchial injuries are often masked in the early phases and may be overlooked at initial presentation. This is unfortunate as the delay may lead to lasting damage. In 10% of cases, there are no suspicious radiological findings. Hemoptysis is a suggestive clinical sign. Bronchoscopy should always be carried out in cases with clinical or radiological suspicion of tracheobronchial injury, particularly in the presence of therapy-resistant pneumothorax or atelectasis. Bronchoscopy is still the modality of choice for diagnosing tracheobronchial injury, though spiral CT may become the primary diagnostic modality in the future.

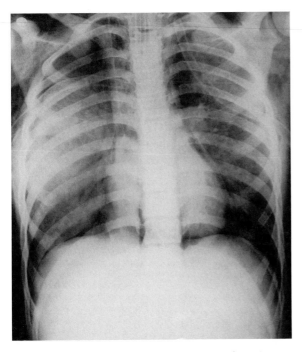

Fig. 5.21. Tracheobronchial tear. The presence of massive mediastinal emphysema, subcutaneous emphysema, and bilateral pneumothorax despite thoracic drains is strongly suggestive of tracheobronchial injury

5.5.4.2 Diagnostic Strategy

The flow chart in Fig. 5.22 shows suitable steps to be followed in patients with persistent and

Table 5.8. Radiological signs suggesting tracheobronchial injury

Therapy-resistant/progressive pneumothorax (60%)
Mediastinal/subcutaneous emphysema (90%)
Lucent bands running parallel to the bronchi (interstitial emphysema)
Therapy-resistant/progressive/massive atelectasis
Misalignment of the bronchial wall outline
Falling lung sign
Associated fractures of the first three ribs

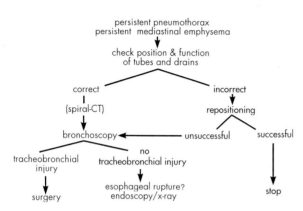

Fig. 5.22. Diagnostic strategy in persistent pneumothorax and/or pneumomediastinum

therapy-resistant penumothorax or mediastinal emphysema. This may help rule out or establish the diagnosis of tracheobronchial injury or esophageal rupture.

5.5.5 Esophageal Injuries

Esophageal injuries may result from perforating injuries, including iatrogenic lesions; they are exceptionally rare with blunt thoracic trauma. They are most often seen as a consequence of profuse and repeated vomiting.

Persistent mediastinal or cervical emphysema (60%) and left-sided pleural effusion are the most common radiological features of esophageal injuries. Widening of the mediastinum and unsharp mediastinal contours are less specific; they are often secondary changes and are an expression of mediastinitis. Esophageal injury should be considered in every patient with unexplained mediastinal emphysema. Diagnosis can be made with the help of an esophagogram using water-soluble nonionic contrast medium or endoscopy; the sensitivity of each is about 90%.

5.6 Diaphragmatic Injury

Diaphragmatic injuries are more common with blunt abdominal injuries (3%–5%) than with blunt chest trauma (1%). Indirect lateral forces resulting from traffic injuries are the predominant mechanism of injury.

Seventy-five percent of diaphragmatic injuries and 95% of transdiaphragmatic organ herniations are on the left side. The tears are mostly radial, often affecting the central tendon or the zone between the tendinous and the muscular part, especially in blunt abdominal injuries. In thoracic trauma, peripheral diaphragmatic tears may also be observed. The organs which herniate most commonly are, in descending order of frequency: the stomach, colon, omentum, small intestine, spleen, liver, pancreas, and kidney.

The various forms of diaphragmatic injury include:

1. Diaphragmatic paresis resulting from injury to the phrenic nerve
2. Diaphragmatic hernia where the pleuroperitoneal layers are intact
3. Diaphragmatic rupture with tears of all tissue layers

Frequent associated injuries are hepatic or splenic ruptures (40%) and pelvic fractures (15%–20%).

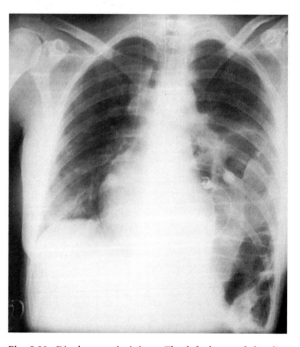

Fig. 5.23. Diaphragmatic injury. The left dome of the diaphragm cannot be delineated. The gas-filled colonic loops have herniated into the thoracic cavity

Table 5.9. Plain film findings in diaphragmatic rupture

Raised dome of the diaphragm with basal plate-like
  atelectasis
Unsharp contours of the diaphragm
Double contour of the diaphragm or irregular "bumps"
  on the diaphragmatic surface
Hemothorax
Unusual shadows resembling hollow viscera
  above the level of the diaphragm (abdominal organ
  herniation)
Mediastinal shift
Amputated fundus sign

Conventional radiography as well as CT or other cross-sectional imaging modalities are often nonspecific. Herniation of abdominal organs into the thoracic cavity is the only proof of diaphragmatic rupture (Fig. 5.23).

The chest radiograph may show a spectrum of findings ranging from irregularity of the diaphragmatic contour to the presence of abdominal organs in the thoracic cavity. The most common findings are listed in Table 5.9. Sharply delineated opacities with air–fluid levels are highly suspicious, especially when occurring in association with shifting of the mediastinum (GELMAN et al. 1991).

It should be noted that thoracic drains are contraindicated in diaphragmatic ruptures as they may cause additional damage.

Fluoroscopy is useful only if combined with a contrast study of the gastrointestinal organs. Ultrasonography is rarely able to directly demonstrate the site of rupture; it is, however, indicated to detect free fluid in the abdominal or thoracic cavity as well as injuries to other organs such as the spleen and liver. CT is only able to detect ruptures involving the diaphragmatic crura or large diaphragmatic defects (Fig. 5.24). Transdiaphragmatic herniations are detected better by the sectional imaging modalities

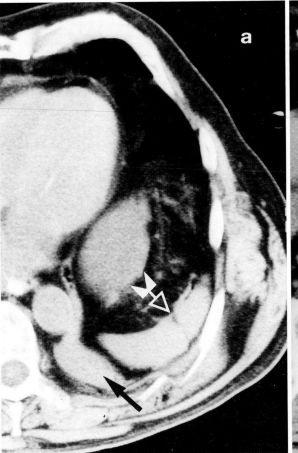
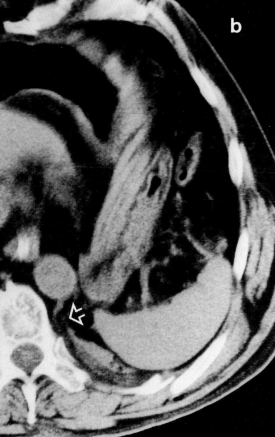

Fig. 5.24a,b. CT scans of diaphragmatic injury. **a** A semilunar hematoma is seen coursing along the diaphragmatic contour (*arrow*), and rib fractures and a linear splenic tear (*open arrow*) are present. **b** The rib fracture is seen, as well as disruption of the left crus of the diaphragm (*arrow*)

than by projection radiography, especially as CT is able to detect herniation of the omental fatty tissue. The same is true for MRI, which may, however, have a certain advantage due to the free choice of the sectional plane.

Apart from clear-cut cases with herniation of the abdominal organs into the thorax, the diagnosis may be difficult irrespective of the diagnostic modality used. In up to 50% of cases, a definitive diagnosis is possible only with operative exploration.

References

Brooks AP, Olson SK (1989) Computed tomography of the chest in trauma patient. Clin Radiol 40:127–132

Conn JH, Hardy JD, Fain WR, Netterville RE (1963) Thoracic trauma: analysis of 1022 cases. J Trauma 3:22–40

Dennis LN, Rogers LF (1989) Superior mediastinal widening from spine fractures mimicking aortic rupture on chest radiographs. AJR 152:27–30

Dunbar RD (1984) Radiologic appearance of compromised thoracic catheters, tubes, and wires. Radiol Clin North Am 22:699–722

Feczko JD, Lynch L, Pless JE, Clark MA, McClain J, Hawley DA (1992) An autopsy case review of 142 nonpenetrating (blunt) injuries of the aorta. J Trauma 33:846–850

Fraser RG, Pare JAP, Pare PD, Fraser RS, Genereux GP (1991) Diagnosis of diseases of the chest. Diseases of the thorax caused by external physical agents. Saunders, Philadelphia, pp 2480–2571

Galanski M, Hartenauer U, Krumme B (1981) Röntgen-diagnostik des Pneumothorax auf Intensivstationen. Radiologe 21:459–462

Gelman R, Mirvis SE, Gens DR (1991) Diaphragmatic rupture due to blunt chest trauma: value of chest radiography. AJR 156:51–57

Gens DR (1992) Imaging priorities in the admitting area. In: Mirvis SE, Young JWR (eds) Imaging in trauma and critical care. Williams & Wilkins, Baltimore, pp 1–22

Glinz W (1981) Chest trauma: diagnosis and treatment. Springer, Berlin Heidelberg New York

Glinz W (1986) Priorities in the diagnosis and treatment of blunt chest injuries. Injury 17:318–321

Goodman PC (1982) CT of chest trauma. In: Federle MP, Brant-Zawadzki M (eds) Computed tomography in the evaluation of trauma. Williams & Wilkins, Baltimore, pp 153–170

Graham JM, Mattox KL, Beall AC (1979) Penetrating trauma of the lung. J Trauma 19:665–669

Groskin SA (1992) Selected topics in chest trauma. Radiology 183:605–617

Harley DP, Mena I (1986) Cardiac and vascular sequelae of sternal fractures. J Trauma 26:553–555

Hauf GH, Lönne E (1989) Herztrauma und Verletzungen der großen thorakalen Gefäße. In: Roskamm H, Raindell H (eds) Herzkrankheiten. Springer, Berlin Heidelberg New York, pp 1422–1432

Healey MA, Brown R, Fleiszer D (1990) Blunt cardiac injury: is this diagnosis necessary? J Trauma 30:137–145

Heiberg E, Wolverson MK, Sundaran M, Shields LB (1983) CT in aortic trauma. AJR 140:1119–1124

Kearns SR, Gay SB (1990) CT of blunt chest trauma. AJR 154:55–60

LoCicero J, Mattox KL (1989) Epidemiology of chest trauma. Surg Clin North Am 69:15

Manson D, Babyn PS, Palder S, Bergman K (1993) CT of blunt chest trauma in children. Pediatr Radiol 23:1–5

Marnocha KE, Maglinte DDT, Woods J, Goodman M, Peterson P (1984) Mediastinal width/chest width ratio in blunt chest trauma. A reappraisal. AJR 142:275–277

Mirvis SE, Bidwell JK, Buddemeyer EU et al. (1987) Value of chest radiography in excluding traumatic aortic rupture. Radiology 163:487–493

Mirvis SE, Rodriguez A (1992) Diagnostic imaging of thoracic trauma. In: Mirvis SE, Young JWR (eds) Imaging in trauma and critical care. Williams & Wilkins, Baltimore, pp 93–144

Moore AV, Putman CE, Ravin CE (1983) Acute thoracic trauma. In: Goodman LR, Putman CE (eds) Intensive care radiology: imaging of the critically ill. Saunders, Philadelphia, pp 141–153

Morgan PW, Goodman LR, Aprahamian C, Foley WD, Lipchik EO (1992) Evaluation of traumatic aortic injury: does dynamic contrast-enhanced CT play a role? Radiology 182:661–666

Moskowitz P, Griscom N (1976) The medial pneumothorax. Radiology 120:143–147

Pais SO (1992) Diagnostic and therapeutic angiography in the trauma patient. Semin Roentgenol 27:211–232

Parmley LF, Manion WC, Mattingly TW (1958a) Nonpenetrating traumatic injury to the heart. Circulation 18:371

Parmley LF, Mattingly TW, Manion WC (1958b) Nonpentrating traumatic injury to the aorta. Circulation 17:1086

Raptopoulos V, Sheiman RG, Phillips DA, Davidoff A, Silva WE (1992) Traumatic aortic tear: screening with chest CT. Radiology 182:667–673

Richardson P, Mirvis SE, Scorpio R, Dunham CM (1991) Value of CT to screen trauma patients with equivocal chest radiographs for great vessel injury. AJR 156:273–279

Smejkal R, O'Malley KF, David E, Cernaianu AC, Ross SE (1991) Routine initial computed tomography of the chest in blunt torso trauma. Chest 100:667–669

Stark P (1990) Radiology of thoracic trauma. Invest Radiol 25:1265–1275

Wagner RB, Crawford WO, Schimpf PP (1988) Classification of parenchymal injuries of the lung. Radiology 167:77–82

Wernecke K, Galanski M, Peters PE, Hansen J (1987) Pneumothorax: evaluation by ultrasound – preliminary results. J Thorac Imaging 2:76–78

Woodring J, Lee C, Jenkins K (1988) Spinal fractures in blunt chest trauma. J Trauma 28:789–793

6 Abdominal Trauma

K.D. Hagspiel

CONTENTS

6.1 Introduction

Accidental trauma is the leading cause of death in the under-38 age group in the United States (Gay and Sistrom 1992). In Switzerland it is the leading cause in the under-45 age group and the third most common for the general population (Todesursachen-Statistik 1991). Because of the young age of the average trauma victim, the actual damage to society, speaking in terms of productivity years, equals the loss from cardiovascular diseases and cancer combined. In the United States, the death rate due to major trauma has increased since 1977. The majority of fatalities are due to injury to the central nervous system, hemorrhage, and multiple organ failure (Trunkey 1988). Although exact figures are not known, injuries of the abdomen comprise a significant portion among the general trauma population.

6.1.1 Classification of Abdominal Trauma

From a clinical standpoint, patients with abdominal injury are grouped into two categories: The first cat-

K.D. Hagspiel, MD, Division of Cardiovascular and Interventional Radiology, Department of Radiology, Brigham and Women's Hospital, Harvard Medical School, 75 Francis Street, Boston, MA 02115, USA

egory separates hemodynamically stable patients from hemodynamically unstable ones. While in hemodynamically stable patients time allows a complete clinical and radiological workup, management of the unstable patient differs significantly and the radiological investigations have to be restricted to the absolute minimum. These patients should immediately undergo either surgical or interventional radiological treatment. ("Don't put the unstable on the x-ray table!"). The second classification of abdominal trauma concerns the mechanism of the trauma. Here, blunt injuries are separated from penetrating injuries. This classification is important because it affects the clinical management as well as the radiological workup of these patients.

6.1.2 Mechanisms of Injury and Injury Patterns

The majority of blunt abdominal injuries are caused by motor vehicle accidents, followed by pedestrian accidents, bicycle accidents, falls, assaults, and falling objects (KINNUNEN et al. 1994). Depending on the location of the major force of the blunt impact, several typical patterns of injuries can be differentiated (FOLEY 1994). Determinants of the injury pattern are the location of the impact, the forces applied, and the intra-abdominal distribution of these forces. The distribution mainly depends on the compression and shearing forces within the abdomen (ANDERSON and BALLINGER 1985).

Several typical injury patterns have been recognized:

1. In patients with midline blunt abdominal trauma there is typically a combination of left hepatic lobe injury, pancreatic, proximal small bowel, and mesentery injury, and central renal pedicle injury. In cases with high forces there may be damage to all viscera including the aorta (see Figs. 6.25, 6.26). These abdominal or retroperitoneal injuries may be accompanied by cardiac contusion and/or tamponade.
2. Right-sided blunt traumata typically result in right liver, right kidney, distal small bowel and mesentery, and right iliac wing injuries (see Fig. 6.4). There may be an accompanying right-sided hemopneumothorax.
3. Left-sided blunt trauma results in splenic and left renal injuries, injuries to the proximal small bowel and mesentery and left iliac wing fractures (see Fig. 6.13). As on the right side there may be a hemopneumothorax.

4. Penetrating injuries in most cases are due to gunshot or stab wounds. Depending on the entrance site, length, and direction of the indwelling force a variety of injury patterns may result that nearly always necessitate surgical exploration of these patients.

6.1.3 Organ Injury Scaling

The American Association for the Surgery of Trauma (AAST) appointed in 1987 an Organ Injury Scaling (OIS) committee. In 1989 this committee published a scaling system for injuries to the spleen, liver, and kidneys (MOORE et al. 1989). The OIS is basically an anatomic description grading injuries to these organs into five groups from the least to the most severe injury. Several other scaling systems have been proposed by other investigators in the field (CROCE et al. 1991). The purpose of these scaling systems has been the establishment of common clinical criteria especially with regard to clinical research. Other scaling systems and indices in use are the Abdominal Trauma Index (ATI), which was introduced by AAST in 1979, the Injury Severity Score (ISS), and the Therapeutic Intervention Scoring System (TRISS) methodology (CULLEN et al. 1974). In addition, several researchers from the radiological field have proposed organ injury scaling systems based on imaging findings (MIRVIS et al. 1989b). A detailed review of all the scaling systems is beyond the scope of this review and the interested reader is referred to the literature (CROCE et al. 1991).

6.1.4 Clinical Evaluation of Patients with Blunt Abdominal Trauma

There is generally no debate about the approach to the hemodynamically unstable abdominal trauma patient, who undergoes immediate explorative laparotomy in most trauma centers around the world. On the other hand, opinions about the best approach to the hemodynamically stable patient vary greatly, especially in regard to whether and when surgery has to be performed, what type of surgery should be applied, and the role of radiological imaging in this group. The clinical evaluation of these patients should always include a thorough clinical examination with special regard to the presence of signs of an acute abdomen, and a laboratory workup including the search for internal blood loss. The evaluation process in hemodynamically stable patients also depends greatly on the injury pattern and the organ most severely injured and will be dicussed in detail in the following sections.

6.1.5 Clinical Evaluation of Patients with Penetrating Abdominal Trauma

As in blunt abdominal trauma, patients are primarily separated into hemodynamically stable and hemodynamically unstable ones. There is generally no debate as to the need for immediate surgery in all unstable patients but the management of those who are stable is somewhat controversial. While some trauma surgeons advocate routine surgical exploration of all patients with potentially penetrating abdominal wounds (MAYNARD and OROPEZA 1968), others see no reason for routine surgical evaluation (DEMETRIADES and RABINOWITZ 1987). DEMETRIADES and RABINOWITZ have published their experience of 651 patients with stab wounds to the anterior abdomen. The decision for or against immediate surgery was based solely on the presence of signs of: an acute abdomen with tenderness, guarding, rebound tenderness, and absent bowel sounds. Of those 651 patients 345 (53%) had the clinical symptoms of an acute abdomen and were immediately operated on. The remaining 306 patients (47%) had no signs or only minimal signs such as mild local tenderness on clinical examinations. This conservative group included 26 patients with intestinal or omental evisceration, 18 patients with air under the diaphragm, 12 patients with a positive peritoneal lavage, and 18 patients with shock on admission. Among these patients, surgery became necessary in only 11 (3.6%), and there was no mortality in this group. In the group that was immediately operated on, there were eight completely negative laparotomies (2.3%), defined as only peritoneal penetration, and another eight laparotomies that were considered unnecessary due to minimal findings. These authors therefore concluded that almost half of the patients with abdominal stab wounds can be managed conservatively with the decision in respect of surgery based solely on careful clinical examination. Even the presence of free intraperitoneal air, a positive pertioneal lavage, and the signs of shock were not absolute indicators for operation in their series. The authors did not evaluate the role of imaging in their study but their results seem to assign a very limited role to radiological imaging in this clinical setting.

Patients with abdominal trauma due to gunshot wounds constitute a different clinical entity and present specific problems. Depending upon the type of firearms and projectiles involved, different types of injuries may be encountered. A thorough discussion of wound ballistics especially with regard to high- and low-velocity projectiles is beyond the scope of this review and the reader is referred to the literature (PHILLIPS 1992). The incidence of hollow organ injury after violation of the peritoneum by a projectile is as high as 90% in some series (MOORE et al. 1980), with the small intestine being the most commonly injured organ. Generally, radiological evaluation is not of prime importance in these patients because in most trauma centers, surgical evaluation is considered mandatory. According to some authors, there may be a small subgroup of patients in whom selective nonsurgical management may be useful and in this subset ultrasonography (US), computed tomography (CT), and angiography might guide treatment (NANCE et al. 1974). RENZ and FELICIANO published their experience in 13 consecutive patients with right thoracoabdominal gunshot wounds and came to the conclusion that hemodynamically stable patients without signs of peritonitis can be treated nonsurgically and that in these cases, which usually present injuries to the right lung and the liver, CT has an important role in both initial diagnosis and follow-up (RENZ and FELICIANO 1994).

6.1.6 Intraperitoneal Hemorrhage: Diagnostic Peritoneal Lavage vs Computed Tomography vs Ultrasonography

The evaluation of intra-abdominal injuries in patients with blunt abdominal trauma based on clinical examination alone is a critical issue. Reported diagnostic accuracies range from 42% to 84% (GOMEZ et al. 1987). Diagnostic peritoneal lavage (DPL) was introduced by ROOT et al. in 1965, and it resulted in a substantial decrease in the incidence of negative laparotomies in these patients. Since the introduction of this method, an extensive body of literature has been accumulated. DPL is now established as a safe, cost-effective, reliable, and easy-to perform technique whose overall diagnostic accuracy has been reported to be as high as 97.8% in a meta-analysis involving 5715 patients (GOMEZ et al. 1987). The complication rate was 1.6%. The studies evaluated in this meta-analysis did not compare CT with DPL. There is still a considerable debate going on about whether DPL or CT should be performed in patients with blunt abdominal trauma. Each modality has its proponents and an extensive body of literature has been accumulated. Three studies comprising a total of 452 patients have been published where CT and DPL have both been performed (Fabian et al. 1986; Goldstein et al. 1986; Meyer et al. 1989) and thus comparison between the two techniques was possible. All three series reported approximately similar results for both methods, with specificities close to 100% and sensitivities between 74% and 95%. CT offered the additional advantage of not only detecting the presence of serious injuries but also defining their extent. In all three studies it was shown that the film reading by experienced trauma radiologists is necessary in order to obtain optimal results whereas the reading of films by residents is significantly less sensitive. On the other hand, DPL does not require the same level of expertise of the performing physician in order to obtain optimal results. The advantages of DPL as compared to CT are, according to Gay and Sistrom (1992), the following: DPL is less expensive, debatably more sensitive, and does not require a very high level of experience on the part of the performing physician in order to yield optimal results. On the other hand, CT is noninvasive, also evaluates the retroperitoneum and osseous structures, and gives a specific diagnosis that might allow a conservative approach. Some authors consider CT as sensitive as DPL for the detection of hemoperitoneum and stress the importance of an initial CT before DPL as a baseline study that enables the follow-up of these patients with regard to rebleeding or resorption of an hematoma. In this way, the presence of delayed intra-abdominal bleeding (Foley et al. 1987) can be detected noninvasively. In order to quantify the amount of intraperitoneal fluid, grading systems for intraperitoneal hemorrhage have been proposed (Federle and Jeffrey 1983). The debate over whether US or CT should be the initial imaging modality is mainly one between American and European groups. While in the United States most centers do not see a role for US in the emergency setting, many European centers successfully use it both for the initial examination and for follow-up. Several papers have now compared US with DPL, and the reported sensitivities, specificities, and accuracies for the detection of free intraperitoneal fluid are usually comparable to those of CT (Marx et al. 1985; Hoffmann et al. 1992; Goletti et al. 1994).

6.2 Radiological Approach to Patients with Blunt Abdominal Trauma

6.2.1 Overview

Today, dynamic, contrast-enhanced CT is considered the imaging method of choice for the evaluation of patients after blunt abdominal trauma in most centers. Nevertheless, several European and Japanese groups, and recently also groups from the United States, have reported excellent results with US. In addition, a variety of other imaging modalities are applied in this clinical setting and it is the aim of this section to give a short overview of the currently available techniques as well as their indications and modes of performance.

6.2.2 Plain Films of the Abdomen

Plain films generally do not provide sufficient information in patients with blunt abdominal trauma. If these films are acquired, there should always be a second film in the horizontal plane in order to detect free intraperitoneal air. Usually, this second film will be a left lateral decubitus film, the other one being a supine film. Indirect signs of organ injury are: elevation of the diaphragm, obliteration of fat planes or the psoas shadow, or presence of a mass displacing other organs (Berk 1970). Fractures (e.g., of the ribs) can be detected, thus giving some information about possible organ injuries. Air in the bile ducts or intrahepatic vessels should be meticulously searched for. The plain film findings in the different clinical entities will be discussed in full in the subsequent sections.

6.2.3 Ultrasonography

There is a vast body of literature showing that there is a role for percutaneous US in the management of blunt abdominal trauma patients (Schlager et al. 1994; Goletti et al. 1994), though in most centers the primary imaging modality is contrast-enhanced CT in hemodynamically stable patients. The great advantage of US is the fact that it can be performed immediately after arrival in the emergency ward, no matter whether the patient is hemodynamically stable or not. A full abdominal examination including the search for free fluid and liver and spleen injuries takes less than 5 min in the hands of experienced sonographers. The time between admission to the emergency department and the completion of the US examination was less than 30 min in 250 cases in GOLETTI et al.'s series. This compares favorably to the 1 h and 19 min from the arrival in the unit until the start of the CT examination reported by GOULD et al. (1988). The specificity of the US examination can be considerably increased by US-guided paracentesis (GOLETTI et al. 1994). One of the disadvantages of US preventing its widespread use is that it is greatly operator-dependent, which limits its acceptance in many trauma centers especially in the United States. In Europe in many cases the US studies are performed by specially trained surgeons and less often by radiologists. Whereas the role of US as the initial imaging method is subject to debate, there is general agreement that US has an important role for the follow-up of patients with abdominal trauma. More detail on the US findings will be given in the following sections.

6.2.4 Computed Tomography

Computed tomography has been shown to be a highly reliable means of evaluating blunt abdominal trauma. Standard protocols involve application of both intravenous and oral contrast. Patients undergoing CT must be hemodynamically stable. Patient monitoring in the CT scanner suite has to be performed by experienced nurses and respiratory technicians and not by radiology technicians. Today, high-speed last-generation scanners which allow rapid, dynamic incremental spiral (helical) scanning are mandatory (FOLEY 1989). The use of oral contrast is optional; if it is applied, it will often have to be given through a nasogastric tube, thus also allowing removal of air and gastric contents from the the stomach. It must be kept in mind that the application of oral contrast on the one hand facilitates analysis of bowel and mesenteric injuries, but on the other hand causes a delay of approximately 30 min before the CT study may be started (KINNUNEN et al. 1994). Generally a 1-cm slice thickness and table increment are accepted. The usually applied dose of intravenous contrast is approximately 150–180 ml; 60% nonionic contrast agents are recommended. Recommended flows are 0.5–1.5 ml/s and scanning should be started 30–45 s after the beginning of the contrast application (GAY and SISTROM 1992). In order to evaluate the urinary bladder, the catheter should be clamped prior to CT. Dis-

tension of the bladder greatly facilitates detection of bladder injuries.

The recent advent of spiral (helical) scanning will probably add additional benefit to the performance of CT in trauma patients due to the fact that it allows scanning of complete volumes within seconds.

6.2.5 GI Tract Studies

Gastrointesinal contrast studies are rarely performed in this clinical situation with the exception of oral contrast-enhanced CT. Only in cases where an injury to a hollow organ is suspected and CT does not allow a definite diagnosis, might a conventional GI tract study using Gastrografin be indicated. In patients with a known intramural hematoma, in whom US gives no definite information, a contrast study may be performed for follow-up to observe resolution of the hematoma. Because of the possibility of subsequent surgery, barium-containing contrast agents are contra-indicated in this clinical setting. The contrast agent recommended is Gastrografin or a similar agent.

6.2.6 Sinography

Sinography can be performed in special clinical situations where fistula tracts (usually due to stab wounds) are looked for (Fig. 6.1). "Stabograms" are usually performed in order to detect peritoneal penetration, but unfortunately have been found to be false-negative in 14% of patients and therefore are not recommended as a routine diagnostic tool in patients after penetrating injuries (ARAGON and EISEMAN 1976; DEMETRIADES and RABINOWITZ 1987).

6.2.7 Angiography and Interventional Radiology

With the advent of US and especially CT, angiography has nearly lost its once predominant role as a diagnostic modality. Instead, due to transcatheter embolization (TCE) techniques, it has turned from a diagnostic into a mostly therapeutic technique. The use of angiography and TCE in abdominal trauma patients differs in hemodynamically stable and unstable patients. In the hemodynamically stable group significant blood loss is usually the indication for angiography; these patients will often

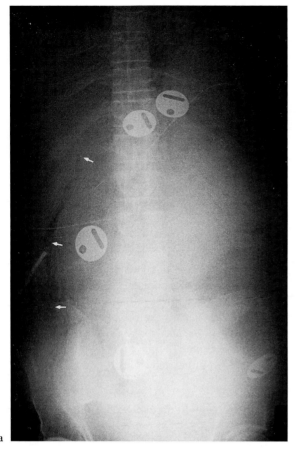

a

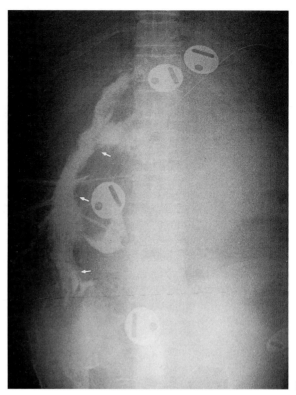

b

Fig. 6.1a,b. Sinogram in a patient who received multiple stab wounds and underwent immediate surgery. Postoperative course was complicated by fever and peritonitis and pus coming from a drain. The sinogram was performed through an intraoperatively placed drain in order to search for fistula tracts and abscesses. **a** Plain film shows gas in the subhepatic space and paracolic area (*arrows*). **b** After the application of a water-soluble contrast agent an extensive fistula tract becomes outlined (*arrows*)

have undergone CT beforehand, and therefore a source of bleeding may already be suspected or identified. These findings will guide angiographic technique. On the other hand, arteriography might be performed immediately in the hemodynamically unstable group, especially in patients with known pelvic fractures. This is done because of the known problems in controlling retroperitoneal bleeding surgically, whereas TCE usually is successful in this clinical setting. In cases with an unknown source of hemorrhage the diagnostic angiographic study should begin with an abdominal aortogram, preferably with cut-film technique. This study provides important information concerning vascular anatomy and also allows detection of vascular and organ pathology. Selective and superselective angiography subsequently are performed to detect and define the site of hemorrhage and finally to perform TCE. The angiographic signs of visceral injury include: con-

trast extravasation, pseudoaneurysms, vessel occlusions, arterioportal or arteriovenous fistulas, subcapsular hematomas, loss of normal parenchymal enhancement, and diffuse vasoconstriction in hypovolemic shock (TEITELBAUM et al. 1994).

The special angiographic and interventional techniques will be discussed in the subsequent sections on the different organs.

6.2.8 Magnetic Resonance Imaging

Magnetic resonance imaging (MRI) plays virtually no role in the acute phase in abdominal trauma patients. This is mainly due to the limited possibilities of monitoring critically injured patients while in the scanner and the relatively long scan times. Nevertheless, MRI plays a role in the diagnosis of diaphragmatic injuries, where it is now considered the modality of choice in the nonacute phase (MIRVIS et al. 1988) (see Fig. 6.27). The role of MRI might change with the advent of ultrafast sequences and the availability of patient monitoring systems that are capable of being used in high magnetic fields.

6.2.9 Scintigraphy

There are only a very few applications for scintigraphic techniques in the evaluation of abdominal trauma patients, with the evaluation of posttraumatic bilomas being the most frequent indication (CARIDE and GIBSON 1982; ZEMAN et al. 1984; WEISSMANN et al. 1979) (see Fig. 6.8). Another indication is the investigation of right-sided diaphragmatic hernias, which can be detected with hepatobiliary scans (KIM et al. 1983).

6.3 Liver

The liver is the second most frequently injured abdominal organ after the spleen and the incidence of hepatic injury in blunt abdominal trauma is reported to be as high as 3%–10% (HANEY et al. 1982). There is a preference for injury to the right lobe of the liver, especially the posterior segment, presumably due to its larger size and its better acessibility to trauma. The mortality from blunt hepatic trauma is relatively high (between 8% and 25%), and refined triage and treatment techniques did not have a dramatic impact on these figures (ANDERSON and BALLINGER 1985). Isolated hepatic injury is rare and in 77%–90% of cases other visceral injuries are present.

6.3.1 Classification and Grading of Liver Trauma

Several grading scales have been proposed for the assessment of traumatic liver injury. Basically, there are two types of grading systems: those relating to laparatomy findings (MOORE et al. 1989) and those based on CT findings (MIRVIS et al. 1989a). Both grading systems take into account the presence and depth of lacerations, the involvement of the capsular surface, the presence of perihepatic blood and hemoperitoneum, and organ disruption (Table 6.1). Surgical grading systems also include the difficulty in operative repair as a parameter. The role of CT is extended to the detection of associated abdominal injuries and the investigation of the healing process or the presence of complications.

6.3.2 Clinical Findings in Liver Injury

The most common clinical symptom in patients with liver trauma is pain in the right upper quadrant, and in some cases also in the right shoulder. Other clinical findings include hypotension and shock in hemorrhage, and symptoms of bile peritonitis like tenderness, guarding, and absent bowel sounds. Singultus can rarely be found in liver injury patients.

6.3.3 Imaging Findings in Liver Injury

From a radiological-pathological standpoint of view, liver traumata can be divided by CT into several groups. These include: periportal tracking, contusions, supcapsular and intraparenchymal hematomas, linear or stellate lacerations, and complete hepatic fractures.

6.3.3.1 Periportal Tracking

The presence of periportal hypodensities or periportal zones of decreased attenuation is well described in the literature. Initially seen in patients after liver transplantation it was soon afterwards seen in patients with blunt abdominal trauma. MACRANDER and co-workers described a series of 51 patients with hepatic trauma in which they retrospectively detected periportal tracking in the majority of cases (62%); indeed, in nine cases it was the only pathological imaging finding. As with all types of liver injury, periportal tracking is found most commonly in the right liver lobe (63% of all tracking patients in this series) (MACRANDER et al. 1989). It is

Table 6.1. Liver trauma grading system (according to MOORE et al. 1989; MIRVIS et al. 1989a)

Grade I	Small capsular laceration and/or parenchymal laceration not deeper than 1 cm, periportal tracking only
	Small subcapsular hematoma smaller than 10% of liver surface
Grade II	Parenchymal laceration 1–3 cm
	Central or subcapsular hematomas 1–3 cm in diameter
Grade III	Parenchymal laceration deeper than 3 cm
	Central or subcapsular hematoma (larger than 3 cm)
Grade IV	Devascularization or destruction of a liver lobe
	Hematoma larger than 10 cm
Grade V	Devascularization or destruction of both liver lobes, hepatic avulsion

believed that periportal tracking in trauma patients represents the presence of blood in the periportal connective tissue sheath (unlike in patients after liver transplantation, in whom it represents perivascular lymphedema) (see Figs. 6.9, 6.26). The sign has not been described in the sonographic literature in trauma patients. Periportal tracking is considered a minimal form of liver trauma. Nevertheless, its presence should indicate hospitalization of the patient even if it is the only finding. A further CT scan before discharge is recommended by some authors in this patient group.

6.3.3.2 Contusion

Hepatic contusions are defined as areas with only minimal intraparenchymal hemorrhage. They are usually ill-defined and of low attenuation on contrast-enhanced CT scans. This entity is not described in the sonographic literature.

6.3.3.3 Hematoma

Lacerations can result in severe intraparenchymal bleeding. The resulting intraparenchymal hematomas are either oval or round. Their CT appearance is hyperdense to normal liver on the initial unenhanced scans and they do not show enhancement after intravenous contrast. Lacerations involving the liver surface may lead to subcapsular hematomas. The radiological appearance of such a subcapsular hematoma is that of a peripherally located, crescentic fluid collection compressing and indenting the underlying liver tissue. Subcapsular hematomas are the least common form of liver injury. The density and echogenicity of these hematomas change with time. Figure 6.2 shows the MRI appearance of a hepatic laceration with a large subcapsular hematoma.

6.3.3.4 Laceration

Lacerations are the most common type of hepatic injury. A blunt injury to the right hepatic lobe usually results in perivascular lacerations (Figs. 6.2–6.5, 6.16). The supposed mechanism of action is probably the presence of shearing forces in close proximity to the central venous structures. This explains why there is a tendency for hepatic lacerations to involve the deep central portions of the liver. Foley describes

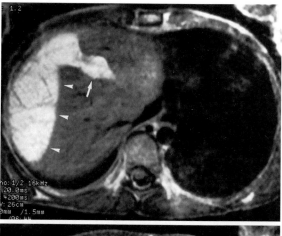

a

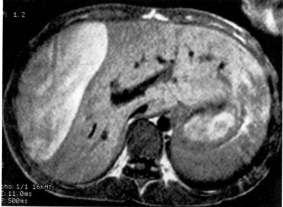

b

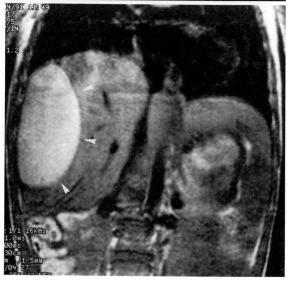

c

Fig. 6.2a–c. Liver laceration and subcapsular hematoma in a child. This boy was treated conservatively after blunt abdominal trauma. MRI 8 days after the trauma shows the large laceration in the right liver lobe (*arrow*) as well as the subcapsular hematoma (*arrowheads*). **a** Axial proton-weighted SE; **b** axial T1-weighted SE after gadolinium i.v.; **c** coronal T1-weighted SE scan

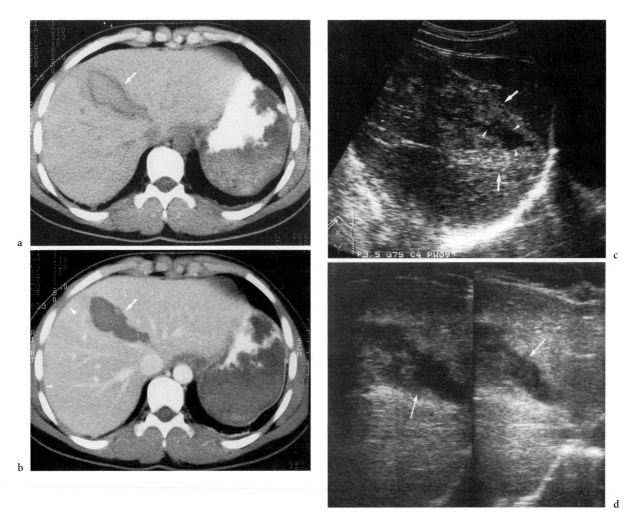

Fig. 6.3a–d. Liver laceration in a 30-year old female patient with blunt abdominal trauma due to a fall from a horse. There is a central liver laceration (*arrow*) on unenhanced CT (**a**) which is somewhat better delineated after intravenous contrast agent (**b**). In addition, there is a minimal amount of perihepatic fluid (*arrowheads*). **c** Sonogram during admission (2 h prior to CT) shows that the laceration is somewhat hyperechoic in relation to the surrounding liver tissue (*arrows*). It contains a central hypoechoic area (*arrowheads*). **d** Follow-up US after 8 days of conservative treatment shows the laceration with sharper demarcation from the surrounding liver. The laceration now has a low echogenicity (*arrows*)

the typical laceration as running parallel to a hepatic vein or the posterior segmental branch of the right portal vein. In massive trauma there may be multiple, complex lacerations which may result in a stellate tear pattern and which may reach the liver capsule. In the majority of cases where the liver capsule is involved, the anterior surface of the liver is lacerated and there is a fluid collection in the right paracolic gutter (FOLEY 1994). Only occasionally do those lacerations involve the liver surface at the bare area between the coronary ligaments. In these cases extraperitoneal hemorrhage may be present, especially around the inferior vena cava and the right adrenal gland, a finding that has been given the name "halo sign" (STALKER et al. 1986). Hepatic fracture is the term for deep lacerations ranging from one liver surface to the other and resulting in lobar or segmental avulsion.

6.3.3.5 Infarction

If the liver injury leads to occlusion of a larger intrahepatic vessel, significant infarction can result. Depending on the vessel occluded, these infarctions may involve segments and even lobes. Infarctions appear as hypodense, nonenhancing, wedge-shaped areas (Fig. 6.6). On contrast-enhanced scans their density is usually lower than that of the paraspinal muscles. Occasionally, these infarctions become superinfected and develop into liver abscesses (ENG et al. 1981).

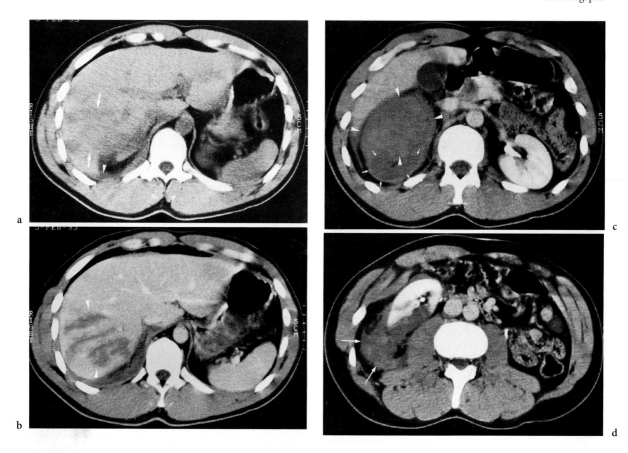

Fig. 6.4a–d. Large liver laceration with perihepatic hematoma and right renal laceration. **a** Unenhanced CT shows poorly delineated hypodense "streaky" lesions within the right liver lobe posteriorly (*arrows*) as well as perihepatic fluid (*arrowhead*). **b** Contrast-enhanced CT clearly demarcates the hepatic laceration (*arrowheads*). **c** Scan at the level of the upper pole of the right kidney shows a large hematoma (*arrowheads*) and no renal perfusion (*arrows*). **d** Scan at the level of the lower pole of the right kidney shows a large renal laceration and anterior displacement of the kidney due to a large hematoma (*arrows*)

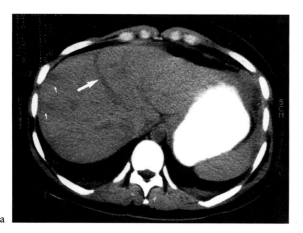

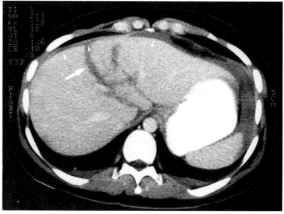

Fig. 6.5a,b. Liver laceration and perihepatic fluid. Unenhanced (**a**) and enhanced CT (**b**) show a liver laceration extending to the liver surface (*arrows*) and perihepatic fluid (*arrowheads*). Note also the rib shadowing artifacts that must not be confused with traumatic lesions (*small arrows*)

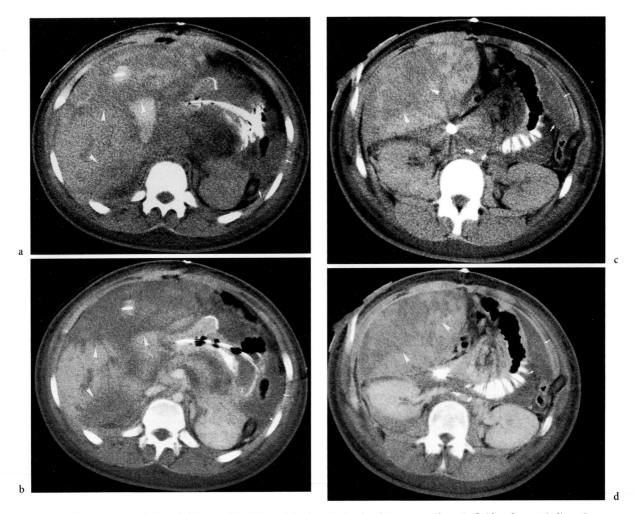

Fig. 6.6a–d. Postraumatic liver infarction. Unenhanced (**a,c**) and contrast-enhanced CT (**b,d**) show large areas of infarcted liver tissue that appear hypodense (*arrowheads*). The patient also underwent splenectomy for laceration of the spleen. The distinction between perihepatic fluid and necrotic liver tissue is difficult to make. Note also the presence of free intraperitoneal fluid (*arrows*)

6.3.3.6 Injuries to the Intrahepatic Biliary Tree and Bilomas

Both intrahepatic and intraperitoneal fluid can represent bile in patients after trauma. The pathomechanism of these injuries is usually a liver parenchyma laceration that extends into a bile duct. Both bile leakage and biloma formation can occur as a result. Bilomas exhibit slow growth over a period of days and weeks and can reach a considerable size if the communication between the bile ducts and the collection persists (Fig. 6.7). Bilomas can be entirely intrahepatic or partly extrahepatic, with loculations anywhere in the peritoneal cavity. Though slow-growing fluid-density lesions usually represent bilomas, CT and US generally cannot differentiate between bilomas, abscesses, cysts, and hematomas.

The diagnosis can be made with certainty by fine-needle aspiration, cholescintigraphy, or oral or intravenous cholangiography/cholangio-CT (Fig. 6.8). Small bilomas (less than 3 cm in diameter) usually do not require treatment unless they become infected. In bilomas over 3 cm some authors recommend percutaneous drainage, which can be performed easily and safely using US or CT guidance. Due to the fact that bilomas usually do not contain debris, the use of small-caliber drainage systems is recommended (VAZQUEZ et al. 1985).

6.3.3.7 Hemoperitoneum in Liver Injury

The amount of free intraperitoneal blood was found to be a powerful prognostic indicator in patients with

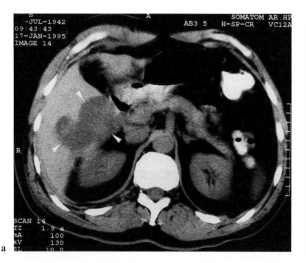 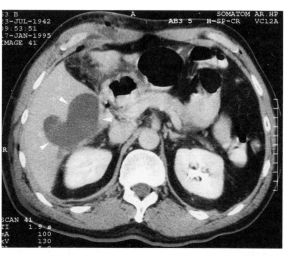

Fig. 6.7a,b. Postraumatic biloma. Unenhanced (**a**) and contrast-enhanced CT (**b**) show a water-density fluid collection in the right liver (*arrowheads*) that developed in this patient with blunt abdominal trauma over a period of several days. There is no marginal contrast enhancement, which is strong evidence against the presence of an abscess or a hematoma

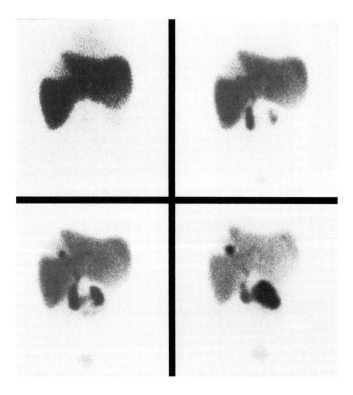

Fig. 6.8. Postraumatic biloma. Hepatobiliary function scintigraphy with ⁹⁹ᵐTc-IODIDA in a 4-year-old child 3 weeks after penetrating gunshot liver trauma. US had demonstrated a cystic lesion within the liver as well as a large defect in the right liver. Two minutes after the radiotracer application the hepatic perfusion defect can be detected (*upper left image*). After 10 min the tracer can be found in the gallbladder and the GI tract (*upper right*). After 20 min (*lower left*) and after 35 minutes (*lower right*) there is a radiotracer collection in the location of the cystic structure, thus proving it to be a biloma. (Case courtesy of Hans C. Steinert, MD, Division of Nuclear Medicine, University Hospital Zurich, Switzerland)

liver trauma. A CT grading system was introduced by FEDERLE and JEFFREY (1983). In one study, it was found that in cases with hemorrhage smaller than 250 ml, surgery usually is not required (MEYER et al. 1985); in another it could be shown that the lack of absorption of the fluid within 1 week after the initial scan usually indicated persistent hemorrhage from liver injury (FOLEY et al. 1987) (Figs. 6.4–6.6).

6.3.3.8 Vascular Complications

6.3.3.8.1 Pseudoaneurysms. The development of pseudoaneurysms is known after both blunt and penetrating trauma. Although their presence sometimes can be proven by contrast-enhanced CT, usually their detection requires angiography. Their location is typically at the laceration margins and

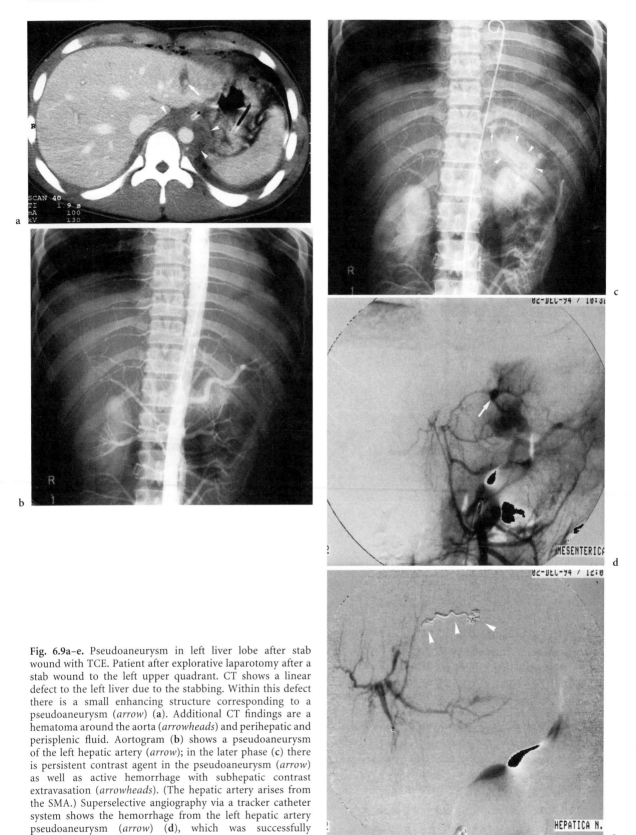

Fig. 6.9a–e. Pseudoaneurysm in left liver lobe after stab wound with TCE. Patient after explorative laparotomy after a stab wound to the left upper quadrant. CT shows a linear defect to the left liver due to the stabbing. Within this defect there is a small enhancing structure corresponding to a pseudoaneurysm (*arrow*) (**a**). Additional CT findings are a hematoma around the aorta (*arrowheads*) and perihepatic and perisplenic fluid. Aortogram (**b**) shows a pseudoaneurysm of the left hepatic artery (*arrow*); in the later phase (**c**) there is persistent contrast agent in the pseudoaneurysm (*arrow*) as well as active hemorrhage with subhepatic contrast extravasation (*arrowheads*). (The hepatic artery arises from the SMA.) Superselective angiography via a tracker catheter system shows the hemorrhage from the left hepatic artery pseudoaneurysm (*arrow*) (**d**), which was successfully embolized with coils (*arrowheads*) (**e**)

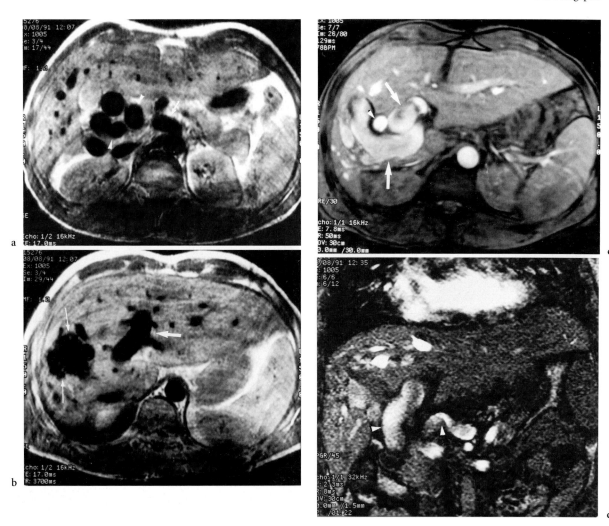

Fig. 6.10a–d. Posttraumatic arterioportal fistula. MRI and MR angiography (**a** and **b** axial long TR/short TE scans, **c** axial gradient echo scan, **d** coronal gradient echo scan) in a male patient many years after blunt abdominal trauma with severe liver injury shows a massively enlarged celiac trunk (*small arrow*) and an enlarged and elongated hepatic artery (*arrowheads*), as well as drastic enlargement of the intrahepatic portal vein branches (*large arrows*) (*long thin arrows*: site of the arterioportal fistula)

their usual clinical presentation is by hemorrhage. Embolization is the treatment of choice and can be performed safely and effectively (Fig. 6.9).

6.3.3.8.2 AV Fistulas. Intrahepatic arteriovenous communications are very rare, with only less than 50 cases reported. The majority of the cases are due to trauma. The three most common are: penetrating trauma, status after biopsies, and blunt trauma (FOLEY 1994). The majority of these fistulas are between the hepatic artery and a branch of the portal vein. In cases with large communications, portal hypertension may develop with all its consequences (Fig. 6.10). In cases with communications between the hepatic artery and the hepatic vein, high-output cardiac failure may develop, depending on the size of the shunt. Therefore, larger fistulas should be embolized or, if embolization is not possible, surgically closed (REDMOND and KUMPE 1988; TARAZOV 1993).

6.3.3.8.3 Juxtahepatic Venous Injuries. Juxtahepatic venous injuries are rare but nearly always fatal. They include rupture or tear of the retrohepatic vena cava or the major hepatic veins (KLEIN et al. 1994). Most patients with this sort of injury do not undergo imaging.

6.3.3.8.4 Hepatic Avulsion. Hepatic avulsion is the most severe liver injury and results in devascularization of the liver. There is no contrast enhancement within the whole organ on CT (GAY and SISTROM 1992).

6.3.3.8.5 Hemobilia. Hemobilia results from a posttraumatic communication between a blood vessel (usually a branch of the hepatic artery) and a bile duct. The most common etiology is rupture of a pseudoaneurysm into a bile duct. Therapy can be either by TCE or surgery. Diagnosis is usually made angiographically (SCHORN and COLN 1977; REUTER et al. 1986).

6.3.4 Management of Posttraumatic Bleeding

The majority of cases of posttraumatic bleeding after blunt liver trauma probably result from transection of central hepatic veins. Because of the surgical difficulty associated with these vessels, the conservative approach to hemodynamically stable patients is preferred. In the unstable group, surgery is usually performed in order to control the hemorrhage. In cases where this proves unsuccessful, TCE may be required. TCE shows the best results in patients bleeding from posttraumatic pseudoaneurysms (see Fig. 6.9).

6.3.5 Role of Imaging in the Follow-up of Patients with Liver Trauma

While in most trauma centers contrast-enhanced CT is the initial radiological modality to assess the extend of liver trauma, US is an excellent modality to monitor the course of the injury and the pattern of healing. VAN SONNENBERG et al. evaluated the sonographic findings of acute trauma to the liver with the initial study taking place less than 24 h following the trauma. Fresh intraparenchymal hemorrhage was found to be echogenic and sometimes very subtle. Within the first week, the hepatic laceration appears more hypoechoic, thus allowing a better delineation from liver parenchyma. This appearance is thought to be the result of reabsorption of devitalized tissue and ingress of interstitial fluid. In about 2–3 weeks the laceration becomes increasingly difficult to detect due to filling of the laceration with granulation tissue (VAN SONNENBERG et al. 1983) (see Fig. 6.3). Follow-up imaging can, of course, also be done using CT, and FOLEY et al. described the findings of serial CT after liver trauma (FOLEY et al. 1987) (Fig. 6.11). One week after the trauma the fluid between

the laceration margins is usually less visible than on the initial posttraumatic scans. There is usually contrast enhancement at the laceration margins, most likely due to granulation tissue. Complete resolution of lacerations and hematomas may take as long as 1–3 months, with a progressive narrowing of the space between the enhancing laceration margins. The routine performance of follow-up imaging studies in patients with abdominal trauma is not recommended because of a lack of impact on the therapeutic strategy. The decision on whether to perform follow-up studies is based solely on the clinical course, with right upper quadrant pain, fever, jaundice, anemia, or melena being the usual indications (MEREDITH et al. 1994).

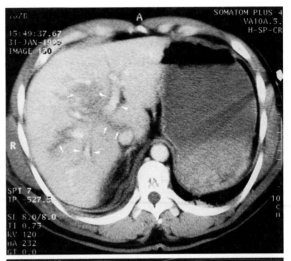

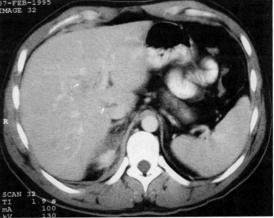

Fig. 6.11a,b. Follow-up CT in liver laceration. **a** Contrast-enhanced CT in a patient with blunt abdominal injury shows a central liver laceration (*arrows*) running towards the vena cava and periportal tracking (*arrowheads*). **b** Follow-up CT 7 days later shows nearly complete healing of the laceration with only minimal residual traumatic changes detectable on contrast-enhanced CT 8 (*arrows*)

6.3.6 Late Sequelae of Hepatic Trauma

6.3.6.1 Posttraumatic Cysts

Occasionally a subcapsular or intraparenchymal hematoma does not resolve. In these cases posttraumatic cysts may develop. Their location may be either subcapsular or anywhere within the liver parenchyma. They show typical features of cysts on all imaging modalities and can be differentiated from congenital or postinflammatory cysts only by reference to the patient's trauma history.

6.3.6.2 Focal Hepatic Fatty Metamorphosis

Focal fatty metamorphosis of the liver parenchyma is a well-recognized phenomenon whose imaging appearance has been described by US, CT, and MRI. It is a nonspecific response of the liver to different insults and can be seen in a variety of metabolic disorders, in infection, in patients undergoing chemotherapy, and also as a result of liver trauma. Pardes and co-workers described three patients with focal fatty liver after trauma. The lesions were of irregular shape with attenuation values around −10 Hounsfield units (PARDES et al. 1982).

6.3.6.3 Portal Hypertension

Portal hypertension is a rare late sequela of hepatic trauma in cases where arterioportal fistulas developed (see text above and Fig. 6.10).

6.3.7 Impact of Imaging Findings on Prognosis and Treatment

The major incentive for the performance of CT in patients with blunt abdominal trauma is, in addition to the detection of organ injury, the establishment of prognostic criteria that allow direction of management in either the operative or the conservative direction. Depending on the trauma center, different approaches are currently used in order to identify the subgroup of patients with liver trauma who are candidates for conservative management. Some centers use CT organ injury scores and estimates of the amount of free intraperitoneal fluid to make this differentiation, while others advocate the conservative approach in all hemodynamically stable patients regardless of the extent of liver injury as assessed by imaging methods.

Several studies have been performed comparing CT with intraoperative findings and evaluating its role in the clinical course of these patients. MIRVIS et al. (1989a) published a paper in which they reviewed 37 cases of blunt abdominal trauma which were hemodynamically stable and in whom liver injury was the only or dominant site of injury. The CT findings (dynamic contrast-enhanced CT) were assigned a score that was developed by these authors based on previously developed surgical-anatomical grading systems. Grading categories were: grade 1: capsular avulsion, superficial laceration, subcapsular hematoma less than 1 cm, or periportal tracking; grade 2: one or several lacerations or parenchymal or subcapsular hematomas 1–3 cm; grade 3: one or several lacerations or parenchymal or subcapsular hematomas more than 3 cm; grade 4: massive parenchymal or subcapsular hematoma larger than 10 cm or lobar tissue maceration or devascularization; grade 5: bilobar tissue maceration or devascularization. In addition, these authors also determined the extent of intraperitoneal hemorrhage according to the method of FEDERLE (FEDERLE and JEFFREY 1983). Thirty-one of these patients (83.7%) (grade 1: 2, grade 2: 6, grade 3: 20, grade 4: 3, grade 5: 0) were successfully treated without surgery. Of the six patients (grade 1: 1, grade 2: 1, grade 3: 4, grade 4: 0, grade 5: 0) who underwent celiotomy, four had nonbleeding liver injuries that required no therapy, one required packing of a stellate liver fracture, and one required repair of a previously undetected rupture of the right hemidiaphragm. The intraoperative liver findings correlated well with the CT findings in these six patients. Indication for surgery was a highly positive DPL in five and a drop in hematocrit in one. The authors concluded that with nonsurgical treatment of blunt hepatic trauma there is a high chance of a favorable outcome even in the presence of higher grades of CT injury in hemodynamically stable patients.

In a study published in 1991, CROCE and colleagues reported their experience in 37 patients with liver injuries who underwent CT prior to celiotomy. These authors used the AAST OIS scaling system, grading liver injury from 1 through 6. A high grade of liver injury found at surgery correlated well with an increasing severity of injury as assessed by higher transfusion requirements and more extensive surgical management. The authors found a poor correlation for the CT grades: 31 (84%) of the CT grades did not correlate with the operative findings. Four patients had intrahepatic hematomas that were not discovered at operation. Twelve lacerations were graded too high by CT and 15 too low. Of these 15, ten CT scores were at least two grades lower than those at operation. The authors concluded that the definition of minimal injury for prospective management of blunt trauma victims by CT findings alone is unreliable and therefore requires extreme caution. This study has been questioned because it is uncertain whether an optimal technique was used for dynamic contrast-enhanced CT.

Meredith and colleagues reviewed 126 patients with blunt liver trauma of whom 92 had CT scans. The aim of this study was to evaluate the role of nonsurgical treatment in blunt liver trauma. They concluded that approximately half of all patients are potential candidates for nonoperative treatment. In addition, they found that CT grading is not a good predictor of the need for surgery (MEREDITH et al. 1994). The study was not designed to evaluate the role of CT in this clinical setting. In addition, CT scans were read in retrospect by nonradiologists and it is unclear whether dynamic CT was applied.

Although its impact on the treatment plan is still being debated, CT does have a role in a conservative management plan as a tool to diagnose hematoma and intraperitoneal fluid resorption or complications such as the development of a biloma. If complete intraperitoneal fluid reabsorption does not occur within the first week, some authors recommend DPL. If this is positive for blood or bile, either surgery or angiography (in the case of hemoperitoneum) is warranted. Some patients bleed from pseudoaneurysms, which are treatable by TCE. Nevertheless most of the posttraumatic hemorrhages (both early and delayed) are probably due to ruptured veins preferentially located in the deep central parts of the liver. These impose great surgical difficulties and are the reason for the preference for the conservative approach in hemodynamically stable patients. Unfortunately CT does not allow identification of patients at risk for delayed hemorrhage from venous lacerations (MEREDITH et al. 1994).

6.3.8 Management and Diagnosis of Blunt Hepatic Trauma in the Pediatric Population

Diagnosis and treatment of children with liver trauma do not differ substantially from those of the adult patient. US and contrast-enhanced CT are the primary imaging modalities in pediatric liver trauma. There are no differences in the imaging appearances of liver trauma in children and adults. The emphasis of treatment is clearly on the conservative approach (KIRKS and CARON 1991).

6.4 Spleen

The spleen is the most commonly injured abdominal organ in blunt trauma (ROSOFF et al. 1972). The spleen has an important role in the defense against bacterial infections and it is known that patients after splenectomy (children as well as adults) are prone to a 50-fold increase in the occurrence of sepsis (especially due to pneumococci) (SEKIKAWA and SHATNEY 1983; GAY and SISTROM 1992). Therefore, the conservative treatment of splenic injury is of considerable interest and various groups have reported their experience with either splenorrhaphy or completely nonsurgical treatment. In children, conservative management was shown to be effective in several studies (BUNTAIN et al. 1985). In adults, the results are not as unequivocal as in the pediatric population and a variety of management plans have been under investigation. US and CT both have been proven to be suitable for diagnosis of splenic injuries, with CT being the superior method. Sensitivities and specificities for CT exceed 95% in some series (JEFFREY et al. 1981; FEDERLE et al. 1987). Only occasionally are subtle parenchymal lacerations not detected during CT and may present later in the course as so-called delayed splenic rupture. It is felt by some authorities that these "delayed ruptures" actually represent missed primary ruptures (PAPPAS et al. 1987). The phenomenon of a delayed rupture can occur as late as 2 weeks after the initial trauma.

6.4.1 Classification and Grading of Splenic Trauma

There are several existing grading systems for splenic injury, the majority of which have been validated by surgical correlation (BUNTAIN, MIRVIS, SCATAMACCHIA). Most of these schemes differentiate four subclasses of injury. The features serving as the basis for classification are: capsular disruption,

Table 6.2. Splenic injury grading system

Grade I	Small capsular laceration and/or parenchymal laceration smaller than 1 cm
	Small subcapsular hematoma smaller than 1 cm
Grade II	Parenchymal laceration 1–3 cm
	Central or subcapsular hematoma 1–3 cm
Grade III	Parenchymal laceration deeper than 3 cm
	Central or subcapsular hematoma larger than 3 cm
Grade IV	Devascularization of the spleen (no contrast enhancement)
	Fragmentation of the spleen

parenchymal lacerations, subcapsular hematomas, and lesions of the vascular pedicle. The splenic injury classification scheme shown in Table 6.2 is a combination of several of the published systems (BUNTAIN et al. 1988; RESCINITI et al. 1988; MOORE et al. 1989; MIRVIS et al. 1989b; GAY and SISTROM 1992):

6.4.2 Clinical Findings in Splenic Injury

The most common findings in severe splenic trauma are signs of systemic blood loss and irrigation of the peritoneum in the left upper quadrant. Sometimes the pain is referred to the left shoulder, which is known as Kehr's sign. Often the patients show no or only unspecific symptoms (HAGSPIEL 1994).

6.4.3 Imaging Findings in Splenic Injury

Generally contrast-enhanced CT is considered the imaging modality of choice in patients with a suspicion of splenic injury. In the following the imaging findings of the different injury patterns will be discussed.

6.4.3.1 Plain Film Findings in Splenic Trauma

Indirect signs of splenic injury are: an elevation of the left hemidiaphragm, fractures of left-sided basal ribs (especially the eighth, ninth, and tenth ribs), and a mass in the region of the left upper quadrant with displacement of neighboring organs (stomach, kidney, left colon). In most cases none of these signs will be present.

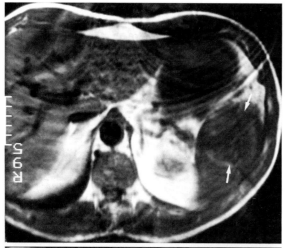

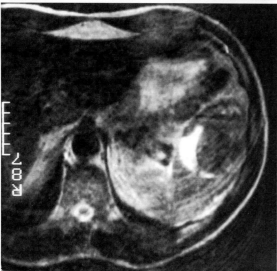

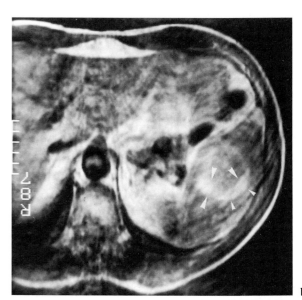

Fig. 6.12a–c. Splenic intraparenchymal hematoma. MRI 5 days after blunt trauma shows an intraparenchymal hematoma (*arrows*) with different signal intensities due to the varying blood products in the hematoma (**a** axial T1-weighted SE scan, **b** axial Gd-enhanced T1-weighted SE scan, **c** axial T2-weighted SE scan). There is peripheral contrast enhancement due to resorption of the hematoma (*arrowheads*)

6.4.3.2 Hematoma

An intraparenchymal or subcapsular hematoma initially presents as an echogenic, nonliquid mass on US. CT shows a high-density mass on unenhanced scans that do not show contrast enhancement. With time the size and echogenicity of the hematoma decrease, as does the density on CT. The MRI appearance of traumatic splenic hematomas depends on the age of the blood clot (Fig. 6.12). Generally, there is no indication for MRI in this clinical setting.

6.4.3.3 Laceration

Small lacerations are sometimes not detectable on US, and they are even less often visualized on contrast-enhanced CT. In some of these cases the only clue to the presence of a splenic laceration may be the presence of perisplenic fluid or a perisplenic blood clot. Perisplenic blood clots show relatively high attenuation values (60–100 HU) which help to differentiate them from unclotted blood or serous fluid. The presence of a blood clot adjacent to the spleen as a sign of splenic injury has been described as the "sentinel clot sign." Lacerations present on CT as low-density linear defects that usually extend from the lateral border of the spleen towards the hilum. In cases with extensive laceration there can be massive hematomas obliterating the splenic contour (Figs. 6.13, 6.14).

6.4.3.4 Infarction

Infarcts generally appear as areas that do not show contrast enhancement on CT. Occasionally, there may be slight rim-like enhancement of the splenic capsule which results from intact vessels of this capsule. The sign is known as the "splenic rim sign." The US diagnosis is somewhat more difficult; usually the splenic parenchyma shows an inhomogeneous echogenicity with large hypoechoic areas (Fig. 6.15).

6.4.3.5 Avulsion

Avulsion is the disruption of the splenic pedicle by traumatic forces. Usually there are large hematomas

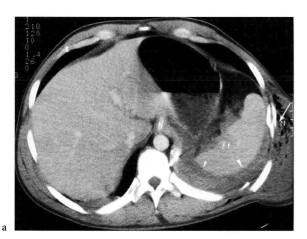

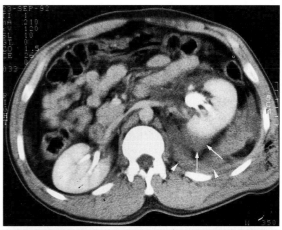

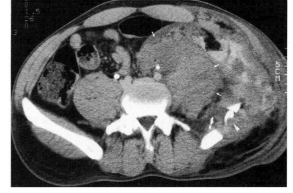

Fig. 6.13a–c. Splenic laceration and perisplenic hematoma. **a** Contrast-enhanced CT shows a medial splenic laceration (*arrows*) and a large perisplenic hematoma (*arrowheads*). Note the fractures of the left-sided ribs (*long arrow*). **b** A lower section at the level of the renal hili shows a hematoma in the posterior pararenal space (*arrowheads*) and the perirenal space (*arrows*) with anterior displacement of the left kidney. **c** A scan at the level of the iliac crest shows an iliac fracture (*arrowhead*) as well as a large hematoma (*arrows*)

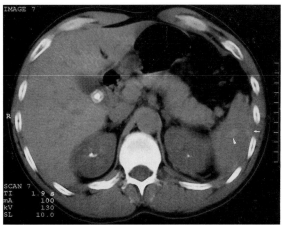

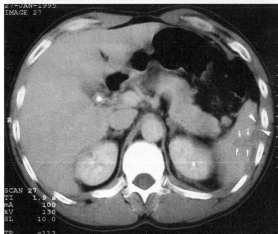

Fig. 6.14a,b. Splenic laceration and sentinel clot. CT shows a classical lateral splenic laceration, a dense intrasplenic hematoma, and a perisplenic clot (sentinel clot sign). There is also perisplenic fluid. **a** Unenhanced CT shows the dense intrasplenic (*arrowhead*) and perisplenic (sentinel) (*arrow*) clot. **b** The laceration (*arrows*) is better visible after intravenous contrast, as is the perisplenic fluid (*arrowheads*). Note also a calcified gallstone and bilateral kidney stones

in the area of the spleen and the organ shows no contrast enhancement on CT.

6.4.3.6 Enlargement of the Spleen on Follow-up CT Scans

Enlargement of the spleen on follow-up scans of patients considered not to be affected by splenic trauma during the initial scan is not a sign of trauma. In most cases it is due to a return of the injury-induced vasoconstriction to a normal state within a few days. This vasoconstriction in shock affects the spleen, among other organs. It might be helpful to correlate this finding with the width of the inferior

vena cava, which can also show an enlarged diameter on follow-up scans as compared to the initial scan where the patient had vasoconstriction due to shock (JEFFREY and FEDERLE 1988; GOODMAN and APRAHAMANIAN 1990).

6.4.3.7 Pitfalls in CT Diagnosis of Splenic Rupture

Two major pitfalls must be kept in mind before making the diagnosis of splenic rupture on CT (Figs. 6.16, 6.17). First, if dynamic CT is performed and the first scans are obtained immediately after initiation of the contrast bolus, a mottled enhancement pattern of the splenic parenchyma is the rule rather than the exception and must not be confused with laceration or infarction. Therefore, it is best to wait at least 45 s after beginning the contrast injection before scanning is initiated. This applies especially to spiral

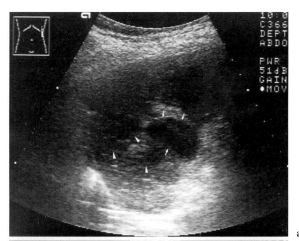

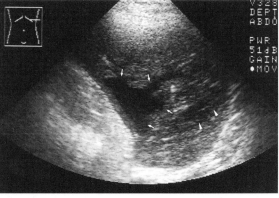

Fig. 6.15a,b. Splenic laceration and infarction. US 10 days after trauma shows a hypodense central intrasplenic lesion (*arrows*) corresponding to the laceration (**a** longitudinal, **b** transverse scan). Around this laceration there are multiple, poorly demarcated hypodense areas corresponding to infarcted splenic tissue (*arrowheads*)

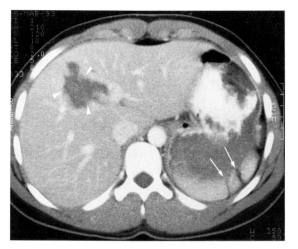

Fig. 6.16. Liver laceration and lobulated surface of the spleen. Contrast-enhanced CT shows a large central liver laceration (*arrowheads*). The surface of the spleen is severely lobulated (*arrows*). The margins of these lobulations are smooth, unlike in splenic lacerations. In addition, there is no evidence of perisplenic fluid. These splenic abnormalities are normal variants and must not be confused with traumatic lesions

scanning, where the whole abdomen is scanned in very short scan times. The second pitfall is the great anatomic variability of the normal spleen, which may show multiple clefts, humps, and lobulations as well as accessory spleens. Laceration outlines are usually

not smooth, unlike clefts and humps. In addition, lacerations usually are located at the outer surface of the spleen whereas clefts are more often medial. Artifacts from patient motion, beam-hardening artifacts from ribs, and streak artifacts originating in the stomach are further possible pitfalls in CT of splenic trauma. In questionable cases scanning must be repeated either with a greater delay after contrast injection or using thinner slices in order to avoid false-positive diagnoses.

6.4.4 Management of Patients with Splenic Trauma

The principal techniques of treatment can be divided into three categories: the conservative, nonsurgical approach where patients are observed and frequently checked for signs of hemodynamic instability, the surgical approach, and the interventional-radiological approach. Each treatment modality has its pros and cons and in the following section these will be discussed briefly.

As previously mentioned, modern therapy for splenic injury aims at the preservation of as much viable splenic tissue as possible. In patients who lack signs of hemodynamic instability, often no surgery is required and supportive measures alone are sufficient.

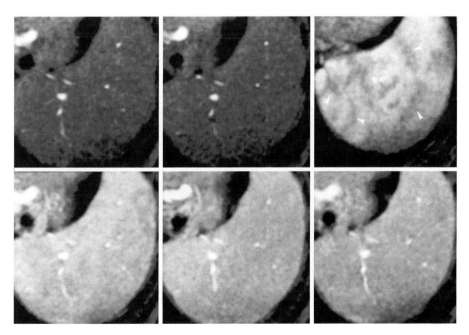

Fig. 6.17. Inhomogeneous enhancement (*arrowheads*) of the spleen 15 s after an intravenous bolus of Gd-DOTA as shown on this fast dynamic gradient echo MR scan must not be confused with splenic laceration. It is a normal finding in the early arterial phase. In order to avoid possible problems with this phenomenon, CT scanning should not be started earlier than 30–45 s after the contrast administration. MRI shows homogeneous enhancement after 30 s

In patients who are hemodynamically unstable and who require surgery, in most cases splenorrhaphy will be possible. There are various surgical techniques which allow the preservation of at least parts of the spleen including: suturing lacerations, cementing lacerations with thrombogenic agents, omental packing, and partial splenectomy (MUCHA et al. 1986). Splenectomy is the maximal surgical treatment option.

SCLAFANI and colleagues published their experience with 44 hemodynamically stable, conscious blunt trauma patients with splenic injuries diagnosed with contrast-enhanced CT. Angiography was performed on all 44 and the patients were divided into three groups according to angiography findings. Group I consisted of patients without extravasation of contrast and bed rest was the treatment. Group II consisted of the patients with contrast extravasation within or beyond the spleen; in these patients, embolization with coils was performed. Clinical control of hemorrhage was accomplished in all patients in group II and the splenic salvage rate was 97%. The third group consisted of the patients who underwent surgical exploration without angiography or embolotherapy because either the patient or the attending surgeon did not agree with the treatment protocol. The authors concluded that CT is a reliable and accurate method for detection of splenic injury and that therapeutic embolization in patients with bleeding from splenic injury may increase both the number of patients who benefit from nonsurgical management and the rate of splenic salvage (SCLAFANI et al. 1991). However, the results of these authors are questioned primarily due to the lack of randomization of the patients in groups with and without angiography. Therefore, it is not known whether a purely conservative approach would have given the same results.

6.4.5 Course of Splenic Injuries

There is not a big difference in the time course of repair of traumatic injuries of the spleen and the liver. Capsular and parenchymal lacerations usually heal over a period of 1–3 months. Hematomas resolve over the same period with the rare exception of the formation of so-called posttraumatic cysts (VAN SONNENBERG et al. 1983).

6.4.6 Late Sequelae of Splenic Trauma

6.4.6.1 Posttraumatic Splenic Cysts

In cases where the subcapsular hematoma does not resolve within several months, posttraumatic splenic cysts may occasionally develop. These may be either subcapsular or, more rarely, intraparenchymal. On US they present as anechogenic masses without a perceptible wall and with through transmission; on CT they have the appearance of low-density fluid collections (HELLER et al. 1982). They can only be differentiated from congenital or postinflammatory cysts by a history of trauma (Fig. 6.18).

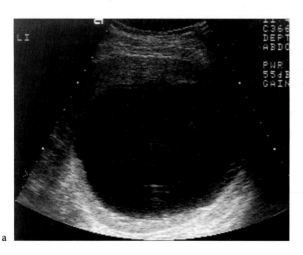 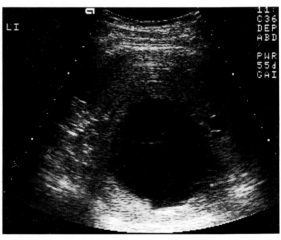

a   b

Fig. 6.18a,b. Posttraumatic splenic cyst. US shows a large posttraumatic cyst with imperceptible wall and posterior enhancement (**a** longitudinal, **b** transverse scan)

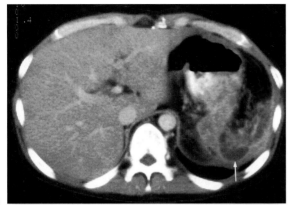

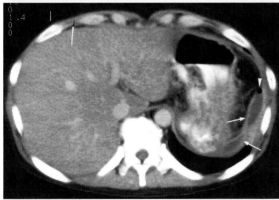

Fig. 6.19a,b. Contrast-enhanced CT with subphrenic abscesses after splenectomy because of blunt trauma to the spleen. **a** There are several loculated fluid collections with peripheral rim enhancement (*arrows* on **a** and **b**). **b** One of the abscesses contains a little air bubble (*arrowhead*)

6.4.6.2 Postoperative Complications

Patients undergoing emergency splenectomy or splenorrhaphy are known to be prone to significant complications. The most common complication is the development of postoperative pancreatic pseudocysts, whose incidence is reported to be as high as 50% (WINSETT et al. 1988). These cysts are susceptible to infection. Another complication is the development of postoperative subphrenic abscesses or pancreatitis (Fig. 6.19). Infected pseudocysts and subphrenic abscesses can be treated by percutaneous catheter drainage.

6.4.6.3 Enlargement of Accessory Spleens

Accessory spleens (splenunculi) are found relatively frequently in the general population and they can enlarge substantially after splenectomy, with diam-

eters of up to 5 cm after 6 months being reported in the literature (DARLING and FLICKINGER 1990). Their presence and function is revealed by technetium-99m sulfur colloid scanning or superparamagnetic ferrite particle-enhanced MRI.

6.4.7 Impact of Imaging Findings on Prognosis and Treatment

Several studies have been conducted with the aim of assessing the impact of CT findings in splenic trauma on the patient's prognosis and treatment (PEITZMAN et al. 1986; BUNTAIN et al. 1988; RESCINITI et al. 1988; SCATAMACCHIA et al. 1989). As has already been mentioned, patients undergoing splenectomy have a much higher risk of developing overwhelming infections, and this greatly influences whether surgical or nonsurgical treatment will be the method of choice. Therefore CT has been suggested in several studies as a good diagnostic tool for evaluating the extent of trauma in hemodynamically stable patients. A variety of grading systems have been proposed and clinically evaluated. Although the value of CT in the detection of splenic injury and definition of its extent is generally acknowledged, its value in predicting the outcome and influencing the treatment option is doubted.

BUNTAIN and RESCINITI developed a CT classification system for splenic injury and applied it to their patients. BUNTAIN et al. (1988) reported on 46 patients and found a good correlation between CT findings and intraoperative findings, although CT had a tendency to underscore the severity of the injury. They concluded that patients with grade I and II injuries without significant intra-abdominal hematomas were candidates for conservative treatment; all others were candidates for surgery in order to obtain optimal results concerning salvage of as much splenic tissue as possible. RESCINITI et al. (1989) devised a grading system consisting of three grades for splenic intraparenchymal hemorrhage and applied it to 60 patients. They found that nonsurgically treated patients had a significantly lower CT score than surgically treated ones and that no patient with a score under 2.5 required surgical treatment.

These favorable results in respect of CT-based grading and its impact on treatment are not without question, however. UMLAS and CRONAN found in their study on 56 patients with splenic trauma that "in most cases, CT is accurate in enabling detection of, and often in quantifying, injury to the spleen, but the extent of injury does not necessarily enable prediction of need for surgical intervention." The authors concluded that the ultimate decision on whether to perform laparotomy should be based on clinical status and not CT findings (UMLAS and CRONAN 1991). MIRVIS and colleagues published their experience in 39 patients with splenic trauma and came to the conclusion that "while CT remains an accurate method of identifying and quantifying initial splenic injury, as well as documenting progression or healing of critical injury, CT cannot reliably help predict the outcome of blunt splenic injury in adults. Treatment choices should therefore be based on the hemodynamic status of the patient and results of serial laboratory and bedside assessments" (MIRVIS et al. 1989b). This statement probably serves as the basis for decision making in most trauma centers worldwide.

6.4.8 Management and Diagnosis of Splenic Trauma in the Pediatric Population

As in adults with splenic trauma, the treatment goal in children should be the preservation of as much viable splenic tissue as possible. Laparotomy is indicated when the rupture leads to severe bleeding with hypotension; in cases with only moderate blood loss (less than 25 ml/kg body weight) during the first 48 h after injury the conservative approach is considered safe. Diagnosis and treatment do not differ between children and adults as do the imaging findings. Contrast-enhanced CT is considered the method of choice, but US has also shown a high sensitivity. In the pediatric population splenectomy in blunt trauma today is exceedingly rare, and conservative treatment is successful in nearly all cases (BUNTAIN et al. 1985). Routine follow-up CT scans are generally not considered necessary.

6.5 Gallbladder

6.5.1 Clinical Presentation of Gallbladder Injuries

Injuries to the gallbladder are extremely rare events. They account for approximately 2% of all visceral injuries and often go undetected during initial workup of the patient with blunt abdominal trauma (PENN 1962). Only in cases of a major hemorrhage due to laceration of the cystic artery are the clinical

signs of the injury obvious, though unspecific. In the majority of cases, the symptoms are relatively minor, and this is true even in cases with extensive leakage of bile into the peritoneal cavity (ELLIS and KRONIN 1960). The most common mechanism of injury is blunt trauma resulting in severe compression of the organ.

6.5.2 Classification of Gallbladder Injuries and Imaging Appearance

The following three types of gallbladder injury are usually distinguished: (a) avulsion of the gallbladder, (b) gallbladder laceration or perforation, and (c) intramural hematoma. Avulsion injuries usually present with severe blood loss and require early surgery (SODERSTROM et al. 1981). CT shows pericholecystic and intraluminal high-density hemorrhage and usually extensive hemoperitoneum. In laceration without hemorrhage the gallbladder is usually collapsed and there may be extensive (water-density) bile throughout the peritoneum (JEFFREY et al. 1986). Fresh intramural hematoma presents as high-density wall thickening on unenhanced scans, and US findings also show wall thickening of different echogenicity depending on the age of the hemorrhage. Occasionally, there may be a mass effect on the duodenum. The injuries most frequently associated with gallbladder trauma are pericholecystic liver lacerations and duodenal hematoma or perforation (ERB et al. 1994).

6.6 Mesentery and Bowel

6.6.1 Clinical Presentation and Diagnosis

Injuries of the gastrointestinal tract rank fourth in frequency among patients with blunt abdominal trauma after injury to the liver, spleen, and kidneys. Approximately 5% of laparotomies following blunt trauma reveal a small bowel injury (ROMAN et al. 1971). The mortality resulting from a delay in diagnosis and surgical treatment of duodenal perforation, for example, is known to increase from 5% to over 65% (SNYDER et al. 1980; GLAZER et al. 1981). The clinical diagnosis of these injuries may be difficult due to the fact that the classical clinical triad of tenderness, rigidity, and absent bowel sounds occurs in as few as one-third of patients. Preoperative diagnosis of these injuries improved with the advent of

DPL, but the method is insensitive to retroperitoneal injuries (duodenum and colon) (DONAHUE et al. 1985). Recently CT was found to be useful in the detection of bowel and mesenteric injuries following blunt abdominal trauma (RIZZO et al. 1989; DONOHUE et al. 1987).

6.6.2 Imaging Diagnosis of Injuries to the Mesentery and the Bowel

6.6.2.1 Plain Film Diagnosis

Signs of injury to the bowel and mesentery include the presence of free air in cases of intraperitoneal perforation and the presence of trapped air in cases of retroperitoneal hollow-viscus perforation (WINEK et al. 1988). Thumb-printing indicates intramural hematoma (see Fig. 6.20), while obliteration of retroperitoneal fat planes indicates retroperitoneal hematomas or abscesses. Scoliosis may be present. Generally, a diagnosis will rarely be possible with

plain films of the abdomen, with only 43% of cases showing any evidence of abdominal trauma (DONAHUE et al. 1985).

6.6.2.2 Ultrasonography

Ultrasonography has no relevant role in this clinical setting because bowel gas severely diminishes the possibility of adequately investigating the patient. Signs of trauma are: thickening of bowel walls, hematomas, and free intraperitoneal fluid. In cases with larger hematomas the assignment of the pathology to a source organ may be difficult.

6.6.2.3 Computed Tomography

Computed tomography is considered the imaging method of choice in this clinical setting. Adequate opacification of the gastrointestinal tract is of utmost importance. Best results are obtained after

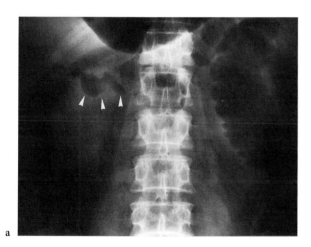
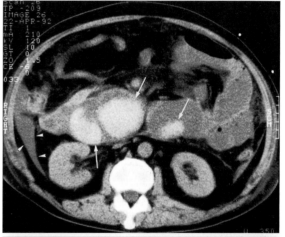
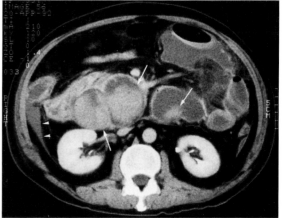

Fig. 6.20a–c. Duodenal hematoma after minimal blunt trauma in a hemophilic patient. **a** The supine abdominal plain film shows irregular thickening of the duodenal wall with thumb-printing (*arrowheads*). Unenhanced (**b**) and contrast-enhanced CT (**c**) show the large high-density hematoma (*arrows*) as well as some free fluid along the left anterior pararenal fascia (*arrowheads*)

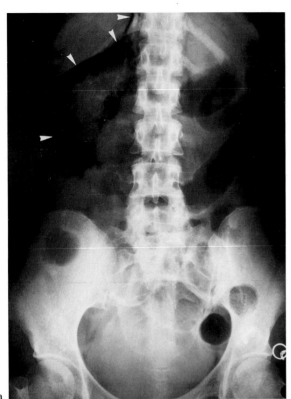

a

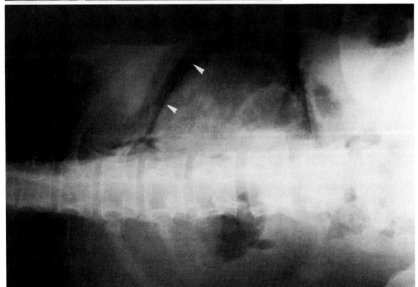

b

Fig. 6.21a,b. Retroperitoneal duodenal rupture due to blunt trauma. Supine (**a**) and left lateral decubitus (**b**) plain abdominal films show free retroperitoneal air (*arrowheads*). There is no evidence of intraperitoneal air

administration of an adequate amount (250–400 ml) of water-soluble (not barium!) contrast agent (Gastrografin) via a nasogastric tube 20–40 min before scanning (Rizzo et al. 1989). CT findings in bowel and mesentery pathologies will be described in the following section.

6.6.2.4 Angiography

The role of angiography is limited to the search for the source of a hemorrhage and its subsequent treatment by TCE.

6.6.2.5 Follow-through Studies

In cases where CT findings are inconclusive, the presence and degree of bowel obstruction by an intramural hematoma or another pathology may be better evaluated using fluoroscopy after Gastrografin. This method is also valuable in the follow-up of the regression of such hematomas (HAGSPIEL and KRESTIN 1994).

6.6.3 Classification of Injuries to the Mesentery and the Bowel

Trauma to the bowel and mesentery can result in intramural, intraperitoneal, or retroperitoneal hematoma, intraperitoneal or retroperitoneal perforation, and mesenteric laceration.

6.6.3.1 Intramural Hematomas

Intramural hematomas effect circumferential or focal bowel wall thickening. Fresh hematomas show relatively high density values on unenhanced CT scans. The duodenum and the proximal jejunum are the most commonly affected bowel segments because of their retroperitoneal fixations (Fig. 6.20). Most patients with this type of injury have automotive steering wheel or seat-belt injuries.

6.6.3.2 Mesenteric Hematomas

Mesenteric hematomas are three times more common than intramural ones (see Fig. 6.23). Usually they do not require surgical intervention.

6.6.3.3 Bowel Perforation

The presence of extraluminal air and the presence of extraluminal contrast agent are the radiological hallmarks of bowel perforation. However, these signs are not always visible.

6.6.3.3.1 Intraperitoneal Perforation. In cases with intraperitoneal perforation free air should

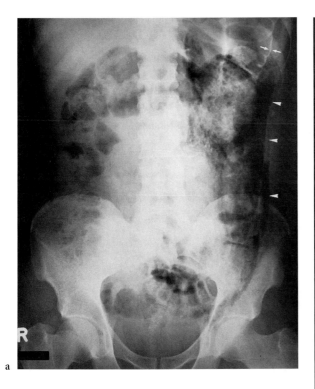
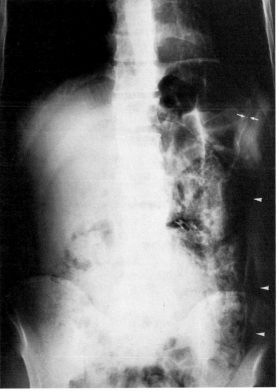

Fig. 6.22a,b. Twenty-four year old patient who was stabbed in the left flank. Plain films shows evidence of left colonic perforation with free air in the retroperitoneal space (*arrowheads*) evidenced by a positive Rigler sign in the area of the left colonic flexure (*arrows*). **a** Supine, **b** erect film. Radiological findings were confirmed at surgery

be carefully searched for on wide CT windows. Preferred localisations are over the liver surface and in the mid-abdomen. Occasionally there will be massive extravasation of oral contrast through the perforation. In some instances only the presence of focal bowel wall thickening may hint at the diagnosis of perforation. Focal mesenteric infiltration together with a large amount of free intraperitoneal fluid must also be considered an indicator of perforation.

6.6.3.3.2 Retroperitoneal Perforation. In retroperitoneal perforation the collection of gas and/or contrast agent may be found in locations adjacent to the perforated hollow organ. In duodenal perforation this is usually the anterior pararenal space (Fig. 6.21). Perforation or hematoma of the large bowel is rare, with the transverse colon, the sigmoid, and the cecum being the most common sites of injury (Fig. 6.22). Sometimes the "sentinel clot sign" may offer a clue as to the localization of suspected perforations.

6.6.3.4 Mesenteric Laceration

Mesenteric lacerations usually occur in massive abdominal trauma. Due to laceration of the mesenteric artery or vein there is severe intraperitoneal bleeding, which in most cases will lead to emergency laparotomy. CT signs include: the presence of hemoperitoneum, a high-density hematoma in the mesenteric root ("sentinel clot sign") (ORWIG and

FEDERLE 1989), and often lack of injury to other organs. Rarely is there direct evidence of contrast extravasation from mesenteric vessels on dynamic contrast-enhanced CT (Fig. 6.23).

6.6.3.5 Posttraumatic Infection

Patients after blunt and especially penetrating abdominal trauma have an increased risk of developing peritonitis. Thickening of the bowel walls, the peritoneum, and the retroperitoneal fascia are signs of infection, as well as the presence of peritoneal fluid. Abscess formation occurs frequently, and interventional radiological drainage has been reported to be helpful in this setting (Fig. 6.24).

6.6.3.6 Posttraumatic Invagination

Traumatic diaphragmatic hernias are sometimes diagnosed by CT. These can be the origin of herniation of bowel or mesentery (GELMAN et al. 1991).

6.6.4 Impact of Computed Tomography on Diagnosis of Injuries to the Mesentery and the Bowel

In the largest study on this subject, Rizzo and colleagues described their experience in 51 patients with suspected bowel or mesenteric injuries after blunt

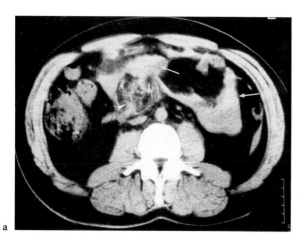

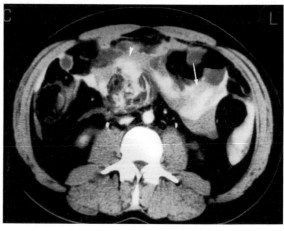

a

b

Fig. 6.23a,b. CT in a 37-year-old male with laceration of the mesenteric root following blunt abdominal trauma. **a** Unenhanced CT shows high-density intraperitoneal blood (*arrows*) and a hematoma in the mesenteric root (*arrowhead*). **b** Contrast-enhanced CT shows high-density contrast agent in the location of the mesenteric root (*arrowhead*) and another contrast collection within the peritoneal cavity (*arrow*) as evidence for active bleeding from the lacerated mesenteric root

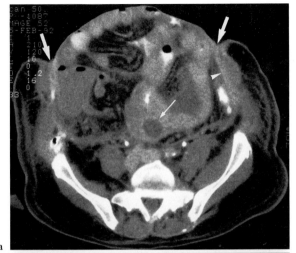

a

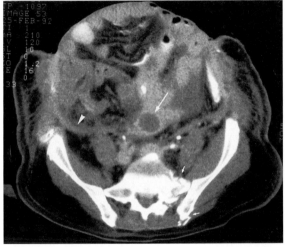

b

Fig. 6.24a,b. Peritonitis and intraperitoneal abscess in a patient after severe blunt trauma. Contrast-enhanced CT shows an abdominal wall defect (*large thick arrows*) resulting from trauma and repeated surgical interventions because of serious mesenteric and bowel injuries. There is thickening of the peritoneum (*arrowheads*) as well as free intraperitoneal fluid. Adjacent to a small bowel loop, there is also an abscess with peripheral rim enhancement (*large thin arrows*). Note fractures of the sacrum and ilium on the left (*small arrows*)

abdominal trauma. Twenty-eight patients underwent laparotomy. CT enabled confirmation of surgically found injuries in 93%. CT findings that correlated with the need for surgery in bowel and mesenteric injury were: free peritoneal fluid (96%), mesenteric infiltration (86%), thick-walled bowel (61%), associated abdominal injuries (43%), and free air (32%). In nonsurgical cases the incidence of bowel wall thickening was 84%, but the incidence of free intraperitoneal fluid was only 21%, that of mesenteric infiltration, 26%, and that of associated injuries, 5% (Rizzo et al. 1989). The authors concluded

that CT helps to distinguish surgical from nonsurgical cases and thereby reduces the rate of nontherapeutic laparotomies. This conclusion is not universally accepted, however, and one study from the surgical literature reported a low sensitivity for CT in this clinical setting which was surpassed by that of DPL (MEREDITH and TRUNKEY 1988).

6.7 Vascular Injury

Vascular injuries to the abdomen may be caused by blunt and penetrating trauma. Most of these injuries will never be evaluated by means of radiological methods because these patients undergo immediate surgical exploration. Nevertheless, there are a number of injuries that are usually diagnosed radiologically and are suitable for primary interventional radiological treatment.

6.7.1 Classification of Abdominal Vascular Injury

Abdominal vascular injuries can be divided into those involving the aorta or its branches and those involving the venous system.

6.7.1.1 Arterial Vascular Injuries

Among arterial injuries, laceration of the aorta and avulsion of its major branches are the most severe forms (Fig. 6.25). These injuries need immediate surgical treatment and time rarely allows the performance of imaging studies.

Occlusion of an artery due to an intimal tear is a rare entity that presents as acute occlusion and not as hemorrhage (Fig. 6.26). These cases also require surgical treatment, but imaging will have been performed preoperatively and in most cases a diagnosis is already at hand.

6.7.1.2 Venous Vascular Injuries

The most severe venous injuries are those to the vena cava inferior. These are subdivided into retrohepatic, suprarenal, pararenal, and infrarenal ones. The retrohepatic injuries show the highest mortality, with the overall mortality for these injuries being between 33% and 66%. Imaging diagnoses are rarely made prior to surgery in these often hemodynamically unstable patients (KLEIN et al. 1994).

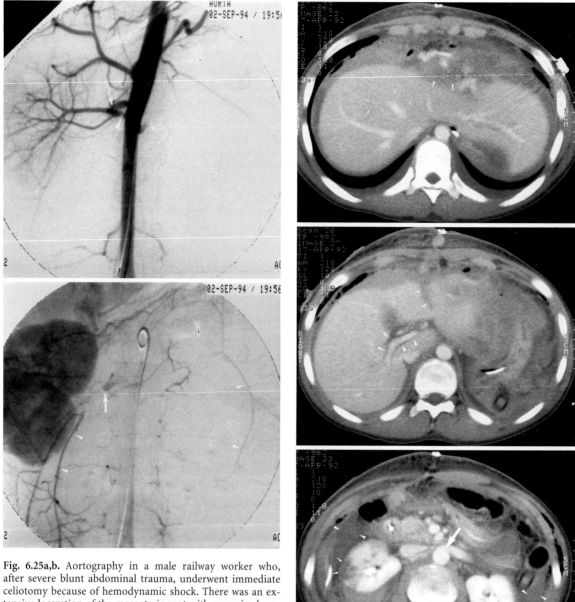

Fig. 6.25a,b. Aortography in a male railway worker who, after severe blunt abdominal trauma, underwent immediate celiotomy because of hemodynamic shock. There was an extensive laceration of the mesenteric root with excessive hemorrhage that could only be controlled by resection of parts of the small bowel and abdominal packing. **a** Control angiogram after surgery showed filling of only the proximal 2 cm of the SMA (*arrow*) with abrupt ending. The same was found in the left renal artery (*small arrow*). Note severe narrowing of the right renal artery due to spasm (*arrowhead*). Later film from the same injection (**b**) shows filling of the ileocolic artery and the right and transverse colonic arteries via collaterals (*arrowheads*), but no evidence of small bowel perfusion). There is no contrast agent in the left kidney. Intraoperative findings during second surgery confirmed the dissection of the SMA and left renal artery and a nephrectomy was performed. Contrary to what was expected from the angiographic findings, the small bowel showed no sign of necrosis and no further resection was necessary

Fig. 6.26a–f. Liver laceration, periportal tracking, and traumatic aortic dissection. **a,b** Contrast-enhanced CT shows a large liver laceration with an infarction in liver segments IV and III (*arrows*). In addition there is periportal tracking (*arrowheads*) and perihepatic fluid. **c** A scan at the level of the renal arteries shows normal contrast enhancement in the aortic lumen (*arrow*), right renal infarctions (*small arrows*), and free intraperitoneal fluid (*arrowheads*). **d** An infrarenal scan shows no contrast enhancement in the aortic lumen (*arrow*). **e,f** Aortography via the brachial artery shows the occlusion of the infrarenal aorta (*arrow*) and filling of the iliac arteries via collaterals (*arrowheads*). On surgery an intimal dissection was found to be the reason for the aortic occlusion

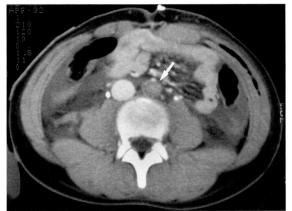

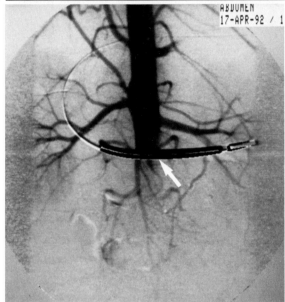

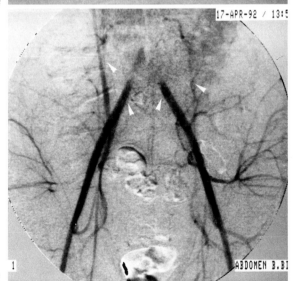

Fig. 6.26d–f

Organ lacerations with extravasation from either the liver, the spleen, the mesenterium, or the kidneys make up a group of cases that are suitable for both surgical and radiological treatments.

A different group consists of patients who are initially stable but develop symptoms days or weeks after the initial trauma. These are the patients who develop complications of traumatic arteriovenous fistulas, pseudoaneurysms, or hemobilia.

6.7.2 Intra-abdominal Hemorrhage: Detection and Treatment

6.7.2.1 Detection of Intraperitoneal Hemorrhage

The primary radiological method for patients with blunt abdominal trauma is contrast-enhanced CT. As previously mentioned, CT is very sensitive in detecting intraperitoneal hemorrhage and often provides information concerning the source of the hemorrhage. It is also of value in the detection of active intra-abdominal arterial hemorrhage, as was shown by Jeffrey and colleagues. They reported on 18 patients in whom active bleeding occurred during the CT examination and concluded that CT is valuable in the diagnosis and localization of active bleeding (see Fig. 6.23). Furthermore, it facilitates the decision on whether surgery or TCE is the preferred method of treatment (JEFFREY et al. 1991).

After CT, angiography can usually be limited to the area identified as the source of hemorrhage. In cases with continuing blood loss and no evident demonstration of a source, the angiographic study has to take all possible sources into consideration. The first step should therefore be an abdominal aortogram, preferentially using a cut-film technique. The films should be centered at the midline and include the diaphragm. This will already exclude aortic pathologies and avulsion of large aortic branches as well as major renal trauma. The complete angiographic workup includes injections in the celiac trunk and a superior mesenteric artery injection. Some authors also perform splenic artery injections. Inferior mesenteric angiograms might become necessary when the other studies are negative and the trauma to the abdomen is low in position.

6.7.2.2 Angiographic Signs of Hepatic and Splenic Injury

In the following, the angiographic signs of hepatic and splenic rupture will be discussed briefly. In the liver, the common hepatic artery or its branches may be displaced by hematomas. Pseudoaneurysms may be present. Other signs include leakage of contrast agent into the liver parenchyma or a mottled appearance of the parenchymal angiographic phase with delayed arterial emptying. AV fistulae between the hepatic artery and the portal vein branches may form, as may connections between the hepatic arteries and the bile ducts. The angiographic findings of splenic injury include extravasation of contrast agent from the splenic arteries in the splenic pulp, early filling of splenic veins during the arterial phase, displacement or occlusion of intrasplenic arteries due to hematomas, and irregular areas of contrast enhancement within infarcted areas or areas with a hematoma (SCHORN and COLN 1977; REUTER et al. 1986; TEITELBAUM et al. 1994).

6.7.2.3 Principles of TCE

Transcatheter embolization (TCE) should only be performed by specially trained interventional radiologists due to the possible harm caused by these procedures if they are not performed properly. Besides having a thorough knowledge of vascular anatomy and pathology, the interventional radiologist should be familiar with the wide array of catheters, embolization materials, and techniques. The latter include hemostatic sponges, coils, balloons, microfibrillar collagen, autologous blood clot, and intentional arterial dissection. Generally, a superselective approach to the target vessel should be the goal in order to save as much viable tissue as possible and to prevent possible side-effects of embolotherapy. A detailed review is beyond the scope of this article. Close cooperation with the surgical team is of utmost importance during TCE in these heavily injured patients who will often require permanent monitoring due to other injuries.

6.7.2.4 TCE of Splenic Hemorrhage

In their series of hemodynamically stable patients with splenic extravasation at angiography, SCLAFANI et al. (1991) reported that TCE of the proximal splenic artery, just distal to the dorsal pancreatic artery, with steel coils showed an excellent success rate in controlling the contrast extravasation. There was no case of splenic infarction or abscess formation in their series; these have been reported to have a high

incidence in distal embolizations, which should therefore be avoided (SCLAFANI et al. 1991).

6.7.2.5 TCE of Hepatic Hemorrhage

Transcatheter embolization in the liver is safer than in the spleen due to the liver's dual blood supply by the hepatic artery and the portal vein. TCE is indicated in cases where the surgical attempt to control the hemorrhage has failed or in cases with arteriovenous fistulas (TEITELBAUM et al. 1994; KAUDE et al. 1969). All embolization procedures should be carried out from a superselective approach using coaxial catheter systems (TEITELBAUM et al. 1994). A report from the literature cited a success rate of 88% for TCE in achieving hemorrhage control in cases of hepatic vascular trauma (SCHWARTZ et al. 1991) (see Fig. 6.9).

6.8 Diaphragmatic Rupture

6.8.1 Types of Diaphragmatic Rupture

The preoperative diagnosis of traumatic diaphragmatic rupture (TDR) is difficult. It may be due to either blunt or penetrating abdominal trauma. From the literature it is known that while 84% of TDRs in penetrating trauma are smaller than 2 cm, the majority in blunt traumas measure more than 10 cm (WISE et al. 1973). The incidence of TDR in blunt trauma is between 0.8% and 1.6% (KEARNEY et al. 1989). TDR can be divided into acute, delayed, and chronic forms (SOLA et al. 1994). Left-sided TDR is encountered clinically far more often than right-sided TDR. This was originally thought to be due to the protective effect of the liver; however, today it is known from autopsy reports that the incidence is actually identical for both sides, but right-sided TDRs are associated with more rapidly fatal injuries. The clinical diagnosis of TDR is exceedingly difficult due to the fact that symptoms are often unspecific and the patients usually have other injuries that mask the TDR. The diagnosis is missed initially in 7%–66% of patients (GELMAN et al. 1991). DPL also proves unreliable, with a false-negative rate of up to 21% in addition to a false-positive rate of 25% (GELMAN et al. 1991).

6.8.2 Diagnosis of Diaphragmatic Injuries

Gelman and colleagues analyzed the sensitivity of plain chest radiographs in 44 patients with left-

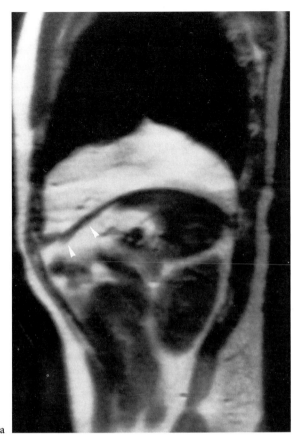

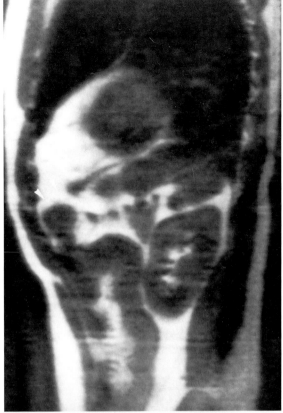

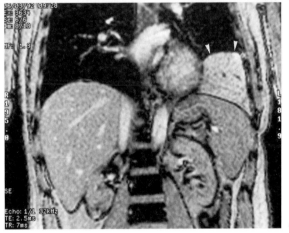

Fig. 6.27a–c. Late posttraumatic left diaphragmatic hernia. MRI 10 years after blunt thoracoabdominal trauma due to a car accident showed a left anterior rupture of the diaphragm with herniation of omental fat in the thoracic cage. Sagittal T1-weighted SE scans show the intact (**a**) and defective (**b**) anterior diaphragm (*arrowheads*). **c** Coronal gradient echo scan shows the intact diaphragm dorsal to the defect as well as the herniated omental fat (*arrowheads*)

sided TDR and six patients with right-sided TDR. Diagnostic or strongly suggestive findings were the presence of air-containing viscera above the hemidiaphragm, which was the most specific sign. This was followed by the presence of the tip of the nasogastric tube above the hemidiaphragm, elevation of the hemidiaphragm not due to atelectasis, and obliteration of a nonelevated hemidiaphragm. These criteria enabled retrospective detection of TDR in 64% of the cases. The diagnosis of right-sided TDR was possible in only one of the six

patients. The authors suggest follow-up radiographs in uncertain cases (GELMAN et al. 1991). In cases with further diagnostic doubt, MRI is currently considered the method of choice due to its multiplanar scanning capabilities (Fig. 6.27). However, to date, no larger series exists to corroborate this opinion. Other methods applied in the workup of TDR are radiographs after nasogastric tube placement, fluoroscopy, gastrointestinal tract contrast examinations, US, CT, peritoneography (using either contrast or air), and liver–spleen

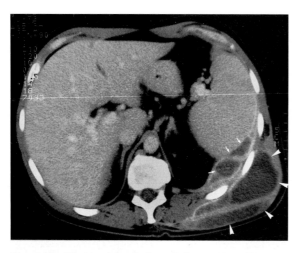

Fig. 6.28. CT in abdominal wall hematoma. Contrast-enhanced CT shows a hematoma in the abdominothoracic wall (*arrows*) and in the posterior pararenal space (*arrowheads*) several days after blunt abdominal trauma. The hematomas show peripheral enhancement due to beginning resorption

scinthigraphy (AMMANN et al. 1983; MIRVIS et al. 1988).

6.9 Abdominal Wall Injuries

Injuries to the abdominal wall include subcutaneous and intramuscular hematomas, and different types of posttraumatic hernias.

Ultrasonography and CT are both appropriate modalities for the detection of abdominal wall hematomas. Fresh hematomas show high density on unenhanced CT scans. Their density varies with age (Fig. 6.28).

Posttraumatic abdominal wall and other hernias may develop, the rarest of which are the intercostal hernias after traumatic diaphragmatic rupture and traumatic lumbar hernias. The CT appearance of both these hernias has been described in the literature (SERPELL and JOHNSON 1994; ESPOSITO and FEDORAK 1994). Diaphragmatic hernias with hernation into the pericardium have been encountered (FAGAN et al. 1979).

6.10 Diagnostic Algorithms

Figures 6.29 and 6.30 show diagnostic algorithms that summarize the information given in this chapter on the appropriate diagnostic response to blunt and penetrating abdominal trauma.

6.11 Summary

The role of radiology has changed dramatically during the last 15 years and a more active function has been assigned to the radiologist, who is now a consistent member of the trauma team in most centers. The central diagnostic tool in hemodynamically stable patients is contrast-enhanced CT, which currently allows the detection of visceral, bowel, and mesenteric injuries. In addition, it detects and quantitates intraperitoneal hemorrhage and is thus a rival to DPL. DPL is used as a triage modality in hemodynamically unstable patients because of the speed, safety, and ease of performance. The role for US is limited in most centers to fast assessment of the presence of hemoperitoneum; only a few centers rely on it for the diagnosis of visceral injuries. In selected cases interventional radiology may allow control of a hemorrhage that is very difficult to control surgically as well as the preservation of viable tissue, which is of special importance in the spleen and the kidneys. The trauma radiologist of the 1990s must be fully trained not only in plain film diagnosis and cross-sectional imaging but also in interventional radiology. Assuming that this prerequisite is met, he will play an active role in both the diagnosis and the treatment of patients with abdominal trauma.

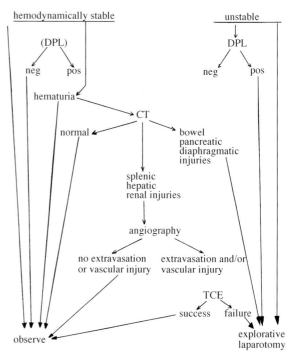

Fig. 6.29. Diagnostic algorithm for cases of blunt abdominal trauma (modified from SCLAFANI et al. 1991)

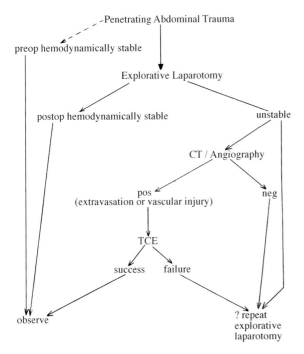

Fig. 6.30. Diagnostic algorithm for cases of penetrating abdominal trauma (modified from TEITELBAUM et al. 1994)

Acknowledgement. I wish to acknowledge the excellent photographic work of Ms. Ursula Schad and Ms. Susanne Hess, both photographers in the Department of Medical Radiology, University Hospital Zurich. University Hospital Zurich, Switzerland.

References

Ammann AM, Brewer WH, Maull KI, Walsh JW (1983) Traumatic rupture of the diaphragm: real-time sonographic diagnosis. AJR 140:915–916

Anderson CB, Ballinger WF (1985) Abdominal injuries. In: Zuidema GD, Rutherford RB, Ballinger WF (eds) The management of trauma, 4th edn. Saunders, Philadelphia

Aragon G, Eiseman G (1976) Abdominal stab wounds: evaluation of sinography. J Trauma 16:792–797

Berk RN (1970) Changing concepts in the plain film diagnosis of ruptured spleen. J Can Assoc Radiol 21:67–70

Buntain WL, Gould HR, Maull KI (1985) Splenic trauma in children and techniques of splenic salvage. World J Surg 9:398–409

Buntain WL, Gould HR, Maull KI (1988) Predictability of splenic salvage by computed tomography. J Trauma 28:24–31

Caride VJ, Gibson DW (1982) Noninvasive evaluation of bile leakage. Surg Gynecol Obstet 154:517–520

Croce MA, Fabian TC, Kudsk KA, Baum SL, Payne LW, Mangiante EC, Britt LG (1991) AAST organ injury scale: correlation with ct-graded liver injuries and operative findings. J Trauma 31:806–812

Cullen DJ, Civetta JM, Briggs BA et al. (1984) Therapeutic intervention scoring system: a method of quantitative comparison of patient care. Crit Care Med 2:57–63

Darling JD, Flickinger FW (1990) Splenosis mimicking neoplasm in the perirenal space: CT characteristics. J Comput Assist Tomogr 14:839–841

Demetriades D, Rabinowitz B (1987) Indications for operation in abdominal stab wounds: a prospective study of 651 patients. Ann Surg 205:129–132

Donahue JH, Crass R, Trunkey DD (1985) Management of duodenal and small intestinal injury. World J Surg 9:904–913

Donahue JH, Federle MP, Griffiths BG, Trunkey DD (1987) Computed tomography in the diagnosis of blunt intestinal and mesenteric injury. J Trauma 27:11–17

Ellis H, Kronin K (1960) Bile peritonitis. Br J Surg 48:166–171

Eng RHK, Tecson-Tumang F, Corrado ML (1981) Blunt trauma and liver abscess. Am J Gastroenterol 76:252–255

Erb RE, Mirvis SE, Shanmuganathan K (1994) Gallbladder injury secondary to blunt trauma: CT findings. J Comput Assist Tomogr 18:778–784

Esposito TJ, Fedorak I (1994) Traumatic lumbar hernia: case report and literature review. J Trauma 37:123–126

Fabian TC, Mangiante EC, White TJ et al. (1986) A prospective study of 91 patients undergoing both computed tomography and peritoneal lavage following blunt abdominal trauma. J Trauma 26:602–608

Fagan CJ, Schreiber MH, Amparo EG, Wysong CB (1979) Traumatic diaphragmatic hernia into the pericardium: verification of diagnosis by computed tomography. J Comput Assist Tomogr 3:405–408

Federle MP, Jeffrey RB (1983) Hemoperitoneum studied by computed tomography. Radiology 148:187–192

Federle MP, Griffiths B, Minagi H et al. (1987) Splenic trauma: evaluation with CT. Radiology 162:69–71

Foley WD (1989) Dynamic hepatic CT scanning. Radiology 170:617–622

Foley WD (1994) Abdominal trauma. In: Freeny PC, Stevenson GW (ed) Margulis and Burhenne's alimentary tract radiology, 5th edn. Mosby, St. Louis, pp 2120–2142

Foley WD, Cates JD, Kellman GM et al. (1987) Treatment of blunt hepatic injuries: role of CT. Radiology 164:635–638

Gay SB, Sistrom CL (1992) Computed tomographic evaluation of blunt abdominal trauma. Radiol Clin North Am 30:367–388

Gelman R, Mirvis SE, Gens D (1991) Diaphragmatic rupture due to blunt trauma: sensitivity of plain chest radiographs. AJR 156:51–57

Glazer GM, Buy JN, Moss AA, Goldberg HI, Federle MP (1981) CT detection of duodenal perforation. AJR 137:333–336

Goldstein AS, Sclafani SJA, Kupferstein NH et al. (1986) The diagnostic superiority of computerized tomography. J Trauma 25:938–946

Goletti O, Ghiselli G, Lippolis PV et al. (1994) The role of ultrasonography in blunt abdominal trauma: results in 250 consecutive cases. J Trauma 36:179–181

Gomez GA, Alvarez R, Plasencia G et al. (1987) Diagnostic peritoneal lavage in the management of blunt abdominal trauma: a reassessment. J Trauma 27:1–5

Goodman LR, Aprahamanian C (1990) Changes in splenic size after abdominal trauma. Radiology 176:629–632

Gould HR, Buntain WL, Maull KI (1988) Imaging in blunt abdominal trauma. In: Advances in trauma. Year Book, Chicago, pp 53–99

Hagspiel KD (1994) Schmerzen im linken Oberbauch. In: Krestin GP (ed) Akutes Abdomen. Thieme, Stuttgart, New York, pp 48–59

Hagspiel KD, Krestin GP (1994) Diffuse abdominelle Schmerzen. In: Krestin GP (ed) Akutes abdomen. Thieme, Stuttgart, pp 89–105

Haney PJ, Whitley NO, Brotman S, Cunat JS, Whitley J (1982) Liver injury and complications in the postoperative trauma patient: CT evaluation. AJR 139:271–275

Heller M, Jend HH, Guertler KF, Lambrecht W (1982) Computertomographische Diagnostik traumatischer Milzlaesionen. Fortschr Roentgenstr 136:243–247

Hoffman R, Nerlich M, Muggia-Sullam L et al. (1992) Blunt abdominal trauma in cases with multiple trauma evaluated by ultrasonography: a prospective analysis in 291 patients. J Trauma 32:452–457

Jeffrey RB, Federle MP (1988) The collapsed inferior vena cava: CT evidence of hypovolemia. AJR 150:431–432

Jeffrey RB, Laing FC, Federle MP et al. (1981) Computed tomography of splenic trauma. Radiology 141:729–732

Jeffrey RB, Federle MP, Laing FC, Wing VW (1986) Computed tomography of blunt trauma to the gallbladder. J Comput Assist Tomogr 10:756–758

Jeffrey RB, Cardoza JD, Olcott EW (1991) Detection of active intraabdominal arterial hemorrhage: value of dynamic contrast-enhanced CT. AJR 156:725–729

Kaude J, Dudgeon DL, Talbert JL (1969) The role of selective angiography in the diagnosis and treatment of hepatoportal arteriovenous fistula. Radiology 92:1271–1272

Kearney PA, Rouhana SW, Burney RE (1989) Blunt rupture of the diaphragm: mechanism, diagnosis and treatment. Ann Emerg Med 18:1326–1330

Kim EE, McConnell BJ, McConnel RW et al. (1983) Radionuclide diagnosis of diaphramatic rupture with hepatic herniation. Surgery 94:36–40

Kinnunen J, Kivioja A, Poussa K, Laasonen EM (1994) Emergency CT in blunt abdominal trauma of multiple injury patients. Acta Radiologica 35:319–322

Klein SR, Baumgartner FJ, Bongard FS (1994) Contemporary management strategy for major inferior vena caval injuries. J Trauma 37:35–41

Kirks DR, Caron KH (1991) Gastrointestinal tract – trauma. In: Kirks DR (ed) Practical pediatric imaging. Little, Brown & Co, Boston, pp 823–840

Lorimer JW, Reid KR, Raymond F (1994) Blunt extraperitoneal rupture of the right hemidiaphragm: case report. J Trauma 36:414–416

Macrander SJ, Lawson TL, Foley WD, Dodds WJ, Erickson SJ, Quiroz FA (1989) Periportal tracking in hepatic trauma: CT features. J Comput Assist Tomogr 13:952–957

Marx JA, Moore EE, Jorden RC, Eule J (1985) Limitations of computed tomography in the evaluation of acute abdominal trauma. A prospective comparison with diagnostic peritoneal lavage. J Trauma 25:933–937

Maynard A, Oropeza G (1968) Mandatory operation for penetrating wounds of the abdomen. Am J Surg 115:307–312

Meredith JW, Trunkey DD (1988) CT scanning in acute abdominal injuries. Surg Clin North Am 68:255–268

Meredith JW, Young JS, Bowling J, Roboussin D (1994) Nonoperative management of blunt hepatic trauma: the exception or the rule? J Trauma 36:529–534

Meyer AA, Crass RA, Lim RC, Jeffrey RB, Federle MP et al. (1985) Selective nonoperative management of blunt liver injury using computed tomography. Arch Surg 120:550–554

Meyer DM, Thal ER, Weigelt JA et al. (1989) Evaluation of computed tomography and diagnostic peritoneal lavage in blunt abdominal trauma. J Trauma 29:1168–1172

Mirvis SE, Keramati B, Buckman R, Rodriguez A (1988) MR imaging of traumatic diaphragmatic rupture. J Comput Assist Tomogr 12:147–149

Mirvis SE, Whitley NO, Wainwright JR, Gens DR (1989a) Blunt hepatic trauma in adults: CT-based classification and correlation with prognosis and treatment. Radiology 171:27–32

Mirvis SE, Whitley NO, Gens DR (1989b) Blunt splenic trauma in adults: CT-based classification and correlation with prognosis and treatment. Radiology 171:33–39

Moore EE, Moore JB, Van Duzer-Moore S et al. (1980) Mandatory laparatomy for gunshot wounds penetrating the abdomen. Am J Surg 140:847–851

Moore EE, Shackford SR, Pachter HL et al. (1989) Organ injury scaling: spleen, liver, and kidney. J Trauma 29:1664–1666

Mucha P, Daly RC, Farnell MB (1986) Selective management of blunt splenic trauma. J Trauma 26:970–979

Nance FC, Wennar MH, Johnson LW et al. (1974) Surgical judgement in the management of penetrating wounds of the abdomen: experience with 2212 patients. Ann Surg 179:639

Orwig D, Federle MP (1989) Localized clotted blood as evidence of visceral trauma on CT: the sentinel clot sign. AJR 153:747–749

Pappas D, Mirvis SE, Crepps JT (1987) Splenic trauma: false-negative CT diagnosis in cases of delayed rupture. AJR 149:727–728

Pardes JG, Haaga JR, Borkowski G (1982) Focal hepatic fatty metamorphosis secondary to trauma. J Comput Assist Tomogr 6:769–771

Peitzman AB, Makaroun MS, Slasky BS, Ritter P (1986) Prospective study of computed tomography in initial management of blunt abdominal trauma. J Trauma 26:585–592

Penn I (1962) Injuries to the gallbladder. Br J Surg 49:636–642

Phillips CD (1992) Emergent radiologic evaluation of the gunshot wound victim. Radiol Clin North Am 30:307–324

Redmond PJ, Kumpe EA (1988) Embolization of an intrahepatic arterioportal fistula: a case report and review of the literature. Cardiovasc Intervent Radiol 11:274–277

Renz BM, Feliciano DV (1994) Gunshot wound to the right thoracoabdomen: a prospective study of nonoperative management. J Trauma 37:737–744

Resciniti A, Fink MP, Raptopoulos V, Davidoff A, Silva WE (1988) Nonoperative treatment of adult splenic trauma: development of a computed tomographic scoring system that detects appropriate candidates for expectant management. J Trauma 28:828–831

Reuter SR, Redman HC, Cho KJ (1986) Trauma (chapter 5). In: Reuter SR, Redman HC, Cho KJ (eds) Gastrointestinal angiography. Saunders, Philadelphia, pp 248–281

Rizzo MJ, Federle MP, Griffiths BG (1989) Bowel and mesentery injury following blunt abdominal trauma: evaluation with CT. Radiology 173:143–148

Roman E, Silva VS, Lucas C (1971) Management of blunt duodenal injury. Surg Gynecol Obstet 132:7–14

Root HD, Hauser CW, McKinley CR (1965) Diagnostic peritoneal lavage. Surgery 57:633–637

Rosoff L, Cohen JL, Telfer N et al. (1972) Injuries of the spleen. Surg Clin North Am 52:667–685

Scatamacchia SA, Raptopoulos V, Fink MP et al. (1989) Splenic trauma in adults: impact of CT grading on management. Radiology 171:725–729

Schlager D, Lazzaareschi G, Whitten D, Sanders AB (1994) A prospective role of ultrasonography in the ED by emergency physicians. Am J Emerg Med 12:185–189

Schorn L, Coln D (1977) Hepatic angiographic changes after trauma. Am J Surg 134:754–757

Schwartz RA, Teitelbaum GP, Finck EJ, Pentecost MJ (1991) Efficacy of transcatheter embolization in control of hepatic vascular injuries (abstract). Radiology 181(P):128

Sclafani SJA, Weisberg A, Scalea TM, Phillips TF, Duncan AO (1991) Blunt splenic injuries: nonsurgical treatment with CT, arteriography, and transcatheter arterial embolization of the splenic artery. Radiology 181:189–196

Sekikawa T, Shatney C (1983) Septic sequelae after splenetomy for trauma in adults. Am J Surg 145:667–673

Serpell JW, Johnson WR (1994) Traumatic diaphragmatic hernia presenting as an intercostal hernia: case report. J Trauma 36:421–423

Snyder WH III, Weigelt JA, Watkins WL, Bietz DS (1980) The surgical management of duodenal trauma: precepts based on a review of 247 cases. Arch Surg 115:422–429

Soderstrom CA, Maekawa K, Dupriest RW, Cowley RA (1981) Gallbladder injuries resulting from blunt abdominal trauma: an experience and review. Ann Surg 193:60–66

Sola JE, Mattei P, Pegoli W, Paidas CN (1994) Rupture of the right diaphragm following blunt trauma in an infant: case report. J Trauma 36:417–420

Stalker HP, Kaufman RA, Towbin R (1986) Patterns of liver injury in childhood: CT analysis. AJR 147:1199–1205

Tarazov PG (1993) Intrahepatic arterioportal fistulae: role of transcatheter embolization. Cardiovasc Intervent Radiol 16:368–373

Teitelbaum GP, Katz MD, Sclafani SJA (1994) Arteriography and therapeutic embolization in abdominal trauma. In: Freeny PC, Stevenson GW (eds) Margulis and Burhenne's alimentary tract radiology, 5th edn. Mosby, St. Louis, p 2143

Todesursachen Statistik 1991 (1992) Info. Bundesamt fuer Statistik, Abteilung Bevölkerung und Beschäftigung, Sektion Gesundheit. Bern

Toombs BD, Sandler CM, Rauschkolb EN, Strax R, Harle TS (1982) Assessment of hepatic injuries with computed tomography. J Comput Assist Tomogr 6:72–75

Trunkey DD (1988) Organization of trauma care. In: Trauma management. Year Book, Chicago, pp 1–10

Umlas S-L, Cronan JJ (1991) Splenic trauma: can CT grading systems enable prediction of successful nonsurgical treatment? Radiology 178:481–487

van Sonnenberg E, Simeone JF, Mueller PR et al. (1983) Sonographic appearance of hematoma in the liver, spleen, and kidney: a clinical, pathologic and animal study. Radiology 147:507–510

Vazquez JL, Thorsen MK, Dodds WJ et al. (1985) Evaluation and treatment of intraabdominal bilomas. AJR 144:933–938

Weissmann HS, Chun KJ, Frank M et al. (1979) Demonstration of traumatic bile leakage with cholescintigraphy and ultrasonography. AJR 133:843–847

Winek T, Moseley H, Grout G, Luallin D (1988) Pneumoperitoneum and its association with ruptured abdominal viscus. Arch Surg 123:709–712

Winsett MZ, Kumar R, Balachandran S et al. (1988) Pseudocysts following splenectomy: impact of CT and ultrasound on its diagnosis and management. Gastrointest Radiol 13:177–179

Wise L, Connors J, Hwang Y, Anderson C (1973) Traumatic injuries to the diaphragm. J Trauma 13:946–950

Zeman RK, Lee CH, Stahl R et al. (1984) Strategy for the use of biliary scintigraphy in non-iatrogenic biliary trauma. Radiology 151:771–777

7 Retroperitoneal Trauma

L. Van Hoe, S. Gryspeerdt, R.H. Oyen, and A.L. Baert

CONTENTS

7.1 Introduction

Injury to retroperitoneal structures can be caused by a variety of blunt, penetrating, and iatrogenic trau-

L. Van Hoe, MD, Department of Radiology, University Hospitals K.U. Leuven, Herestraat 49, 3000 Leuven, Belgium
S. Gryspeerdt, MD, Department of Radiology, University Hospitals K.U. Leuven, Herestraat 49, 3000 Leuven, Belgium
R.H. Oyen, MD, PhD, Professor, Adjunct Clinic Head, Department of Radiology, University Hospitals K.U. Leuven, Herestraat 49, 3000 Leuven, Belgium
A.L. Baert, MD, PhD, Professor and Chairman, Department of Radiology, University Hospitals K.U. Leuven, Herestraat 49, 3000 Leuven, Belgium

mata. While injuries involving the kidney are among the most frequent of all abdominal injuries, injuries of other retroperitoneal structures such as the pancreas, duodenum, adrenal glands, ureter, bladder, and great vessels are relatively uncommon. As in other injuries, early diagnosis and determination of the severity of retroperitoneal injuries is mandatory for optimal treatment selection. Unfortunately, specific symptoms and signs of trauma to a retroperitoneal organ are often absent or delayed (Maull et al. 1987; Lang 1990). Therefore, imaging studies, in particular computed tomography (CT), play an increasingly important role in planning and management of injuries.

7.2 Pancreas

7.2.1 Mechanisms, Mechanics, and Classification

Pancreatic injury is relatively uncommon and accounts for 1%–12% of all abdominal injuries (Jeffrey et al. 1983; Dodds et al. 1990). It may result from penetrating or from blunt trauma. The classic mechanism in blunt pancreatic trauma is a sudden force compressing the pancreatic body or neck against the first lumbar vertebra. In the adult this form of injury most frequently follows motor vehicle accidents, whereas in children bicycle accidents are more common. The clinical diagnosis of acute pancreatic injury can be difficult. Pancreatic injury results in liberation of pancreatic enzymes, autodigestion, and posttraumatic pancreatitis. As a result, pancreatic inflammatory changes evolve over time and the clinical manifestations of a pancreatic injury appear slowly: the patient can remain asymptomatic for hours, days, or even weeks after the injury. Elevated serum amylase levels are found in 14%–71% of patients with blunt pancreatic trauma (Wilson and Moorehead 1991; Berni et al. 1982). High mortality rates (up to 20%) have been reported (Jones 1985; Wilson and Moorehead 1991; Jeffrey et al. 1983). Death is usually due to concurrent major vascular or visceral injury rather than to pancreatic trauma itself (CARR et al. 1989). Organs or structures commonly affected in association with blunt pancreatic injury are: spleen (28%–62%), liver (24%–47%), diaphragm (0%–12%), abdominal vessels (12%–41%), kidney (12%–23%), and duodenum (9%–19%) (COGBILL et al. 1991; JOHANET et al. 1991).

A number of classifications exist to describe pancreatic injuries (LUCAS 1977; JEFFREY 1990). The classification proposed by JEFFREY can be simplified as follows:

Grade I: parenchymal contusion or minor hematoma
Grade II: small parenchymal laceration
Grade III: parenchymal laceration with rupture of the main pancreatic duct
Grade IV: severe crush injury

The most important task in clinical practice is to differentiate between grade I/II lesions and grade III/IV lesions. The reason is that grade I or grade II lesions usually resolve with conservative or minimal surgical treatment (drainage). In the case of a grade III or grade IV lesion (ductal injury), however, surgery is always required, because such injury is associated with a high degree of morbidity unless partial pancreatectomy is performed (STONE et al. 1990; SUKUL et al. 1992; CARR et al. 1989). A distal pancreatectomy is used for injuries involving the distal 80% of the pancreas. If the injury involves the proximal 20% of the pancreas (pancreatic head), pancreatoduodenectomy may be required, particularly in cases of severe pancreatic crush or devascularization.

7.2.2 Examination Methods

7.2.2.1 Ultrasonography

Most authors agree that ultrasonography (US) is not as accurate as state of the art CT for detection of small pancreatic injuries (JEFFREY et al. 1986). However, pancreatic injuries can be detected using US if the pancreas is clearly visible (VAN STEENBERGEN et al. 1987; GOTHI et al. 1993) (Fig. 7.1a). US also can be useful in identifying the development of a pancreatic pseudocyst in patients with previous pancreatic injury.

7.2.2.2 Computed Tomography

Because pancreatic injuries are relatively rare, the sensitivity and specificity of CT for detection of the different types of pancreatic injury are not well known. False-negative CT studies have been described in the literature (JEFFREY et al. 1983; SIVIT et al. 1992a; COOK et al. 1986). In the acute phase of the injury, detection of parenchymal laceration or contusion may be difficult because the affected paren-

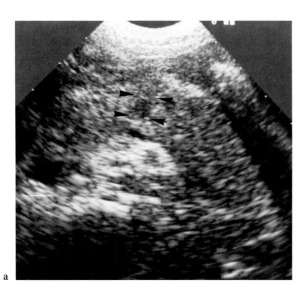
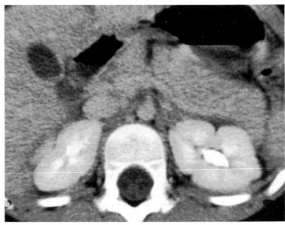

Fig. 7.1a,b. US and CT features in main pancreatic duct rupture. **a** US showing a band-like hypoechoic lesion involving the entire thickness of the pancreatic gland at the junction of the pancreatic neck and pancreatic body (*arrowheads*). **b** CT reveals a hypodense band-like lesion in the same area

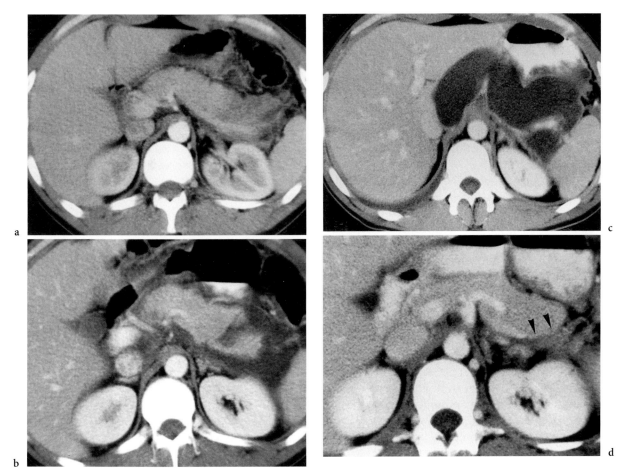

Fig. 7.2a–d. Utility of repeated CT in the detection of pancreatic duct rupture. **a** Contrast-enhanced CT study obtained 2 h after blunt abdominal trauma. The pancreatic tail is hypodense relative to the pancreatic body. However, a fracture line cannot be demonstrated. **b** Contrast-enhanced CT image obtained 3 days later. The laceration of the pancreatic tail is clearly demonstrated, due to separation of the fractured fragments. This scan also shows an important fluid collection in the left anterior pararenal space. **c** Follow-up study 2 weeks later shows a large pseudocyst in the omental bursa. **d** Image obtained 2 months later, after percutaneous drainage of the pseudocyst: there is only limited residual infiltration of the peripancreatic fat (*arrowheads*)

chyma may be nearly isodense to the surrounding parenchyma, and there may be little separation of fractured pancreatic fragments. When a repeat CT examination is performed after 12 or 24 h, pancreatic injury may be easier to detect, probably because of more extensive intra- and peripancreatic hemorrhage and secondary pancreatitis (Fig. 7.2). Direct signs of pancreatic trauma may be particularly difficult to identify on CT in children (SIVIT et al. 1992a). This may be attributed in part to the relative paucity of surrounding retroperitoneal fat and the smallness of the organ.

Despite the previously reported limitations of CT in the detection of pancreatic injuries, a recent report described a sensitivity of 100% (LANE et al. 1994). A further improvement in the detection of small pan-

creatic lesions can be expected with the introduction of spiral (helical) scanners, because this technique allows scanning of the entire pancreas during the phase of "peak" parenchymal enhancement after intravenous (IV) contrast injection. Besides scan speed, other important technical factors for optimization of lesion detection are a sufficiently low slice thickness (e.g., 5 mm), rapid injection of IV contrast material (e.g., 3–4 ml/s), and adequate bowel opacification (COOK et al. 1986).

7.2.2.3 Magnetic Resonance Imaging

Magnetic resonance imaging (MRI) currently has no role in the clinical setting of acute pancreatic trauma.

In the future, MR cholangiopancreatography may become a valuable noninvasive alternative to endoscopic retrograde cholangiopancreatography (ERCP) in the diagnosis of pancreatic duct rupture in stable patients (Soto et al. 1994).

7.2.2.4 Endoscopic Retrograde Cholangiopancreatography

The importance of pre- and intraoperative endoscopic cholangiopancreatography for the staging of pancreatic injury resides in the fact that (a) demonstration of pancreatic duct anatomy is the most important element guiding the therapeutic approach and (b) pancreatic duct injury can be missed on CT (Blind et al. 1994; Barkin et al. 1988; Stone et al. 1990). Several authors have suggested that an ERCP should be performed in stable trauma patients with suspected pancreatic injury; intraoperative cholangiopancreatography can be helpful in unstable patients who require emergency surgery (Johanet et al. 1991; Blind et al. 1994; Barkin et al. 1988; Lewis et al. 1993). Berni et al. (1982) noticed a significant decrease in postoperative morbidity following the introduction of intraoperative pancreatography. ERCP also aids in the treatment of late complications by delineating ductal anatomy (Stone et al. 1990).

7.2.3 Trauma Pattern

7.2.3.1 Ultrasonography

Pancreatic lacerations appear as hypoechoic band-like lesions that are usually located in the neck of the pancreas (Van Steenbergen et al. 1987; Gothi et al. 1993) (Fig. 7.1a). The sonographic demonstration of pancreatic duct rupture has also been reported (Gothi et al. 1993).

7.2.3.2 Computed Tomography

A pancreatic contusion may be seen as a hypodense area after administration of intravenous contrast medium. Usually, the CT picture is dominated by the signs of secondary pancreatitis: peripancreatic fluid, focal enlargement, increased density of the anterior pararenal fat, and thickening of the perirenal fascia (Jeffrey et al. 1983; Sivit et al. 1992a). Lane et al. (1994) stressed the importance of recognizing fluid

between the splenic vein and the pancreas. This sign was seen on CT scans in 90% of patients with pancreatic trauma.

A pancreatic laceration (fracture) most frequently involves the pancreatic neck or body ventral to the lumbar spine. It is seen as a hypodense line, nearly always oriented perpendicular to the long axis of the pancreas (Figs. 7.1b, 7.3a). The fracture may be very thin and hardly visible. Associated features are infiltration of the peripancreatic fat and thickening of the left anterior perirenal fascia (Dodds et al. 1990). The pancreatic parenchyma surrounding the fracture line usually does not show any changes in density (Douws et al. 1994). Rupture of the pancreatic duct is not directly visible. It can be suspected when a laceration is demonstrated that involves the entire thickness of the pancreas (Figs. 7.1b, 7.3a). Moreover, the presence of peripancreatic fluid collections may be a useful marker for major ductal injury (Sivit et al. 1992a). However, as mentioned above, a normal appearance of the pancreas on CT does not exclude the presence of pancreatic duct rupture, particularly if the study is performed early after trauma.

7.2.3.3 Endoscopic Retrograde Cholangiopancreatography

In the acute setting, the diagnosis of the rupture of the pancreatic duct is easy and is based on demonstration of extravasation of contrast material (Berni et al. 1982). ERCP and intraoperative cholangiopancreatography show not only the presence but also the exact location of the disruption of the duct, which aids in the selection of the optimal surgical approach. Although the classic site of pancreatic injury lies over the vertebral column, ductal rupture can occur in any of the anatomical subdivisions of the gland and more than one region may be involved (Carr et al. 1989). ERCP can also be used for evaluation of pancreatic duct integrity in patients with relapsing pancreatitis or pseudocyst formation after blunt pancreatic injury. In these patients, continued leakage or stricutre formation can be demonstrated (Fig. 7.3b,c).

7.2.4 Follow-up and Late Complications

Injury to the main pancreatic duct is the principal determinant of the development of significant complications after pancreatic injury (Sivit et al. 1992a). The presence of pseudocysts, abscesses, and fistulae

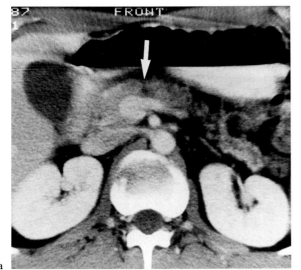

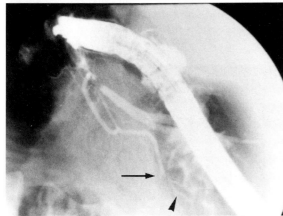

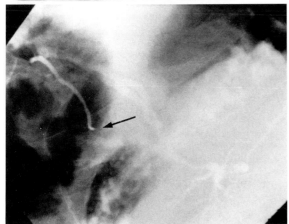

Fig. 7.3a–c. ERCP in pancreatic duct rupture. **a** CT scan because of relapsing pancreatitis 2 years after blunt abdominal trauma. Fracture line at the junction of the pancreatic neck and pancreatic body involving the entire thickness of the parenchyma suggests (previous) duct rupture (*white arrow*). There is atrophy of the pancreas distal to the tear. **b** Anteroposterior and **c** lateral views during ERCP display the occlusion of the main pancreatic duct (*arrows*). Note filling of side branches of the pancreatic duct (*arrowhead*). (Courtesy of E. Ponette)

on follow-up studies suggests continued leakage and thus rupture of the pancreatic duct. In one series, pseudocysts occurred in 36% of patients with pancreatic injury (SIVIT et al. 1992a). Another long-term complication of ductal trauma (most common in cases of incomplete duct transection) is fibrosis and stricture formation. This may cause recurrent episodes of acute pancreatitis (CARR et al. 1989). Furthermore, duct stenosis may induce fibrosis and atrophy of the parenchyma, with atrophy of the exo- and endocrine glands (Fig. 7.4). However, functional pancreatic insufficiency is extremely rare after trauma, even after partial pancreatectomy (WILSON and MOOREHEAD 1991). Although the latter procedure is generally considered the treatment modality of choice in many cases of duct rupture, complications are not rare in patients who survive surgery. In a series of 74 patients who were managed by distal pancreatic resection, intra-abdominal abscess was found in 32%, pancreatic fistula in 14%, pancreatitis in 8%, and pseudocyst formation in 3% (COGBILL et al. 1991).

Computed tomography and US play a role not only in the detection and follow-up of complications, but also in the guidance of percutaneous puncture and drainage of posttraumatic pseudocysts (Fig. 7.2c,d). Complications of pseudocyst formation such as secondary infection, spontaneous perforation, and massive hemorrhage can be avoided by percutaneous drainage (JAFFE et al. 1989).

7.3 Duodenum

7.3.1 Mechanisms

Duodenal injury occurs in approximately 4% of all patients with abdominal trauma (ASENSIO et al. 1993). Overall, penetrating injuries are the most common cause of duodenal trauma. The second and third parts of the duodenum are most commonly affected. The mid duodenum crosses the vertebral column and is therefore relatively easily compressed against the spine by a direct blow. Isolated duodenal injury is relatively rare (5%). Organs commonly injured in cases of duodenal injury are the liver (16%), the pancreas (11%), and the small bowel (11%) (ASENSIO et al. 1993). Duodenal injury may be classified into duodenal hematoma and duodenal perforation. Differentiation has profound therapeutic implications because perforation warrants surgical treatment while hematoma can be treated conservatively (KUNIN et al. 1993). Avulsion of the papilla of

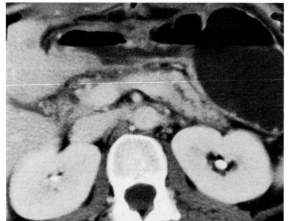

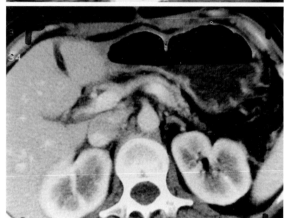

Fig. 7.4a,b. Atrophy of the pancreatic tail after trauma. **a** CT image 1 year after blunt pancreatic trauma. While the patient was initially treated conservatively, surgical drainage was subsequently required because of pseudocyst formation. The pancreatic tail has a normal size. **b** CT scan obtained 2 years later reveals the marked atrophy of the pancreatic tail

Vater is a rare complication of duodenal rupture that requires more complex surgery (SCHIMPL et al. 1992). Making the specific diagnosis of this latter condition is extremely difficult unless ERCP is performed. The combination of signs of progressive pancreatitis, peritonitis, and obstructive jaundice is typical. Irrespective of the exact nature of the duodenal lesion, early diagnosis is important. A delay in diagnosis and repair of duodenal perforation dramatically increases the morbidity and mortality (HOFER and COHEN 1989).

7.3.2 Examination Method/Trauma Pattern

7.3.2.1 Ultrasonography

There is no role for US in the detection of duodenal perforation. However, US can be used as a

noninvasive tool for the follow-up of duodenal hematomas (Fig. 7.5a).

7.3.2.2 Upper Abdominal Series with Gastrografin

In the acute phase, an upper abdominal study with Gastrografin may demonstrate contrast extravasation, gastric outlet obstruction, or duodenal narrowing (Fig. 7.6c). In a more delayed phase, fibrosis occurring after duodenal wall hematoma may lead to segmental duodenal narrowing.

7.3.2.3 Computed Tomography

Computed tomography is the method of choice for demonstration of duodenal hematoma and per-

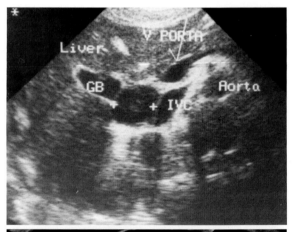

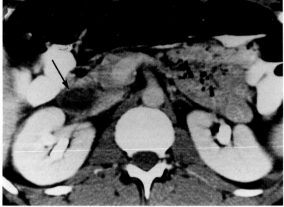

Fig. 7.5a,b. Old hematoma in the duodenal wall (images obtained 1 month after blunt abdominal trauma). **a** On US the hematoma is seen as a hypoechoic mass lesion located between the gallbladder (*GB*) and inferior vena cava (*IVC*). **b** On CT the hematoma remains hypodense on contrast-enhanced images (*arrow*)

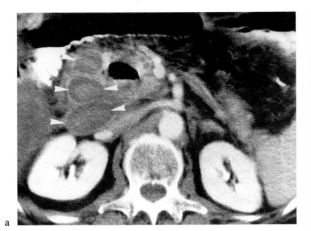

a

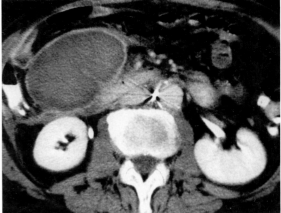

b

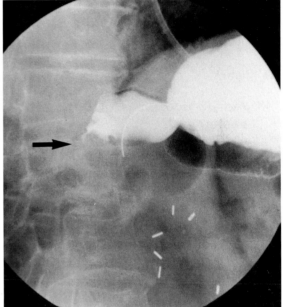

c

Fig. 7.6a–c. Hematoma in the duodenal wall after iatrogenic trauma (repair of aortic aneurysm). **a** CT at the level of D2. The hematomas in the lateral wall of the duodenum appear as lesions with a hyperdense center and hypodense peripheral rim (*white arrowheads*). **b** CT at the level of D3. A large hematoma with pseudocystic features is present in the right anterior pararenal space. **c** Gastrografin study reveals obstruction at the level of D2 (*arrow*)

foration. While large hematomas are easily detected (Fig. 7.6a,b), it has been stressed by several authors that the CT findings of duodenal perforation rely heavily on the use of oral contrast medium. If no oral contrast medium is used, adequate distention of the duodenum cannot be achieved and significant duodenal injuries can be missed (HOFER and COHEN 1989). Acute duodenal hematoma can be recognized as high-density wall thickening of the duodenum on CT scans (Fig. 7.6). Older hematomas are more hypodense (Fig. 7.5b). In the presence of duodenal perforation (rupture), collections of extraluminal gas and/or contrast material adjacent to the ruptured duodenum can be seen (KUNIN et al. 1993). Fluid or air can sometimes be observed in the right pararenal space, the mesocolon, and the mesenteric

fat (HOFER and COHEN 1989). Because of the retroperitoneal location of the second and third portions of the duodenum, peritoneal fluid or air is not typically associated with duodenal trauma. It should be streessed that the amount of retroperitoneal free air can be subtle and therefore the radiologist interpreting the CT study of a patient with blunt or penetrating abdominal trauma should pay special attention to this body area. On the other hand, the demonstration of periduodenal fluid or air is not 100% specific for duodenal rupture; similar findings have been described in cases of bladder rupture and pneumothorax (COOK et al. 1986). Therefore, an upper gastrointestinal study with water-soluble contrast material should be performed following CT to confirm a suspected diagnosis of duodenal perforation (COOK et al. 1986).

7.3.2.4 Magnetic Resonance Imaging

Although MRI is rarely required in the clinical setting, it may provide the specific diagnosis of duodenal hematoma based on the presence of a typical three-layered appearance on T1- and T2-weighted images ("ring sign") (Hahn et al. 1986).

7.3.2.5 Complications

Hemorrhagic shock is the most common cause of early mortality after duodenal trauma. Duodenal fistula is the most important complication following surgical repair, with an incidence of 2%–14% (Weigelt 1990).

7.4 Kidney

7.4.1 Mechanisms, Mechanics, and Classification

The kidney differs from other organs in that the vascular pedicle is the primary point of intra-abdominal fixation. As a result, horizontal as well as vertical acceleration and deceleration injuries can produce tearing of the renal arteries.

Posteriorly, approximately the lower two-thirds of each kidney rests on the quadratus lumborum muscle. Medially the psoas muscle and laterally the aponeurosis of the transversus abdominis muscle form the remainder of the kidney bed. The transverse processes of the first and second lumbar vertebrae are close to both kidneys along the lateral edge of the psoas, while the right kidney is crossed by the twelfth rib, and the left by both the eleventh and twelfth ribs. There posterior close relationships explain the significance of fractures of the ribs and/or transverse processes, as well as loss of psoas shadow in patients with blunt abdominal trauma.

The principal anterior relationship of the kidneys is with the peritoneum and those organs which, during fetal development, have come to lie in close relationship to the kidney. On the right, the hepatic flexure of the colon, and on the left, the tail of the pancreas and splenic flexure of the colon have lost their serosa. The areas of both kidneys in direct contact with these organs are the so-called bare areas. The left kidney is furthermore in close relationship to the spleen, the stomach, and the small bowel on the superolateral, superomedial, and inferomedial peritoneal covered areas, respectively. The right kid-

ney extends upward to the level at which the paretal peritoneum reflects onto the liver as the right coronary ligament. Below this point, the anterior aspect of the right kidney is covered by peritoneum which forms the posterior wall of the pouch of Morison. The suprarenal gland lies in a layer of connective tissue close to the superior and medial aspect of each kidney. The intimate relationship of the kidneys to all these organs explains the high percentage of associated injuries in patients with blunt or penetrating renal trauma.

The renal parenchyma is enclosed in a thin membrane: the true capsule. Outside this capsule is the perirenal fat, separated from the pararenal fat by the renal fascia, also known as the fibrous renal fascia of Gerota. Cranially and inferiorly, the renal fascia is fairly closed, except inferomedially, where the ureteral sheaths descend as caudal extensions of the renal fascia, explaining the possible presence of periureteral fluid collections in cases of reanl trauma. The perinephric space contains bridging septa between the true renal capsule and the fasica of Gerota. These septa might explain why retroperitoneal bleeding from renal injuries is frequently self-limiting, and only 2.6% of all patients presenting with renal trauma require surgery (McAninch and Carroll 1989).

7.4.1.1 Blunt Trauma

Blunt trauma is responsible for the vast majority (80%) of renal injuries (Pollack and Wein 1989). Significant renal injury is found in approximately 8%–10% of all cases of abdominal trauma (Bretan et al. 1986). In 1%–3% a significant renal artery injury occurs after blunt renal trauma (Lupetin et al. 1989). There are several mechanisms of closed renal injury. The kidney may be injured by a direct blow, it may be lacerated by the lower ribs, or it may be torn by rapid acceleration and deceleration. Injury of the liver, the spleen, and less often the pancreas and the bowel is present in approximately 20% of patients who have sustained closed renal trauma (Bretan et al. 1986). Associated pancreatic lesion is an infrequent finding that should be suspected in cases of left renal injury.

Classification of renal trauma provides a guide to both treatment and prognosis. An often used and practical classification includes (Federle 1989):

Category I lesions (80%): contusions and parenchymal lacerations that do not communicate with the collecting system.

Category II lesions (15%): parenchymal lacerations that communicate with the renal collecting system.

Category III lesions (5%): shattered kidney or injuries to the renal vascular pedicle.

Category IV lesions (rare): ureteropelvic junction avulsion; laceration of the renal pelvis.

Renal pedicle injuries can be divided into lesions of the renal artery (thrombosis, avulsion, intimal flap, spasm, pseudoaneurysm), lesions of the renal vein (laceration, avulsion, thrombosis), and arteriovenous fistulae. Venous injuries have a worse prognosis because of the poor ability of the veins to contract (LANG et al. 1992).

Hematomas may be present in any of these categories, and are categorized as intrarenal, perirenal, or pararenal. The size of the hematoma is usually, but not necessarily, directly proportional to the extent of the underlying renal injury.

There is general agreement on the management of category I, III, and IV lesions (GUERRIERO 1988): category I lesions do not require surgical treatment, whereas category III and IV lesions warrant immediate surgery. Controversy, however, exists on the appropriate management of category II lesions: while some surgeons advocate early surgical repair, others defend a conservative approach (PETERSON 1977; WEIN et al. 1977; EVINS et al. 1980).

7.4.1.2 Penetrating Renal Injury

Penetrating injuries (20%) can be divided primarily into gunshot wounds and stab wounds. There is general consensus that gunshot wounds need to be treated surgically, mainly because of the likelihood of associated injuries and contamination by foreign material. Stab wounds, on the other hand, may be managed conservatively if there is no associated intraperitoneal injury (CARROLL and McANINCH 1985).

7.4.1.3 Iatrogenic Trauma

Iatrogenic conditions constitute an important subgroup of renal trauma. Percutaneous nephrostomy may cause renal injuries similar to those seen after penetrating trauma. Internal ureteral stents may cause perforation of the renal pelvis (SALAZAR et al. 1984). Subcapsular or (more rarely) intraparenchymal hematomas may be expected in up to 15%–24% of patients after extracorporeal shock

wave lithotripsy (ESWL) (RUBIN et al. 1987). Renal hemorrhage is to be expected in 90% of patients who undergo renal biopsy. Severe hemorrhage requiring blood transfusion occurs in approximately 2%–6% of these cases (CASTOLDI et al. 1994).

Other causes of direct or indirect iatrogenic renal trauma are retroperitoneal surgery and radiation therapy.

7.4.1.4 Predisposing Anomalies

It is well recognized that the presence of any renal abnormality such as hydronephrosis, ectopia, horseshoe kidney, and renal tumor increases the vulnerability of the kidney to trauma (EL MRINI et al. 1993; RHYNER et al. 1984). It is also well known that the kidney is more susceptible to injury in childhood than in adulthood, mainly because of its relatively large size and its inadequate protection by perinephric fat, ribs, and muscle.

7.4.1.5 Indications for Imaging

There is no agreement on the question as to which trauma victims require which radiological investigation for suspected renal injury, and this is especially true for blunt renal trauma. Several reports have shown that the presence or absence of macroscopic hematuria is associated with the severity of renal injury. While 25% of patients with gross hematuria have significant renal damage, important renal injury is seen in only 1%–2% of patients with microscopic hematuria. However, gross hematuria may be absent in up to 30% of patients with renal pedicle injury. These patients, however, in whom there is no gross hematuria despite the presence of severe renal injury, almost always present with shock. Recent studies therefore advocate radiological investigation in cases of macroscopic hematuria or microscopic hematuria associated with shock, whereas patients without hematuria or microscopic hematuria without shock are considered not to need radiological investigations (HERSCHORN et al. 1991; EASTHAM et al. 1992; MEE et al. 1989; McANDREW and CORRIERE 1994). These findings are in contrast to those of STABLES et al. (1976), who reported that in up to 24% of patients with renal pedicle injury, there was no hematuria at all. It thus remains an open question whether it can be justified to refuse imaging studies to the victims of blunt abdominal trauma based on the presence or absence of hematuria. Similarly, with respect to penetrating trauma, while TANG and BERNE (1993) suggested that intravenous urography (IVU) is not needed in the absence of hematuria, FEDERLE et al. (1987) did not find any correlation between hematuria and extent of trauma.

Intravenous urography or US can be used as a triage modality. In cases where emergent surgery is required, US may be the only imaging study that is likely to be performed without considerable time loss. Intraoperative urography, too, may provide valuable information to the surgeon who faces an unsuspected retroperitoneal hematoma during emergency laparotomy. It is, however, advocated that CT should be performed whenever possible for evaluation of associated injuries (LANG 1990).

Whilst there is no consensus about patient selection for imaging, there is general agreement that whenever there is evidence suggestive of vascular or parenchymal injury, further investigations should be performed without delay. The rationale is based on the observation that in the presence of complete arterial occlusion, renal function is irreversibly lost after 2h of ischemia in more than 90% of cases.

7.4.2 Examination Methods

7.4.2.1 Ultrasonography

Ultrasonography has attracted increasing interest in the initial workup of blunt renal trauma because of its noninvasiveness, its low cost, and the fact that it can be performed in the emergency department (FURTSCHEGGER et al. 1988). US will easily identify the presence or absence of abdominal bleeding (though it fails to identify the origin of the bleeding) and has been used instead of peritoneal lavage (ROCHE et al. 1992). Limitations of US include the fact that hematomas may be nearly isoechoic to the renal parenchyma or the perirenal fat (depending on their age), and that infarctions and even injuries to the renal pedicle may be completely invisible on gray-scale US (ROSALES et al. 1992). Therefore, in order to obtain essential functional information, it is necessary to perform a (color) Doppler examination.

7.4.2.2 Intravenous Urography

Intravenous urography was used as the first-line screening procedure before the introduction of US and CT. The reported accuracy of this technique for the detection of severe renal trauma varies widely.

While some authors report up to 90% accuracy in the staging of renal injury (MAHONEY and PERSKY 1968), others state that the technique is of only slight value (WILSON and ZIEGLER 1987; HERSCHORN et al. 1991). In any case, most posttraumatic changes seen on IVU are nonspecific and can be mimicked by a variety of preexisting conditions. Nevertheless, normal findings on IVU virtually exclude severe renal trauma, particularly in hemodynamically stable patients (BERGREN et al. 1987). Nonvisualization indicates severe injury and 97% of IVUs are positive in patients with vascular injuries. Delayed or incomplete filling is inconclusive and requires further investigation (KRISTJANSSON and PEDERSON 1993). Despite the fact that IVU is less accurate than CT for staging of renal trauma, the technique may be valuable in emergency situations because it is simple, quick, and readily available. Limited IVU may be performed in the operating room when a retroperitoneal hematoma of unknown origin is encountered during exploration of the abdomen.

7.4.2.3 Computed Tomography

In many centers, CT is the examination of choice for the study of renal injuries (KISA and SCHENK 1986; BRETAN et al. 1986). Compared with IVU and US, CT more readily identifies the location and extent of renal contusions and lacerations and extrarenal hematomas (McANINCH and FEDERLE 1981; FEDERLE et al. 1981). In cases of trauma to an abnormal kidney (e.g., neoplasm, hydronephrotic kidney, polycystic disease, horseshoe kidney, or simple renal cyst), CT is more specific than IVU (RHYNER et al. 1984). In addition, CT provides detailed and accurate information on the hematoma size, allowing calculation of the "average bleeding rate," expressed by the size of the hematoma divided by the time elapsed since injury. This average bleeding rate provides a dynamic picture of the trauma and may indicate whether a hematoma is enlarging rapidly (TONG et al. 1991). Moreover, injuries to other parenchymatous organs, such as the liver and the spleen, and the central nervous system can also be demonstrated. Thus, repeat administration of contrast medium in a patient with potentially compromised renal function can be avoided (PEITZMAN et al. 1986).

Whereas the value of CT in establishing renal parenchymal injury is well accepted, this does not hold true for renal pedicle injuries. While FEDERLE et al. (1987) completely relied on CT for the detection of renal pedicle injury, LANG et al. (1985) reported on potential false-negative diagnoses of renal artery injury. Such false-negative findings might be caused by incomplete occlusion of the renal artery (POLLACK and WEIN 1989). Although detailed comparative studies are not available, there is no doubt that the detection of small parenchymal and vascular injuries has been improved by the introduction of the new generation of rapid CT scanners, in particular spiral CT. Using the "two-phase" technique, a first scan can be performed in the "arterial" or "renal cortical" phase, while a second scan can be obtained during the phase of peak medullary enhancement. While scanning during the arterial phase allows direct visualization of arterial lesions such as pseudoaneurysms, scannng during the phase of peak enhancement of the renal cortex provides functional information concerning the integrity of the renal arteries: side-to-side differences in cortical enhancement may point to the diagnosis of unilateral arterial injury (LANG et al. 1992). Finally, scanning in the intravenous phase should always be performed in patients who have sustained renal trauma in order to (a) demonstrate integrity or damage of the excretory system and (b) detect abnormal staining of the renal parenchyma, a sign suggestive of renal vein thrombosis (LANG et al. 1992). Multiplanar CT imaging can be useful for accurate demonstration of the extent of intra- and perirenal lesions such as infarction and hematoma (Fig. 7.7a).

7.4.2.4 Magnetic Resonance Imaging

The cost and availability of MRI preclude its routine use in the setting of acute renal trauma. MRI has been used effectively to demonstrate small renal contusions and hematomas after ESWL (BAUMGARTNER et al. 1987).

7.4.2.5 Angiography

Angiography is not used in the assessment of all blunt renal injuries. It is not indicated for subcapsular hematomas or for small perinephric or intrarenal hematomas. The information on CT is augmented by angiography when CT is suspicious for (major) vascular injury (e.g., large perirenal retroperitoneal hematoma or major renal fracture) (Fig. 7.7b; see also Fig. 7.14c). Angiography is also used in patients with persistent or recurrent posttraumatic gross hematuria or delayed complications,

such as hypertension (LANG 1975; SCLAFANI et al. 1985). There is no consensus concerning the optimal imaging modality when a non-functioning kidney is identified at IVU. While some authors state that angiography is required for definite demonstration of arterial injuries such as an intimal flap, progressive arterial thrombosis, severance of the main renal artery, or renal vein thrombosis, others believe that (spiral) CT is as accurate (POLLACK and WEIN 1989).

Currently, the major indication for angiography is supraselective transcatheter embolization of bleed-

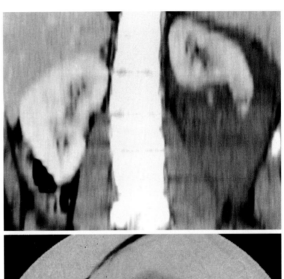

a

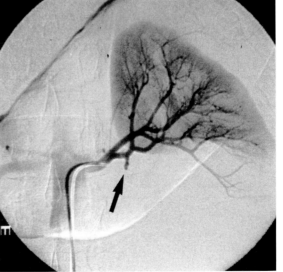

b

Fig. 7.7a,b. Posttraumatic infarction due to occlusion of a lower pole artery. **a** CT (coronal reformatted image) reveals infarction of the lower pole of the left kidney and extensive hematoma in the perirenal space. The devascularized renal parenchyma has the same attenuation numbers as the hematoma. **b** On angiography occlusion of the lower pole artery (*arrow*) is observed; no active bleeding site could be demonstrated

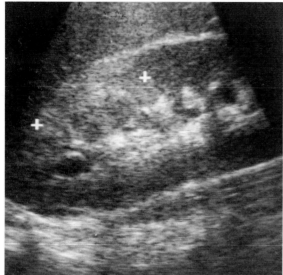

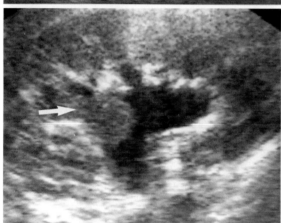

Fig. 7.8a,b. US appearance of fresh parenchymal (**a**) and pelvicaliceal hematoma (**b**). **a** Intrarenal hematoma after ESWL: A well-delineated hyperechoic area is present, involving the upper part of the renal parenchyma. **b** Blood clot in the upper part of the slightly dilated collecting system 24 h after ureterorenoscopy (*white arrow*). Repeat US may be necessary for differentiation from urothelial carcinoma

ing renal vessels (FISHER et al. 1989; KANTOR et al. 1989).

7.4.3 Trauma Pattern

7.4.3.1 Ultrasonography

The sonographic appearance of renal contusion and hematoma varies widely with the age of the lesion (KAY et al. 1980). In general, a hyperacute hematoma is relatively hypoechoic but it gradually becomes more echogenic with blood clot formation (Fig. 7.8).

With aging, the hematoma becomes hypoechoic and easily visible (liquefaction) (Fig. 7.9a). Lacerations present as band-like defects in the parenchyma. Multiple mobile fragments can be observed in cases of shattered kidneys. Subcapsular hematomas may be rather difficult to recognize in the acute phase because they tend to be completely isoechoic to the renal parenchyma. Indirect signs, such as deformity of the renal contour, indicate the presence of such a subcapsular collection. Even large subcapsular hematomas completely disappear spontaneously over time. Extrarenal fluid collections are usually

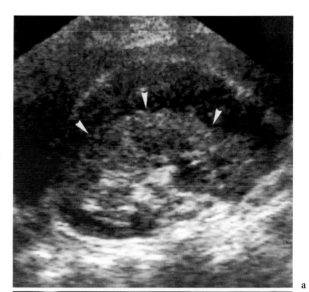

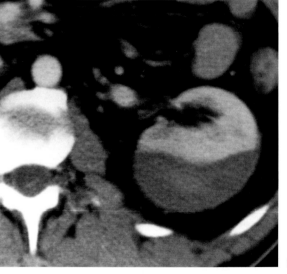

Fig. 7.9a,b. Subcapsular hematoma (after ESWL). **a** US shows a hypoechoic mass lesion of lenticular shape compressing the outer renal surface (*white arrowheads*, renal surface). **b** On CT the subcapsular hematoma is seen to compress the renal parenchyma

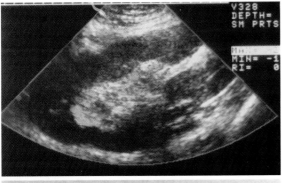

a

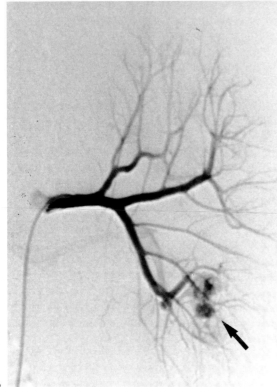

b

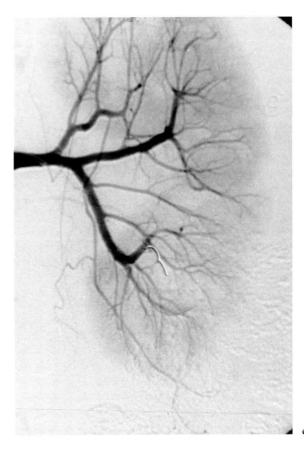

c

Fig. 7.10a–c. Pseudoaneurysm after renal biopsy. a Color Doppler study shows turbulent flow in the pseudoaneurysm. b Angiogram showing pooling of dye at the lower pole (*arrow*). c Angiogram after successful embolization with BOD coils. (b and c by courtesy of G. Wilms and L. Stockx)

well visualized, although in the acute phase they are sometimes hardly visible and their size may be underestimated.

Ultrasonography fails to visualize ureteral or pelvic injury, but the diagnosis might be suspected in the presence of a urine collection next to the renal pelvis (JAKSE et al. 1986).

Vascular lesions such as pseudoaneurysms are easily identified with the systematic application of color Doppler US (Fig. 7.10a). Power Doppler US is a new technique that will probably increase the ability to demonstrate renal perfusion disorders, in particular complete or segmental renal infarction.

7.4.3.2 Intravenous Urography

7.4.3.2.1 Grade I.
Mild renal enlargement, faint renal opacification, and a striated nephrogram, although atypical, may suggest renal contusion (RUBIN and SCHLIFTMAN 1979). A patchy nephrogram suggests perfusion defects from segmental infarctions or multiple parenchymal injuries. Intra- and perirenal hematoma caused by laceration is seen as a mass lesion in the parenchyma.

7.4.3.2.2 Grade II.
Extravasation of opacified urine indicates laceration of the collecting system (Fig. 7.11a). Extravasation with an otherwise normal renal

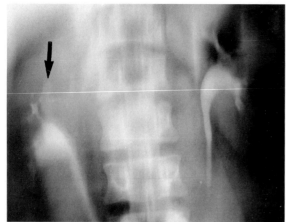

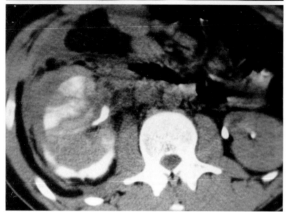

Fig. 7.11a,b. Grade II renal trauma (rupture of collecting system). **a** Urogram showing subtle signs of contrast leakage at the upper pole of the right kidney (*arrow*). **b** CT clearly demonstrates the urinoma that extends into the perirenal space. Note the hematoma at the anterolateral aspect of the kidney

parenchyma and distal ureter suggests rupture of a caliceal fornix; rapid involution of the extravasation and normalization within 3–5 days support this diagnosis (CASS et al. 1993).

7.4.3.2.3 Grade III.
A unilateral afunctional kidney is an indication of a severe renal injury, most commonly arterial occlusion or avulsion. The differential diagnosis includes severe contusion, pedicle injury, subcapsular hematoma, traumatic arteriovenous fistula, preexisting renal disease, renal agenesis, shock, and a posttraumatic state of nonexcretion (TODD 1994).

7.4.3.2.4 Grade IV.
Massive accumulation of contrast material in the presence of normal renal parenchyma and absence of opacification of the ureter suggests ureteropelvic disruption (see Fig. 7.21) (POLLACK and WEIN 1989).

7.4.3.3 Computed Tomography

7.4.3.3.1 Grade I.
On contrast-enhanced CT images, renal contusions are seen as areas of hypoattenuation (WOLFMAN et al. 1992). Minor contusions can be difficult to appreciate. LANG et al. (1985) described the appearance of small collections of contrast medium in the renal interstitium on delayed scans as a sign of contusion.

Intrarenal hematoma, defined as a well-demarcated interstitial collection of blood, may be seen as a high-density lesion on unenhanced images and as a low-density area on contrast-enhanced series (Fig. 7.12) (POLLACK and WEIN 1989).

Renal lacerations are visualized as bank-like hypoattenuating lesions typically paralleling intervascular tissue planes. The margins of the renal lacerations may have an inhomogeneous, mottled appearance (SCLAFANI et al. 1985).

Segmental renal infarcts (caused by injury to small renal vessels) are seen as wedge-shaped hypodense defects. A cortical rim sign may be observed (see Sect. 7.4.3.3.3).

7.4.3.3.2 Grade II.
Deep lacerations extend into the medulla and may transect the collecting system. The presence of urine outside the confines of the collecting system (urinoma) is easily demonstrated on CT, confirming transection of the collecting system (Fig. 7.11b).

Delayed images are an important prerequisite in the differential diagnosis between hematoma, cysts, and pelvic rupture.

7.4.3.3.3 Grade III.
The shattered kidney contains multiple lacerations, some of which may shear across

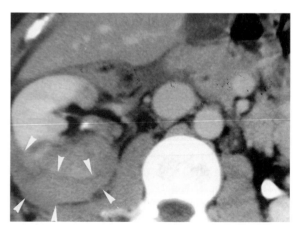

Fig. 7.12. CT showing renal hematoma and perirenal hemorrhage of characteristic shape and location (*white arrowheads*)

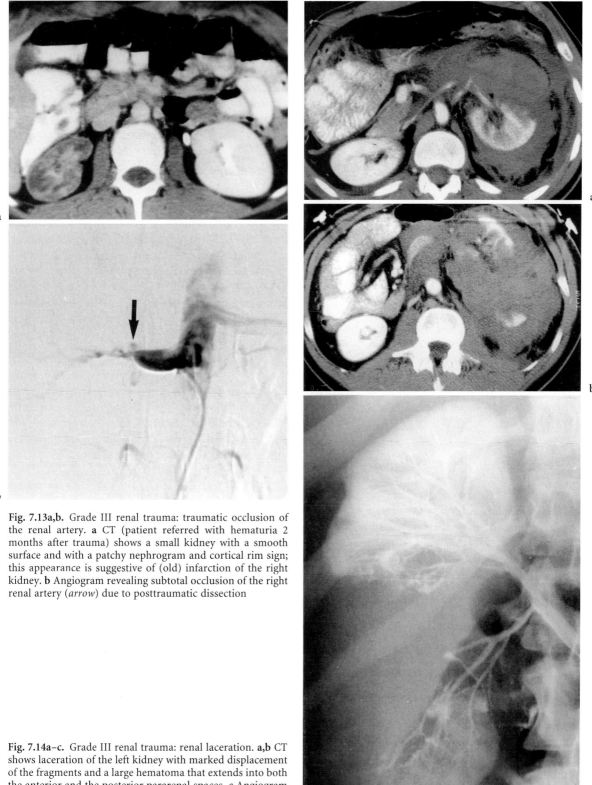

Fig. 7.13a,b. Grade III renal trauma: traumatic occlusion of the renal artery. **a** CT (patient referred with hematuria 2 months after trauma) shows a small kidney with a smooth surface and with a patchy nephrogram and cortical rim sign; this appearance is suggestive of (old) infarction of the right kidney. **b** Angiogram revealing subtotal occlusion of the right renal artery (*arrow*) due to posttraumatic dissection

Fig. 7.14a–c. Grade III renal trauma: renal laceration. **a,b** CT shows laceration of the left kidney with marked displacement of the fragments and a large hematoma that extends into both the anterior and the posterior pararenal spaces. **c** Angiogram (in another patient) revealing laceration with residual perfusion in only a small fragment of the lower pole. The separation of the renal fragments is an indication of the volume of the hematoma

the vascular planes and produce devascularized fragments (WOLFMAN et al. 1992) (Fig. 7.13).

The most specific features of renal pedicle injuries include the absence of renal contrast enhancement, the presence of the cortical rim sign (as a result of collateral blood flow from the capsular arteries), the presence of a hematoma surrounding the renal pedicle, and visualization of an abrupt cut-off of the contrast-filled renal artery (TONG et al. 1991) (Fig. 7.14a,b). Additional observations include central retroperitoneal hematoma associated with limited perinephric hematoma causing lateral displacement of the kidney. When the renal artery is only partially occluded, a patchy nephrogram may be observed and the CT diagnosis of pedicle injury may be difficult (LANG et al. 1992). Demonstration of renal vein injury is more difficult than demonstration of arterial injury (MCANINCH 1987). Classic signs are unilateral renal enlargement, a cortical rim sign (especially a thick cortical rim), and the demonstration of a thrombus within the dilated renal vein (LANG et al. 1992). Also suggestive for venous injury is massive bleeding with preserved contrast uptake by the affected kidney. Another important sign is unilateral increase in the density of the renal parenchyma on delayed images (LANG et al. 1992).

7.4.3.3.4 Grade IV. When an unusual large extravasation is observed in the medial part of the perirenal space, the diagnosis of an isolated ureteral or renal pelvic laceration should be strongly considered, particularly when the extravasation is associated with a non-opacified ureter and an intact renal parenchyma (see Fig. 7.21).

7.4.3.3.5 Patterns of Renal Hematoma. Hematomas may be intrarenal, subcapsular, perirenal, or pararenal, or any combination thereof (POLLACK and WEIN 1989). A subcapsular hematoma is easily recognized by its eccentric location, its semicircular or lenticular shape, and the deformity of the renal contour (Fig. 7.9b). Perirenal hematomas spread preferably posterolateral to the kidney (Fig. 7.12). Due to fascial fusions in the retroperitoneum, renal hematoma usually does not cross the midline; therefore, the finding of such a hematoma should prompt the search for injuries of the aorta, its branches, or other midline structures (SCLAFANI et al. 1985). In the event of severe arterial damage, the hematoma may spread into the pararenal space and may even reach the contralateral side.

7.4.3.3.6 Trauma Patterns in the Presence of Predisposing Factors. Renal cysts or pyelocaliceal diverticula may rupture after blunt trauma. Following rupture of a diverticulum, perirenal extravasation of urine may be observed. The specific diagnosis of bleeding caliceal diverticulum may be difficult unless delayed images are obtained. Renal or perirenal hemorrhage found after minor trauma arouses suspicion of an underlying parenchymal tumor. The detection of fatty components may be the key to the dagnosis of a bleeding angiomyolipoma (Fig. 7.15).

7.4.3.3.7 Extracorporeal Shock Wave Lithotripsy. Post-ESWL scans may demonstrate subcapsular, intrarenal, or perirenal hematomas (Fig. 7.9) (RUBIN et al. 1987). Subcapsular hematomas are seen in up to 15%–24% of patients. An increase in renal size has also been observed after ESWL. Other findings are perirenal soft tissue stranding (in fact thickening of the bridging lamellae) and thickening of the renal fascia.

7.4.3.3.8 Renal Biopsy. Intrarenal, perirenal, subcapsular, and pararenal hematomas may be observed. Vascular injuries such as pseudoaneurysms and fistula can be detected with dynamic incremental CT and in particular with spiral CT.

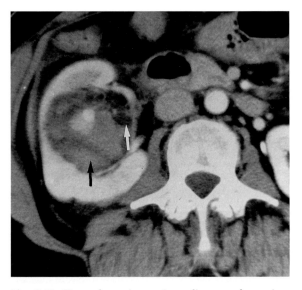

Fig. 7.15. Hemorrhage in angiomyolipoma after minor trauma. CT image after IV contrast injection, showing pseudoaneurysm in a renal mass, surrounded by a fresh hematoma (*arrow*) and fat (*white arrow*) Hemorrhage in angiomyolipoma was confirmed at surgery

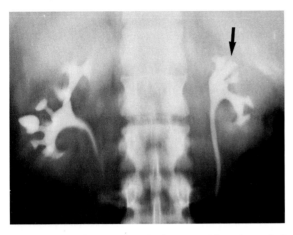

Fig. 7.16. Atrophy as a sequel of trauma. There is marked atrophy of the renal parenchyma at the upper pole of the left kidney after traumatic avulsion (*arrow*)

7.4.3.4 Angiography

In cases of renal contusion, the affected kidney may appear swollen, and angiography shows slow arterial flow but is otherwise normal. Intrarenal hematomas are suggested by stretching of the arteries; subcapsular and extrarenal hematomas can usually be differentiated by the fact that the latter are less well confined and produce renal displacement rather than renal deformity. Stretching and displacement of lumbar or other retroperitoneal arteries suggest retroperitoneal hematoma.

In cases of renal artery injury, extravasation is seen as puddles of high-density contrast; opacification of the renal vein or pelvicaliceal system in the early phase of the arteriogram suggests arteriovenous or arteriocaliceal fistulae, while thrombosis of the renal artery is depicted as a cut-off of the affected vessel. Occasionally, active bleeding sites can be demonstrated.

Angiographic findings in case of renal vein injury are renal enlargement, poor visualization of renal parenchyma and the pelvicaliceal system, splaying of the intrarenal arteries, a faint or prolonged nephrographic opacification, and nonvisualization of the renal vein.

7.4.4 Transcatheter Arterial Embolization

There is only a limited role for interventional angiography in the setting of acute renal trauma because while patients with renal pedicle injuries are treated surgically, those with minor renal laceration, contusion, or bleeding from peripheral renal

vessels do well with nonsurgical management. Nevertheless, an important indication for transcatheter embolization is persistent hematuria associated with arteriovenous fistulization or pseudoaneurysm (Fig. 7.10b,c). Although embolization of renal vessels may result in renal infarction, embolization is justified because less loss of renal substance is to be expected from catheter embolization than from an attempt at operative repair. Indeed, substantial improvements in catheter and guide wire design permit superselective embolization, thus minimizing the loss of renal substance. Particles such as Gelfoam can be used for small-vessel occlusion. Large emboli such as steel coils and detachable balloons are usually employed for treatment of arteriovenous fistulae and pseudoaneurysms.

7.4.5 Follow-up and Long-term Complications

Ultrasonography can be considered as the imaging modality of choice for initial follow-up of patients, for instance in cases of perirenal hematoma. Follow-up CT or US studies are particularly important in injuries that are managed conservatively. It has been observed experimentally that fibrosis occurs at the site of a laceration about 1 month after the trauma (Gerlaugh et al. 1960). Fibrosis and scarring can easily be detected on follow-up CT studies. Isolated parenchymal fragments without blood supply also develop fibrosis and scarring (Fig. 7.16). In the presence of adequate residual blood supply and minor laceration or contusion a morphological and functional restitutio ad integrum may be the final outcome (Rassweiler et al. 1984).

Follow-up studies may be necessary to document the following complications after nonsurgical treatment: urinoma, abscess formation, hydronephrosis, stone or cyst formation, aneurysm or arteriovenous fistula, and fistulization (Fig. 7.17). Another long-term complication of renal trauma, observed both after blunt renal trauma and after ESWL, is hypertension (Williams et al. 1988). One of the probable causes of hypertension after renal trauma is infarction. CT and US can be used for the evaluation of renal size and integrity in these patients.

7.5 Adrenal Gland

7.5.1 Mechanisms

There is no agreement on the frequency of posttraumatic hemorrhage of the adrenal glands. In autopsy

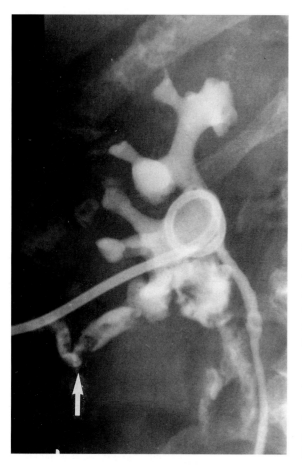

Fig. 7.17. Fistula after percutaneous nephrolithotripsy. A residual stone fragment in the proximal ureter is causing persistent leakage at the course of the previous percutaneous nephrolithotomy (*white arrow*). A percutaneous nephrostomy tube was inserted again and the ureteral calculus was treated by ureteroscopy

There are at least three possible mechanisms for adrenal hemorrhage after blunt trauma (MURPHY et al. 1988):

1. The adrenal gland becomes compressed against the spine by direct trauma.
2. The bleeding arises from an acute increase in intra-adrenal venous pressure due to compression of the inferior vena cava.
3. Hemorrhage is secondary to deceleration forces which cause tearing of small vessels that perforate the adrenal capsule.

Pathologically, the hemorrhage is located in the adrenal medulla and probably originates from the intramedullary sinusoids which receive blood from the subcapsular vascular plexus after it passes through the cortex. The cortex thins as it becomes stretched around the hematoma (SEVITT 1955). In cases of bilateral bleeding, the differential diagnosis includes hemorrhage due to anticoagulant therapy, stress, surgery, sepsis, and hypotension.

7.5.2 Examination Methods/Trauma Pattern

The relative value of US, CT, and MRI for the detection of adrenal hemorrhage has not yet been established. Most lesions are detected on abdominal CT studies that are routinely performed in many centers after a severe blunt abdominal trauma.

7.5.2.1 Ultrasonography

In acute adrenal hemorrhage, a hyperechoic mass lesion is seen in the adrenal area (Fig. 7.18a). In the subacute stage the hemorrhage becomes hypoechoic (WILMS et al. 1987; MURPHY et al. 1988) (Fig. 7.18b). Very rarely, in the chronic stage a hyperechoic fibrotic mass persists (Fig. 7.18c).

7.5.2.2 Computed Tomography

Typical features of acute posttraumatic adrenal hemorrhage on CT are enlargement of the gland, high attenuation numbers before intravenous contrast administration (>50 HU), and relative hypodensity after contrast administration. Associated features are infiltration of the periadrenal fat and thickening of the adjacent right diaphragmatic crus (WILMS et al. 1987; MURPHY et al. 1988; BURKS et al. 1992; SIVIT et al. 1992b). While in most patients the hematoma

series, adrenal injury is reported in up to 25% of patients with significant abdominal trauma (SEVITT 1955). Adrenal hemorrhage was detected with CT in 2%–3% of posttraumatic patients in two recent reports (BURKS et al. 1992; SIVIT et al. 1992b). Posttraumatic adrenal bleeding is usually unilateral; the right side is most commonly affected. Bilateral bleeding occurs in approximately 20% of cases (WILMS et al. 1987). The majority of adrenal injuries (up to 95%) are associated with ipsilateral thoracic, abdominal, or retroperitoneal trauma (SEVITT 1955). Thus, careful inspection of the ipsilateral adrenal gland is warranted when significant injury of adjacent structures is present, particularly in the lower chest, the liver, the spleen, and the kidneys (BURKS et al. 1992). Adrenal hemorrhage has also been described after liver transplantation (SOLOMON and SUMKIN 1988).

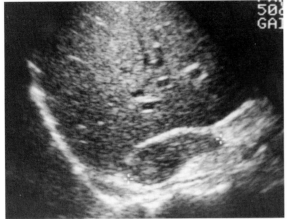

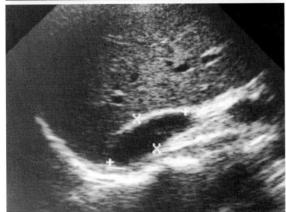

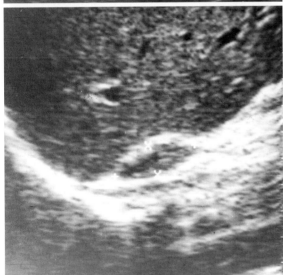

Fig. 7.18a–c. US of adrenal injury. a On the initial sonogram the enlarged right adrenal gland is isoechoic with the liver parenchyma. b Sonogram 3 weeks later: Liquefaction is decreasing the echogenicity of the adrenal hematoma. c Follow-up sonogram after 4 months shows a residual echogenic mass, probably due to residual fibrosis. (Courtesy of G. Wilms)

appears as a discrete rounded lesion, it sometimes presents as a diffuse irregular mass, obscuring the adrenal gland (BURKS et al. 1992).

Rarely, a fluid-fluid level may be observed in the acute stage (Fig. 7.19). The density of the adrenal gland on precontrast studies depends on the age of the hematoma. Over time, both the size and the attenuation numbers of the hematoma decrease (WILMS et al. 1987). Occasionally, an adrenal pseudocyst (seroma) persists.

7.5.2.3 Magnetic Resonance Imaging

As for CT and US, the signal intensity on MRI depends on the age of the hemorrhage, and therefore a wide variability of signal intensities on T2- and T1-weighted images can be expected. Typically bright signal intensity is observed on T2-weighted images in the subacute stage because of the formation of methemoglobin (Fig. 7.20). In the chronic stage the signal intensity decreases on T2- and T1-weighted images due to hemosiderin deposition.

7.5.3 Follow-up and Sequelae

Acute adrenal hemorrhage usually has no clinical importance when it is unilateral. In the presence of bilateral hemorrhage, however, adrenal insufficiency may occur, which usually is permanent and requires continued steroid replacement therapy (FEUERSTEIN and STREETEN 1991). Occasionally, the adrenal insufficiency only becomes obvious after a long period,

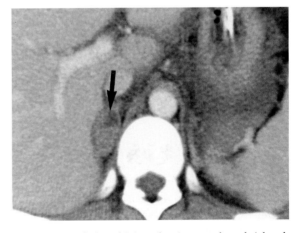

Fig. 7.19. CT of adrenal injury showing an enlarged right adrenal gland, with fluid-fluid level; this is diagnostic of post-traumatic hemorrhage (arrow)

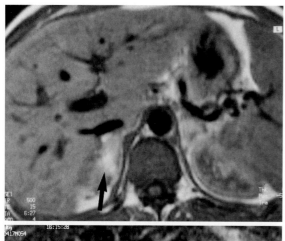

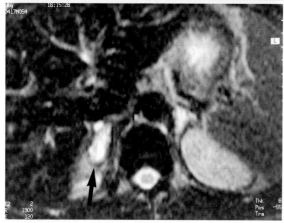

Fig. 7.20a,b. MRI of adrenal injury. The enlarged adrenal appears as a hyperintense mass on T1- (**a**) and T2- (**b**) weighted images, which is typical for acute hemorrhage (methemoglobin) (*arrows*)

and the link with the initial trauma may be forgotten. Follow-up with imaging can be used for monitoring the expected decrease in size of the hematoma after a few weeks (Fig. 7.18). Follow-up is particularly important for the differential diagnosis between posttraumatic hemorrhage and adrenal tumor. Some tumors indeed look exactly alike adrenal hematomas at the time of the initial presentation (MURPHY et al. 1988).

7.6 Ureter

7.6.1 Mechanisms

About 3%–5% of genitourinary injuries involve the ureter (KENNEY et al. 1987). The clinical diagnosis of ureteral injury is often difficult and delayed. Hematuria is an unreliable symptom as it is seen in only 15%–66% of patients (CAMPBELL et al. 1992).

Early recognition is important, however, since delayed surgical repair may result in a significant increase in morbidity (KENNEY et al. 1987).

Ureteral injuries can be divided into iatrogenic and noniatrogenic injuries. The first group is by far the most important. Common causes of iatrogenic injury include ligation or transection of the ureter during pelvic surgery, injury from ureteroscopic manipulations, and injury caused by indwelling ureteral stents (SALAZAR et al. 1984; KAUFMAN JJ 1984). Noniatrogenic injuries can be divided into blunt and penetrating trauma. In the group of penetrating trauma, gunshot wounds are the most common. Blunt trauma is a rare cause of ureteral injury. The mechanism proposed for this type of injury includes sudden deceleration and acceleration associated with hyperextension. Other possible mechanisms are a direct blow to the second or third lumbar vertebra or compression of the renal pelvis and proximal ureter against a transverse process. Blunt ureteral injury is more often discovered in children and the large majority of cases occur at the ureteropelvic junction or (more rarely) the proximal ureter (REDA and LEBOWITZ 1986; TOPOROFF et al. 1993). The diagnosis of ureteropelvic junction (UPJ) disruption should be considered when the historical findings reveal a rapid deceleration injury (BOONE et al. 1993). Patients with chronic ureteral obstruction are at increased risk for ureteral rupture after a minimal trauma.

7.6.2 Examination Methods

Radiological methods that have been used are intravenous urography (IVU), CT, retrograde pyelography, and antegrade (percutaneous) pyelography. While some authors could detect all injuries using IVU (ROBER et al. 1990), others have reported serveral where IVU missed the diagnosis of ureteral rupture (CAMPBELL et al. 1992; PRESTI et al. 1989; BRANDES et al. 1994). If the ureter is only incompletely filled or the renal function is poor, retrograde or antegrade pyelography may be necessary for ultimate diagnosis. The relative value of CT and IVU is not clearly established. CT has proven to be of value for the demonstration of UPJ rupture (KENNEY et al. 1987). In any case, CT is often used as an initial study in traumatized patients and many ureteral lesions will first become manifest on CT. It has to be emphasized that delayed CT images must be obtained at least 10–15 min after contrast administration in order to detect small amounts of extra-

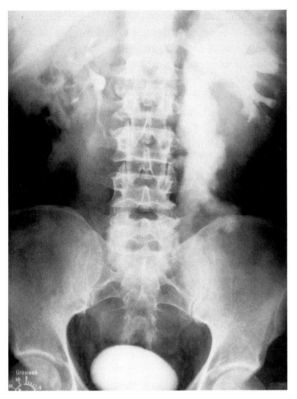

Fig. 7.21. UPJ avulsion. On the urograma large urinoma is observed at the inferomedial site of the renal pelvis and extending distally along the course of the ureter. There is no opacification of the distal ureter

vasation from the collecting system (TOPOROFF et al. 1993).

7.6.3 Trauma Pattern

The most reliable direct urographic sign of ureteral rupture is contrast extravasation and no filling of the distal ureter. Sometimes there is only dilation of the proximal ureter or ureteral deviation (CAMPBELL et al. 1992).

The IVU and CT findings in cases of UPJ disruption include: intact renal parenchyma, no perirenal hematoma, no opacification of the ureter distal to the disruption, and contrast medium extravasation (Fig. 7.21). Of good diagnostic value is pooling of contrast-opacified urine almost exclusively in the medial perirenal space (KENNEY et al. 1987). If the UPJ disruption is incomplete, medial perirenal extravasation occurs, but the ureter is opacified (KENNEY et al. 1987). It is obvious that CT can identify the complications related to ureteral injury: urinoma, abscess formation, and hydronephrosis.

Fistulization and ureteral fibrosis as sequelae of trauma can be demonstrated using IVU (Figs. 7.22a, 7.23); occasionally, CT may be indicated for demonstration of the specific underlying cause (Fig. 7.22b).

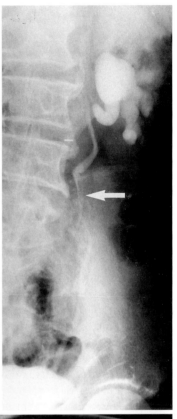

a

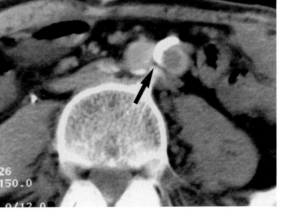

b

Fig. 7.22a,b. Stricture of the left ureter detected 6 months after aortic bypass surgery. **a** Urography was performed because of suspicion of stone disease in the left ureter. The urogram shows a stenosis of 2 cm in length involving the middle third of the left ureter (*white arrow*). **b** CT image obtained 30 min after contrast injection. The contrast-filled left ureter is trapped between the bifurcation of the aortoiliac graft (*arrow*). The stricture is probably caused by a combination of mechanical compression and fibrosis

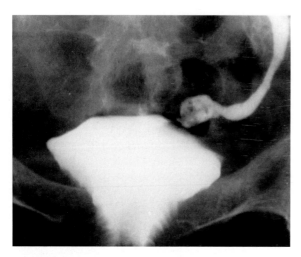

Fig. 7.23. Ureterovaginal fistula after pelvic surgery

7.7 Bladder

7.7.1 Mechanisms

The bladder is bordered by both peritoneal and extraperitoneal spaces. The anterior aspect of the bladder is separated from the symphysis pubis by an extraperitoneal space known as the perivesical space or Retzius' space. The superior aspect of the bladder (bladder dome) is covered by peritoneum. The caudal extent of the peritoneal reflections on the anterior and posterior surfaces of the bladder is variable (SANDLER et al. 1986).

Bladder trauma is present in approximately 10% of patients with pelvic fracture. Another common cause of bladder rupture is blunt trauma. The chance of rupture increases if the bladder is (over-) distended. Rare causes of bladder injury are penetrating injury, iatrogenic injury such as rupture after cystoscopic clot evacuation or biopsy, electrocoagulation or lasering (SMITH et al. 1994), and perforation caused by a migrating intrauterine device. Finally, perforation of the bladder wall related to long-term indwelling catheters has been reported as a rare cause of peritonitis (MERGUERIAN 1985). Bladder rupture can be submucosal (intramural), intraperitoneal, or extraperitoneal (MIRVIS 1989). The differentiation between intra- and extraperitoneal rupture is important because the former usually requires surgical treatment. Intraperitoneal rupture (10%–20% of cases) is associated with blunt trauma and usually occurs at the bladder dome. It is more frequently seen after alcohol abuse and in children. In children the bladder is in fact an abdominal structure rather than a pelvic one, and therefore is more susceptible to blunt trauma to the

lower abdomen (BRIJS et al. 1992). "Secondary" tears of the bladder can occur after minor trauma if a locus of minor resistance exists; a classic example is a bladder wall hematoma after previous trauma (BRIJS et al. 1992). Extraperitoneal rupture (80%–90% of cases) is an anterior bladder base injury that is usually due to separation of the symphysis pubis and pelvic fracture. There may be associated rupture of the urogenital diaphragm, allowing extravasation to extend to the scrotum, thigh, and penis (CORRIERE and SANDLER 1988). From time to time, herniation of the bladder into the fractured pelvic rim is observed.

7.7.2 Examination Methods

Until recently cystography has been considered the gold standard for evaluation of bladder trauma (SANDLER et al. 1986; CASS 1989; TUCHSCHMID and ROHNER 1993). However, since many of these patients are also suspected of having other organ injuries (e.g., pelvic fractures), CT is currently the method for initial evaluation. Recent reports show that CT may be as sensitive as cystography provided that the CT technique is adapted to the purpose (KANE et al. 1989; HORSTMAN et al. 1991). Adaptation of the CT technique includes delayed pelvic imaging with a full bladder, infusion of contrast material through the Foley catheter, delayed scanning, and scanning of the pelvis both before and after bladder drainage. Scanning after drainage allows the detection of subtle amounts of extravasated contrast material beyond the confines of the bladder, which otherwise may be obscured by the full bladder (SANDLER et al. 1986). IVU is a third technique that can be used for demonstration of bladder rupture (see Fig. 7.25a). Comparative studies have shown that this technique is less accurate than cystography, presumably because of decreased density of the contrast medium (SANDLER et al. 1986). Irrespective of the technique used, adequate distention of the bladder is required. Cystograms can be false-negative if less than 250 ml contrast material is instilled (CASS 1989). Both in IVU and in cystography, images should be obtained both with the bladder filled and after emptying.

7.7.3 Trauma Pattern

7.7.3.1 Extraperitoneal Rupture

In cases of extraperitoneal rupture there is streaky contrast extravasation inferior, anterior, or lateral to the bladder (Fig. 7.24). The extraluminal contrast re-

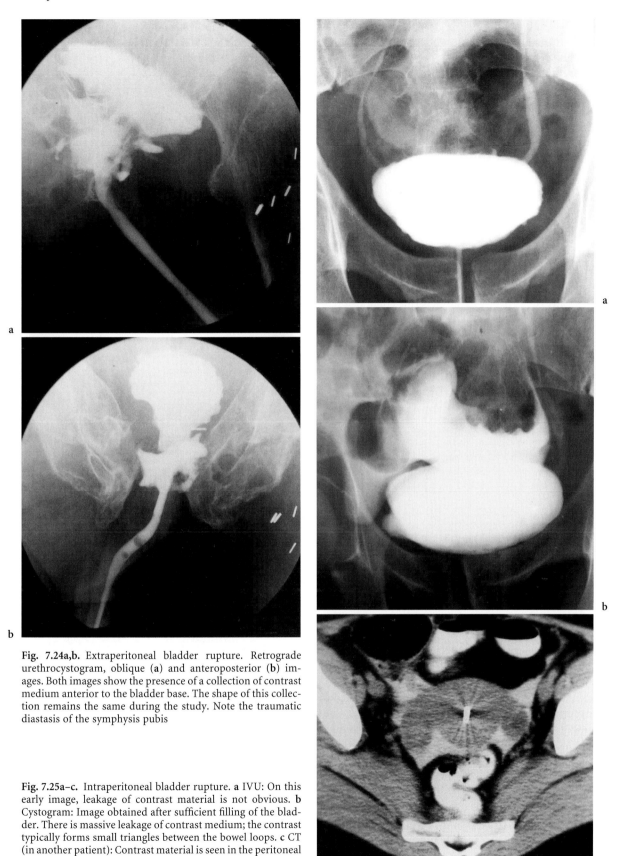

Fig. 7.24a,b. Extraperitoneal bladder rupture. Retrograde urethrocystogram, oblique (**a**) and anteroposterior (**b**) images. Both images show the presence of a collection of contrast medium anterior to the bladder base. The shape of this collection remains the same during the study. Note the traumatic diastasis of the symphysis pubis

Fig. 7.25a–c. Intraperitoneal bladder rupture. **a** IVU: On this early image, leakage of contrast material is not obvious. **b** Cystogram: Image obtained after sufficient filling of the bladder. There is massive leakage of contrast medium; the contrast typically forms small triangles between the bowel loops. **c** CT (in another patient): Contrast material is seen in the peritoneal space

mains in the same area over a period of time. The bladder may have a teardrop configuration because of compression by a perivesical hematoma. If the injury is severe, extravasation of contrast material may extend beyond the perivesical space. Upward extension into the perinephric space has been described (SANDLER et al. 1986). In the event of rupture of the urogenital diaphragm, contrast may be identified within the scrotum and penis. In these patients, the differentiation with urethral rupture may be difficult.

7.7.3.2 Intraperitoneal Rupture

In intraperitoneal rupture there is leakage of urine and/or contrast material into the peritoneal cavity. Typically the contrast material forms small triangles between the bowel loops (Fig. 7.25b). Contrast can also be pooled in dependent parts of the abdominal cavity, such as the Douglas' space or the paracolic gutter (Fig. 7.25c).

7.7.3.3 Submucosal Rupture

Submucosal rupture results in irregularities of the bladder wall on cystograms, without frank extravasation of contrast material.

7.8 Retroperitoneal Hematoma

7.8.1 Mechanisms

Retroperitoneal hematoma is usually part of a spectrum of multisystem injuries (GOINS et al. 1992). Hematomas without associated organ injury are rare. The causes of retroperitoneal hematoma can be classified as blunt trauma, penetrating trauma, and iatrogenic injury. Blunt injuries of the abdominal aorta are rare. Mechanisms of injury include motor vehicle crashes. The spectrum of aortic lesions ranges from simple contusion or intramural hematoma to intimal disruption, false aneurysm, and frank rupture (BRATHWAITE and RODRIGUEZ 1992). Injury to the thoracic aorta is much more common than injury to the abdominal aorta (WILLIAMS et al. 1994). Another rare entity after blunt trauma is isolated injury to the inferior vena cava. The overwhelming majority (85%–95%) of inferior vena cava injuries are due to penetrating

trauma, mostly gunshot and stab wounds. Vascular injuries, either arterial or venous, are also associated with pelvic fractures (Fig. 7.26). There is a higher incidence of vascular injury in patients with pelvic fractures with posterior ring disruption. Hemorrhagic complications after percutaneous femoral angiography are uncommon (0.25%–5%) (KAUFMAN JL 1984) (Fig. 7.27).

The primary aim in the management of patients with retroperitoneal hematoma is stabilization of the circulation by early recognition and treatment of the bleeding source.

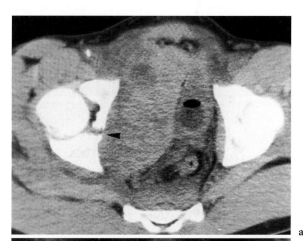

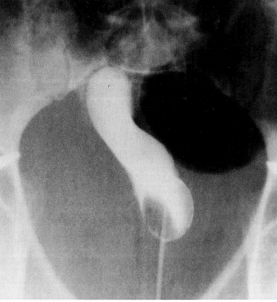

Fig. 7.26a,b. Extraperitoneal pelvic hematoma. **a** CT image showing dense acute posttraumatic hematoma that displaces the bladder. Note the fracture of the right acetabulum (*arrowhead*). **b** (Another patient.) Note the teardrop shape of the bladder at retrograde cystogram, caused by a pelvic hematoma

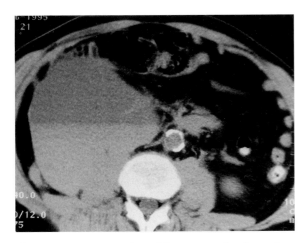

Fig. 7.27. Acute retroperitoneal hematoma after femoral artery catheterization. Non-enhanced CT scan shows a large hematoma with a fluid-fluid level

7.8.2 Examination Methods and Trauma Pattern

Computed tomography is the technique of choice for demonstration of retroperitoneal hematoma (Fig. 7.28). Major vascular injury can usually be detected on CT. Arterial injury is easily seen after contrast administration because of contrast extravasation. Fast scanning and fast contrast injection are crucial for detection of arterial lesions. Acute hematomas are seen as dense structures on non-contrast-enhanced CT images (Figs. 7.26, 7.28a). Occasionally, a fluid-fluid level may be observed (Fig. 7.27). CT findings in cases of inferior vena cava injury following blunt trauma are a retroperitoneal hematoma with a paracaval epicenter, an irregular contour of the inferior vena cava, and extravasation of contrast-enhanced blood from the inferior vena cava (PARKE et al. 1993).

Angiography is the best technique for specific visualization of arterial lesions. The following findings may be observed: frank extravasation of contrast material, arterial occlusion, pseudoaneurysm formation, formation of arterial venous fistula, and dissection. Transcatheter embolization plays an important role in the control of persisting retroperitoneal hemorrhage, e.g., after pelvic fracture (HOELTING et al. 1992; KLEIN et al. 1992; KANTOR et al. 1989).

7.9 Diagnostic Flow Chart (Fig. 7.29)

There is no doubt that CT is the technique of choice for initial evaluation of abdominal injuries. US can be reserved for hemodynamically unstable patients

who cannot be transported to the CT department or can be used for a first triage. While US is valuable for detection of conditions such as splenic and hepatic laceration, renal rupt lure and hemoperitoneum, visualization of injuries confined to the retroperitoneum may be impossible. Two other techniques that have proven their value in cases of emergency laparotomy are (limited) IVU and intraoperative cholangiography. Emergency IVU can answer the vital question as to whether or not a normal functioning contralateral kidney is present, in patients in whom an injured kidney has to be re-

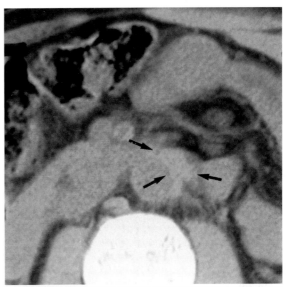

a

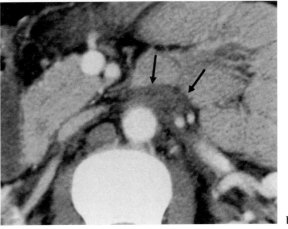

b

Fig. 7.28a,b. Small retroperitoneal hematoma after blunt trauma. **a** Non-contrast-enhanced CT image obtained 2 h after trauma shows a hyperdense mass adjacent to the aorta (*arrows*), representing acute hematoma. **b** CT image obtained after contrast injection: the hematoma is hypodense relative to the surrounding vessels (*arrows*); no active site of bleeding could be demonstrated with CT. The patient did well after conservative treatment

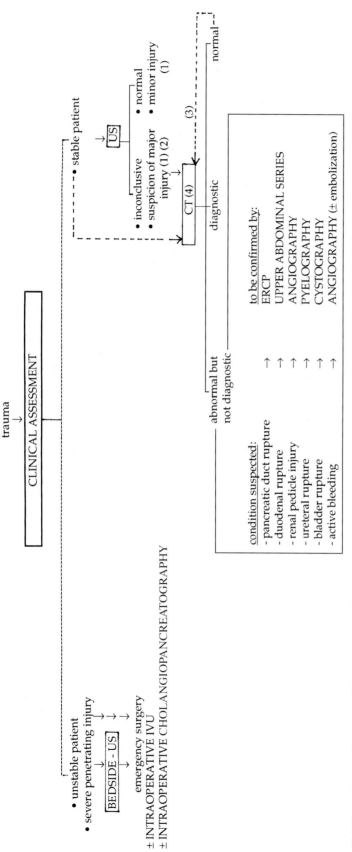

Fig. 7.29. Diagnostic flow chart

(1) IVU may be used instead of CT in cases of mild, isolated renal injury

(2) Cystography is the preferred diagnostic modality in cases of isolated bladder injury

(3) Repeat CT after 12 – 24 h may be required in patients with suspected pancreatic injury

(4) Technical specifications: see text

moved. IVU may also be used as a first-line imaging tool in stable patients who are under suspicion for isolated renal injury. Intraoperative cholangiography can be used to exclude pancreatic duct rupture when the surgeon suspects pancreatic injury.

CT in abdominal injuries must be performed with meticulous technique to achieve high diagnostic accuracy. Intravenous contrast medium should be used in every case unless specific contraindications exist. Administration of oral contrast medium is mandatory for detection of duodenal and small bowel injury and for avoiding misinterpretation of small bowel loops as hematoma or hemorrhage. Water-soluble contrast should be administered if the possibility of perforation exists; on the other hand, barium suspension may be preferred if the fear of vomiting and aspiration is high (RAPTOPOULOS 1994). Fast intravenous injection of contrast material and dynamic (or spiral) scanning is required to achieve optimal organ enhancement.

In spiral CT, the time delay between the start of contrast injection and scanning should be carefully selected. For instance, when contrast is injected at a rate of 2.5–3 ml/s, a delay of approximately 70–80 s is required (HEIKEN et al. 1993) to achieve peak enhancement of liver, spleen, and kidneys. When biphasic spiral CT is available, 5-mm collimation scanning of the pancreas can be performed during the phase of peak enhancement of the pancreatic parenchyma (approximately 30–40 s after contrast injection), while the entire upper abdomen can be examined with a second 5- or 8-mm collimation scan. A delay of approximately 90–150 s is required for evaluation of pelvic (venous) structures and the inferior vena cava. When spiral CT is used, the entire abdomen is examined during two consecutive breathhold periods of 20–25 s. Alternatively, the scans can be performed during (quiet) breathing. The slice thickness and pitch (i.e., the ratio of table feed to slice thickness) used in spiral CT typically vary between 5 and 8 mm and 1 and 1.5, respectively. Delayed images are needed whenever injury to the renal pelvis, ureters, and bladder is suspected. If there is specific suspicion of bladder rupture, the study should be completed by obtaining images after bladder evacuation (see Sect. 7.4.2). When clinical data or US findings suggest the presence of arterial lesions (active hemorrhage, pseudoaneurysm), a first spiral scan can be performed early after contrast injection, in the so-called arterial phase. Thin-section scanning and tailored bolus timing are required for accurate demonstration of arterial anomalies (VAN HOE et al. 1995).

The usefulness of imaging studies other than US and CT depends on the type of trauma, the clinical signs, the data obtained with CT, and the general condition of the patient. Upper abdominal series with water-soluble contrast are useful for confirmation of duodenal perforation. ERCP (or intraoperative cholangiopancreatography) is the modality of choice for demonstration of pancreatic duct rupture. Angiography may be indicated for confirmation of vascular injury and for therapeutic embolization of active bleeding sites. Ascending or descending pyelography may be necessary for demonstration of ureteral lesions. Cystography remains the gold standard for demonstration of bladder trauma. In all cases the successful diagnosis and treatment of retroperitoneal injury require close cooperation between radiologists and referring clinicians.

Acknowledgments. The authors thank E. Ponette, G. Wilms, and L. Breysem for their advice, I. Liboton and B. Verbist for assistance in the preparation of the manuscript, and W. Desmedt for preparation of the figures.

References

Asensio J, Feliciano D, Britt LD, Kerstein M (1993) Management of duodenal injuries. Curr Probl Surg 30:1023–1049

Barkin JS, Ferstenberg RM, Panullo W, Manten HD, Davis C (1988) Endoscopic retrograde cholangiopancreatography in pancreatic trauma. Gastrointest Endosc 34:102–105

Baumgartner BR, Dickey KW, Ambrose SS, Walton KN, Nelsen RC, Bernardino ME (1987) Kidney changes after extracorporeal shock wave lithotripsy: appearance on MR imaging. Radiology 163:531–534

Bergren CT, Chan FN, Bodzin JH (1987) Intravenous pyelogram results in association with renal pathology and therapy in trauma patients. J Trauma 27:515–518

Berni GA, Bandyk DF, Oreskovich MR, Carrico CJ (1982) Role of intraoperative pancreatography in patients with injury to the pancreas. Am J Surg 143:602–605

Blind J, Mellbring G, Hjertkvist M, Sandzén B (1994) Diagnosis of traumatic pancreatic duct rupture by on-table endoscopic retrograde pancreatography. Pancreas 3:387–389

Boone TB, Gilling PJ, Husmann DA (1993) Ureteropelvic junction disruption following blunt abdominal trauma. J Urol 150:33–36

Brandes SB, Chelsky MJ, Buckman RF, Hanno PM (1994) Ureteral injuries from penetrating trauma. J Trauma 36:766–769

Brathwaite CEM, Rodriguez A (1992) Injuries of the abdominal aorta from blunt trauma. Am Surg 58:350–352

Bretan PN, McAninch JW, Federle MP, Jeffrey RB (1986) Computerized tomographic staging of renal trauma: 85 consecutive cases. J Urol 136:561–565

Brijs S, Oyen R, Brijs A, Swinnen E (1992) Spontaneous rupture of the bladder: an uncommon finding on excretory urography. J Belge Radiol 75:486–488

Burks DW, Mirvis SE, Shanmuganathan K (1992) Acute adrenal injury after blunt abdominal trauma: CT findings. AJR 158:503–507

Campbell EW, Filderman PS, Jacobs SC (1992) Ureteral injury due to blunt and penetrating trauma. Urology 40:216–220

Carr ND, Cairns SJ, Lees WR, Russell RCG (1989) Late complications of pancreatic trauma. Br J Surg 76:1244–1246

Carroll PR, McAninch JW (1985) Operative indications in penetrating renal trauma. J Trauma 25:587–593

Cases AS (1989) Diagnostic studies in bladder rupture: indications and techniques. Urol Clin North Am 16:267–273

Cass AS, Lee JY, Smith CS (1993) Perirenal extravasation with blunt trauma of a caliceal fornix. J Trauma 35:20–22

Castoldi MC, Del Moro RM, D'Urbano ML et al. (1994) Sonography after renal biopsy: assessment of its role in 230 consecutive cases. Abdom Imaging 19:72–77

Cogbill TH, Moore EE, Morris JA et al. (1991) Distal pancreatectomy for trauma: a multicenter experience. J Trauma 31:1600–1606

Cook DE, Walsh JW, Vick CW, Brewer WF (1986) Upper abdominal trauma: pitfalls in CT diagnosis. Radiology 159: 65–69

Corriere JN, Sandler CM (1988) Mechanisms of injury, patterns of extravasation and management of extraperitoneal bladder rupture due to blunt trauma. J Urol 139:43–44

Dodds WJ, Taylor AJ, Erickson SJ, Lawson TL (1990) Traumatic fracture of the pancreas: CT characteristics. J Comput Assist Tomogr 14:375–378

Douws C, Grenier N, Brichaux JC (1994) Pancreatic trauma. In: Baert AL (ed) Radiology of the pancreas. Springer, Berlin Heidelberg New York, pp 247–253

Eastham JA, Wilson TG, Ahlering TE (1992) Radiographic evaluation of adult patients with blunt renal trauma. J Urol 148:266–267

El Mrini M, Aboutaieb R, Benjelloun S (1993) Tumeur de la voie excrétrice sur rein en fer à cheval découverte lors d'un traumatisme rénal. Ann Urol 27:90–92

Evins SC, Thomason WB, Rosenblaum R (1980) Non-operative management of severe renal lacerations. J Urol 123:247–249

Federle M (1989) Evaluation of renal trauma. In: Pollack HM (ed) Clinical urography. Saunders, Philadelphia, pp 1472–1494

Federle MP, Kaiser JA, McAninch JW, Jeffrey RB, Mall JC (1981) The role of computed tomography in renal trauma. Radiology 141:455–460

Federle MP, Brown TR, McAninch JW (1987) Penetrating renal trauma: CT evaluation. J Comput Assist Tomogr 11:1026–1030

Feuerstein B, Streeten DHP (1991) Recovery of adrenal function after failure resulting from traumatic bilateral adrenal hemorrhages. Ann Intern Med 115:785–786

Fisher RG, Ben-Menachem Y, Whigham C (1989) Stab wounds of the renal artery branches: angiographic diagnosis and treatment by embolization. AJR 152:1231–1235

Furtschegger A, Egender G, Jakse G (1988) The value of sonography in the diagnosis and follow-up of patients with blunt renal trauma. Br J Urol 62:110–116

Gerlaugh RL, DeMuth WE, Rattner WH, Murphy JJ (1960) The healing of renal wounds. 2. Surgical repair of contusions and lacerations. J Urol 83:529

Goins WA, Rodriguez A, Brathwaite CEM (1992) Retroperitoneal hematoma after blunt trauma. Surg Gynecol Obstet 174:281–290

Gothi R, Bose NC, Kumar N (1993) Case report: ultrasound demonstration of traumatic fracture of the pancreas with pancreatic duct disruption. Clin Radiol 47:434–435

Guerriero WG (1988) Genitourinary trauma. In: Guerriero WG (ed) Problems in urology, vol II. Lippincott, Philadelphia, pp 186–187

Hahn PF, Stark DD, Vici LG, Ferruci JT (1986) Duodenal hematoma: the ring sign in MR imaging. Radiology 159: 379–382

Heiken JP, Brink JA, McClennan BL, Sagel SS, Forman HP, Di Croce J (1993) Dynamic contrast-enhanced CT of the liver: comparison of contrast medium injection rates and uniphasic and biphasic injection protocols. Radiology 187:327–331

Herschorn S, Radomski SB, Shoskes DA, Mahoney J, Hirshberg E, Klotz L (1991) Evaluation and treatment of blunt renal trauma. J Urol 146:274–277

Hoelting T, Buhr HJ, Richter GM, Roeren T, Friedl W, Herfarth C (1992) Diagnosis and treatment of retroperitoneal hematoma in multiple trauma patients. Arch Orthop Trauma Surg 11:323–326

Hofer GA, Cohen AJ (1989) CT signs of duodenal perforation secondary to blunt abdominal trauma. J Comput Assist Tomogr 13:430–432

Horstman WG, McClennan BL, Heiken JP (1991) Comparison of computed tomography and conventional cystography for detection of traumatic bladder rupture. Urol Radiol 12:188–193

Jaffe RB, Arata JA, Matlak ME (1989) Percutaneous drainage of traumatic pancreatic pseudocysts in children. AJR 152: 591–595

Jakse G, Furtschegger A, Egender G (1986) Ultrasound in patients with blunt renal trauma managed by surgery. J Urol 138:21–23

Jeffrey RB (1990) Pancreas, retroperitoneal duodenum, colon and vascular trauma. In: McCort JJ (ed) Trauma radiology. Churchill Livngstone, New York, pp 215–230

Jeffrey RB, Federle MP, Crass RA (1983) Computed tomography of pancreatic trauma. Radiology 147:491–494

Jeffrey RB, Laing FC, Wing VW (1986) Ultrasound in pancreatic trauma. Gastrointest Radiol 11:44–46

Johanet H, Fasano JJ, Marmuse JP, Fichelle A, Saint-Marc O, Benhamou G, Charleux H (1991) Traumatismes du pancréas: urgence diagnostique et thérapeutique. Chirurgie 128:337–342

Jones RC (1985) Management of pancreatic trauma. Am J Surg 150:698–704

Kane NM, Francis IR, Ellis JH (1989) The value of CT in the detection of bladder and posterior urethral injuries. AJR 153:1243–1246

Kantor A, Sclafani SJA, Scalea T, Duncan AO, Atweh N, Glanz S (1989) The role of interventional radiology in the management of genitourinary trauma. Urol Clin North Am 16:255–265

Kaufman JJ (1984) Ureteral injury from ureteroscopic stone manipulation. Urology 23:267–269

Kaufman JL (1984) Pelvic hemorrhage after percutaneous femoral angiography. AJR 143:335–336

Kay CJ, Rosenfield AT, Armm M (1980) Grayscale ultrasonography in the evaluation of renal trauma. Radiology 134:461–466

Kenney PJ, Panicek DM, Witanowski LS (1987) Computed tomography of ureteral disruption. J Comput Assist Tomogr 11:480–484

Kisa E, Schenk WG III (1986) Indications for emergency intravenous pyelography (IVP) in blunt abdominal trauma: a reappraisal. J Trauma 26:1086–1089

Klein SR, Saroyan RM, Baumgartner F, Bongard FS (1992) Management strategy of vascular injuries associated with pelvic fractures. J Cardiovasc Surg 33:349–357

Kristjansson A, Pederson J (1993) Management of blunt renal trauma. Br J Urol 72:692–696

Kunin JR, Korobkin M, Ellis JH, Francis IR, Kane NM, Siegel SE (1993) Duodenal injuries caused by blunt abdominal trauma: value of CT in differentiating perforation from hematoma. AJR 160:1221–1223

Lane MJ, Mindelzun RE, Sandhu JS, McCormick VD, Jeffrey RB (1994) CT diagnosis of blunt pancreatic trauma: importance of detecting fluid between the pancreas and the splenic vein. AJR 163:833–835

Lang EK (1975) Arteriography in the assessment of renal trauma: the impact of arteriographic diagnosis on preservation of renal function and parenchyma. J Trauma 15:553–566

Lang EK (1990) Intra-abdominal and retroperitoneal organ injuries diagnosed on dynamic computed tomograms obtained for assessment of renal trauma. J Trauma 30:1161–1168

Lang EK, Sullivan J, Fretz G (1985) Renal trauma: radiological studies. Comparison of urography, computed tomography, angiography and radionuclide studies. Radiology 154:1–6

Lang EK, Schild HH, Schweden FJ, Alken P (1992) Renal trauma. In: Schild HH, Schweden FJ, Lang EK (eds) Computed tomography in urology. Thieme, Stuttgart, pp 116–134

Lewis G, Krige JEJ, Bornman JC, Terblanche J (1993) Traumatic pancreatic pseudocysts. Br J Surg 80:89–93

Lucas CE (1977) Diagnosis and treatment of pancreatic and duodenal injury. Surg Clin North Am 57:49–65

Lupetin AR, Mainwaring BL, Daffner RH (1989) CT diagnosis of renal artery injury caused by blunt abdominal trauma. AJR 153:1065–1068

Mahoney SA, Persky L (1968) Intravenous drip nephrotomography as an adjunct in the evaluation of renal injury. J Urol 99:513–516

Maull KI, Rozycki GS, O'Neal Vinsant G, Pedigo RE (1987) Retroperitoneal injuries: pitfalls in diagnosis and management. South Med J 80:1111–1115

McAndrew JD, Corriere JN (1994) Radiographic evaluation of renal trauma: evaluation of 1103 consecutive patients. Br J Urol 73:352–354

McAninch JW (1987) Renal injuries. In: Gillenwater JY, Grayhack JT, Howard SS, Duckett JW (eds) Adult and pediatric urology, vol I. Year Book Medical Publishers, Chicago, p 427

McAninch JW, Carroll PR (1989) Renal exploration after trauma. Indications and reconstructive techniques. Urol Clin North Am 16:203

McAninch JW, Federle MP (1981) Evaluation of renal injuries with computerized tomography. J Urol 128:456–460

Mee HL, McAninch JW, Robinson AL, Auerbach PS, Carroll PR (1989) Radiographic assessment of renal trauma: a 10-year prospective study of patient selection. J Urol 141:1095–1098

Merguerian PA (1985) Peritonitis and abdominal free air due to intraperitoneal bladder perforation associated with indwelling catheter drainage. J Urol 143:747

Mirvis SE (1989) Diagnostic imagng of the urinary system following blunt trauma. Clin Imaging 13:269–280

Murphy BJ, Casillas J, Yrizarry JM (1988) Traumatic adrenal hemorrhage: radiological findings. Radiology 169:701–703

Parke CE, Stanley RJ, Berlin AJ (1993) Infrarenal vena caval injury following blunt trauma: CT findings. J Comput Assist Tomogr 17:154–157

Peitzman AB, Makaroun MS, Slasky BS, Ritter P (1986) Prospective study of computed tomography in initial management of blunt abdominal trauma. J Trauma 26:585–592

Peterson NE (1977) Intermediate-degree blunt renal trauma. J Trauma 17:425–435

Pollack HM, Wein AJ (1989) Imaging of renal trauma. Radiology 172:297–308

Presti JC, Carroll PR, McAninch JW (1989) Ureteral and pelvic injuries from external trauma: diagnosis and management. J Trauma 29:370–374

Raptopoulos V (1994) Abdominal trauma: emphasis on computed tomography. Radiol Clin North Am 32:969–987

Rassweiler J, Eisenberger F, Buck J, Miller K (1984) Das stumpfe Nierentrauma: eine differenziertere Klassifikation als Grundlage einer stadiengerechten Therapie. Akt Urol 15:60

Reda EF, Lebowitz RL (1986) Traumatic ureteropelvic disruption in the child. Pediatr Radiol 16:164–166

Rhyner P, Federle MP, Jeffrey RB (1984) CT of trauma to the abnormal kidney. AJR 142:747–750

Rober PE, Smith JB, Pierce JM (1990) Gunshot injuries of the ureter. J Trauma 30:83–86

Roche BG, Bugmann PH, Le Coultre C (1992) Blunt injuries to liver, spleen, kidney and pancreas in pediatric patients. Eur J Pediatr Surg 2:154–156

Rosales A, Arango O, Coronado J, Vesa J, Maristany J, Gelabert A (1992) The use of ultrasonography as the initial diagnostic exploration of blunt renal trauma. Uron Int 48:134–137

Rubin BE, Schliftman R (1979) The striated nephrogram in renal contusion. Urol Radiol 1:119–121

Rubin JI, Arger PH, Pollack HM, Banner MP, Coleman BG, Mintz MC, VanArsdalen KN (1987) Kidney changes after extracorporeal shock wave lithotripsy: CT evaluation. Radiology 162:21–24

Salazar JE, Johnson JB, Scott RL (1984) Perforation of renal pelvis by internal ureteral stents. AJR 143:816–818

Sandler CM, Hall JT, Rodriguez MB, Corriere JN (1986) Bladder injury in blunt pelvic trauma. Radiology 158:633–638

Schimpl G, Sauer H, Schober PH, Weber G (1992) Rupture of the duodenum with avulsion of the papilla of Vater due to blunt trauma in a child, and review of the literature. Eur J Pediatr Surg 2:291–294

Sclafani SJA, Goldstein AS, Panetta T, Phillips TF, Golueke P, Gordon DH, Glanz S (1985) CT diagnosis of renal pedicle injury. Urol Radiol 7:63–68

Sevitt S (1955) Posttraumatic adrenal apoplexy. J Clin Pathol 8:185–194

Sivit CJ, Eichelberger MR, Taylor GA, Bulas DI, Gotschall CS, Kushner DC (1992a) Blunt pancreatic trauma in children: CT diagnosis. AJR 158:1097–1100

Sivit CJ, Ingram J, Taylor GA, Bulas DI, Kushner DC, Eichelberger MR (1992b) Posttraumatic adrenal hemorrhage in children: CT findings in 34 patients. AJR 158:1299–1302

Smith DP, Goldman SM, Fishman EK (1994) Rupture of the urinary bladder following cystoscopic clot evacuation: report of two cases diagnosed by CT. Abdom Imaging 19:177–179

Solomon N, Sumkin J (1988) Right adrenal gland hemorrhage as a complication of liver transplantation: CT appearance. J Comput Assist Tomogr 12:95–97

Soto JA, Yucel EK, Barrish M, Chuttani R, Ferruci JT, Shah J (1994) MR cholangiopancreatography: correlation with endoscopic retrograde cholangiopancreatography. Radiology 193(P):133

Stables DP, Fouche RF, De Villiers Van Niekerk JP, Cremin JB, Holt SA, Peterson ME (1976) Traumatic renal artery occlusion. J Urol 115:229–233

Stone A, Sugawa C, Lucas C, Hayward S, Nakamura R (1990) The role of endoscopic retrograde pancreatography (ERP) in blunt abdominal trauma. Am Surg 56:715–720

Sukul K, Lont HE, Johannes EJ (1992) Management of pancreatic injuries. Hepatogastroenterology 39:447–450

Tang E, Berne TV (1993) Intravenous pyelography in penetrating trauma. Am Surg 60:384–386

Todd A (1994) Radiological management of renal trauma. Br J Hosp Med 51:512–515

Tong YC, Chun JS, Tsai HM, Yu CY, Lin JSN (1991) Use of hematoma size on computerized tomography and calculated average bleeding rate as indications for immediate surgical intervention in blunt renal trauma. J Urol 147:984–986

Toporoff B, Scalea TM, Abramson D, Sclafani SJA (1993) Ureteral laceration caused by a fall from a height: case report and review of the literature. J Trauma 34:164–166

Tuchschmid Y, Rohner S (1993) Les ruptures vésicales: traitement chirurgical ou conservateur. J Chir (Paris) 130:343–348

Van Hoe L, Marchal G, Baert AL, Gryspeerdt S, Mertens L (1995) Determination of scan delay time in spiral CT

angiography: utility of a test bolus injection. J Comput Assist Tomogr 19:216–220

Van Steenbergen W, Samain H, Pouillon M et al. (1987) Transection of the pancreas demonstrated by ultrasound and computed tomography. Gastrointest Radiol 12:128–130

Weigelt JA (1990) Duodenal injuries. Surg Clin North Am 70:529–539

Wein AJ, Murphy JJ, Mulholland SG, Chait AW, Arger PH (1977) A conservative approach to the management of blunt renal trauma. J Urol 117:425–427

Williams CM, Kaude JV, Newman RC, Peterson JC, Thomas WC (1988) Extracorporeal shock-wave lithotripsy: long-term complications. AJR 150:311–315

Williams JS, Graff JA, Uku JM, Steining JP (1994) Aortic injury in vehicular trauma. Ann Thorac Surg 57:726–730

Wilms G, Marchal G, Baert A, Adisoejoso B, Mangkuwerdojo S (1987) CT and ultrasound features of post-traumatic adrenal hemorrhage. J Comput Assist Tomogr 11:112–115

Wilson RF, Ziegler DW (1987) Diagnostic and treatment problems in renal injuries. Am Surg 53:399–402

Wilson RH, Moorehead RJ (1991) Current management of trauma to the pancreas. Br J Surg 78:1196–1202

Wolfman NT, Bechtold RE, Scharling ES, Meredith JW (1992) Blunt upper abdominal trauma: evaluation by CT. AJR 158:493–501

8 The Shoulder Girdle

K.-F. Kreitner and R. Löw

CONTENTS

8.1 The Shoulder and Proximal Humerus

8.1.1 General Considerations

The shoulder girdle is an anatomically complex structure consisting of the scapula, clavicula, proximal humerus, and their articular connections. The wide range of motion is provided by the glenohumeral joint and the two shoulder girdle joints, the acromioclavicular and sternoclavicular joints.

Injuries of the shoulder region occur at all ages, but the spectrum of injuries varies with age. The glenohumeral joint is especially prone to soft tissue injuries because of its complex anatomy (NEER and WELSH 1977). It is the most mobile joint of the human body, this being made possible by the shallow glenoid, the large spherical head of the humerus, and the stability provided by soft tissue. Forces that exceed the tolerance of the stabilizing soft tissue structures frequently lead to subluxation or dislocation of the joint. The subacromial space, which functions as a second joint cavity, is predisposed to derangements of repetitive loading which result in impingement lesions. Fractures of the proximal humerus are more often seen in older patients. However, with unusual violence any type of fracture or fracture dislocation can occur at any age.

Although the clavicle is part of the shoulder girdle, injuries of the clavicle and its articular connections will be discussed separately.

8.1.2 Anatomy and Biomechanics

According to the physeal lines, the proximal end of the humerus can be divided into four parts: the humeral head with the articular surface, the greater tuberosity, the lesser tuberosity, and the proximal shaft (BERQUIST 1992). The anatomic neck is located at the margin of the articular surface and separates the tuberosities from the humeral head segment. The greater tuberosity has three facets for insertion of the supraspinatus, infraspinatus, and teres minor muscles. The intertubercular sulcus lies between the greater and the lesser tuberosities and contains the long biceps tendon. The lesser tuberosity lies medial to the intertubercular sulcus and serves as the insertion of the subscapularis muscle (BIGLIANI et al. 1991). The blood supply of the proximal humerus is derived from the anterior and posterior circumflex humeral arteries. The most important source of circulation to the humeral head is the ascending branch of the anterior circumflex artery that enters the bone in the vicinity of the bicipital groove. This artery may be severely damaged by four-part frac-

K.-F. KREITNER, MD, Klinik und Poliklinik für Radiologie, Johannes-Gutenberg-Universität Mainz, Langenbeckstraße 1, 55131 Mainz, Germany
R. Löw, MD, Klinik und Poliklinik für Radiologie, Johannes-Gutenberg-Universität Mainz, Langenbeckstraße 1, 55131 Mainz, Germany

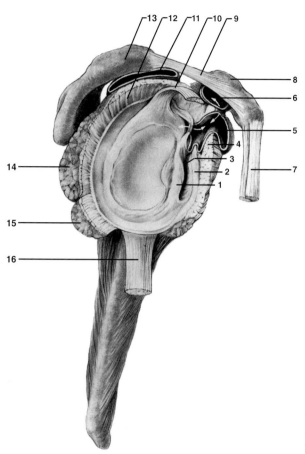

Fig. 8.1. Lateral view of the right shoulder after removal of the humerus, demonstrating a direct view of the glenoid fossa and surrounding soft tissue stabilizing structures. *1*, Glenoid labrum; *2*, joint capsule reinforced by glenohumeral ligaments; *3*, recess between labrum and joint capsule; *4*, subscapularis tendon; *5*, subscapular bursa; *6*, subcoracoid bursa; *7*, short biceps and coracobrachialis tendons; *8*, coracoid process; *9*, coracoacromial ligament; *10*, long biceps tendon; *11*, subacromial bursa; *12*, supraspinatus muscle; *13*, acromion; *14*, infraspinatus muscle; *15*, teres minor muscle; *16*, long triceps tendon. (Adapted from Tillmann and Tichy 1986)

tures of the proximal humerus, and has to be preserved during open reduction procedures (Gerber et al. 1990).

The scapula lies dorsal to the chest wall. It can be divided into the body, the neck, and the glenoid fossa. The body is a large, flat, triangular bone that is almost entirely covered with muscles dorsally and ventrally (Zuckerman et al. 1993). The subscapularis muscle covers the ventral surface; dorsally the scapular spine separates the origin of the supraspinatus from that of the infraspinatus muscle. The teres minor and major muscles originate from the inferior scapula. Laterally the scapular spine

blends with the acromion, which together with the coracoid process and the coracoacromial ligament forms the fornix humeri (Fig. 8.1). The glenoid fossa is deepened by a fibrocartilaginous rim, the glenoid labrum. It consists mainly of dense fibrous tissue and extends around the entire peripheral margin of the glenoid fossa.

Despite minor discrepancies the glenohumeral joint can be regarded as a ball-and-socket joint, where the shallow glenoid fossa articulates with the spherical humeral head. The humeral head is nearly hemispheric and has four times the surface area of the glenoid (Neer 1970). As a consequence, bony restraint of the joint is minimal, but this fact allows for the wide range of motion.

The synovium-lined joint capsule is normally large and loose, and it attaches proximally to the glenoid labrum or the scapular neck and extends distally to the anatomic neck of the humerus. Its volume is nearly twice that of the humeral head. Reinforcement of the glenohumeral joint capsule is achieved by surrounding ligaments, tendons, and muscles (Fig. 8.1).

The glenohumeral ligaments are focal thickenings of the ventral joint capsule which arise from the anterior glenoid and extend to the lesser tuberosity. According to experimental studies, these ligaments vary considerably in size and thickness (Mosely and Övergaard 1962; Turkel et al. 1981). Among them, the inferior glenohumeral ligament is considered to be the major stabilizing ligament anteroinferiorly.

The shoulder joint is guided predominantly by the muscles of the rotator cuff, which help to center the humeral head in the glenoid fossa during motion of the glenohumeral joint. Anterior reinforcement of the shoulder joint is provided by the subscapularis muscle, superior reinforcement by the supraspinatus muscle, and posterior reinforcement by the infraspinatus and teres minor muscles.

These stability-providing soft tissues can be summarized under the term "capsular mechanism" (Moseley and Övergaard 1962; Pappas et al. 1983). They can be divided into anterior and posterior parts that are separated superiorly by the coracohumeral ligament and the long tendon of the biceps muscle, and inferiorly by the long tendon of the triceps muscle. Since the open face of the glenoid fossa is directed anterolaterally, the glenohumeral joint is inherently more stable posteriorly than anteriorly. This explains why anterior instabilities occur far more often than posterior instabilities (Fig. 8.2).

Anterior

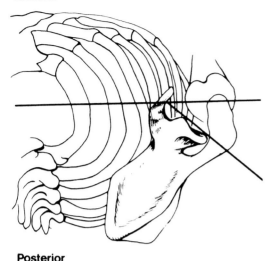

Posterior

Fig. 8.2. View from the top showing that the open face of the glenoid fossa is directed anterolaterally, making the glenohumeral articulation more stable posteriorly than anteriorly

There are numerous bursae about the shoulder which help to facilitate the movements of the shoulder. The two most important are the subscapularis and subacromial-subdeltoid bursae. The subscapularis bursa is an outpouching of the synovial membrane of the glenohumeral joint between the superior and middle glenohumeral ligaments. It is situated anteriorly beneath the coracoid process and lies dorsal to the subscapularis tendon.

The subacromial-subdeltoid bursa lies in the subacromial spatium. The roof is formed by the undersurface of the acromion, coracoacromial arch, and deltoid muscle. The floor of the bursa is the greater tuberosity and the tendons of the rotator cuff. Anteriorly the bursa extends to the subcoracoid position. The bursa acts as a gliding mechanism between these structures (TILLMANN and TICHY 1986). It also lubricates motion between the rotator cuff muscles and the overlying acromion and acromioclavicular joint, thus preventing pressure forces between the fornix and caput humeri. As it functions as a secondary joint it is often called the "secondary subacromial joint" (Fig. 8.1).

Another gliding structure that is important for the free mobility of the shoulder girdle is the "scapulothoracic joint" (TILLMANN and TICHY 1986). It refers to the spatium between the serratus anterior and subscapularis muscle and is filled with soft connective tissue. It enables movement between the scapula and the thoracic cage. Complete abduc-

tion, flexion, or elevation is dependent on the free motion in all joints of the shoulder girdle.

8.1.3 Examination Methods

8.1.3.1 Conventional Radiography

Despite the increasing availability of computed tomography (CT) and magnetic resonance imaging (MRI), plain radiography still plays an important role in the evaluation of shoulder trauma. Numerous views have been described for shoulder examinations, especially for the glenohumeral joint and proximal humerus. For clinical routine, however, it seems to be more practical to be familiar with some elementary projections that can be summarized as the "trauma series" (GUTJAHR 1983; NEER 1990; ROCKWOOD et al. 1991a). This series includes the anteroposterior view in the plane of the glenoid fossa ("true AP view" or tangential-glenoidal projection), true lateral views of the scapula ("Y-view" or transscapular projection), axillary views, and AP views of the humerus in internal and external rotation (Fig. 8.3).

On the tangential-glenoidal radiograph of the shoulder, there is normally no overlap between the articular surface of the humeral head and the glenoid fossa (Fig. 8.4). Any overlapping of these two struc-

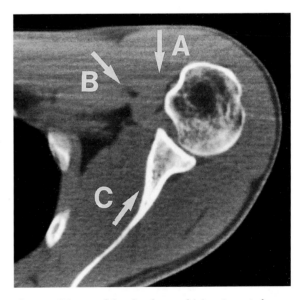

Fig. 8.3. CT scan of the glenohumeral joint. *A*, central x-ray beam in AP view of the shoulder; *B*, central x-ray beam in tangential-glenoidal view ("true" AP view) of the shoulder; *C*, central x-ray beam in transscapular view ("true" lateral view) of the shoulder

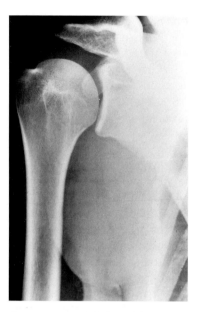

Fig. 8.4. Tangential-glenoidal view of the glenohumeral joint: there is no overlap between the humeral head and the glenoid fossa; postreduction radiograph after anterior shoulder dislocation

tures on this projection proves a glenohumeral dislocation; its direction must be determined on transscapular radiographs. On true AP views, the anterior and posterior glenoid rims are superim-posed, thus facilitating the detection of glenoid rim fractures.

The transscapular or Y-view is perpendicular to the tangential-glenoidal projection and therefore represents the true lateral view of the glenohumeral joint (Fig. 8.5). The characteristic Y-configuration is formed by the wing of the scapula caudally, the scapula spine dorsally, and the coracoid process ventrally. The glenoid fossa is the center of the "Y" and is covered by the humeral head. Any dislocation of the humeral head in an anterior-posterior or superior-inferior direction can easily be detected by this projection. The supraspinatus view, which allows for evaluation of the acromion and subacromial space, can be obtained by angling the beam 5° caudally (Fig. 8.6) (KILCOYNE et al. 1989).

The true AP and lateral views of the glenohumeral joint are the two most important projections for evaluation the glenohumeral joint in acute trauma. In proximal fractures of the humerus, it is essential to define the fractured segments and to determine their degree of displacement. Glenohumeral dislocations can be exactly determined.

The axillary view, which has to be done carefully in the acutely injured patient, requires abduction of the involved arm by 60–90°. This view may provide

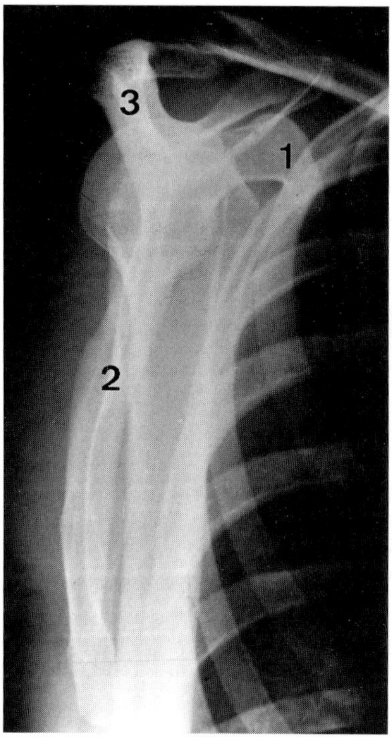

Fig. 8.5. Transscapular view of the glenohumeral joint with the characteristic Y-configuration of the scapula. *1*, Coracoid process; *2*, wing of the scapula; *3*, scapular spine

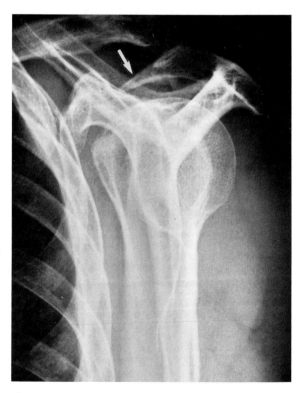

Fig. 8.6. Supraspinatus-outlet view in a patient with rotator cuff tear and a "hooked" acromion (*arrow*)

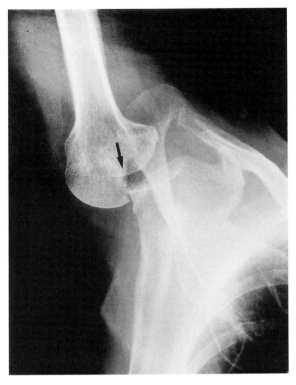

Fig. 8.7. Axillary view of the shoulder in a patient with posterior dislocation and an impression fracture (*arrow*) of the anteromedial humeral head ("reverse" Hill-Sachs deformity)

additional information in patients with fractures and dislocations of the humeral head and glenoid fossa and with injuries of the acromion and acromioclavicular joint (Fig. 8.7).

Anteroposterior views of the proximal humerus are often used to obtain a first overview of the injured shoulder. Nevertheless, they must not replace the aforementioned projections as they are not sufficient for classifying especially glenohumeral dislocations or proximal humeral fractures. Additional views in internal and external rotation may clarify the presence of a fracture of the tuberosities and their degree of dislocation (Fig. 8.8).

Stress views of the glenohumeral joint may demonstrate the amount of glenohumeral translation with loading in various directions. They may be helpful in evaluating subtle forms of atraumatic instabilities where normally no apparent dislocation can be documented (Fig. 8.9) (ROCKWOOD et al. 1991a).

There exist numerous other projections for evaluating the glenohumeral joint, such as the Stryker notch, Didiee, Hermodsson, and Westpoint views or variations of the axillary projection. They serve to detect fixed abnormalities after glenohumeral dislocations like the Hill-Sachs and reverse Hill-Sachs de-

formity of the humeral head or glenoid rim fractures (ROCKWOOD et al. 1991a). In the era of widespread CT and MRI and owing to their degree of impracticability, however, there seems to be no further need to perform them.

8.1.3.2 Arthrography

Standard arthrography, with either the single- or double-contrast technique, can be used to evaluate the possibility of rotator cuff tears and to demonstrate the presence of adhesive capsulitis. The latter is characterized by a diminished capacity of the glenohumeral joint (<7 ml), small or absent capsular recesses, and irregularity of capsular insertion (RESNICK 1981). The diagnosis of a complete rotator cuff tear is based upon the identification of an abnormal communication between the glenohumeral joint cavity and the subacromial-subdeltoid bursa (Fig. 8.10). In partial tears of the articular surface, there is a collection of contrast material in the inferior substance of the rotator cuff without extension into the subacromial bursa. The sensitivity and specificity of conventional arthrography for full-thickness tears lie between 85% and 100% and between 90% and 100%, respectively. There are limitations in the detection of partial tears, especially of the bursal surface of the rotator cuff (RESNICK 1981).

If the presence or absence of a complete rotator cuff tear influences further therapy, then conventional arthrography remains an easy and cost-effective way to make the diagnosis. Arthrography can distinguish between massive and small tears. However, assessment of the exact size of the tear and of the quality of the torn edges is not possible (STILES and OTTE 1993).

8.1.3.3 Ultrasonography

There exist numerous studies concerning the accuracy of ultrasonography in the evaluation of rotator cuff tears (STILES and OTTE 1993). Tears of the rotator cuff can be diagnosed by focal thinning of the cuff, nonvisualization, discontinuity in echo patterns, and a central echogenic band within the cuff substance. Large tears may show regions of diminished echo density. The values for sensitivity and specificity range from 33% to 100% and from 50% to 94%, respectively (MISAMORE and WOODWARD 1991; WIENER and SEITZ 1993). These results may explain why, generally, the technique has

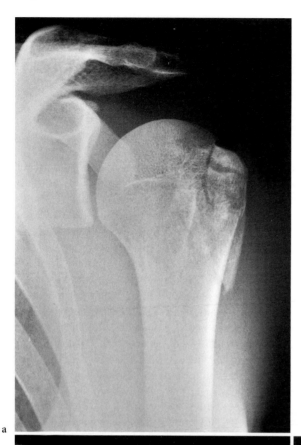

Fig. 8.8a–c. Fracture of the greater tuberosity after anterior glenohumeral dislocation. The real extent of fracture displacement is better demonstrated on the AP views. a "True" AP view of the shoulder (tangential-glenoidal projection); b "normal" AP view of the humerus; c AP view in internal rotation of the humerus

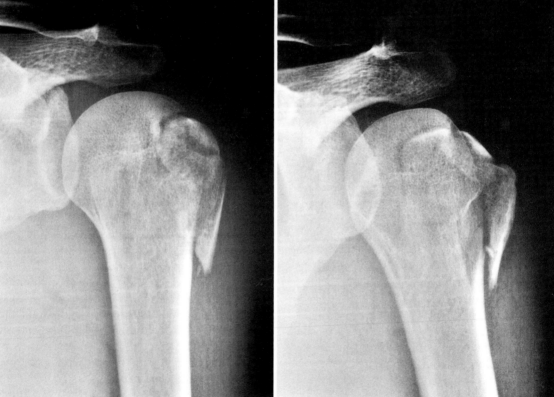

Fig. 8.9a,b. Inferior translation of the humeral head in a patient with atraumatic multidirectional instability. Note the vacuum phenomenon in the glenohumeral joint in **a**. **a** AP view of the shoulder; **b** stress radiograph of both shoulders

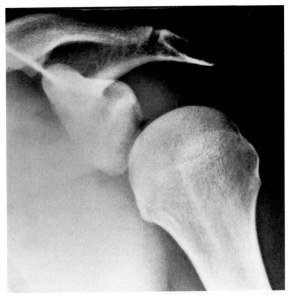

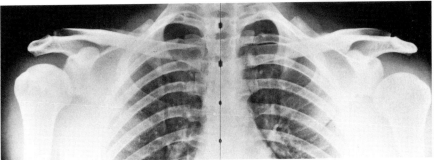

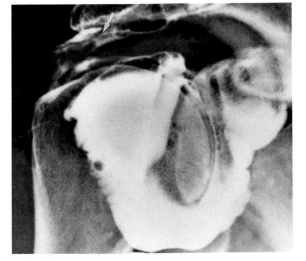

Fig. 8.10. Complete tear of the supraspinatus tendon with broad communication between the glenohumeral joint and the subacromial-subdeltoid bursa (*arrow*)

not become widely accepted. However, when performed by dedicated examiners, ultrasonography enables the diagnosis of rotator cuff tears with a high accuracy.

8.1.3.4 Computed Tomography

In the preoperative evaluation of patients with proximal humeral fractures, the amount of displacement or rotation of fragments may be difficult to determine even on plain radiographs of the "trauma series". Specific cases in which the plain films may underestimate displacement include fractures of the greater or lesser tuberosity, impression fractures of the humeral head, head-splitting fractures, or loose bodies in the shoulder joint (CASTAGNO et al. 1987; KILCOYNE et al. 1990). CT can be helpful in these cases (Figs. 8.11, 8.24, 8.32). Furthermore, CT has proved to be useful for better definition of glenoid fractures and displaced fractures of the scapula. Multiplanar reformation of CT data and 3D

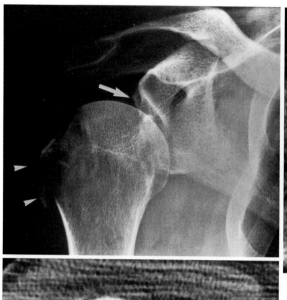

a

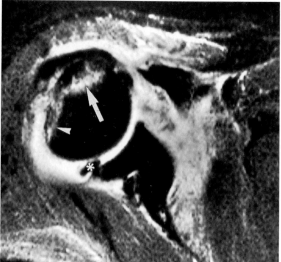

c

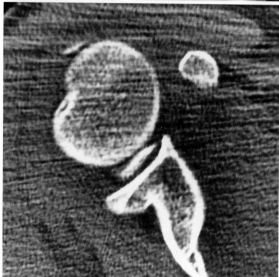

b

Fig. 8.11a–c. Loose body in the shoulder joint after anterior dislocation. **a** The postreduction AP view of the shoulder shows a double contour of the posterior glenoid rim (*arrow*) and a fracture of the greater tuberosity (*arrowheads*). **b** The CT scan clearly depicts the large intra-articular loose body. **c** Besides the loose body (*asterisk*), MRI shows the fracture of the greater tuberosity (*arrow*) and a defect of the posterolateral humeral head (*arrowhead*); axial STIR image

reconstructions help to display the complexity of these fractures and ease the surgical planning (Fig. 8.34).

In combination with double-contrast arthrography CT can be used to define the extent of labral and capsular abnormalities in patients with glenohumeral instability (Fig. 8.12). It seems to be more accurate than standard MRI in young patients as injuries of the rotator cuff are uncommon at this age (KREITNER et al. 1992). Bony lesions, especially of the anteroinferior glenoid rim and of the posterolateral humeral head, are demonstrated with great accuracy (Figs. 8.20, 8.21). CT-arthrography also depicts tears of the rotator cuff, but it is not the imaging modality of choice in defining these lesions (BLUM et al. 1993; KREITNER et al. 1993).

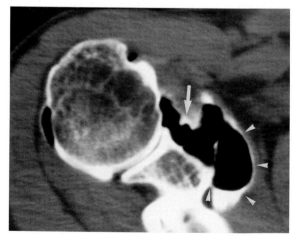

Fig. 8.12. Avulsion of the anterior glenoid labrum and glenohumeral ligament (*arrow*) and stripping of the anterior joint capsule from the scapular neck (*arrowheads*)

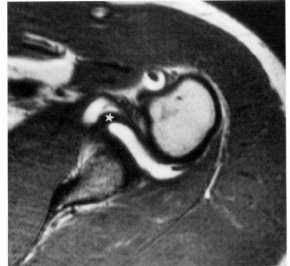

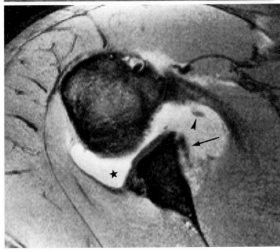

Fig. 8.13. a T1-weighted axial MR-arthrogram showing a normal inferior glenohumeral ligament (*asterisk*) and capsulolabral complex. **b** T2*-weighted gradient-echo image showing avulsion of the inferior labrum (*arrow*) and tear of the inferior glenohumeral ligament (*arrowhead*) after traumatic dislocation; the *asterisk* denotes joint effusion

8.1.1.3.5 Magnetic Resonance Imaging

Since its introduction into clinical routine, MRI has become an important technique for evaluating suspected shoulder abnormalities, especially rotator cuff disorders and instability. Improvements in diagnostic accuracy could be achieved by combining MRI with single-contrast arthrography using a 2-mM solution of Gd-DTPA as contrast agent (CHANDNANI et al. 1995; PALMER et al. 1994). MR-arthrography allows for visualization and evaluation of the labral-ligamentous complex, which plays an important role in glenohumeral instability (Fig. 8.13). The role of MR-arthrography in delineating SLAP lesions (lesions of the superior labrum, anterior posterior), however, remains yet to be determined (Fig. 8.14) (HODLER et al. 1992).

Magnetic resonance-arthrography detects complete and partial tears of the articular surface of the rotator cuff with a high accuracy (Fig. 8.15). Furthermore, it enables assessment of the size of the tear and the quality of the torn edges (IANOTTI et al. 1991; QUINN et al. 1995). Up to now, it is unclear from the existing literature whether or not MRI can reliably differentiate – except for tears of the rotator cuff – the various stages of the impingement syndrome, and in particular between degeneration and tendinitis (KJELLIN et al. 1991; ROBERTSON et al. 1995). MRI clearly depicts tears and dislocations of the long biceps tendon, which often accompany dislocations and rotator cuff tears in the elderly (ERICKSON et al. 1992; TUCKMAN 1994).

Magnetic resonance imaging is very sensitive for the detection of bone bruises and occult fractures. It may prove the presence of non-displaced fractures (especially of the greater tuberosity) that are missed on conventional radiographs. It is highly sensitive for the detection of early signs of osteonecrosis of the humeral head after fracture.

For the successful use of MRI of the shoulder, some technical factors warrant mention. The shoulder must be imaged with a surface coil. T2-weighted spin-echo images with and without fat suppression are required for evaluating the rotator cuff. Labral abnormalities are best demonstrated on

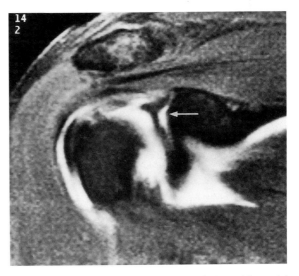

Fig. 8.14. Arthroscopically proven SLAP lesion with partial avulsion of the superior labrum (*arrow*); T1-weighted coronal MR-arthrogram with fat saturation

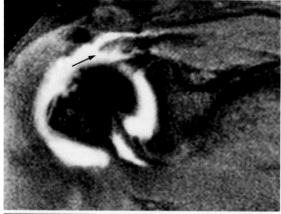

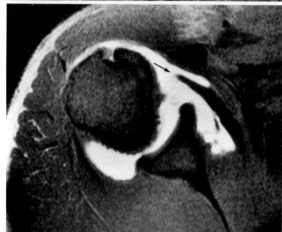

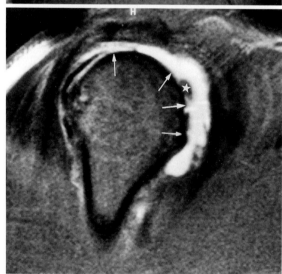

Fig. 8.15a–c. Large tear of the rotator cuff: T1-weighted MR-arthrograms with fat saturation. **a** Retraction of the supraspinatus tendon (*arrow*), coronal plane. **b** Retraction of the torn subscapularis tendon (*arrow*), axial plane. **c** Large defect of the rotator cuff superiorly and anteriorly (*arrows*), best demonstrated on sagittal images. The *asterisk* denotes the long biceps tendon

T2*-weighted gradient-echo images. For MR-arthrography with diluted Gd-DTPA solutions, T1-weighted spin-echo images with and without fat suppression are recommended (MASSENGILL et al. 1994; PALMER et al. 1995). The field of view should be 180 mm or less to gain sufficient spatial resolution.

8.1.3.6 Angiography

Angiography may become necessary after dislocated scapular fractures and, rarely, after glenohumeral dislocations with major injury to the subclavian and axillary vessels (Fig. 8.16).

8.1.4 Subluxations and Dislocations of the Glenohumeral Joint

8.1.4.1 General Considerations

As stability of the glenohumeral joint is mainly provided by the supporting soft tissues, glenohumeral dislocation is the most common dislocation among the greater joints: it accounts for 50% of all dislocations. Most dislocations (about 97% of all cases) are anterior; posterior dislocations occur in 1.5%–2.5% of patients. Superior and inferior dislocations (luxatio erecta) are rare (ROCKWOOD et al. 1991a). The incidence of primary anterior dislocations is estimated to be around 10/100 000 per year (HOELEN et al. 1990). Up to now, no data exist concerning the

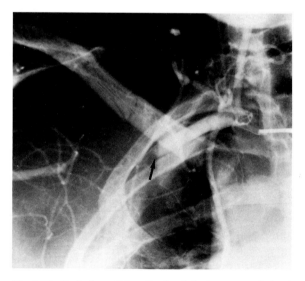

Fig. 8.16. Occlusion of the distal subclavian artery (*arrow*) after severe shoulder trauma due to intimal tear

real incidence of atraumatic instabilities, which is estimated to be higher than that of traumatic instabilities (ROCKWOOD et al. 1991a).

Glenohumeral dislocations are more often induced by indirect than by direct forces (GUTJAHR et al. 1993). Anterior dislocations are often the result of a combination of abduction, extension, and external rotation forces applied to the arm, which then indirectly transfers the force to the anterior capsule and ligaments. Conversely, a combination of internal rotation, adduction, and flexion forces may cause posterior dislocations. They are most commonly produced by accidental electrical shocks and convulsive seizures. Anterior and posterior glenohumeral dislocations are rarely caused by direct forces.

8.1.4.2 Classification, Trauma Pattern, and Pathomorphology

Glenohumeral instabilities can be classified according to their degree, frequency, cause, and direction and the anatomic location of the humeral head.

A glenohumeral dislocation is a complete separation of the articular surfaces; immediate spontaneous relocation does not occur. A subluxation is defined as a translation of the humeral head in relation to the glenoid without complete separation of the articular surfaces; the humeral head quickly returns to its normal position in the glenoid fossa. Glenohumeral subluxations are transient and commonly momentary, and are most often felt by the patient. However, in the "dead arm syn-

drome," which is characterized by a sudden sharp or "paralyzing" pain when the shoulder subluxates, more than 50% of patients are not aware of their shoulder instability (ROWE and ZARINS 1981). Like dislocations, subluxations may be traumatic or atraumatic, anterior, posterior or inferior, acute or recurrent.

The frequency of glenohumeral dislocations may be acute, recurrent, or fixed, the direction anterior, posterior or multidirectional. The cause of shoulder instability may be traumatic or atraumatic. The distinction between traumatic and atraumatic cause of instability is of importance for therapeutic decisions (GERBER and GANZ 1986). Atraumatic instabilities are commonly associated with voluntary, multidirectional and bilateral instability and respond very often to a rehabilitation program. They mostly affect young females. Surgical procedures, in the form of inferior capsular shift operations, are rarely required (NEER and FOSTER 1980). A hint for atraumatic instability may be the glenohumeral translation documented by stress radiographs (Fig. 8.9) Traumatic shoulder instabilities are commonly unilateral, and anterior with a Bankart lesion, for which surgery is usually required, and mainly affect young males.

Anterior dislocations are classified according to the location of the humeral head into subcoracoid, subglenoid, subclavicular and intrathoracic dislocations. The subcoracoid dislocation is the most common type of dislocation a major joint in the body: it is far more common than the subglenoid type of anterior dislocation (Fig. 8.17). Subclavicular and intrathoracic dislocations are rare.

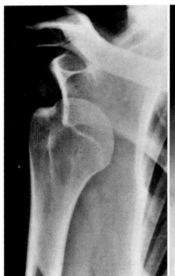 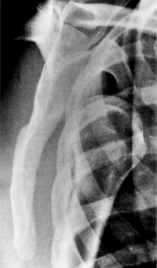

Fig. 8.17a,b. Anterior, subcoracoid dislocation of the shoulder. **a** Tangential-glenoidal (true AP) view; **b** transscapular (true lateral) view

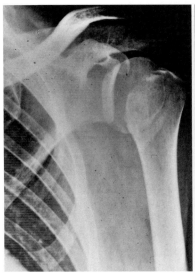 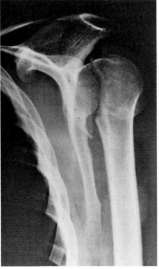

a   b

Fig. 8.18a,b. Posterior, subacromial dislocation of the shoulder. **a** Tangential-glenoidal view; **b** transscapular view

In posterior dislocations, the humeral head may be in a subacromial (head behind the glenoid and beneath the acromion), subglenoid (head behind and beneath the glenoid), or subspinous position. The subacromial dislocation is by far the most common (Fig. 8.18).

In inferior dislocations, the humeral head is below the glenoid fossa, with the humerus turned upside down. In superior dislocations, there is upward displacement of the humeral head, often accompanied by fractures of the acromion, clavicle, coracoid process, or tuberosities. The soft tissue of the fornix humeri is severely damaged (BERQUIST 1992).

In acute dislocations, the direction can be easily assessed by the tangential-glenoidal ("true anterior") and transscapular ("true lateral") views of the glenohumeral joint (Fig. 8.17, 8.18). They precisely document any dislocation in any direction (GUTJAHR 1983). Normal AP views of the shoulder alone are insufficient for classifying glenohumeral dislocations. Classically, posterior dislocations are easily overlooked on AP radiographs of the shoulder as the humeral head apparently articulates with the glenoid fossa (Figs. 8.19, 8.32, 8.34). There may be several signs that lead to the correct diagnosis, such as the absence of the normal elliptical overlap of the humeral head and the glenoid fossa, the vacant glenoid sign, and the "trough line" which is the result of an impaction fracture of the anteromedial humeral head caused by the posterior glenoid rim ("reverse Hill-Sachs lesion").

Postreduction radiographs have to be analyzed for adequate reduction and accompanying osseous lesions of the humeral head and glenoid rim

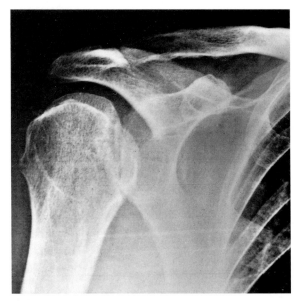

Fig. 8.19. Normal AP view of the shoulder with a posterior dislocation. Note the absence of the normal elliptical overlap between the humeral head and glenoid fossa, and the trough line

(ROCKWOOD et al. 1991a). The most common lesion after anterior dislocations is the impression fracture of the posterolateral aspect of the humeral head, resulting from the impaction of the humeral head onto the ventral glenoid rim (HILL and SACHS 1940). The reported incidence of the Hill-Sachs deformity ranges from 46% to 90% (Fig. 8.20). The corresponding lesion in posterior dislocations is the impression fracture of the anteromedial aspect of the humeral head that is produced by the posterior glenoid rim. It is often called the reverse Hill-Sachs deformity. Its

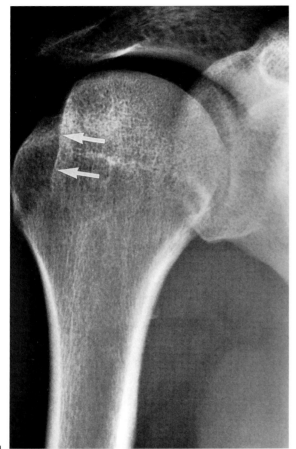

a

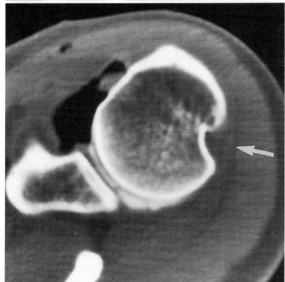

b

Fig. 8.20a,b. Typical posterolateral impression fractures of the humeral head (*arrows*). **a** Normal AP view of the humerus in internal rotation. **b** Axial CT scan

dimensions are best appreciated on axillary views or CT scans (Figs. 8.7, 8.32); its size may be a cause of recurrence in posterior dislocations.

Bony lesions of the anterior or posterior glenoid rim should be detected on tangential-glenoidal views of the glenohumeral joint. However, like impression fractures of the humeral head, they are best assessed by CT scans (Fig. 8.21) (MADLER et al. 1988).

Fractures of the greater tuberosity accompany anterior shoulder dislocations in up to 35% of cases (KREITNER et al. 1987). They most commonly occur beyond the age of 40. Fractures of the lesser tuberosity may be seen after posterior dislocations; these are avulsion fractures of the subscapularis muscle and are best seen on axial views or CT scans (Fig. 8.24).

Lesions of the so-called capsulolabral complex are regarded as the major cause of recurrence in traumatic instabilities and are best assessed by CT- or MR-arthrography (Figs. 8.12–8.14). The latter allows for evaluation of the integrity of the glenohumeral ligaments in anterior instability, thus influencing the therapeutic regimen (PALMER et al. 1994; SCHWEITZER 1994).

8.1.4.3 Complications

Recurrent dislocation is the most common complication following acute traumatic anterior dislocations of the shoulder, with reported recurrence rates of up

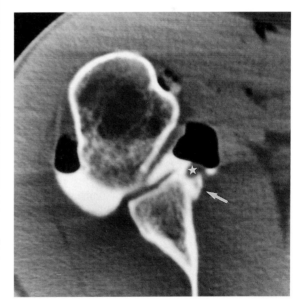

Fig. 8.21. CT scan clearly showing the avulsion of the anterior glenoid rim (*arrow*) and anteroinferior glenoid labrum (*asterisk*)

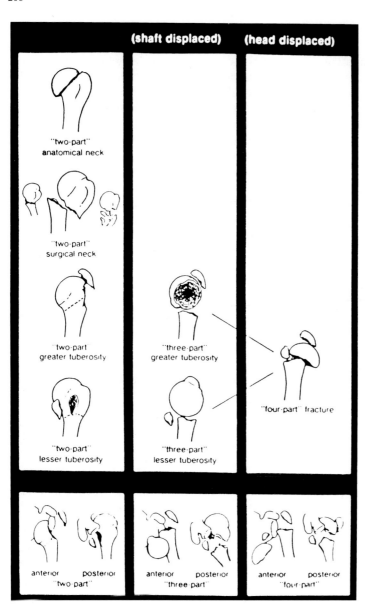

Fig. 8.22. Neer's classification of proximal humeral fractures (modified from NEER 1990)

to 90% in younger patients (HOELEN et al. 1990; NEER and WELSH 1977). At present, the age of the patient at the time of initial dislocation seems to be the most important prognostic factor rather than the treatment of the initial dislocation and associated fractures. In younger patients, avulsions of the glenohumeral ligaments and capsule are relatively unlikely to heal in a manner yielding a stable shoulder (ROCKWOOD et al. 1991a). In older patients, stretching of the capsule or avulsion of the greater tuberosity heal, leaving a stable shoulder.

Direct complications of glenohumeral dislocations are rotator cuff tears and vascular and neural injuries. Rotator cuff tears most commonly occur in patients older than 40 years (HOELEN et al. 1990).

They may severely impair shoulder function after glenohumeral dislocation (Fig. 8.15). Neural injuries mostly affect the axillary nerve and may be present in up to 30% of patients with anterior dislocations (KREITNER et al. 1987). Vascular injuries are rare, affect the axillary artery, and should be confirmed by angiography.

8.1.5 Fractures of the Proximal Humerus

8.1.5.1 General Considerations

Fractures of the proximal humerus are common and account for about 4%–5% of all fractures. They occur more frequently in older patients, after the cancellous bone of the humeral neck has become weakened by osteoporosis (NEER 1990). However, fractures of the humeral head are seen in patients of all ages; they involve the proximal epiphysis in up to 80% of cases during childhood. Newer epidemiologic studies indicate that there is an increase in incidence, with age-adjusted incidences of 104–105 per 100 000 person-years, due to the increased average life span. Further analysis reveals that most proximal humeral fractures are osteoporosis-related and an important source of morbidity among the elderly population (BENGNER et al. 1988).

In older patients, the fractures often result from a minor fall on the outstretched arm or from a direct blow on the lateral side of the arm, and are usually minimally displaced. In younger individuals and athletes, the strength of the proximal humerus normally is greater than that of the surrounding soft tissues so that dislocations usually occur instead of fractures. However, with unusual violence any type of displaced fracture or fracture dislocation can occur at any age (BERQUIST 1992).

8.1.5.2 Classification, Trauma Pattern, and Pathomorphology

Fractures of the proximal humerus tend to follow the physeal lines that divide the proximal end of the humerus into four parts: the articular segment of the humeral head, the lesser tuberosity, the greater tuberosity, and the shaft (level of the surgical neck). NEER, in 1970, proposed the most widely accepted classification for adult fractures of the proximal humerus, which combines morphologic with functional and vascular considerations. The classification is based on the accurate identification of the status of the four parts, the number of fragments, and their degree of displacement. A fracture is considered to be displaced when any of the four major segments is displaced more than 1.0 cm or angulated more than 45°. Lesser displacement is categorized as minimal, regardless of the number and level of the fracture lines. Fissure lines or hairline fractures are not to be considered displaced. A fragment may have several undisplaced components, and these should not be considered separate fragments since they are in continuity and are held together by soft tissue.

A modification of Neer's classification incorporates the differentiation between fracture and fracture-dislocation according to whether the articular segment of the humeral head is dislocated or not

(Fig. 8.22) (NEER 1990; GUTJAHR et al. 1993). Correct assessment of proximal humeral fractures before and after closed or open reduction and internal fixation requires proper plain radiographs, including the aforementioned "trauma series". CT scans may be helpful in identifying loose intra-articular bodies, and in all cases where the degree of fracture displacement remains unclear.

Approximately 70%–80% of proximal humeral fractures are minimally displaced (Fig. 8.23). These fractures most commonly involve the surgical neck. The rotator cuff, capsule, and periosteum remain mostly intact, and assist in maintaining the position of the fragments. As there is no disturbance of blood supply, the prognosis of the injury is generally good.

In a two-part fracture, the displaced fragment can be the greater or the lesser tuberosity, the shaft, or the articular segment (Figs. 8.24, 8.25). In the last-mentioned case, the blood supply to the humeral

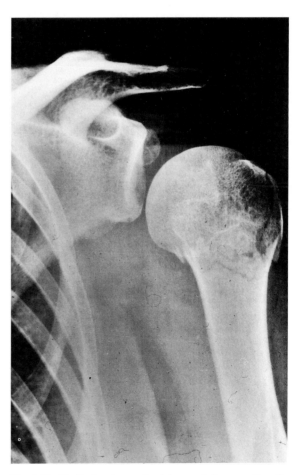

Fig. 8.23. Undisplaced, proximal humeral fracture. Despite several fracture lines, there is no displacement greater than 1 cm or angulation of more than 45°

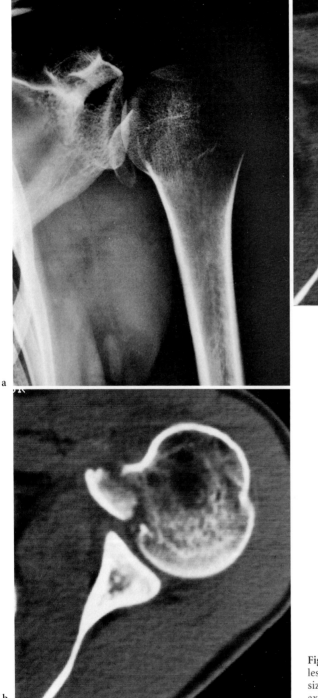

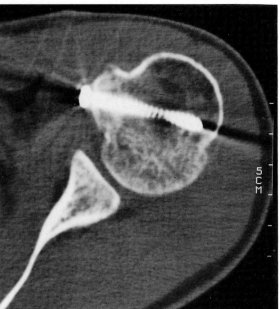

Fig. 8.24a–c. Two-part fracture with displacement of the lesser tuberosity. **a** AP view of the shoulder. **b** The fragment size and the degree of displacement are best demonstrated on axial CT scans. **c** CT scan after internal screw fixation

head may be damaged with a risk of secondary osteonecrosis.

In a three-part fracture, two fragments are displaced in relationship to each other and the other two undisplaced fragments (Fig. 8.26). The articular segment of the humerus remains in contact with the glenoid. Its blood supply may be maintained by one of the tuberosities and parts of the shoulder capsule. There are longitudinal tears in the rotator cuff. Closed reduction is not possible in these cases.

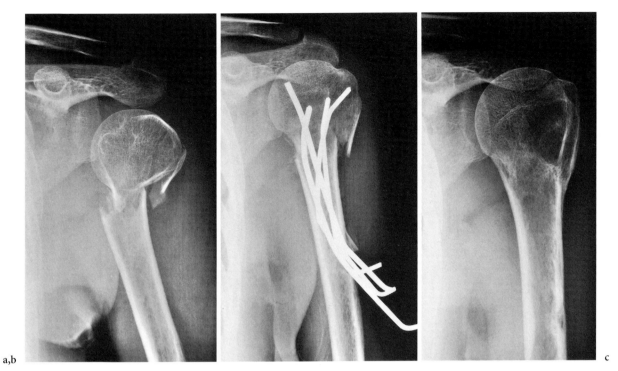

Fig. 8.25a–c. Two-part fracture with displacement of the shaft. **a** AP view of the shoulder. **b** Control radiograph after internal fixation with several pins. **c** Normal healing of the fracture

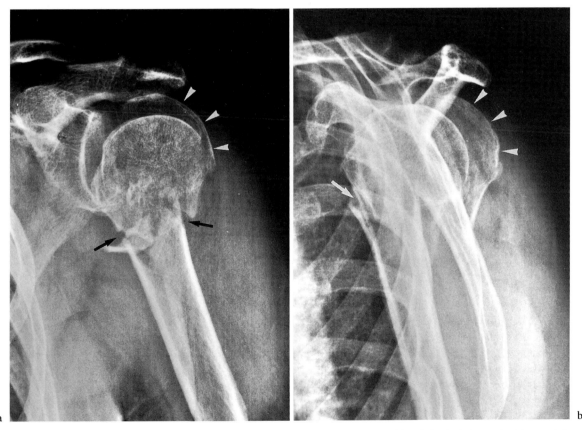

Fig. 8.26a,b. Three-part fracture with displacement of the greater tuberosity (*arrowheads*) and the shaft (*arrows*). **a** Tangential-glenoidal projection; **b** transscapular projection

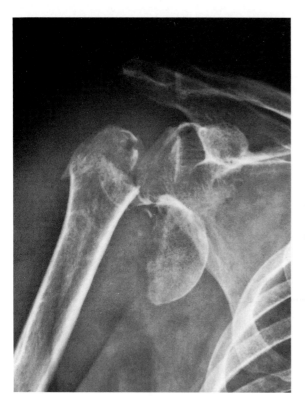

Fig. 8.27. Two-part fracture-dislocation with anterior dislocation of the humeral head segment

rim. They are graded according to the percentage of the involved articular surface and can be assessed best on axillary views or CT scans. Head-splitting fractures are uncommon. They are the result of violent trauma and are normally combined with other fractures of the proximal humerus.

The AO classification (MÜLLER et al. 1992) centers on the vascular supply to the head segment as this plays an important role in the prognosis of the in-

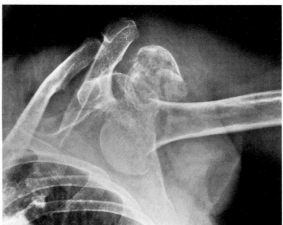

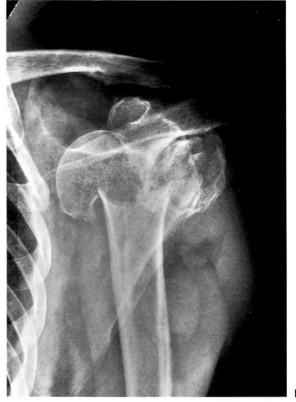

Fig. 8.28a,b. Four-part fracture dislocation of the proximal humerus. **a** AP view of the shoulder. **b** Transscapular view delineating the anterior dislocation of the humeral head

In a four-part fracture, all four fracture fragments are displaced. The head segment is detached from both tuberosities and may be angulated laterally, anteriorly, posteriorly, inferiorly, or superiorly. Normally, there is a loss of blood supply to the humeral head.

In fracture-dislocations there is – in addition to a fracture – a dislocation of the head segment outside the joint space rather than intra-articular rotation or subluxation (Figs. 8.27, 8.28). Fracture-dislocations can be classified according to the direction – usually anterior or posterior – as well as to the number of fracture fragments. It is of clinical value to note that anterior dislocation are mostly associated with displacement of the greater tuberosity, whereas posterior dislocations are associated with displacements of the lesser tuberosity. Due to the dislocation of the head segment, the extent of soft tissue damage and the risk of osteonecrosis exceed that associated with single fractures (GUTJAHR et al. 1993).

Special fractures are the so-called head-splitting and impression fractures. The impression fractures result from acute (usually posterior) dislocations with severe impact of the head against the glenoid

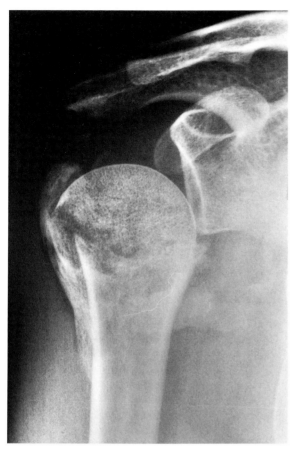

Fig. 8.29. Myositis ossificans in a chronic unreduced fracture with impaction of the humeral head onto the shaft

jury, with avascular necrosis being a common complication. Nevertheless, the AO classification has not gained a degree of acceptance comparable to the Neer classification.

8.1.5.3 Complications

Avascular necrosis of the humeral head is a common complication in three- and four-part fractures, with reported incidences of 13%–34% (HAGG and LUNDBERG 1984). Beside the severity of the fracture, extensive damage and traumatization of soft tissue has proved to be a major contributing factor (BIGLIANI et al. 1991). Myositis ossificans is a rare complication in chronic unreduced fracture-dislocations (Fig. 8.29). A frozen shoulder may be the result of inadequate rehabilitation after fracture or operative repair. Malunion occurs after an inadequate closed reduction or failed open reduction and internal fixation. Malunion may lead to posttrau-

matic osteoarthritis with considerable loss of shoulder motion, and to impingement syndromes, if a significant dislocation of the tuberosities remains (BIGLIANI et al. 1991).

Vascular complications after proximal humeral fractures are infrequent; however, they have an incidence of up to 5% in displaced fractures (STABLEFORTH 1984). Most commonly the axillary artery is involved and the injury should be confirmed by angiography. Injuries of the brachial plexus are encountered in 6% of displaced fractures.

8.1.6 Fractures of the Scapula

8.1.6.1 General Considerations

Fractures of the scapula are relatively uncommon injuries. They account for 3%–5% of all shoulder fractures and only 0.5%–1% of all fractures. They occur most frequently in males between 30 and 40 years of age (ZUCKERMAN et al. 1993). Due to the surrounding muscle mass, which provides a significant amount of protection, scapular fractures are usually the result of major, direct traumas, most commonly motor vehicle accidents, falls from heights, or other types of high-energy injuries. In up to 80% of cases, scapular fractures are associated with injuries to the ipsilateral lung, chest wall, and shoulder girdle. The most commonly associated injuries are rib fractures in 27%–54% of cases, followed by pulmonary contusions (11%–54%), pneumothorax (11%–38%), and clavicular fractures (23%–39%) (for more details, see Chap. 5). Because of the gravity of these injuries, fractures of the scapula may be missed initially (NEER 1990; ZUCKERMAN et al. 1993). Scapular fractures also occur from indirect trauma, e.g., avulsion fractures caused by muscle contraction (electroshock therapy, seizures, high-voltage injuries) (SCHUNK et al. 1993).

8.1.6.2 Classification, Trauma Pattern, and Pathomorphology

Scapular fractures are commonly classified according to the anatomic location (Fig. 8.30). Fractures of the body are most commonly encountered, followed by neck, glenoid, acromion, spine, and coracoid fractures. In many cases, there is a combination of these different types, e.g., fractures of the body with an extra-articular extension into the neck, or intra-articular glenoid fractures that extend into the neck and body.

Fractures of the scapular body and spine are mostly caused by direct violence and, therefore, have the highest incidence of associated injuries (Fig. 8.31). Despite comminutions and displacements, there is usually no need for surgical intervention.

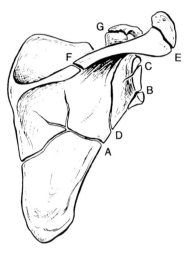

Fig. 8.30. Anatomic classification of scapular fractures. *A*, Body; *B*, glenoid rim; *C*, glenoid fossa; *D*, scapular neck; *E*, acromion; *F*, spine; *G*, coracoid

Fractures of the neck are the second most common fractures of the scapula; they are often impacted and the fracture pattern extends from the suprascapular notch across the neck to the lateral border of the scapula. For therapeutic reasons, it is essential to decide whether the fracture has to be considered stable or unstable (BIGLIANI et al. 1991). In stable fractures there is no additional injury of the ipsilateral clavicle or acromioclavicular ligaments, the latter preventing further displacement and enhancing stability. Ipsilateral fractures of the clavicle or acromiclavicular ligament tears are indicators of instability in scapular neck fractures ("humeroscapular dissociation") and require open reduction and internal fixation (Fig. 8.32) (LEUNG and LAM 1993; LEUTENEGGER and RÜEDI 1993).

Glenoid fractures are intra-articular fractures; they can be divided into five types (Fig. 8.33) (IDEBERG 1987). Type I represents an avulsion fracture from the glenoid rim occurring most probably from dislocations. Type II comprises transverse and oblique fractures exiting inferiorly. Type III refers to transverse fractures exiting superiorly, and type IV to fractures exiting through the medial border of the scapula. Type V combines a type II and type IV pattern. It is of great importance to define the extent of

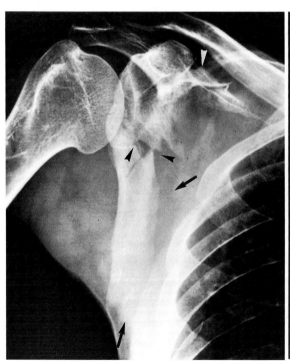

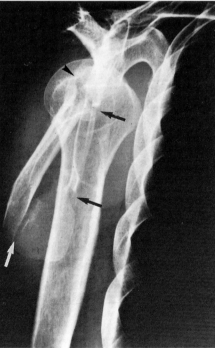

a   b

Fig. 8.31a,b. Fracture of the body of the scapula (*arrows*) with extension into the neck and the glenoid fossa (*arrowheads*). **a** AP view of the shoulder; **b** transscapular view. The real extent of fragment displacement is seen only on the transscapular view. There is no accompanyling dislocation of the glenohumeral joint

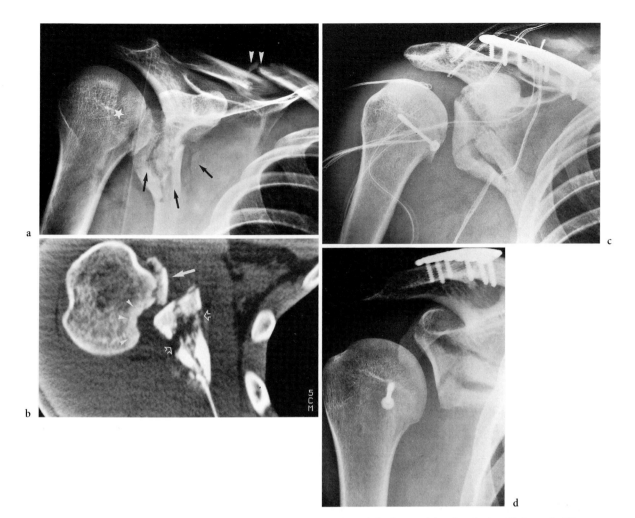

Fig. 8.32a-d. Complex shoulder girdle injury in a polytraumatized patient with a comminuted fracture of the scapular neck extending into the glenoid fossa (*arrows* in **a**). There are an associated fracture of the clavicle (*arrowheads* in **a**) and a posterior dislocation of the humeral head (*asterisk* in **a**) with avulsion fracture of the lesser tuberosity and a small anteromedial impression fracture of the humeral head (two-part fracture dislocation of the proximal humerus, according to the Neer classification). **a** AP radiograph of the shoulder girdle. Note the apparent articulation of the humeral head, but there is a vacant glenoid anteriorly and a lack of the elliptical overlap of the humeral head and glenoid fossa. **b** CT scan clearly delineating the posterior dislocation of the humeral head and the avulsion fracture of the lesser tuberosity (*arrow*). Note the impression fracture of the humeral head (*arrowheads*) and the comminution of the scapular neck extending into the glenoid fossa (*open arrows*). The fracture is about 2 weeks old and shows the onset of callus formation. **c,d** Postoperative radiographs in the AP and tangential-glenoidal projections revealing a normal articulation in the glenohumeral joint, no incongruency of the glenoid fossa, and an internal plate fixation of the clavicle

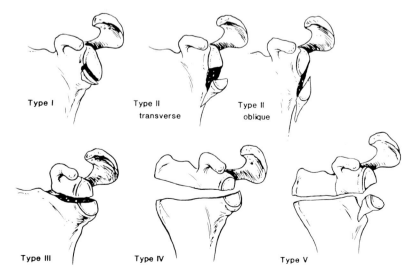

Fig. 8.33. Classification of glenoid fractures after IDEBERG (1987) (see text)

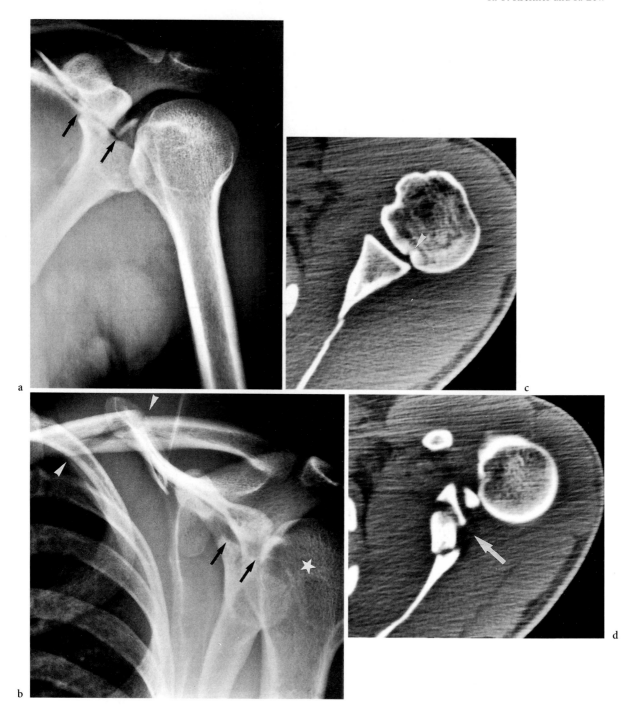

a

b

c

d

Fig. 8.34a–g. Complex shoulder girdle injury with dislocated fracture of the glenoid fossa extending through the base of the coracoid, with posterior subluxation of the humeral head and fracture of the clavicle. **a,b** AP and transscapular views of the shoulder clearly showing the glenoid fracture extending through the base of the coracoid (*arrows*), the fracture of the clavicle (*arrowheads*), and the posterior subluxation of the humeral head (*asterisk*). **c,d** Axial CT scans showing the rotation, posterior subluxation, and small impression fracture of the humeral head (*arrowhead*) and the fracture of the glenoid (*arrow*). **e–g** 3D reconstructions of CT data with and without electronic subtraction of the humeral head (**e** AP view, **f** lateral view, **g** view from behind). The 3D reconstructions clearly reveal the extent of dislocation of the superior half of the glenoid (*arrows*), an additional fragment of the posterior glenoid fossa (*asterisk*), and posterior subluxation of the humeral head

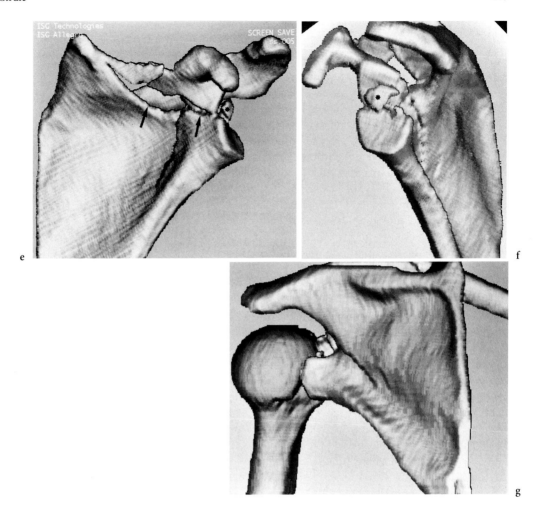

Fig. 8.34e-g

glenoidal incongruity either on proper plain radiographs or on CT scans with secondary or 3D reconstructions (Fig. 8.34).

Acromial fractures usually result from direct violence and are mostly nondisplaced. Sometimes, they have to be differentiated from a persistent apophysis and an os acromiale that is bilateral in about 60% of cases (ZUCKERMAN et al. 1993).

Coracoid fractures typically are avulsion fractures caused by pull of the inserting muscles, as in a seizure. The coracoid can also be fractured by the impact of a dislocating humeral head or by direct trauma. Coracoid fractures account for 2%–5% of all scapular fractures, and can be easily seen on true lateral views of the scapula. They should not be confused with secondary ossification centers that may occur at the proximal and distal aspects of the coracoid process. Involvement of the body of the scapula or the glenoid fossa may indicate an unstable fracture that requires surgical stabilization (Fig. 8.34) (EYRES et al. 1995).

8.1.6.3 Complications

Scapular fractures are isolated in only 2%–18% of cases, i.e., significant associated injuries occur in up to 98%. This figure reflects the degree of trauma necessary to fracture the scapula, so the detection of a scapular fracture should be regarded as a warning (BIGLIANI et al. 1991; SCHUNK et al. 1993).

Beside injuries of the clavicle and the upper torso, scapular fractures lead to brachial plexus injuries in up to 13% of patients; in 11% of cases, there are associated arterial injuries. Supravascular nerve injuries can occur in association with body, neck, or coracoid fractures that involve the suprascapular notch. Twenty-four percent of patients with scapular fractures present with skull fractures, and 20% of patients have closed head injuries. The associated injuries are responsible for a mortality of up to 15%. Half of these deaths are related to severe pulmonary contusion and sepsis (THOMPSON et al. 1985; ZUCKERMAN et al. 1993).

8.1.7 Miscellaneous

Besides the proximal femur, the proximal humerus is a common site for pathologic fractures. These fractures usually result from local disease, such as bone tumors and metastases (NEER 1990). They may also be caused by osteonecrosis after radiation therapy. The most common locations are the surgical neck and proximal shaft (Fig. 8.35). Metastatic tumors and infiltrations due to a plasmacytoma occur more often than primary tumors such as bone cysts, giant cell tumors, chondrosarcomas, osteosarcomas, and Ewing's sarcoma. Radiographically, most lesions can be clearly depicted; MRI, on the other hand, superiorly delineates the extent of soft tissue and bone marrow infiltration.

8.1.8 Special Features of Trauma in Children and Adolescents

In children, dislocations of the glenohumeral joint are extremely rare. They usually do not occur before the age of 12 and commonly have an atraumatic cause. Atraumatic instabilities may be due to an abnormal congenital or acquired laxity of the joint capsule or dysplasia or hypoplasia of the glenoid fossa, and may be associated with emotional instability and psychiatric problems. The latter are characterized by voluntary dislocations and reductions.

After the age of 6 years, the centers of the humeral head and the greater and the lesser tuberosities coalesce to form one epiphysis. As the epiphysis is the weakest point of the proximal humerus, fractures occur instead of dislocations, which are so common during adult life. In childhood, these fractures involve the proximal epiphyseal plate in up to 80% of cases (DAMERON and ROCKWOOD 1984). As the fracture lies distally to the attachment of the rotator cuff, the proximal segment is held in a neutral position. Dislocations of the distal shaft fragment are the result of a pull of the inserting pectoralis major muscle. The latter acts to displace the shaft anteriorly and medially (NEER 1990). Radiographically, the extent of fracture and displacement are clearly demonstrated on true AP and true lateral views of the glenohumeral joint. Characteristically, the epiphyseal growth contributes to the correction of deformities ("epiphyseal remodeling") so that closed reductions are only required if the deforming angle exceeds 40° (NEER 1990).

Fractures of the scapula are rare in children. They mainly occur in polytraumatized patients. Occasion-

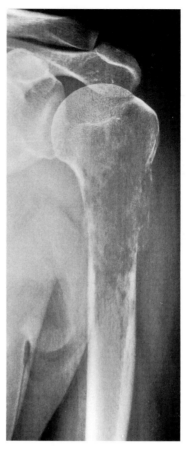

Fig. 8.35. Metastasis of a bronchial carcinoma destroying the surgical neck and proximal shaft

ally, secondary ossification centers may be misinterpreted as fractures.

8.1.9 Diagnostic Algorithm

Plain radiography remains the most important imaging modality in the evaluation of fractures and dislocations of the shoulder and proximal humerus. The initial diagnostic step includes radiographs in the plane of the scapula ("true" AP and lateral views) and an axillary view that may be supplemented by normal AP views in internal and external rotation ("trauma series") (Fig. 8.36). CT should be done if plain films do not allow for sufficient fracture classification; it is recommended in patients with impression fractures of the humeral head, head-splitting fractures, loose bodies in the shoulder joint, or displaced fractures of the glenoid and scapula. Multiplanar reformation and 3D reconstructions may ease the surgical planning. CT-arthrography displays the labral-capsular complex and demon-

Fig. 8.36. Diagnostic algorithm with respect to fractures and dislocations of the shoulder and proximal humerus

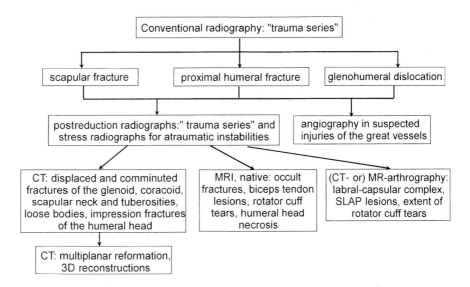

strates bony lesions after dislocations with great accuracy. MRI is the most sensitive modality for the detection of occult fractures and associated soft tissue injuries, and for the diagnosis of humeral head necrosis. MR-arthrography is well suited to document the status of the labral-capsular complex and the extent of rotator cuff tears.

8.2 The Clavicle and Its Articular Connections

8.2.1 General Considerations

The clavicle is the first bone which begins to ossify during embryonal life. It is the bone most frequently fractured while passing through the birth canal, the incidence being up to 3.2% (WALLE and HARTIKAINEN-SORRI 1993). Fractures of the clavicle account for about 10% (6%–16%; during childhood: 25%) of all fractures, and they are therefore one of the most frequent fractures in man (ALLMAN 1967). Seventy percent of these fractures occur in patients under the age of 40. During adult life, they occur most frequently in males. Eighty percent of all clavicular fractures are caused by indirect forces, the typical mechanism being a fall on an outstretched hand. Direct traumas usually lead to fractures of the distal or inner third of the clavicle.

Injuries of the acromioclavicular joint occur less commonly than glenohumeral dislocations. In a review of dislocations about the shoulder, 85% were reported to concern the glenohumeral joint and 12%, the acromioclavicular joint (BERQUIST 1992). The injury more often involves males in a ratio of 5:1 up to

10:1, and is more often incomplete than complete (ratio 2:1). More than 60% of patients are younger than 40 years (ROCKWOOD et al. 1991b) The most common cause of acromioclavicular dislocation is a direct force produced by the patient falling onto the point of the shoulder with the arm at the side in the adducted position. Dislocations due to direct forces are rare.

Dislocations of the sternoclavicular joint are uncommon injuries; they account for about 3% of all dislocations of the shoulder girdle; however, they are not as rare as posterior dislocations of the glenohumeral joint (ROCKWOOD 1991). The most common causes of sternoclavicular dislocations are motor vehicle accidents, followed by sports trauma.

8.2.2 Anatomy and Biomechanics

The clavicle is the sole bony strut connecting the trunk to the shoulder girdle, and it is the only bone of the shoulder that forms a synovial joint with the trunk. The shape and configuration of the clavicle are important to its function (BIGLIANI et al. 1991). Though appearing nearly straight on AP views, the clavicle is actually a slightly curved, "S"-shaped bone with a concavity laterally and ventrally and a convexity medially and ventrally when seen from above. Its cross-section varies from flat along the outer third to prismatic along the inner third. The junction between these two cross-sections lies within the middle third of the bone and, together with the curvature of the bone, represents a weak spot, particularly with respect to axial loading. This may explain why fractures of the clavicle occur so commonly in the midportion of the bone; another reason may be the lack of muscle and ligamentous attachments in this area (SCHUNK et al. 1988).

Medially the clavicle articulates with the manubrium and the cartilaginous portion of the first rib through the sternoclavicular joint. It is the only true articulation between the upper extremity and the axial skeleton. Because of the paucity of articular contact between the medial clavicle and the upper sternum, the joint has the least amount of bony stability of the major joints of the body (COPE et al. 1991). Stability is provided by the surrounding ligaments: the interclavicular ligament superiorly, the costoclavicular ligament inferiorly, and the sternoclavicular ligaments anteriorly and posteriorly. The intra-articular disk extends from the upper clavicle to the cartilage of the first rib, dividing the joint into medial and lateral compartments. It functions like a buffer and is stabilized by the joint capsule and the anterior and posterior sternoclavicular ligaments. The sternoclavicular joint is freely movable and functions almost like a ball-and-socket joint. It is probably the most frequently moved joint because almost any motion of the upper extremity is transferred proximally to it.

Laterally the clavicle articulates with the medial portion of the acromion. Since the joint capsule is rather thin, the acromioclavicular joint is reinforced by the acromioclavicular ligaments, which are strongest superiorly, where they blend with the fibers of the deltoid and trapezius muscles (ROCKWOOD et al. 1991b).

The coracoclavicular ligament is a very strong ligament running from the outer, inferior surface of the clavicle to the base of the coracoid process of the scapula. It consists of two components, the medial conoid and the lateral trapezoid ligaments. Its primary function is to strengthen the acromioclavicular articulation and to couple glenohumeral motion to scapular rotation on the thorax. Experimental studies have shown that the acromioclavicular ligaments provide horizontal, and the coracoclavicular ligaments vertical stability of the acromioclavicular joint.

8.2.3 Classification of Injuries

8.2.3.1 Classification of Clavicular Fractures

Fractures of the clavicle are classified according to the localization of the fracture (ALLMAN 1967). Group I encompasses the most common fractures of the middle third (Fig. 8.37).

Fractures of the distal third constitute group II (NEER 1968). These fractures can be further subclassified according to their position relative to the coracoclavicular ligaments (Fig. 8.38): Type I refers to fractures with intact coracoclavicular ligaments, the fracture side being lateral between the acromioclavicular and coracoclavicular ligaments. In type II fractures the coracoclavicular ligaments are detached from the medial fracture fragment, and may be partially torn. Type III distal clavicular fractures involve the articular surface of the acromioclavicular joint alone, without any ligamentous injury.

Fractures of the medial third of the clavicle constitute group III.

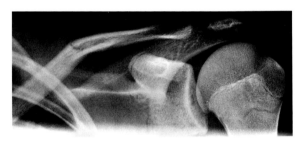

Fig. 8.37. Clavicular fracture of the middle third

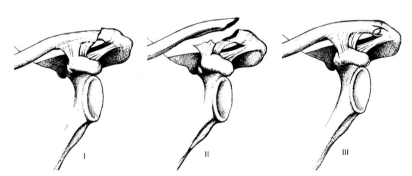

Fig. 8.38. Classification of lateral clavicular fractures (see text)

8.2.3.2 Classification of Acromioclavicular Dislocations

Injuries of the acromioclavicular joint are classified according to the extent of injury to the acromioclavicular and coracoclavicular ligaments (ALLMAN 1967). In "Tossy I" injuries, the acromioclavicular ligaments are sprained, but intact. In "Tossy II" injuries, these ligaments are completely torn, and the coracoclavicular ligaments are sprained but intact. "Tossy III" refers to a complete acromioclavicular dislocation with disruptions of both the acromioclavicular and coracoclavicular ligaments (Fig. 8.41).

8.2.3.3 Classification of Sternoclavicular Dislocation

Dislocations of the sternoclavicular joint can be classified into anterior and posterior dislocations (COPE et al. 1991). Corresponding to the injuries of the acromioclavicular joint, three types of dislocation can be differentiated. In type I, there is sprain, but no disruption of the ligaments. In type II, there is partial disruption of the sternoclavicular and costoclavicular ligaments resulting in a subluxation of the joint. Type III is characterized by complete disruption of the ligaments leading to complete luxation of the sternoclavicular joint.

8.2.4 Examination Methods

Plain radiography plays the most important role in evaluating injuries of the clavicle and the acromiclavicular joint. Generally, two views at right angles are recommended (COPE et al. 1991). For fractures of the shaft of the clavicle, an anteroposterior view and a 45° cephalic tilt view ("tangential view" after ZIMMER-BROSSY 1992) should be performed. The latter more accurately assesses the anteroposterior relationship of the fracture fragments.

Distal clavicular fractures and acromioclavicular injuries requires proper exposure of the plain radiographs (Fig. 8.39) (SCHUNK et al. 1988). AP and cephalic tilt views, however, may not be sufficient for assessment of type II distal clavicular fractures. Additional anterior and posterior 45° views and stress radiographs of both shoulders have been proposed (NEER 1968). Axillary views of the shoulder can be used to document the extent of fracture-dislocation in the anterior-posterior direction. While stress radiographs are necessary to determine the extent of acromioclavicular dislocation, there is a risk of further displacement of otherwise minimally displaced type II distal clavicular fractures. Stress radiographs should be done with the weights hanging from the wrists rather than held by the patient, to encourage complete muscle relaxation.

If articular surface fractures of the distal clavicle are suspected, but not evident on conventional x-rays, CT scans may demonstrate the presence and extent of an articular surface injury.

Fractures of the medial third and injuries of the sternoclavicular joint are difficult to detect because of the overlap of ribs, vertebrae, and mediastinal shadows (ROCKWOOD 1991). Fractures are often revealed by cephalic tilt views of 40–45°. In unclear cases conventional, or better, computed tomography clarifies the situation and helps to differentiate fracture-dislocations of the medial clavicle third from sternoclavicular dislocations (Fig. 8.40).

In the acute setting, angiography may become necessary if a major injury to a great vessel, especially the subclavian vein and artery, is suspected. Compression syndromes of these vessels can develop after clavicular fractures because of abundant

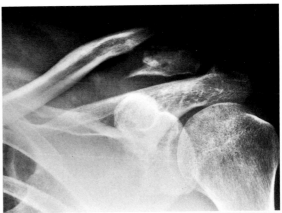

a

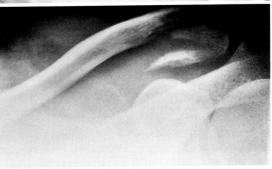

b

Fig. 8.39a,b. Fracture of the lateral third of the clavicula. a Normal AP view; b cephalic tilt ("tangential") view

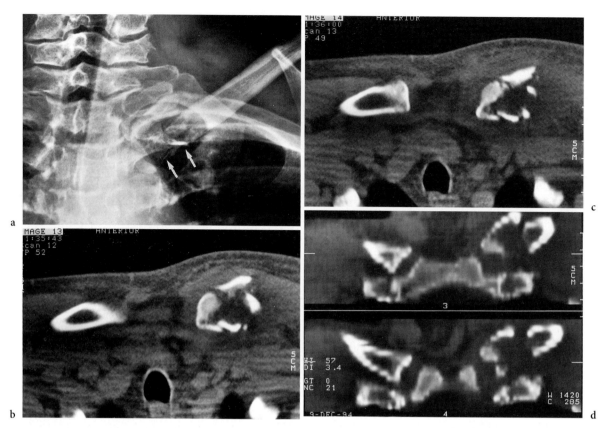

Fig. 8.40a–d. Fracture of the medial clavicular third with subluxation of the sternoclavicular joint. **a** Normal AP view shows medial clavicular fracture (*arrows*) overlapped by ribs, mediastinal vessels, and lateral processes of the thoracic spine. **b,c** CT clearly delineates the comminuted fracture of the medial clavicular third. **d** Secondary coronal reformatted images demonstrate a slightly superior subluxation of the left sternocavicular joint

callus formation or significant fracture deformity (MNAYMNEH et al. 1980). For planning appropriate therapy, these lesions should be definitively assessed by angiography.

8.2.5 Trauma Pattern and Pathomorphology

8.2.5.1 Clavicular Fractures

Fractures of the medial third of the clavicle account for about 80% of all clavicular fractures in adults. Displacement of these fractures is common: the proximal fragment is elevated by the sternocleidomastoid muscle and pulled dorsally by the trapezius muscle. The distal segment is pulled downward by the weight of the arm and inward by the pectoralis major and latissimus dorsi muscles. Rotation of the distal fragment is caused by motion of the scapula and humerus through the intact coracoclavicular and acromioclavicular ligaments. These factors result in a superior tented radiographic

appearance (Fig. 8.37). Undisplaced fractures can occasionally be missed unless radiographs at right angles are performed.

Fractures of the distal third account for about 10%–18% of all clavicular fractures (Fig. 8.39). They should not be confused with acromioclavicular dislocation type II or III in adults.

Fractures of the inner third of the clavicle account for 5%–6% of clavicular fractures (Fig. 8.40). As the sternal epiphysis of the clavicle is the last to close (normally between ages 22 and 25 years), epiphyseal fractures in adolescents and young adults can be mistaken for sternoclavicular dislocations (WEBB and SUCHEY 1985). Unclear findings should be further evaluated by CT.

8.2.5.2 Dislocations of the Acromioclavicular Joint

In Tossy I lesions, radiographs, including stress radiographs, remain normal when compared with those of the normal shoulder (ROCKWOOD et al.

1991b). In a Tossy II injury, the acromioclavicular joint appears to be widened compared with the unaffected side. The distance between the upper aspect of the coracoid and the undersurface of the clavicle is increased by about 25%–50% compared with the unaffected shoulder. Stress views document the integrity of the coracoclavicular ligaments. In Tossy III lesions, the lateral end of the clavicle is completely above the superior border of the acromion, and the distance between the upper aspect of the coracoid and the undersurface of the clavicle is greater than 50% or increased by more than 5 mm, compared with the unaffected side (Fig. 8.41). Concomitant dorsal dislocations of the lateral clavicle should be assessed by axillary views of the shoulder.

8.2.5.3 Dislocations of the Sternoclavicular Joint

Anterior dislocations are much more common than posterior dislocations. Because of overlying structures, radiographic evaluation of the sternoclavicular joints remains difficult. In the case of a suspected injury, any asymmetry of the joint on conventional radiographs should be clarified by CT (COPE et al. 1991).

8.2.6 Miscellaneous

The clavicle can be the site of neoplastic or infectious destruction of bone. Pathologic fractures have also been described following radiation of a neoplastic area or in association with arteriovenous malformations (MNAYMNEH et al. 1980).

8.2.7 Complications

Complications from clavicular fractures are usually rare. Clavicular fractures may be associated with rib fractures, scapular fractures, acromioclavicular dislocations, and head and neck injuries in up to 10% cases (SCHUNK et al. 1988). However, these statistics are from centers with a higher portion of severe fractures. Injuries of the neurovascular bundle are rare and occur in about 1% of clavicular fractures. In the majority of cases, they are the sequelae of excessive callus formation and consist of thrombosis, aneurysms, arteriovenous fistulae, and compressions mainly of the subclavian vein and artery (BIGLIANI et al. 1991).

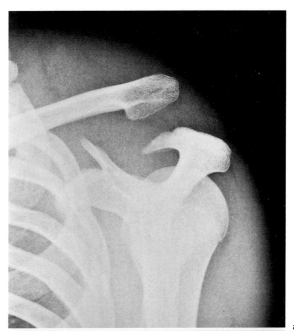

a

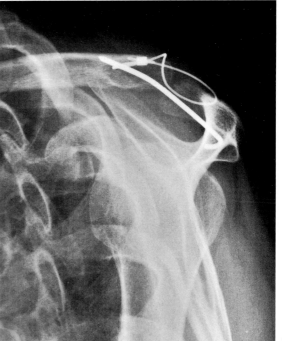

b

Fig. 8.41. Type III acromioclavicular dislocation before (**a**) and after (**b**) internal fixation; transscapular view

Injuries of the pleura with subsequent pneumothorax are estimated to have an incidence of about 3%. Nonunion of clavicular fractures occurs in 1%–2% (Fig. 8.42). Predisposing factors are inadequate immobilization, severity of trauma, refracture, fractures of the distal third, marked displacement, and primary open reduction

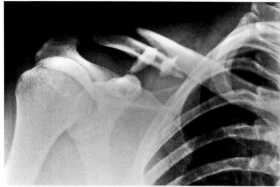

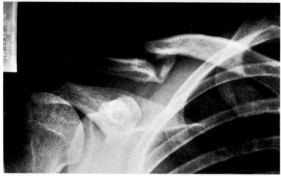

Fig. 8.42a,b. Nonunion of a clavicular fracture after severe trauma and initially marked displacement. **a** AP radiograph at the time of the initial trauma. **b** One year after the accident, there is nonunion of the fracture, requiring operation with internal fixation and bone grafting

of shaft fractures may be more difficult, especially in newborns or infants. An indirect sign of a fracture can be the loss of the accompanying soft tissue shadow. In uncertain cases, control radiographs 5–10 days after the injury will reveal callus formation.

Trauma to the child's clavicle may result in plastic bowing alone, without evidence of cortical disruption. This injury has to be differentiated from other causes of bowing (i.e., metabolic disorders). Characteristically, these fractures show healing with obvious callus formation and thickening of the compacta.

Lateral clavicular fractures occurring below the age of 16 may be confused with complete acromioclavicular separations. The distal clavicle fractures, and, due to a loose attachment between bone and periosteum, the proximal fragment ruptures through the thin periosteum ("banana peeling," FALSTIE-JENSEN and MIKKELSEN 1982). It may be displaced upward by muscular force; the coracoclavicular ligaments, however, remain intact (Fig. 8.43). If plain radiographs do not identify a small fracture fragment, differentiation from acromioclavicular separation is not possible.

As the medial epiphysis of the clavicle normally fuses between 22 and 25 years of age (WEBB and SUCHEY 1985), many misdiagnosed sternoclavicular dislocations are in fact epiphyseal fractures of the

(HERBSTHOFER et al. 1994). Posttraumatic osteoarthritis may follow intra-articular injuries of both sternoclavicular and acromioclavicular joints. The latter often result from an unrecognized intra-articular fracture of the distal clavicle.

Posterior dislocations of the sternoclavicular joint may be potentially fatal because of involvement of the trachea and great mediastinal vessels.

8.2.8 Special Features of Trauma in Children and Adolescents

Fractures of the clavicle account for about 25% of all fractures during childhood, with nearly half the fractures occurring before 7 years of age. As in adults, they usually result from either a direct or an indirect blow, such as a fall on an outstretched hand. Some fractures, however, may be due to a battered child syndrome.

Direct or indirect trauma more often results in incomplete or greenstick rather than in displaced fractures (BIGLIANI et al. 1991). Thus, the diagnosis

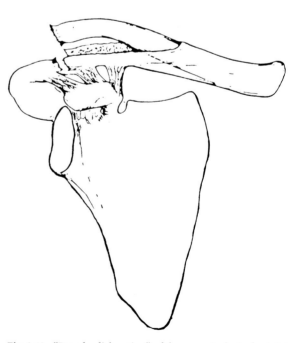

Fig. 8.43. "Pseudo-dislocation" of the acromioclavicular joint during childhood (see text)

Fig. 8.44. Diagnostic algorithm with respect to fractures and dislocations of the clavicle and its articular connections

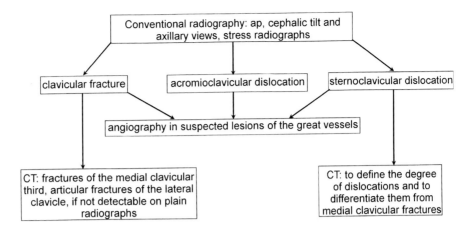

medial third. As already mentioned, CT is the imaging modality of choice in these cases.

8.2.9 Diagnostic Algorithm

Overall, plain radiography is sufficient to evaluate trauma of the clavicle and its articular connections. The initial evaluation should include AP and cephalad tilted views of the clavicle (Fig. 8.44). All fractures should be documented in at least two projections. Additional oblique and axial-axillary views may be helpful in clarifying the degree of dislocation in fractures of the lateral third. Stress radiographs help to differentiate type II and type III acromioclavicular dislocations and may be necessary to identify type II fractures of the lateral clavicle. CT should be performed in patients with fractures and dislocations of the medial clavicle and sternoclavicular joint as it provides superior differentiation and delineation of these injuries. It enables detection of nondisplaced fractures of the acromion and lateral clavicle that are missed by conventional radiographs.

References

Allmann FL (1967) Fractures and ligamentous injuries of the clavicle and its articulations. J Bone Joint Surg [Am] 49:774–784

Bengner U, Johnell O, Redlund-Johnell I (1988) Changes in the incidence of fracture of the upper end of the humerus during a 3-year period. A study of 2125 cases. Clin Orthop 231:179–182

Berquist T (1992) Shoulder and arm. In: Berquist T (ed) Imaging of sports injuries. Aspen, Gaithersburg, pp 221–264

Bigliani U, Craig EV, Butters KP (1991) Fractures of the shoulder. In: Rockwood CA, Green DP, Bucholz RW (eds)

Rockwood and Green's fractures in adults, vol 1, 3rd edn. Lippincott, Philadelphia, pp 871–1020

Blum A, Boyer B, Regent D, Simon JM, Claudon M, Mole D (1993) Direct coronal view of the shoulder with arthrographic-CT. Radiology 188:677–681

Castagno AA, Shuman WP, Kilcoyne RF, Haynor DR, Morris ME, Matsen FA (1987) Complex fractures of the proximal humerus: role of CT in treatment. Radiology 165:759–762

Chandnani VP, Gagliardi JA, Murname TG, Bradley YC, DeBerardino TA, Spaeth J, Hansen MF (1995) Glenohumeral ligaments and shoulder capsular mechanism: evaluation with MR arthrography. Radiology 196:27–32

Cope R, Riddervold HO, Shore JL, Sistrom CL (1991) Dislocation of the sternoclavicular joint: anatomic basis, etiologies, and radiologic diagnosis. J Orthop Trauma 5:379–384

Dameron TB, Rockwood CA (1984) Fractures and dislocations of the shoulder. In: Rockwood CA, Wilkins KE, King RE (eds) Fractures in children, vol 3, 2nd edn. Lippincott, Philadelphia, pp 577–623

Erickson SJ, Fitzgerald SW, Quinn SF, Carrera GF, Black KP, Lawson TL (1992) Long bicipital tendon of the shoulder: normal anatomy and pathologic findings on MR imaging. AJR 158:1091–1096

Eyres KS, Brooks A, Stanley D (1995) Fractures of the coracoid process. J Bone Joint Surg [Br] 77:425–428

Falstie-Jensen S, Mikkelsen P (1982) Pseudodislocation of the acromioclavicular joint. J Bone Joint Surg [Br] 64:368–369

Gerber C, Ganz R (1986) Diagnostik und kausale Therapie der Schulterinstabilitäten. Unfallchirurg 86:418–428

Gerber C, Schneeberger A, Vinh TS (1990) The arterial vascularization of the humeral head. J Bone Joint Surg [Am] 72:1486–1494

Gutjahr G (1983) Die Röntgendiagnostik der Schulterluxation und ihrer knöchernen Begleitverletzungen. Röntgen blätter 36:225–233

Gutjahr G, Weigand H, Schunk K (1993) Schultergürtel. In: Thelen M, Ritter G, Bücheler E (eds) Radiologische Diagnostik der Verletzungen von Knochen und Gelenken. Thieme, Stuttgart, pp 273–330

Hagg O, Lundberg B (1984) Aspects of prognostic factors in comminuted and dislocated proximal humeral fractures. In: Bateman JE, Welsh RP (eds) Surgery of the shoulder. Dekker, Philadelphia, pp 51–59

Herbsthofer B, Schütz W, Mockwitz J (1994) Indikation zur operativen Behandlung von Klavikulafrakturen. Akt. Traumatol 24:263–268

Hill HA, Sachs MD (1940) The grooved defect of the humeral head. Radiology 35:690-700

Hodler J, Kursunoglu-Brahme S, Flannigan B, Snyder SJ, Karzel RP, Resnick D (1992) Injuries of the superior portion of the glenoid labrum involving the insertion of the biceps tendon: MR imaging findings in nine cases. AJR 159:565-568

Hoelen MA, Burgers AMJ, Rozing PM (1990) Prognosis of primary anterior shoulder dislocation in young adults. Arch Orthop Trauma Surg 110:51-54

Ianotti JP, Zlatkin MB, Esterhai JL, Kressel HY, Dalinka MK, Spindler RP (1991) MR imaging of the shoulder: sensitivity, specificity and predictive value. J Bone Joint Surg [Am] 73:17-29

Ideberg R (1987) Unusual glenoid fractures: a report on 92 cases. Acta Orthop Scand 58:191-192

Kilcoyne RF, Reddy PK, Lyons F, Rockwood CA (1989) Optimal plain film imaging of shoulder impingement syndrome. AJR 153:795-797

Kilcoyne RF, Shuman WP, Matsen FA, Morris M, Rockwood CA (1990) The Neer classification of displaced proximal humeral fractures: spectrum of findings on plain radiographs and CT scans. AJR 154:1029-1033

Kjellin I, Ho CP, Cervilla V, Haghighi P, Kerr R, Vangness CT, Friedman RJ, Trudell D, Resnick D (1991) Alterations in the supraspinatus tendon at MR imaging: correlation with histopathologic findings in cadavers. Radiology 181:837-841

Kreitner KF, Schild H, Becker HR, Müller HA, Ahlers J (1987) Die Schulterluxation. Eine klinisch-radiologische Spätuntersuchung. Fortschr Röntgenstr 147:407-413

Kreitner KF, Runkel M, Grebe P et al. (1992) MR-Tomographie versus CT-Arthrographie bei glenohumeralen Instabilitäten. Fortschr Röntgenstr 157:37-42

Kreitner KF, Schweden F, Mildenberger P, Schwickert H, Schild HH (1993) CT-Arthrographie des Schultergelenkes. Aktuel Radiol 3:105-111

Leung KS, Lam TP (1993) Open reduction and internal fixation of ipsilateral fractures of the scapular neck and clavicle. J Bone Joint Surg [Am] 79:1015-1018

Leutenegger A, Rüedi T (1993) Frakturen der Scapula und Verletzungen des Acromioclaviculargelenkes. Z Unfallchir Versicherungs Med 86:22-26

Madler M, Mayr B, Baierl P, Klein C, Habermeyer R, Huber R (1988) Wertigkeit von konventioneller Röntgendiagnostik und Computertomographie im Nachweis von Hill-Sachs-Defekten und knöchernen Bankart-Läsionen bei rezidivierender Schultergelenkluxation. Fortschr Röntgenstr 148:384-389

Massengill AD, Seeger LL, Yao L, Gentili A, Shnier RC, Shapiro MS, Gold RH (1994) Labrocapsular ligamentous complex of the shoulder: normal anatomy, anatomic variation, and pitfalls of MR imaging and MR arthrography. Radiographics 14:1211-1223

Misamore GW, Woodward C (1991) Evaluation of degenerative lesions of the rotator cuff. J Bone Joint Surg [Am] 73:704-706

Mnaymneh W, Vargas A, Kaplan J (1980) Fractures of the clavicle caused by arteriovenous malformation. Clin Orthop 148:256-258

Mosely HF, Övergaard B (1962) The anterior capsular mechanism in recurrent anterior dislocation of the shoulder. J Bone Joint Surg [Br] 44:913-927

Müller ME, Allgöwer M, Schneider R, Willenegger H (eds) (1992) Manual der Osteosynthese, 3rd edn. Springer, Berlin Heidelberg New York

Neer CS (1968) Fractures of the distal third of the clavicle. Clin Orthop 58:43-50

Neer CS (1970) Displaced proximal humeral fractures. I. Classification and evaluation. J Bone Joint Surg [Am] 52:1077-1089

Neer CS (1990) Shoulder reconstruction. Saunders, Philadelphia

Neer CS, Foster CR (1980) Inferior capsular shift for involuntary inferior and multidirectional instability of the shoulder. J Bone Joint Surg [Am] 62:897-908

Neer CS, Welsh RP (1977) The shoulder in sports. Orthop Clin North Am 8:583-591

Palmer WE, Brown JH, Rosenthal DI (1994) Labral-ligamentous complex of the shoulder: evaluation with MR-arthrography. Radiology 190:645-651

Palmer WE, Caslowitz PL, Chew FS (1995) MR arthrography of the shoulder: normal intraarticular structures and common abnormalities. AJR 164:141-146

Pappas AM, Goss TP, Kleinman PK (1983) Symptomatic shoulder instability due to lesions of the glenoid labrum. Am J Sports Med 11:279-288

Quinn SF, Sheley RC, Demlow TA, Szumowski J (1995) Rotator cuff tendon tears: evaluation with fat-suppressed MR imaging with arthroscopic confirmation in 100 patients. Radiology 195:497-501

Resnick DR (1981) Shoulder arthrography. Radiol Clin North Am 19:243-253

Robertson PL, Schweitzer ME, Mitchell DG, Schlesinger F, Epstein RE, Frieman BG, Fenlin JM (1995) Rotator cuff disorders: interobserver and intraobserver variation in diagnosis with MR imaging. Radiology 194:831-835

Rockwood CA (1991) Injuries to the sternoclavicular joint. In: Rockwood CA, Green DP, Bucholz RW (eds) Rockwood and Green's fractures in adults, vol 1, 3rd edn. Lippincott, Philadelphia, pp 1253-1307

Rockwood CA, Thomas SC, Matsen FA (1991a) Subluxations and dislocations about the glenohumeral joint. In: Rockwood CA, Green DP, Bucholz RW (eds) Rockwood and Green's fractures in adults, vol 1, 3rd edn. Lippincott, Philadelphia, pp 1021-1180

Rockwood CA, Williams GR, Young DC (1991b) Injuries to the acromioclavicular joint. In: Rockwood CA, Green DP, Bucholz RW (eds) Rockwood and Green's fractures in adults, vol 1, 3rd edn. Lippincott, Philadelphia, pp 1181-1251

Rowe CR, Zarins B (1981) Recurrent transient subluxation of the shoulder. J Bone Joint Surg [Am] 63:863-872

Schunk K, Strunk H, Lohr S, Schild H (1988) Klavikulafrakturen: Einteilung, Diagnose, Therapie. Röntgenblätter 41:392-396

Schunk K, Werner M, Strunk H, Schild H (1993) Verletzungen des Thoraxskelettes. Aktuel Radiol 3:75-83

Schweitzer ME (1994) MR arthrography of the labral-ligamentous complex of the shoulder. Radiology 190:641-643

Snyder SJ, Karzel RP, Del Pizzo W, Ferkel RD, Friedman MJ (1990) SLAP lesions of the shoulder. Arthroscopy 18:229-234

Stableforth PG (1984) Four-part fractures of the neck of the humerus. J Bone Joint Surg [Br] 66:104-108

Stiles RG, Otte MT (1993) Imaging of the shoulder. Radiology 188:603-613

Thompson D, Flynn T, Miller P, Fischer R (1985) The significance of scapular fractures. J Trauma 25:974-977

Tuckman GA (1994) Abnormalities of the long head of the biceps tendon of the shoulder: MR imaging findings. AJR 163:1183-1188

Turkel SJ, Panio MW, Marshall JL, Girgis FG (1981) Stabilizing mechanisms preventing anterior dislocations of the glenohumeral joint. J Bone Joint Surg [Am] 63:1208–1217

Tillmann B, Tichy P (1986) Funktionelle Anatomie der Schulter. Unfallchirurg 89:389–397

Walle T, Hartikainen-Sorri AL (1993) Obstetric shoulder injury. Associated risk factors, prediction and prognosis. Acta Obstet Gynecol Scand 72:450–454

Webb PA, Suchey JMM (1985) Epiphyseal union of the anterior iliac crest and medial clavicle in a modern multiracial sample of American males and females. Am J Phys Anthropol 68:457–466

Wiener SN, Seitz WH (1993) Sonography of the shoulder in patients with tears of the rotator cuff: accuracy and value for selecting surgical options. AJR 160:103–107

Zimmer-Brossy M (1992) Lehrbuch der röntgenologischen Einstelltechnik, 4th edn. Springer, Berlin Heidelberg New York

Zuckerman JD, Koval KJ, Cuomo F (1993) Fractures of the scapula. Instructional Course Lectures 42:271–281

9 Elbow

S. Palmié and M. Heller

CONTENTS

9.1 Conditions and Epidemiology of Elbow Trauma

The main function of the elbow articulation is the precise positioning of the hand in conjunction with the shoulder. Any elbow injury followed by chronic pain and restriction of motion limits the use of the whole extremity for daily activities (like writing), for more complex tasks at the workplace, and especially for greater functional demands in sports.

Approximately 6% of all fractures and dislocations involve the elbow articulation (Eppright and Wilkins 1975). Fractures of the radial head and neck account for approximately one-third of all elbow fractures (corresponding to 1%–2% of all fractures). Another common injury is the medial elbow tension stress syndrome encountered in baseball pitchers or the lateral one in tennis players (Priest and Jones 1974; Mirowitz and London 1992). Capitellar fractures and Monteggia lesions are rare and respectively account for only 1% and 0.7% of all elbow injuries (DeLee et al. 1984; Beck and Dabezies 1984).

In all age groups trauma to the elbow region is common. In general, fractures of the elbow are the result of indirect trauma, either transmitted through the forearm or as a direct force to the radius and ulna against the articular margins of the humerus. Especially in childhood trauma to the elbow is frequent: first while learning to stand and walk in infancy, and later during play and athletic activities in childhood and young adolescence. For example, about 80% of distal humeral fractures occur in children by falling on the outstretched hand (Morrey 1985).

S. Palmié, MD, Klinik für Radiologische Diagnostik, Klinikum der Christian-Albrechts-Universität, Arnold-Heller-Straße 9, 24105 Kiel, Germany
M. Heller, MD, PhD, Professor and Direktor der Klinik für Radiologische Diagnostik, Klinikum der Christian-Albrechts-Universität zu Kiel, Arnold-Heller-Straße 9, 24105 Kiel, Germany

9.2 Anatomy of the Elbow and Mechanisms of Elbow Trauma

9.2.1 Anatomy of the Elbow Articulation

9.2.1.1 Introduction

Knowledge of the anatomic relationships of the elbow is essential for diagnostic examination and proper interpretation of possible trauma manifestations. The elbow articulation is one of the most congruent and complex in the human body. It is composed of three distinct joints (MORREY 1985) – the humeroulnar, humeroradial, and proximal radioulnar – which are contained within a common fibrous and synovial joint capsule. The flexion and extension movements of the forearm are preponderantly based within the humeroulnar joint. This hinged articulation, with about 150° versatility, permits little medial or lateral motion (HENLEY 1987). The musculus triceps brachii is the extensor, while the musculi biceps, brachioradialis, and brachialis are the group of elbow flexors. Strength and stability are provided by the congruent hinged articulation supported by thickenings of the fibrous joint capsule, which are the ulnar and radial collateral ligaments. The humeroradial and the proximal and distal radioulnar joints allow 90° of pronation and supination. The movement of the radius's head within the radial notch of the ulna is restricted to pure rotation by the annular ligament.

9.2.1.2 Anatomy of the Distal Humerus

The distal humerus shaft flares to form a more prominent medial and a lateral condyle (Fig. 9.1). These bony columns, each triangular shaped, bear an epicondyle and a distal articular surface. The articular portion of the distal humerus is subdivided by the trochlear ridge. The medial surface, i.e., the cylindrical trochlea, articulates with the ulna. The lateral, more hemispherically formed surface is termed the capitellum and articulates with the radial head. The flexor and pronator muscles arise from the medial epicondyle, and the extensor muscles of the forearm from the lateral epicondyle. Depressions in the anterior and posterior surfaces between the condyles and above the trochlea form the coronoid, radial, and olecranon fossae.

9.2.1.3 Anatomy of the Proximal Radius

The proximal radius consists of the head, neck, and tuberosity (Fig. 9.1). The concavity of the disk-shaped head articulates with the hemispherical capitellum humeri. The proximal radioulnar joint is formed by the border of the radial head and the lateral base side of the coronoid process. The proximal neck lies within the joint, encircled by the annular ligament. Distal to the neck the extra-articular radial tuberosity serves as the insertion for the biceps tendon. At this level the neck is angulated about 15° with the shaft.

9.2.1.4 Anatomy of the Proximal Ulna

The proximal articulating surface consists of the sigmoid notch with an arc of approximately 180° accounting for the stability of this joint. The anterior margin is formed by the coronoid process (Fig. 9.1) and serves as the insertion for the musculus brachialis at its distal surface. The triceps muscle inserts with a broad tendinous expansion at the posterior margin of the notch, the olecranon. It is notable that in approximately 95% of patients no articular cartilage is present at the midportion of the olecranon trochlear notch. On the lateral base side of the coronoid process a depression, the radial notch, serves as an articulation for the radial head.

9.2.1.5 Joint Capsule and Ligaments of the Elbow Joint

The joint capsule, consisting of an inner synovial and an outer fibrous capsule, is interspersed with ligaments. Between the two distinct layers, fat is interposed anteriorly and posteriorly, corresponding to the coronoid and the olecranon fossae. These fat layers are termed fat pads.

The joint capsule is attached to the humeral epicondyles but inserts more proximally along the proximal margins of the coronoid and olecranon fossae. Distally the capsule envelops the entire articulation. On the medial and anterior surface the ulna is attached distally to the trochlear notch. The capsule continues laterally to the radial neck, covering the radial head, and intersperses with the annular ligament. Like the collateral ligaments, this ligament represents a circumscribed thickening of the joint capsule.

Fig. 9.1. a Anteroposterior plain film of a normal elbow articulation. The arteries are added to the figure. **b** Lateral projection of a normal left elbow. The arteries are added to the figure. The anterior tilt of the humeral condyles ("hockey stick" appearance) is obvious. Note that this is not a true lateral projection and that the elbow is not flexed 90°

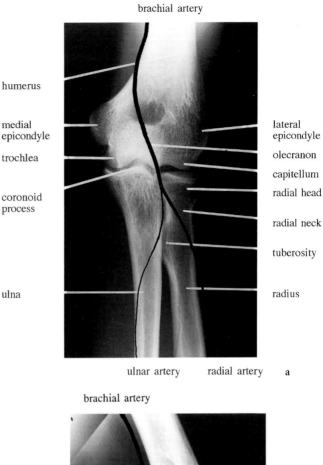

The medial collateral band complex consists of an anterior and a posterior bundle, both of which originate from the ulnar epicondyle, and a small transverse bundle. The anterior ligament inserts at the medial surface of the coronoid. The posterior bundle is attached to the medial surface of the olecranon and is taut only in elbow flexion. The medial complex, in particular the anterior bundle, provides stability to the elbow articulation, even after resection of the proximal olecranon.

The radial/lateral collateral ligaments arise from the radial epicondyle of the humerus, branching out distally into a radial and a lateral ulnar portion. They are both intertwined with the annular ligament. The annular ligament provides stability to the radioulnar joint but does not impair rotation in the radiocapitellar joint.

9.2.1.6 Arteries and Nerves of the Elbow Region

The brachial artery passes into the anticubital fossa after following the dorsomedial borderline of the biceps brachii muscle. At the level of the radial head the brachial artery divides into the radial and ulnar arteries (Fig. 9.1). The brachial artery runs with the median nerve, also crossing the anticubital fossa. Lateral to the capitellum the radial nerve crosses the elbow articulation. The ulnar nerve lies on the posterior surface of the medial condyle with direct bony contact to the medial epicondyle and also the medial surface of the olecranon. This region is sometimes termed the "funny bone."

9.2.2 Mechanisms of Elbow Trauma

9.2.2.1 Introduction

Usually soft tissue injuries, dislocations, and fractures of the elbow result from indirect trauma. The forces are transmitted through the forearm to the angulated articular structures, resulting in bending fractures or direct bony impact. Only a small number of fractures and dislocations are caused by direct blows. The most common injuries in adults are: fractures of the radial head or neck (30%–50%), olecranon fractures (ca. 20%), dislocations and fracture-dislocations (ca. 15%), and supracondylar fractures of the humerus (ca. 10%). It is notable that the apportionment of fractures in children is quite different (see Sect. 9.6.1).

9.2.2.2 Soft Tissue, Ligament, and Tendon Injuries

Soft tissue injuries normally result from falling on the outstretched hand. Combined with hyperextension or valgus stress, this mechanism can cause stretching of the capsule and collateral ligaments, resulting in at least a hemarthrosis indicated by a fat pad sign (see Fig. 9.11 and Sect. 9.5.3) (PITT and SPEER 1990). Soft tissue injuries also may occur secondary to fractures caused by sharp fragments. Traumatic tendon injuries or avulsion are rare and usually due to preexisting degenerative changes.

9.2.2.3 Distal Humeral Fractures

9.2.2.3.1 Supracondylar and Transcondylar Fractures. The typical mechanism is a fall on the outstretched hand causing an extension type of supracondylar fracture. This extra-articular fracture type is frequently associated with intense pain, a volar compartment syndrome, and brachial artery and nerve injuries. Most frequently the radial nerve is affected. This fracture type is usually unstable.

The much less common flexion injury mainly occurs in older people (preponderantly women) and is caused by direct dorsal forces towards the flexed elbow joint. This type is often combined with a sharp proximal fragment responsible for soft tissue and tendinous injuries resulting in an open fracture (SOLTANPUR 1978).

Transcondylar fractures have the same mechanisms as supracondylar fractures but the fractures lie within the joint capsule. This injury is more common in elderly patients with osteoporosis.

9.2.2.3.2 Avulsion Fractures of an Epicondyle. These fractures occur by valgus or varus stress and are unusual in adults as an isolated fracture (see Fig. 9.7) (KEON-COHEN 1966).

9.2.2.3.3 Medial and Lateral Condyle Fractures. Fractures involving a single condyle are the result of angular or shearing forces caused by a fall on the flexed elbow with the forearm in a valgus or varus angulation.

9.2.2.3.4 Intercondylar T- or Y-fractures. These fracture types are caused either by a violent direct force to the proximal ulna or by falling on the flexed elbow. Displacement and rotation of fragments are frequent and result from their muscular attachments (see Fig. 9.9).

9.2.2.3.5 Capitellum Fractures. The mechanism of this rare fracture type is a fall on the outstretched hand (see Fig. 9.8). Resulting shearing forces are transmitted by the radial head and explain the association with fractures of the radial head.

9.2.2.4 Proximal Radius Fractures

Proximal radius fractures are common and result from a fall on the outstretched hand. Typically the elbow joint is partially flexed and the forearm partially pronated. The resulting axial force presses the radial head against the congruent capitellum. Radial head fractures (see Fig. 9.10) are often associated with ligamentous injury and a rupture of the interosseous membrane.

9.2.2.5 Proximal Ulna Fractures

9.2.2.5.1 Olecranon Fractures. The classical mechanism is a direct blow to the prominent olecranon process caused by falling on the flexed articulation (see Fig. 9.12). Increasing forces result in a comminuted fracture (see Fig. 9.13). Another possible fracture mechanism results from indirect violence to the flexed elbow: either by falling onto the outstretched hand during a strong triceps contraction or through a hyperextension injury.

9.2.2.5.2 Coronoid Fractures. Coronoid fractures result from the impaction of the ulna against the humerus in the event of a posterior dislocation and indicate severe instability (see Fig. 9.15). Isolated coronoid fractures are unusual (see Fig. 9.14) (REGAN and MORREY 1992).

9.2.2.6 Elbow Dislocation

The common posterior dislocation occurs when falling onto the outstretched hand with coincident hyperextension and valgus stress. This injury is commonly associated with fractures especially of the tip of the coronoid, ligament/capsule avulsions, and vascular and nerve injuries (see Fig. 9.15).

9.2.2.7 Monteggia's Fractures

Each type of Monteggia lesion (types I–IV) can be caused by a direct blow, hyperpronation, or hyperex-

tension (with regard to the pathomorphology, see Sect. 9.5.9). The common mechanism is a fall on the outstretched hand with forced pronation of the forearm.

9.3 Classifications of Fractures of the Elbow Region

9.3.1 Fractures of the Distal Humerus

There is no generally accepted method of classification of fractures but the most comprehensive and commonly utilized is that of Mueller (Fig. 9.2) (MUELLER et al. 1987). Mueller's AO/ASIF classification of fractures of the distal humerus in adults should be complemented by the classification of T- and Y-shaped condylar fractures proposed by Riseborough and Radin (Fig. 9.3) (RISEBOROUGH and RADIN 1969).

The above classifications are used to determine the severity of the injury and guide in therapy planing. Since about 50% of distal humeral fractures are T- or Y-shaped bicondylar or intercondylar fractures, their classification is discussed below.

Mueller's classification divides the distal humeral fractures into three major groups labeled A, B and C, each consisting of three subgroups 1–3 (Fig. 9.2). *Group A* is composed of extra-articular fractures: A1 is an avulsion of the medial epicondyle, A2 a supra- or transcondylar fracture, and A3 a comminuted supracondylar fracture. *Group B* consists of intra-articular and unicondylar fractures: B1 is a fracture of the lateral condyle, B2 a fracture of the medial condyle, and B3 a fracture of the capitellum. *Group C* consists of intra-articular bicondylar fractures: C1 is a T- or Y-shaped intercondylar fracture, C2 an intercondylar fracture with comminution of the distal humeral shaft, and C3 a comminuted intercondylar fracture involving both the joint surface and the distal shaft.

Riseborough and Radin's classification of T- and Y-shaped condylar fractures distinguishes four types of fracture: Type I is an undisplaced fracture, while type II consists of a fracture with displacement but without significant condylar fragment rotation. Type III fractures are dislocated with medial and lateral condylar fragment rotation caused by flexor and extensor muscles. Type IV fractures are displaced and rotated fractures with marked comminution (Fig. 9.3).

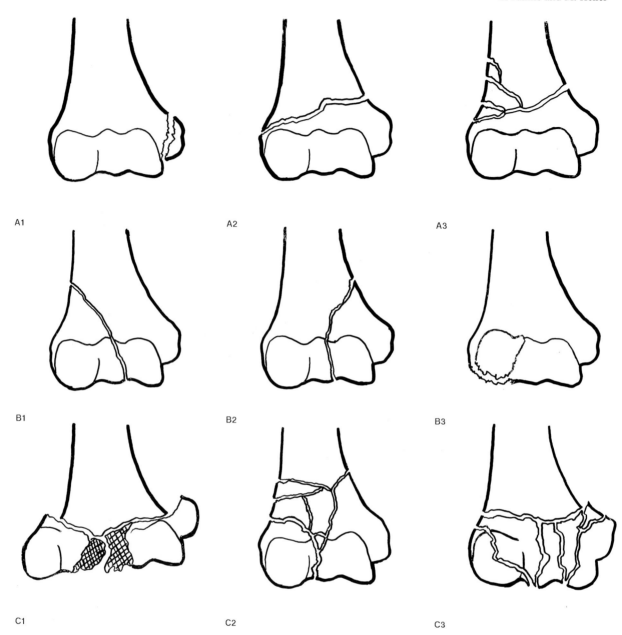

A1   A2   A3

B1   B2   B3

C1   C2   C3

Fig. 9.2. Mueller et al.'s (AO/ASIF) classification of fractures of the distal humerus in adults. The fractures are divided into three major groups (A–C), each with three subgroups (1–3). Type A consists of extra-articular fractures. Type B are intra-articular, unicondylar fractures. Type C are intra-articular, bicondylar fractures

9.3.2 Fractures of the Proximal Radius

Fractures of the radial head and neck are commonly described using Mason's classification (Fig. 9.4). The original classification consisted of three fracture types; Johnston added a type IV in 1962. Type I is a fissure or marginal fracture with less than 2 mm displacement, as seen in approximately 50% of all fractures of the proximal radius. In reference to the radial neck the angulation of the fragments is less than 20–30°. Type II fractures involve approximately one-third of the radial head, with a displacement of more than 2 mm or radial neck angulation above 20–30°. Type III fractures are comminuted fractures of the whole radius head or a neck angulation of more than 60° or a complete dislocation of the neck. Type IV, added by Johnston, includes any type I–III fracture in combination with an elbow dislocation, usu-

Fig. 9.3. Classification of T- and Y-shaped bicondylar fractures. Type I is an undisplaced bicondylar fracture of the distal humerus. Type II is a displaced, but not rotated bicondylar fracture. Type III is a displaced fracture with rotated condylar fragments. Type IV is a displaced, rotated, and comminuted bicondylar fracture

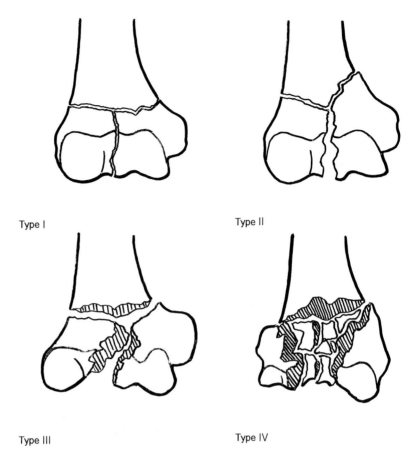

Type I

Type II

Type III

Type IV

ally of the humeroradial joint (Fig. 8.4). None of the existing classifications take account of injuries of the interosseous membrane that are commonly associated with injuries of the distal radioulnar joint or an articular mechanical blockage. This is noteworthy since it affects treatment. A careful physical examination should reveal these important diagnostic factors.

9.3.3 Fractures of the Proximal Ulna

Other than for the distal humerus there is no generally accepted classification of olecranon fractures. That most commonly used was published by COLTON (1973), who simply differentiated displaced and undisplaced fractures (Fig. 9.5). It is notable that a fracture of the olecranon must meet three criteria to be considered undisplaced. First, the displacement has to be less than 2 mm. Second, it may not increase in 90° elbow flexion. Third, the ability to extend the elbow articulation actively against gravity must be maintained. The group of displaced fractures is subdivided into avulsion fractures, oblique and trans-

verse fractures, comminuted fractures, and fracture-dislocations (Fig. 9.5). Both comminuted fractures and fracture-dislocations involve not only the midportion but also the proximal portion of the olecranon. If located distally, both fractures typically involve the collateral ligaments, resulting in a more unstable type of fracture associated with difficulties for surgical treatment and influencing the outcome (see Fig. 9.13). All types of displaced fractures usually require open reduction and internal fixation.

Coronoid fractures are classified after REGAN and MORREY (1992) into three types (see Fig. 9.13), each subdivided into a type A without and a type B with associate elbow dislocation. Type I is an avulsion fracture of the coronoid tip. Type II fractures involve up to and type III fractures more than 50% of the coronoid process.

9.3.4 Monteggia's Fractures

A simple and commonly used classification is that described by BADO (1967), which consists of four types. Since surgical intervention is the treatment of

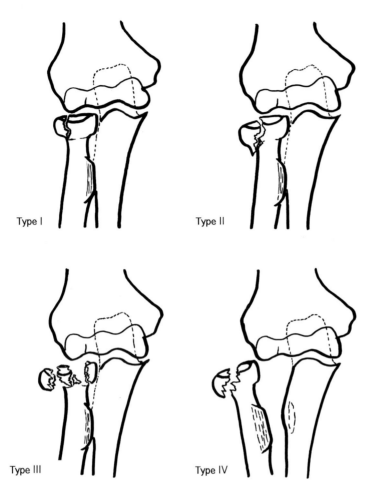

Type I

Type II

Type III

Type IV

Fig. 9.4. Classification of proximal radius fractures. Mason's classification of radial head and neck fractures consists of three different types. Type I is an undisplaced fracture (neck angulation <20–30°). Type II is a displaced (more than 2 mm) fracture (neck angulation <60°). Type III consists of comminuted fractures of the whole radial head or a neck angulation of more than 60° or a neck dislocation. Type IV consists of any type I–III fracture in combination with an elbow dislocation (mainly of the humeroradial joint)

choice and since the different types fail to influence the therapy, a description is dispensable.

9.4 Examination Methods

9.4.1 Plain X-ray

The standard projections for evaluating the elbow are an AP and a lateral view. These views, taken at 90° angles, are the essential minimum (see Fig. 9.1). The AP view should be obtained with full extension of the elbow and a supinated hand (as in Fig. 9.1a). The lateral view is obtained with the elbow in 90° flexion and the forearm midway between pronation and supination (cf. Fig. 9.1b).

Oblique views provide visualization of regions which are overlapped in the standard projections: the radiocapitellar articulation, epicondyles, radioulnar articulation, and coronoid tubercle. If an injury in one of the regions listed above is suspected, additional oblique views should obtained.

Suspected injuries of the proximal radius which are not depicted in the standard films require a radial head view projecting the radius away from the ulna (PAGE 1986).

The axial projection demonstrates both epicondyles, the sulcus of the ulnar nerve and the joint compartment between the olecranon and trochlea.

Stress views are used in cases of suspected ligamentous instabilities. Varus and valgus stress views should be obtained of both elbows for comparison using fluoroscopy for positioning. When compared with the unaffected side, widening of the joint space of 2 mm or more indicates a ligamentous instability.

9.4.2 Arthrography

Arthrography is a rare examination in clinical routine. It is most commonly indicated for the evaluation of entrapped bony fragments or chondral bodies

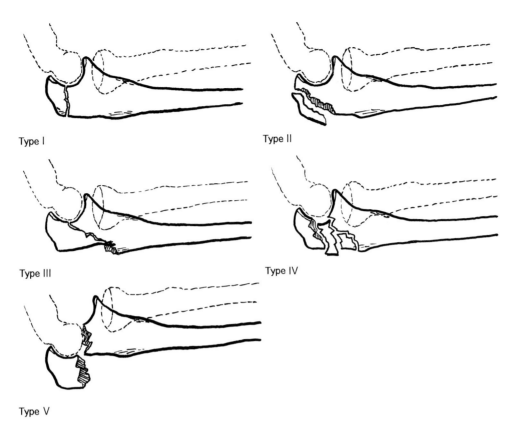

Type I   Type II

Type III   Type IV

Type V

Fig. 9.5. Classification of olecranon fractures. The classification of Colton simply classifies olecranon fractures as undisplaced (type I) or displaced (types II–IV). Type I usually results from a direct blow, with the fragments separated less than 2 mm. The fracture may or may not involve the articular joint. Type II is a fracture involving avulsion and a transverse or oblique fracture line. Type III is a transverse or oblique olecranon fracture, usually in the midportion of the olecranon and commonly caused by a more indirect mechanism of injury. Type IV is a comminuted fracture and type V is a fracture dislocation

within the joint. Arthrography is either performed as double-contrast CT or augmented by conventional polytomography. It also may be useful in demonstrating complex injuries and capsule ruptures (SINGSTON et al. 1986).

9.4.3 Tomography

Tomography is used to evaluate posttraumatic complications such as nonunion and secondary infection, especially if osteosynthetic material overlaps the region of interest on the plain x-ray film.

9.4.4 Ultrasound

Ultrasound examinations have no significant indication in the evaluation of the elbow articulation.

9.4.5 Computed Tomography

Computed tomography (CT) is most frequently used in conjunction with elbow arthrogaphy, preferably in double contrast. CT may be superior to MRI in the evaluation of intra-articular bodies and in demonstrating the radial head and the radioulnar articulation. Some consider CT to be helpful in the evaluation of complex and comminuted articular fractures by virtue of its ability to demonstrate to the surgeon the fragment positions and relationships; in this context CT may be especially useful if augmented by three-dimensional reconstructions (BLICKMAN et al. 1990). In clinical routine CT of the elbow is rarely performed due to the lack of indications as well as the lack of the mobility of the injured extremity that is required for positioning in the CT gantry.

9.4.6 Magnetic Resonance Imaging

Magnetic resonance imaging (MRI) has become a valuable technique for evaluating elbow disorders. MRI can evaluate acute traumatic soft tissue injuries involving ligaments, tendons, muscles, and neurovascular structures, as well as soft tissue derangements caused by chronic overuse, which are a common source of dysfunction (TEHRANZADEH et al. 1992). MRI is well known for its superior soft tissue contrast and its sensitivity in demonstrating bone edema and hemorrhage, especially in fat-suppressed imaging. T1-weighted images can help to delineate morphologic features of non-displaced fractures and unsuspected subcortical infraction. The questionable cost-effectiveness of MRI might be solved by the new generation of extremity scanners. In view of the radiation dose associated with tomography, arthrotomography, and CT, MRI is to be preferred for the evaluation of complex epiphyseal fractures in younger patients when the extension of the fracture cannot be determined with radiographic techniques (BELTRAN et al. 1994 BLICKMAN et al. 1990). It should also be mentioned that compared with arthrography, MRI is noninvasive and avoids the rare but disastrous complication of articular infection.

9.5 Trauma Pattern and Pathomorphology

9.5.1 Introduction

A detailed and thorough analysis of the standard radiographs of any injured elbow articulation significantly decreases the chance of missing subtle injuries. The analysis should include a study of the fat pads (see Fig. 9.7), the supinator fat stripe (Fig. 9.6), and the specific anatomic relationships (especially in children the anterior humeral and radiocapitellar lines and also the presence and positions of ossification centers) and be completed by a search for common injuries such as radial and olecranon fractures. The analysis and interpretation should relate to clinical findings and injury mechanism. There are two common pitfalls: first, an obvious fracture of the proximal ulna may be associated with a dislocation of the proximal radius and this may be overlooked if the interpretation ends with the recognition of the obvious fracture. Second, fractures of the proximal radius frequently show only subtle bony changes which may be superimposed by the ulna so that in many cases only indirect signs, as described below, indicate this common fracture.

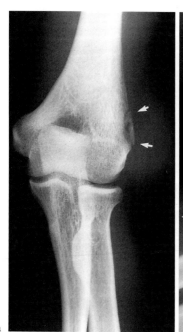 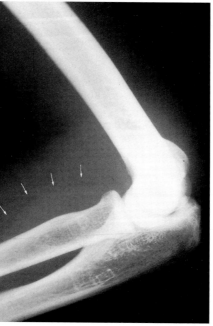

Fig. 9.6a,b. Extra-articular fracture in a 29-year-old man. **a** An uncommon example of an extra-articular distal humeral fracture: a fractured supracondylar ridge (*arrows*) without evident displacement. **b** The lateral view looks essentially normal, with a clearly visible normal supinator fat stripe (*arrows*) and without fat pad signs

a   b

9.5.2 Soft Tissue Alterations

Soft tissue alterations are often the most obvious pathomorphologic finding in elbow trauma. Extracapsular soft tissue swelling may be diffuse, but the supinator fat stripe and the intra-articular fat pads are of unique diagnostic importance (DIHLMANN et al. 1992).

The supinator fat stripe lies on the supinator muscle parallel to the radial head and neck (Fig. 9.6). A ventral displacement, blurring or obliteration of the fat stripe is typical in fractures of the radial head and neck (see Fig. 9.11) and was also reported by ROGERS and MACEWAN (1969) to be present in about 80% of other elbow fractures. Since fractures of the proximal radius may not be obvious or visualized on standard projections, alterations of the supinator fat stripe should suggest further investigations such as a radial head view or oblique projections.

The olecranon bursa lies directly adjacent to the olecranon and extended hemorrhage into the bursa is often associated with an olecranon fracture. Swelling or hemorrhage of the olecranon bursa should therefore initiate a detailed search for subtle bony irregularities indicating an oblique or undisplaced fracture, especially through the trochlear notch.

9.5.3 The Fat Pad Sign

The fat pads are, as described above (see Sect. 9.2.1.5), thin layers of fat between the synovial and fibrous joint capsule corresponding to the distal humeral fossae. Any intra-articular fluid collection, especially hemorrhage, causes a distention of the capsule with secondary elevation of the fat pads ventrally out of the coronoid and radial fossae (see Fig. 9.11). Dorsally the posterior fat pad is displaced out of the olecranon fossa. The lateral radiograph shows triangular radiolucent shadows anterior and posterior to the distal humerus, which are termed "fat pad signs" (HALL-CRAGGS et al. 1985). For the interpretation of the fat pads on the lateral elbow view, it is important to recognize a number of specific features (DIHLMANN et al. 1992; MURPHY and SIEGEL 1977):

1. The anterior fat pad is normally seen in a typical shape (Fig. 9.7).
2. A "normal" fat pad does not exclude a fracture in the elbow articulation.
3. The normal posterior fat pad is invisible in 90° flexion; in any other degree of extension, however, the olecranon may displace the fat pad out of the fossa.
4. Small joint effusions may elevate the anterior fat pad earlier than the posterior one.
5. The signs are not specific for trauma because any fluid collection could be associate with fat pad signs, e.g., inflammatory changes or activated arthrosis.
6. Fat pads may be invisible due to extended soft tissue edema, corpulence, or hematoma.
7. Rupture of the capsule will negate the fat pad sign because the fluid spreads into the surrounding soft tissue and muscular compartments (see Figs. 9.7, 9.15).
8. Between 70% and 90% of children with a fat pad sign have an intra-articular fracture
9. The fat pad sign is less frequent in adults.

In conclusion, it can be stated that, if a fat pad sign is missing in a child, the probability of a significant articular injury is low. If, on the other hand, a positive fat pad sign is present in an injured adult elbow, there is a great likelihood of an articular fracture.

9.5.4 The Anterior Humeral Line

The anterior humeral line is drawn along the anterior cortex of the distal humerus and its prolongation passes through the middle third of the capitellum. This imaginary line is useful to check for the typical "hockey stick" appearance of the distal humerus on the lateral view and serves as a satisfactory index of its angulation with the humeral shaft (see Fig. 9.1). In the presence of a supracondylar fracture, which typically occurs in children and results from a hyperextension mechanism, the line passes through the anterior third of the capitellum or, if the dislocation is larger, entirely anteriorly to it. Especially the common supracondylar greenstick fractures with or without only a subtle fracture line are much more easily detectable with the help of the anterior humeral line. In the uncommon flexion type fractures, the condylar fragment dislocates anteriorly and the anterior humeral line passes through the posterior third of the capitellum or entirely posteriorly. The use of the anterior humeral line in adults is of minor relevance.

9.5.5 The Radiocapitellar Line

The radiocapitellar line confirms articulation between the radial head and the capitellum. The line is

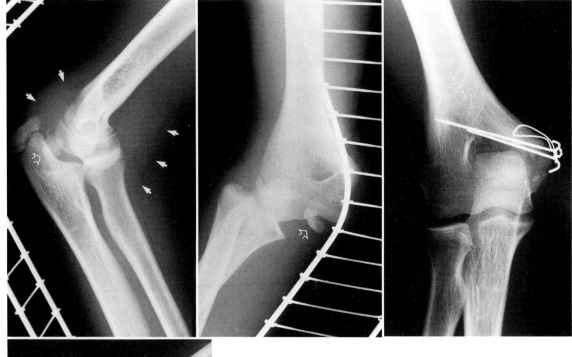

a   b,c

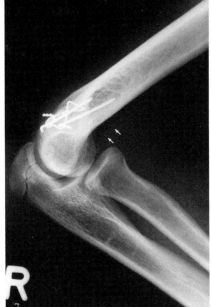

Fig. 9.7a–d. Articular distal humeral fracture in a 16-year-old boy. **a,b** Avulsed medial epicondyle with displacement (*open arrows*) in a case of a lateral dislocation. Note the considerable periarticular hematoma (*arrows*). **c,d** Because the avulsed medial epicondyle was displaced more than 3 mm, open reduction and internal fixation were performed. After treatment the radiographs show an accurate reduction and fixation of the medial epicondyle. Note the distinct but normal anterior fat pad (*arrows*)

d

drawn by bisecting the proximal radius proximally to the tuberosity and it usually passes through the middle three-fifths of the capitellum on every radiographic view. Since this artificial construct does not fit all variants, interpretation should be careful. The radiocapitellar line fails to pass through the capitellum if the radial head is dislocated by a fracture or as a component of Monteggia's lesion. If the proximal radius is normal and the line fails, a frac-

ture of the lateral condyle or, in children, a displacement of the capitellar ossification center is likely.

9.5.6 Fractures of the Distal Humerus

Fractures and fracture lines extending into the distal humerus as well as the site of origin of the fracture fragments are usually obvious on the AP projection.

Hence, the classification of the fracture types is usually demonstrated on the AP view, the single exception to this general rule being a fracture of the capitellum (cf. Fig. 9.8).

The articular surface is involved in 95% of all distal humeral fractures. The remaining 5% of extra-articular fractures consist of transcondylar fractures involving both condyles or either the medial or lateral epicondyle alone as a result of avulsions (see Fig. 9.6). The transcondylar fractures are similar to the common supracondylar fractures in childhood and appear as a single transverse fracture line. Undisplaced fractures may be difficult to identify.

Avulsion fractures of the epicondyles, especially lateral ones, are rare in adults. The medial epicondyle provides stability to the joint since the ligamentous integrity of the joint depends upon its normal position. If the fragment, which is typically flake shaped, is dislocated it becomes clearly visible on the AP view, except if it becomes entrapped in the joint space (cf. Fig. 9.7).

An isolated condyle is chiselled off by angular forces transmitted within the trochlear notch by the ulna or by the radial head against the capitellum. The fracture line separates the medial or lateral condyle obliquely. Depending on the position of the fracture line, the fracture may be stable or unstable. Fractures of a singular condyle account for 5% of all fractures of the distal humerus.

Bicondylar or intercondylar fractures of the distal humerus normally occur from a direct blow to the proximal ulna. These fracture types are obvious and account for about 80% of all humeral articular frac-

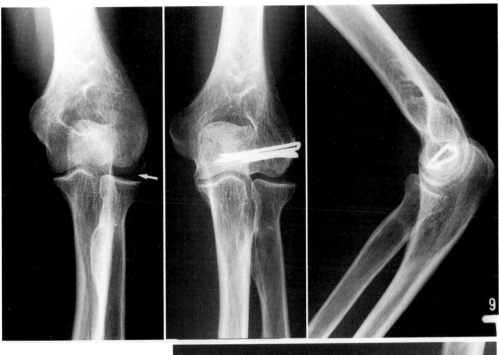
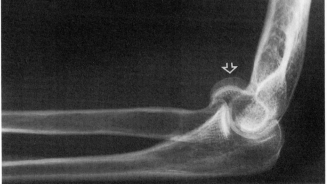

Fig. 9.8a–d. Fracture of the capitellum in a 66-year-old woman. **a** The articular margin of the capitellum shows an abnormal arc of cortical bone (*arrow*), which represents the articular surface of the displaced capitellum. **b** The fat pads are invisible due to extended soft tissue edema. The displaced capitellar fragment (*arrow*) lies proximal to the radial head. Note the upward facing articular surface. The position and appearance are characteristic of fractures of the capitellum. **c,d** After open reduction and internal fixation, the radiographs show an accurate position and fixation of the capitellum

tures. The fracture line, which originates in the central groove of the trochlea, propagates across the olecranon and coronoid fossa, branches, and then emerges across the supracondylar bony columns. The most common pattern formed by the fracture lines is T- or Y-shaped and accounts for about 50% of articular humeral fractures. With increasing forces additional comminution is frequent, sometimes with multiple fragments and fracture lines running in many different directions (Fig. 9.9). The condylar

fragments tend to be displaced and rotated by their muscular attachments (Fig. 9.9a,b). A special bicondylar fracture has been termed "sideswipe fracture" because of its mechanism of injury. This injury happens when the arm is held in flexed position out of a car window and is sideswiped by another car or a standing object. The injury is also known as "floating elbow," referring to the resulting extended articular instability (KUUR and KJAERSGAARD-ANDERSON 1988). The "floating" results from a com-

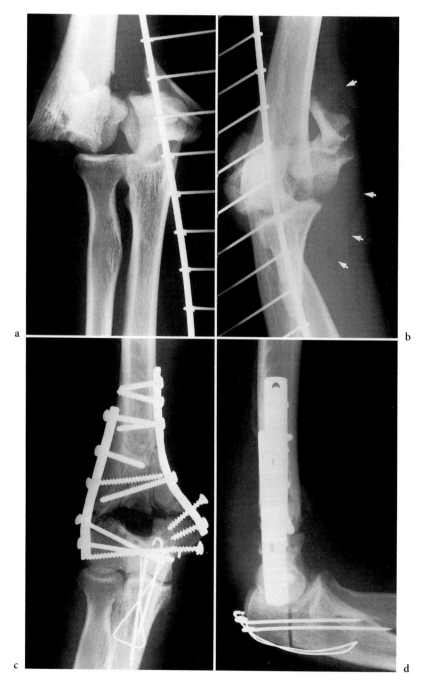

Fig. 9.9a–d. Displaced intercondylar fracture in a 26-year-old man. **a,b** Type IV T-condylar fracture with various fragments. The fragments are displaced, rotated, and subluxated. Note the considerable periarticular hematoma (*arrows*). **c,d** After open reduction and internal fixation the articular congruity is well reconstructed through a transolecranon approach. The preexisting foramen olecrani is now obvious. Note that the important intercondylar portion of the fracture is kept in position with crossed screws

plex dislocated bicondylar fracture usually combined with fractures of the proximal radius and ulna.

Shearing forces transmitted by the radial head result in a fracture of the capitellum. The fragment is obvious on the lateral view and is typically shaped like a half circle or "half moon" and is displaced proximally to the radial head (see Fig. 9.8). Frequently the fragment rotates 90° so that the articular surface points ventrally and the fragment's origin is invisible (as in Fig. 9.8b). The AP view often shows only a lack of definition of the articular cortex of the capitellum (cf. Fig. 9.8a). It is notable that fractures of the capitellum occur in association with fractures of the radial head and the fragments are smaller under these circumstances, but proximal dislocation of the radial head fracture fragments is rare (cf. Fig. 9.11). Hence a confusion of the fragments can be avoided and the capitellum fracture will not be overlooked.

9.5.7 Fractures of the Proximal Radius

The proximal radius may be fractured in the region of either the head or the neck by impaction against the capitellum of the humerus. The mechanism is similar to other depression fractures and results in either angulation of the neck or fragmentation of the head.

Fractures of the radius head range from single line fractures to severe comminution with increasing

force (Fig. 9.10). More angulated forces transmitted through the humerus may result in an additional fracture of the capitellum. The single line fractures are typically vertically oriented to the radial aspect of the joint surface and show a disruption of the cortex at the peripheral margin of the radial head. Frequently the fragment is slightly depressed, as indicated by the appearance of a double line of cortical bone. If the fragment is not displaced the fracture line may not be visualized on standard projections and radial head or oblique views are frequently necessary to depict the fracture. It is notable that fragments of the radial head are rarely displaced proximally (Fig. 9.11). Fractures of the radial neck are best visualized on the lateral projection by an abrupt step-off between the radial head and neck. Normally the radial head forms a concave curve with a smooth transition to the radial neck. The AP view sometimes shows a line of increased density or a slight angulation between the radial head and neck.

9.5.8 Fractures of the Proximal Ulna

9.5.8.1 Olecranon Fractures

Fractures of the proximal ulna are characterized by the involved anatomic area: the olecranon or the coronoid process. Fractures of the olecranon account for 20% of all elbow injuries in adults and occur

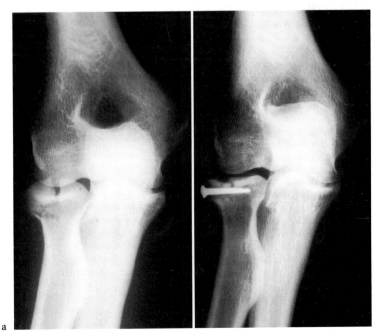

Fig. 9.10a,b. Displaced type II fracture of the radial head in a 25-year-old man. **a** The single fracture line and its extent are obvious. The fracture of the radial head involves more than one-quarter of the head, and some would consider a resection necessary. **b** The fracture was treated by open reduction and internal fixation with two AO (ASIF) minifragment screws. This procedure is technically difficult and should be undertaken with care. The result shows a slight depression of the fragment with a small step in the articular surface

a

b

242
S. Palmié and M. Heller

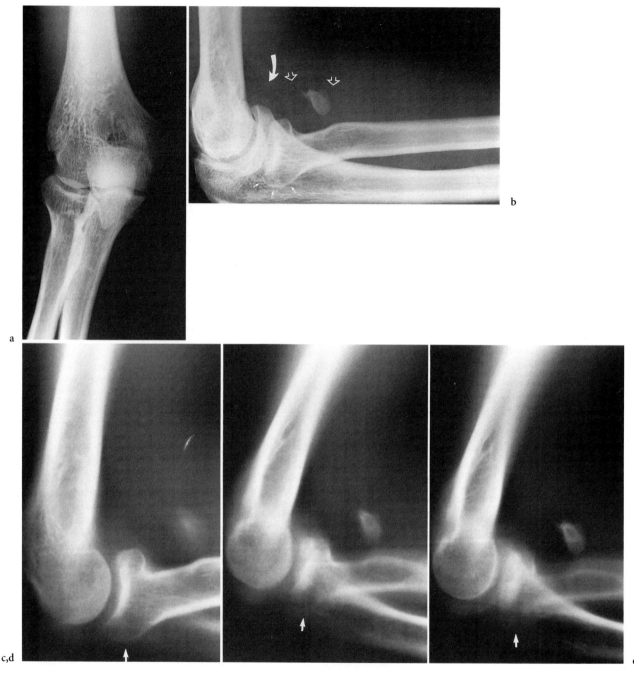

Fig. 9.11a–e. Displaced, uncommon radial head fracture (type II) in a 27-year-old man. **a** The AP view looks essentially normal. **b** The lateral view shows a fragment ventrally to the tuberosity. The fragment's origin is not clearly visible and questionable (*arrows*). Typically the supinator fat stripe is blurred, as shown here (*open arrows*). An abnormal anterior fat pad indicates the intra-articular injury (*curved arrow*), although the joint capsule had been ruptured. **c–e** Conventional polytomography shows the fragment's origin (*arrows*)

either indirectly or directly. The fracture line is typically apparent in the lateral projection because most fractures are oriented transversely to the long axis of the ulna, extending to the depth of the trochlear notch and disrupting the posterior cortex (Fig. 9.12).

Fragments are separated by the traction of the triceps if the periosteum is completely torn.

Comminuted fractures, typically resulting from a direct blow and often associated with dislocated fragments, also are readily apparent on the lateral view

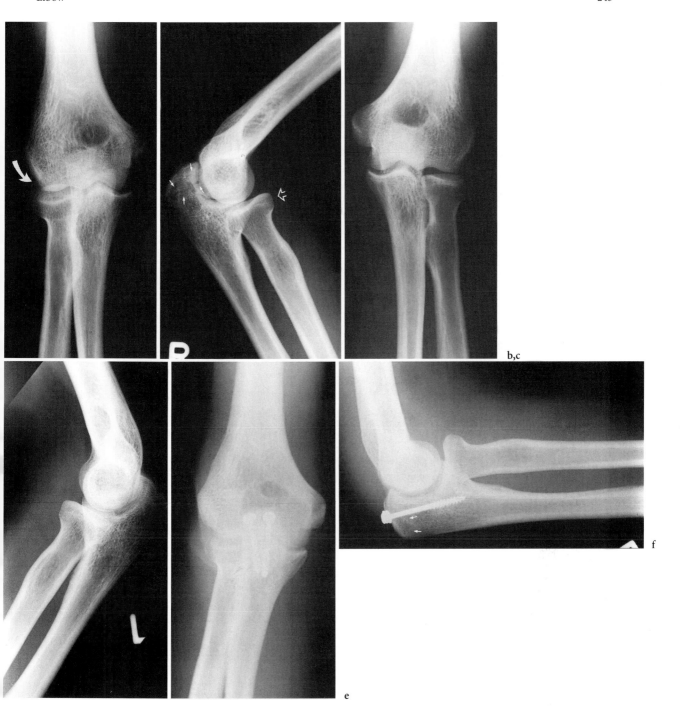

Fig. 9.12a–f. Undisplaced articular olecranon fracture in a 19-year-old young man. **a,b** The fracture line (*arrows*) was suspected to be an epiphyseal line. Note that the epiphyseal lines of the radial head (*open arrow*) and the capitulum (*curved arrow*) are already closed. **c,d** Radiographs of the opposite elbow "for comparison" show no epiphyseal lines in any site. In this case obtaining radiographs of the opposite elbow could have been avoided. **e,f** Proper osteosynthetic result by screw fixation with only a partially visible fracture line dorsally (*arrows*) and without dislocation. Such an "incomplete fracture line" can be confused with a partially persisting epiphyseal line as a variant at initial presentation

(Fig. 9.13). The typical oblique fracture may be difficult to visualize on radiographs if the fracture is undisplaced. This fracture type is usually caused by valgus forces while the extended elbow is locking the olecranon in its humeral fossa. The resulting oblique fracture line extends from proximal and medial to distal and lateral and is open or gapped medially. Conversely, the fracture line runs from proximal and

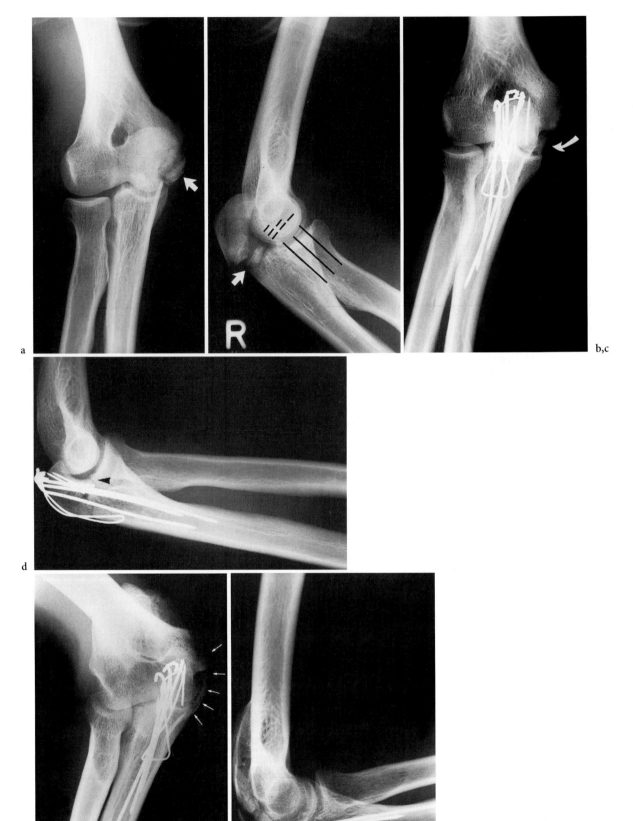

a

b,c

d

e

f

lateral to distal and medial if the injury is caused by varus forces. Sometimes it is necessary to obtain variable angulated lateral projections to demonstrate the fracture, which is indicated by soft tissue swelling in the olecranon bursa and fat pad signs. Fracture lines extending from the anterior portion of the trochlear notch towards the coronoid process are often associated with an anterior displacement of the distal ulnar fragment and a disrupted radiocapitellar joint termed an anterior fracture dislocation (cf. Fig. 9.5).

9.5.8.2 Coronoid Process Fractures

Isolated fractures of the coronoid process are rare and difficult to visualize on standard projections due to superimposition of other bony structures (Fig. 9.14). This fracture type is normally associated with a posterior dislocation of the elbow caused by impaction against the trochlear or sometimes by avulsion of the brachial muscle (Fig. 9.15) (REGAN and MORREY 1992). The fracture line is typically obscured by the radius but can be depicted on the lateral view. The nondislocated fracture type can best be visualized on oblique views. In cases of posterior elbow dislocation the tip of the coronoid process is depicted as a free fragment of unknown origin but with a typical triangular shape (Fig. 9.15).

9.5.9 Monteggia's Fracture

The typical Monteggia's fracture consists of a fracture of the ulna and a luxation of the radial head. The fracture can either run slightly oblique in the ulnar shaft, be located in the proximal ulna, or, even more proximally, involve the olecranon. The fracture line of the ulna extends from proximal and radial to distal and ulnar. With growing forces, dislocations and the

---

Fig. 9.13a–f. Displaced oblique and comminuted olecranon fracture in a 31-year-old man. **a,b** The fracture involves the proximal portion of the olecranon and the region of the collateral ligament attachments. Note the medially displaced fragment and its shape on the AP view (*arrows*). The lateral radiograph of the elbow demonstrates the three types of coronoid fractures. **c,d** Proper osteosynthetic fixation in a typical manner: AO-recommended tension band wiring. Note the minimal step of the articular surface (*arrowhead*) and an additional differently shaped fragment that is displaced medially (*curved arrow*). **e,f** One year later a marked capsule calcification had developed. The AP view demonstrates the restricted extension and the calcifications of the posterior bundle of the medial collateral ligaments (*arrows*)

number of fragments increase. The luxation of the radial head may be associated with a sloping fracture of the radial neck.

9.6 Special Features of Elbow Trauma in Children and Adolescents

9.6.1 Introduction

As in adults, fractures and dislocations of the pediatric elbow are usually the result of indirect trauma transmitted through the forearm. The injury patterns in childhood are generally dominated by the intrinsic weakness of the epiphyseal lines, the separate ossification centers, and also a prevailing bending mechanism. However, it is notable that an isolated epiphysiolysis without a bony fragment is a rare event. During growth the distal humerus consists of four separate ossification centers.

The most common fractures are supracondylar, accounting for approximately 60% of all fractures in childhood. Less common, accounting for about 15%, are fractures of the lateral condyle (a rare isolated injury in adults) followed by separation of the medial epicondyle's ossification center (about 10%).

9.6.2 Subluxation of the Radial Head

A subluxation of the radial head is caused by forcible traction on the extended and pronated forearm. In reference to the mechanism, the injury has been called pronation doloreux (or pronation doloreuse Chassaignac), "pulled elbow," or "nursemaid elbow" (SALTER and ZALTZ 1971). Typically, the extremity is extended over the head and the child is lifted by his hand, resulting in an entrapment of the proximal part of the annular ligament between the radius head and the capitellum. This injury is relatively common between the ages of 2 and 4 years. The diagnosis is based on clinical findings. The radiographic examination typically fails to reveal any pathomorphologic finding and some consider a radiographic examination dispensable if the history of injury is quite typical, as described above. Beyond the age of 6 years the annular ligament is fixed to the radial head so that entrapment of the ligament within the joint space becomes impossible.

9.6.3 Supracondylar Fractures

Supracondylar and transcondylar fractures are most common in the pediatric elbow. If only minimally

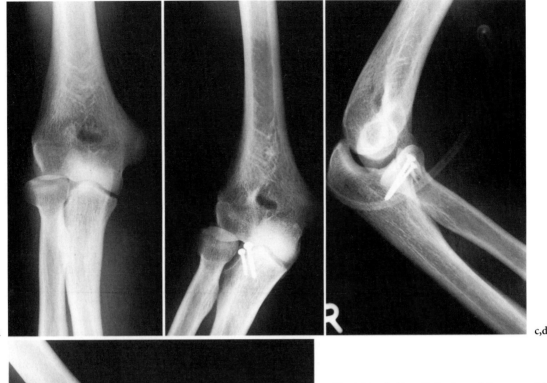

a

c,d

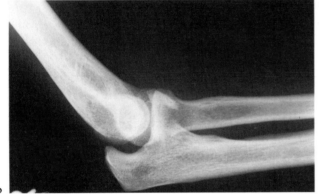

b

Fig. 9.14a–d. Type II fracture of the coronoid process in a 63-year-old man. **a** It is usually impossible to identify the fracture on the AP view. **b** The coronoid fracture is typically obscured on the lateral routine radiograph. In most cases the fragment is triangular and avulsed upward by muscular traction. Note the enlarged humeroulnar joint space. **c,d** AP and lateral views of the elbow with a slightly angulated fragment after AO screw fixation. The fragment must be large enough to accommodate the large end of the screws without further fragmentation. Refixation is often technically difficult and frequently results in slight incongruities, as shown here

displaced, they are difficult to detect on plain films. Fat pad signs and soft tissue swelling are obviously pathologic and typically they are the only radiographic manifestations of these fractures. The fracture itself is sometimes only visible as a subtle distal abnormality of the humerus. The typical mechanism is a fall on the outstretched hand resulting in hyperextension that breaks the region of weakness. Displaced fractures are typical; they are usually clearly visible and the fragments dislocate posteriorly. Secondarily, the median nerve and the brachial artery are stretched and compressed (diminished blood flow) or primarily damaged by sharp margins of the fracture fragments. Immediate fracture reduction and internal fixation are necessary to reduce the likelihood of the disastrous Volkmann's ischemic contracture. The postreduction radiographs accurately depict the alignment of the fragments. The

presence or recurrence of a strong radial pulse is essential for successful therapy. In some cases an angiographic evaluation is necessary before carrying out an open reduction.

9.6.4 Epiphyseal Fractures

The second most common humeral fracture involves the lateral condyle followed by separations of the medial epicondyle's ossification center. The typical injury mechanism is a fall on the outstretched hand with the forearm in supination. Classification of these fractures is based on the extent of the fracture line through the distal humerus (Salter-Harris). Identification of the fracture relies on knowledge of sequential appearance, age, and normal position (on AP and lateral projections) of the distal humeral os-

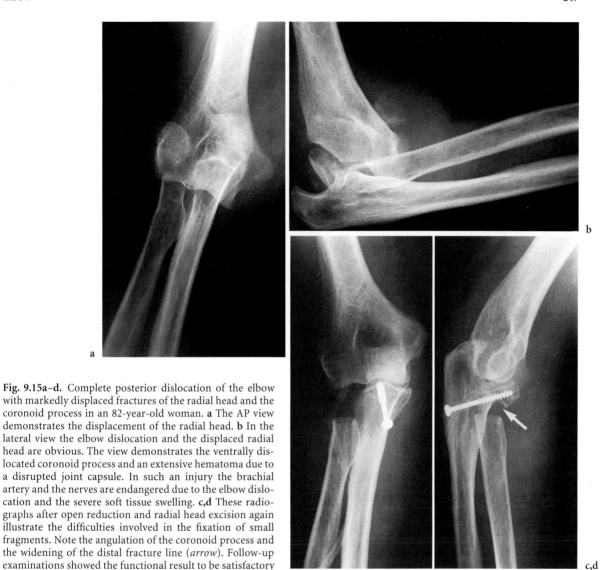

Fig. 9.15a–d. Complete posterior dislocation of the elbow with markedly displaced fractures of the radial head and the coronoid process in an 82-year-old woman. **a** The AP view demonstrates the displacement of the radial head. **b** In the lateral view the elbow dislocation and the displaced radial head are obvious. The view demonstrates the ventrally dislocated coronoid process and an extensive hematoma due to a disrupted joint capsule. In such an injury the brachial artery and the nerves are endangered due to the elbow dislocation and the severe soft tissue swelling. **c,d** These radiographs after open reduction and radial head excision again illustrate the difficulties involved in the fixation of small fragments. Note the angulation of the coronoid process and the widening of the distal fracture line (*arrow*). Follow-up examinations showed the functional result to be satisfactory

sification centers. Incomplete epiphyseal fractures (types I and II) may represent an indication for MRI in order to exclude type III fractures (unstable joint area lesions) which require open reduction and internal fixation. Fractures of the lateral condyle are normally complete fractures of the metaphysis and epiphysis that cross the epiphyseal line (type IV) and tend to dislocate through muscular traction.

9.7 Sequelae and Complications

9.7.1 Introduction

In general the current philosophy of treatment for the majority of elbow articular fractures, as for proximal humeral fractures, emphasizes early kinesitherapy. Prolonged castings and immobilization are associated with an increased risk of permanently diminished versatility. Early mobilization as the treatment of choice for specific fractures and dislocations demands open fragment reduction and internal fixation with rigid devices to protect and stabilize damaged structures while permitting as much active motion as pain and swelling allow.

Soft tissue calcifications and scarring around the elbow articulation are common even with minimal trauma in overuse syndromes (PATTEN 1995). More severe intra-articular injuries are associated with a higher degree of scarring and calcification (see Fig. 9.13) that can be disastrous, especially in the case of hopelessly comminuted fractures and sometimes after elbow dislocation.

Nerve palsy is normally associated with severe injuries. Supracondylar humeral fractures usually involve the ulnar nerve but also may involve the median and radial nerves. Dislocated fractures of the radial head and neck may cause radial nerve palsy as well as a dislocation of the radial head in the case of a Monteggia injury. Cross-union of the ulnar and radial shafts is another known complication after a Monteggia injury. The ulnar nerve passing the ulnar ridge, also termed "the funny bone," is endangered in olecranon fractures and during fracture healing by hypertrophic callus.

9.7.2 Fractures of the Distal Humerus

The most common fracture type of the distal humerus is a T- or Y-shaped bicondylar fracture. Sometimes, hypertrophic callus either posteriorly or anteriorly obliterates the radial, the coronoid, or the olecranon fossa, resulting in limitations of flexion or extension. The most drastic complication in the region of the elbow results from a dislocated or comminuted supracondylar fracture and is termed Volkmann's ischemic contracture. Reduced circulation, most commonly caused by high pressure in the soft tissue compartment due to severe swelling, is the primary pathophysiological insult. Other mechanisms based on a more direct involvement of the brachial artery, e.g., laceration, arterial rupture or occlusion, arterial spasm combined with a reflex spasm of collateral arteries, or even entrapment between fracture fragments occurring primarily or after reduction also subsequently impede the circulation. The disastrous results are ischemic muscle and nerve degeneration with flexion contractures of the hand and wrist, impairment of sensation, and finally a functional loss of the whole extremity.

9.7.3 Fractures of the Proximal Radius

Especially in type III and IV fractures the area of the radial head is known for multiple complications due to the injury but also due to sequelae of treatment. Calcification of the capsule and ligaments, ectopic ossifications, and shortening of the interosseous membrane may be due to the injury itself. After radial head resection (see Fig. 9.15c,d), joint instability (usually only slight) can cause symptoms at the wrist due to axial forces. Local overgrowth of the radial neck stump extending to apparent regrowth of

the radial head and ectopic ossifications are well-known complications of surgery. Finally, it should be mentioned that the treatment of radial fractures is a controversial topic in orthopedic surgery. Today, most surgeons prefer conservative functional treatment.

9.7.4 Fractures of the Proximal Ulna

Depending on the extent of an olecranon fracture, there may be reduction of motion, involvement of the ulnar nerve with a resulting neuropathy, and posttraumatic arthritis and arthrosis caused by a loss of articular congruency. The usually low number of complications, such as articular instability or nonunion, rises sharply in cases of comminuted distal humeral fractures (cf. the case in Fig. 9.13).

9.8 Diagnostic Algorithm and Flow Chart

9.8.1 Diagnostic Strategy

In any patient who has sustained an adequate trauma to the elbow, a minimum of two projections (AP and lateral views) are necessary to evaluate the bony and soft tissue structures of the elbow articulation (Fig. 9.16). In the absence of a suspected fracture no further radiographic investigations are indicated. Unfortunately, patients with elbow injuries are frequently unable to position the elbow as needed and the standard views have to be approximated by tube angulation.

Since the elbow articulation is a complex joint and superimposition of critical regions is inevitable on the standard views, additional projections are necessary if the clinical examination provides evidence of a fracture (Fig. 9.16). The region of the lateral epicondyle is best visualized on an external oblique view and is also partially demonstrated by an axial view. The medial epicondyle requires an internal oblique view and can also be demonstrated on an axial view. A suspected radial head fracture in a typical position is preferably visualized on a radial head view and is also demonstrated on an external oblique view (PAGE 1986). The capitellum is also best demonstrated on the radial head view (GREENSPAN and NORMAN 1987). Suspected fractures of the coronoid process are visible on the radial head view but are especially well demonstrated on an internal oblique view. Complex fractures of the elbow articulation such as side swipe injuries and comminuted frac-

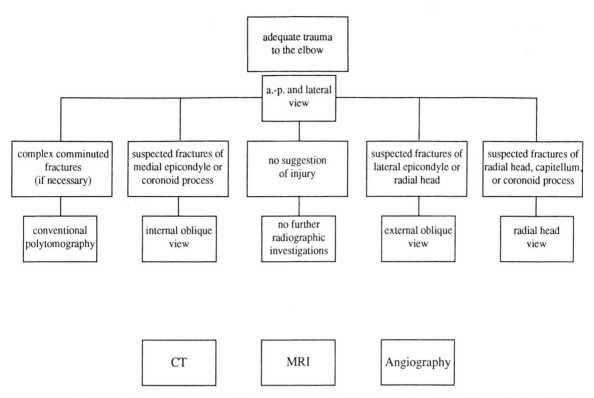

Fig. 9.16. Diagnostic algorithm with respect to adequate trauma to the elbow. Indications for ancillary techniques for the evaluation of injury, sequelae, and complications are given in the text

tures require conventional tomography to assess the position of comminuted or dislocated fragments (see Fig. 9.11). In some cases CT and CT reconstructions are superior in demonstrating the injury and supply additional information about the surrounding soft tissues. Tomography is also indicated in cases of nonunion and secondary infections, especially when metallic osteosynthetic material superimposes bony structures. Arthrography with single or double contrast augmented by tomography or CT has rare and similar indications: capsular ruptures, chondral and osteochondral fractures, free bodies within the joint space, and subtle abnormalities of the synovia and the articular cartilage. MRI is superior for demonstrating soft tissue injuries of ligaments, capsule, nerves, tendons, and musles (TEHRANZADEH et al. 1992). Joint effusions and hematomas are visible, and subtle alterations such as bone edema and contusions as well as epiphyseal fractures in children are well demonstrated without radiation exposure (BELTRAN et al. 1994). It is notable that CT requires good mobility of the injured extremity for positioning in the CT gantry. MRI, typically performed with surface coils (designed for the shoulder or knee), is possible if extension of the injured elbow is

feasible. MRI is generally difficult to perform due to positioning problems, an exception being so-called open MRI.

9.8.2 Important Points to Remember in Adults

1. Indirect fracture signs, e.g., positive fat pad signs, alterations of the supinator fat stripe, and hemorrhage into the olecranon bursa, are strong indicators of a fracture. Occult fractures or subtle changes require additional views of the clinically suspicious regions.

2. Fractures of the radial head and neck are the most common elbow fractures in adults, accounting for about one-third of cases. The fractures are best demonstrated with a radial head view and require classification of the fracture type, extension of the fracture lines, degree of fragment dislocation, and articular displacement in order to permit selection of the appropriate course of therapy. Due to the common axial injury mechanism, radial head fractures may be associated with capitellum fractures, luxations of the distal radioulnar joint, and scaphoid fractures.

3. Fractures of the coronoid process are rare as an isolated injury; commonly they are associated with articular dislocations (see Figs. 9.14, 9.15). The fracture is preferably demonstrated on the radial head view. The fragment tends to dislocate proximally (in contrast to radial head fragments) (cf. Figs. 9.11, 9.15) or into the joint space. If the fracture is missed or nonunion occurs, complications such as an unstable elbow joint or the very rare condition of a recurrent dislocation might ensue (REGAN and MORREY 1992).

4. Distal olecranon fractures, ulnar fractures, and radial head dislocations have to be suspected to be a part of a Monteggia injury in all cases and demand further, appropriate radiographic investigation (GIUSTRA et al. 1974).

9.8.3 Important Points to Remember in Children

1. In childhood trauma to the elbow articulation is frequent, usually occurring via an indirect mechanism transmitted through the forearm. Evaluation of the radiographic films is among the most critical and difficult tasks in trauma radiology.

2. The most common fracture type (accounting for 60% of all fractures) is a supracondylar fracture of the distal humerus. In this case the lateral projection shows a loss of the typical "hockey stick" appearance.

3. Knowledge and assessment of sequential appearance, age, normal positions, and the variable, sometimes irregular shape of the ossification centers, supported by evaluation of the anterior humeral line, the radio-capitellar line, and soft tissue alterations will usually lead to a satisfactory interpretation. Routinely obtaining radiographs of the opposite elbow "for comparison" does not meet today's standard of radiologic care and should be substituted by "comparison with the literature" (cf. Fig. 9.12) (RICKETT and FINLAY 1993).

References

Bado JL (1967) The Monteggia lesion. Clin Orthop 50:71–86
Beck C, Dabezies EJ (1984) Monteggia fracture-dislocation. Orthopedics 7:329–331
Beltran J, Rosenberg ZS, Kawelblum M, Montes L, Bergman AG, Strongwater A (1994) Pediatric elbow fractures: MRI evaluation. Skeletal Radiol 23:277–281
Blickman JG, Dunlop RW, Sanzone CF, Franklin PD (1990) Is CT useful in the traumatized pediatric elbow? Pediatr Radiol 20:184–185
Colton CL (1973) Fractures of the olecranon in adults: classification and management. Injury 5:121–127

DeLee JC, Green DP, Wilkins KE (1984) Fractures and dislocations of the elbow. In: Rockwood CA Jr, Green DP (eds) Fractures in adults, vol 1, 2nd edn., Lippincott, Philadelphia
Dihlmann SW, Meenen NM, Wolf L, Jungbluth KH (1992) Fat pad signs and supinator fat line in cubital trauma. Unfallchirurgie 18:148–153
Eppright RH, Wilkins KE (1975) Fractures and dislocations of the elbow. In: Rockwood CA Jr, Green DP (eds) Fractures, vol I. Lippincott, Philadelphia
Giustra PE, Kiloran PJ, Furman RS, Root JA (1974) The missed Monteggia fracture. Radiology 110:45–48
Greenspan A, Norman A (1987) Radial head-capitellum view: an expanded imaging approach to elbow injury. Radiology 164:272–274
Hall-Craggs MA, Shorvon PJ, Chapman M (1985) Assessment of the radial head-capitellum view and the dorsal fat-pad sign in acute elbow trauma. AJR 145:607–609
Henley MB (1987) Intra-articular distal humeral fractures in adults. Orthop Clin North Am 18:11–23
Keon-Cohen BT (1966) Fracture at the elbow. J Bone Joint Surg 48:1623–1639
Kuur E, Kjaersgaard-Anderson A (1988) Side-swipe injury to the elbow. J Trauma 28:1397–1399
Mirowitz SA, London SL (1992) Ulnar collateral ligament injury in baseball pitchers: MR imaging evaluation. Radiology 185:573–576
Morrey BF (1985) The elbow and its disorders. Saunders Philadelphia
Mueller ME, Allgöwer M, Schneider R, Willeneigger H (1979) Manual of internal fixation. Techniques recommended by the AO group, 2nd edn. Springer, New York Berlin Heidelberg
Murphy WA, Siegel MJ (1977) Elbow fat pads with new signs and extended differential diagnosis. Radiology 124:659–665
Page AC (1986) Critical evaluation of the radial head-capitellum view in elbow trauma. AJR 146:81–82
Patten RM (1995) Overuse syndromes and injuries involving the elbow: MR imaging findings. AJR 164:1205–1211
Pitt MJ, Speer DP (1990) Imaging of the elbow with an emphasis on trauma. Radiol Clin North Am 28:293–305
Priest JD, Jones HH, Nagel DA (1974) Elbow injuries in highly skilled tennis players. J Sports Med 2:137
Randal PM (1995) Overuse syndromes and injuries involving the elbow: MR imaging findings. AJR 164:1205–1211
Regan W, Morrey BF (1992) Classification and treatment of coronoid process fractures. Orthopedics 15:845–848
Rickett AB, Finlay DB (1993) An audit of comparative views in elbow trauma in children. Br J Radiol 66:123–125
Riseborough EJ, Radin EL (1969) Intracondylar T-fractures of the humerus in adult. A comparison of operative and nonoperative treatment in 29 cases. J Bone Joint Surg 51:130–141
Rogers LF, McEwan DW (1969) Changes due to trauma in the fat plane overlying the supinator muscle: a radiologic sign. Radiology 92:954
Salter RB, Zaltz C (1971) Anatomic investigations of the mechanism of injury and pathologic anatomy of "pulled elbow" in young children. Clin Orthop 77:134–136
Singston RD, Feldman F, Rosenberg ZS (1986) Elbow joint: assessment with double-contrast CT arthrography. Radiology 160:167–169
Soltanpur A (1978) Anterior supracondylar fracture of the humerus (flexion type). J Bone Surg 60:383–386
Tehranzadeh J, Kerr R, Amster J (1992) Magnetic resonance imaging of tendon and ligament abnormalities. I. Spine and upper extremities. Skeletal Radiol 21:1–9

10 Distal Forearm, Wrist, and Hand

V.M. METZ

CONTENTS

10.1 Distal Forearm

10.1.1 General Considerations

The distal fifth of the forearm is one of the most common sites of fracture. Fractures of the distal forearm account for 17% of all emergency room fractures (WOOD and BERQUIST 1992) and are ten times more frequent than fractures of the carpal bones. The nature of the injury depends on several factors such as the severity of the forces involved, the degree of flexion or extension and supination or pronation of the wrist, the degree of radial or ulnar deviation, and the age of the patient. Most fractures of the distal fore-

V.M. METZ, MD, Associate Professor, Universitätsklinik für Radiodiagnostik, Allg. Krankenhaus Wien, Währinger Gürtel 18-20, 1090 Wien, Austria

arm are the result of a fall on the outstretched hand; they are most often seen in patients above the age of 50 years and are more frequent in women than in men.

10.1.2 Anatomy

The distal radius is largely composed of spongious bone and has a relatively thin cortex. On the lateral margin of the distal radius there is a predominant bony projection, the styloid process (Fig. 10.1). The articular surface of the radius has two fossae, one at the radial aspect for the articulation with the scaphoid bone, and one at the ulnar aspect for the articulation with the lunate bone. On the medial border of the distal radius is a concavity, the sigmoid or ulnar notch, for the articulation with the head of the ulna. The articular joint surface of the distal radius is angulated 10–25° in the palmar (volar) direction, which is called the "palmar tilt" (Fig. 10.1b) (TALEISNIK 1985). In addition, the distal radius is angled in the ulnar direction (= radial angulation) (Fig. 10.1a). This radial angulation is between 16° and 28°, averaging around 20°. Loss of these angles indicates a distal radius fracture with impaction or overlap of fragments in most cases.

The distal ulna is also composed of cancellous bone but has a thicker cortex than the distal radius. It consists of the styloid process and the head of the ulna; latter articulates with the distal radius and the triquetral and the lunate bones (Fig. 10.1). The length of the radius relative to that of the ulnar head is defined by the term "ulnar variance." In most patients the length of the distal ulna and the distal radius is equal (neutral) or the ulnar head is about 1 mm shorter than the distal radius. If the ulna is short (more than 1 mm shorter than the distal radius), the term "negative ulnar variance" is used. Conversely, ulnar variance is positive if the ulnar head ends more distally than the radius. However, it must be noted that measurement of ulnar variance is only reliable if the arm and forearm are in a neutral

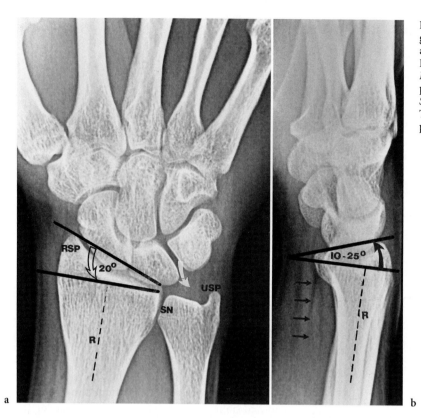

Fig. 10.1. PA (**a**) and lateral (**b**) radiographs of a normal wrist. Radial angulation (**b**) averages around 20°. Palmar tilt (**a**) is between 10° and 25°. *R*, Radial axes; *RSP*, radial styloid process; *USP*, ulnar styloid process; *SN*, sigmoid notch; *white arrow*, TFCC; *arrows*, pronator quadratus fat pad

position (see later in this chapter) (HARDY et al. 1987).

In the distal radioulnar joint rotation (pronation and supination) of the radius about the ulna takes place. This rotation is supported by the proximal radioulnar joint as a functional unit. Normally a range of rotation of 160–180° is possible (HARDY et al. 1987).

The triangular fibrocartilage complex (TFCC) consists of the fibrous articular disk as an extension of the articular surface of the radius, the meniscus homologue, the ulnar collateral ligament, the tendon sheath of the extensor carpi ulnaris tendon, and poorly defined volar and dorsal radioulnar ligaments. This complex arises from the ulnar side of the lunate fossa of the radius and is attached at the ulnar head and the styloid process of the ulna. Proximally the TFCC articulates with the ulnar head, and distally it articulates with the triquetral bone and the ulnar aspect of the lunate bone. The function of the TFCC is to absorb axial loading and to provide stability of the distal radioulnar joint.

10.1.3 Fractures and Dislocations

Fractures of the distal forearm include Colles' fracture, Smith's fracture, Barton's fracture, chauffeur's or Hutchinson's fracture, fracture of the ulnar styloid, and transverse fracture of the distal radius.

The most common fracture of the distal radius is *Colles' fracture* (Fig. 10.2). It occurs in older patients and is more common in women than in men. Above the age of 60 years, Colles' fracture is six times more frequent in women than in men (ALFFRAM and BAUER 1962) due to postmenopausal osteoporosis. By definition, Colles' fracture is a fracture of the distal radial epiphysis or metaphysis, with or without intra-articular involvement, with the distal fracture fragment displaced or angulated in the dorsal direction (DOBYNS and LINSCHEID 1984; JUPITER 1991). In many cases there is dorsal cortical comminution and in the majority of cases there is intra-articular involvement of either the radiocarpal or the radioulnar joint or both joints (KNIRK and JUPITER 1986). In 60% of cases there is an associated fracture of the ulnar styloid. The mechanism of injury is a fall on the outstretched hand (SHORT et al. 1987). The patient lands on the thenar eminence, which places the dorsal surface of the distal radius in compression and the ventral surface of the radius in tension. The compression force leads to comminution of the posterior cortex of the distal radius and tension forces result in gapping of the anterior cortex. Numerous classification systems have been reported. However, the classification described by FRYKMAN (1967) has

Fig. 10.2. PA (**a**) and lateral (**b**) radiographs of a patient with a Colles' fracture. Typically, as depicted on the lateral radiograph (**b**), the distal fracture fragment is angulated dorsally (*curved arrow*). There is an associated fracture of the ulnar styloid process (*open arrow* in **a**)

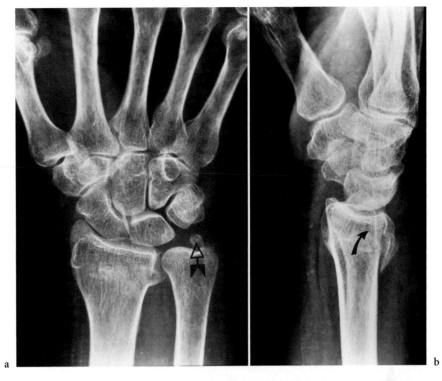

Fig. 10.3. PA (**a**) and lateral (**b**) radiographs of a patient with Smith's fracture. In this fracture the distal fracture fragment displays volar angulation (*curved arrow* in **b**). As shown in **a** (*arrow*), the distal radioulnar joint is widened, indicating associated subluxation of this joint. Note that there is additional fracture of the ulnar styloid

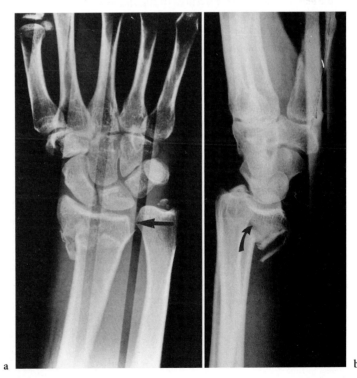

gained wide acceptance. This classification divides Colles' fractures into eight types and is based on the presence of intra-articular involvement of either the radiocarpal or the distal radioulnar joint and the presence or absence of an associated fracture of the distal ulna.

Smith's fracture, also called reverse Colles' fracture, is a fracture of the distal radius epiphysis or metaphysis with volar displacement or angulation of the distal fracture fragment (Fig. 10.3). Similarly to Colles' fractures, Smith's fractures may occur with or without intra-articular involvement of the radiocarpal and/or the distal radioulnar joint, and with or without an associated fracture of the ulnar styloid. The mechanism of injury is hyperflexion from a fall on the volar flexed wrist but may also occur from a direct blow to the back of the wrist or from a fall one the outstretched wrist impacting the supinated forearm against the dorsiflexed wrist (DOBYNS and LINSCHEID 1984). THOMAS (1957) classified Smith's fractures into three types. Type 1 is an extra-articular fracture of the distal radial metaphysis with the classic volar displacement or angulation of the distal fragment. This type is often comminuted and there is frequently a fracture of the ulnar styloid. Type 1 usually occurs in older patients. Type 2, more commonly seen in younger men, is an anterior marginal fracture of the lower articular end of the radius with volar and proximal displacement of the distal fracture fragment (volar Barton fracture, discussed later). Type 3 is described as an oblique juxta-articular fracture approximately 3 cm proximal to the radiocarpal joint. The distal end of the radius is displaced and tilted anteriorly. Type 3 fractures are more unstable than type 1 fractures and are frequently associated with fractures of the metacarpals. They commonly occur in motorcyclists.

Barton's fracture (DE OLIVEIRA 1973) is defined as an intra-articular fracture of the posterior or anterior rim (= reverse Barton fracture) of the distal radius *with* accompanying palmar and dorsal

dislocation of the carpus, respectively (Fig. 10.4). The dislocation or subluxation of the carpus distinguishes these fractures from intra-articular fractures of the Smith and Colles types. Anterior rim fractures are more common than dorsal rim fractures and occur by a mechanism similar to that described for Smith's fractures. They are frequently encountered in younger patients as a result of motorcycle accidents. Posterior rim fractures, more common in the elderly, result from a fall on the outstretched hand that produces wrist extension and forearm pronation under compressive axial loading.

Another type of fracture of the distal radius is the radial styloid fracture of *chauffeur's fracture* (Fig. 10.5) (eponym: Hutchinson's fracture) (DOBYNS and LINSCHEID 1984). By definition it is an intra-articular fracture with the fracture line usually originating from the junction of the scaphoid and lunate fossae of the distal articular surface of the radius and coursing laterally in a transverse or oblique direction. This type of fracture may be simple or comminuted and undisplaced or displaced (more common), but without any evidence of radiocarpal subluxation. The mechanism of injury is a direct blow or impaction (axial compression) of the scaphoid bone against the radial styloid.

Dislocation or subluxation of the distal radioulnar joint commonly occurs in association with fractures of the distal radius and ulna and has been referred to

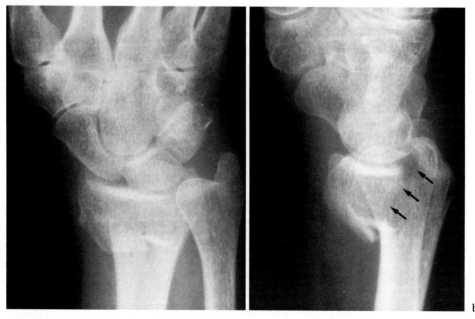

a   b

Fig. 10.4. PA (**a**) and lateral (**b**) radiographs of a young man with a Barton's fracture, defined as an intra-articular fracture (*arrows* in **b**) of the posterior rim of the distal radius

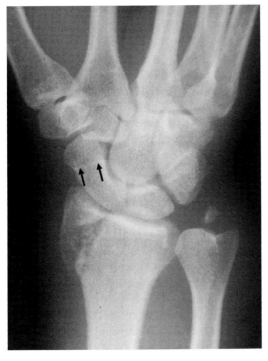

Fig. 10.5. Chauffeur's fracture is defined as an oblique intra-articular fracture of the radial styloid process. There is no displacement of the fracture fragments. An additional fracture of the scaphoid bone at its distal third can be identified as a dense line (*arrows*). There is also a fractured ulnar styloid process

as Moore's fracture (DOBYNS and LINSCHEID 1984). Less commonly, isolated subluxations or dislocations of the distal radioulnar joint occur (HEAD 1971). According to the position of the ulnar head in relation to the distal radius, subluxations/dislocations are classified as dorsal, volar, or rotational. In most cases the subluxation/dislocation is in the dorsal direction (DAMERON 1972; HEAD 1971). Posterior dislocation is the result of a severe hyperpronation trauma (Fig. 10.6). The radiological diagnosis can be made on a true lateral radiograph showing dorsal displacement of the ulna with respect to the radius. On the posteroanterior (PA) radiograph the distal radioulnar joint space is widened in many cases. The less common anterior dislocation is thought to be due to a severe supinating stress from a fall on the outstretched hand. On the PA radiograph the ulnar head overlaps the distal radius (in contrast to posterior dislocation) and on the lateral view the head of the ulna is projected anterior to the anterior aspect of the radius. In rotational subluxation the head of the ulna is fixed within the sigmoid notch in an abnormal position due to hyperpronation or hypersupination stress (GRAHAM et la. 1985). In this case the radius rotates about the ulna abnormally widely, and the ulnar head becomes entrapped in the ulnar notch because incongruity of the joint surfaces

Fig. 10.6. PA (**a**) and lateral (**b**) radiographs in a patient with a fracture of the shaft of the radius. On the PA view the distal radioulnar joint seems normal. On the lateral radiograph, however, the ulnar head is severely displaced dorsally, indicating subluxation of the distal radioulnar joint (*arrow*)

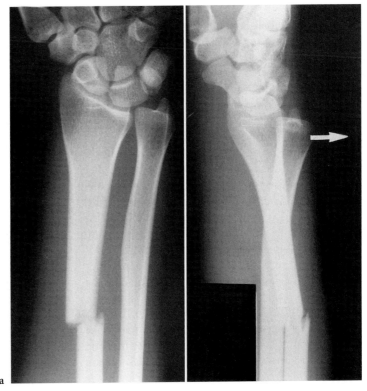

a   b

does not allow a derotation of the radius. The key to radiographic diagnosis of rotational subluxation is the position of the ulnar styloid process (SNOOK et al. 1969). On the PA view the ulnar styloid process lies on the lateral margin of the ulnar head, and on the lateral view it projects on the dorsal aspect of the ulnar head. In cases of rotational subluxations, however, the ulnar styloid process projects on the midportion of the ulnar head on the PA view and does not lie dorsal of the ulnar head on the lateral radiograph. However, subtle changes of any types of subluxation or dislocation may be overlooked on conventional radiographs, and inadequate positioning of the wrist on the PA and lateral radiographs may lead to misdiagnosis (discussed later in this section).

10.1.4 Examination Methods

10.1.4.1 Plain Film Radiography

In most cases of distal forearm fractures, routine radiographs are sufficient for correct diagnosis and adequate treatment. The minimum routine evaluation requires two views: PA and lateral. The PA view should be performed with the humerus abducted 90° from the chest wall, so that the elbow is at the same level as the shoulder, and with the elbow flexed 90° degrees (YIN et al. 1996b). Under these conditions the distal radioulnar joint is in true neutral position and therefore allows precise measurement of ulnar variance. For the lateral view the humerus is adducted against the chest wall and the elbow flexed 90°.

When considering the PA and lateral radiographs, at least two radiographic measurements may be important for accurate treatment and adequate radiological follow-up after fractures of the distal radius (MANN et al. 1992; YIN et al. 1996b). Radial angulation is the relative angle of the distal radial articular surface on the PA view to a line perpendicular to the long axis of the radius (Fig. 10.1a). This angle should be between 16° and 28°, averaging around 20°. As mentioned, loss of this angle indicates a radial fracture, with impaction or overlap of fragments in most cases. A second measurement of the distal articular surface of the radius is the palmar tilt, measured on the lateral radiograph (Fig. 10.1b). This is the angle created between the articular surface of the distal radius and a line perpendicular to the long axis of the radius, and is between 10° and 25° (mean, 15°).

Routine radiographic views other than the PA and lateral views, such as a 30–45° semipronated oblique view, are helpful to evaluate more clearly certain fracture patterns and the extent of fracture lines. Indeed, some fracture lines will not be discernible on the routine PA and lateral views.

Since fractures of the distal radius and ulna may be occult, exact evaluation of the soft tissues of the distal forearm and wrist can be the key to correct diagnosis and be useful in preventing misdiagnosis (CURTIS et al. 1984). The deep fat pad of the pronator quadratus, constantly seen on the lateral view (Fig. 10.1b), lies between the pronator quadratus muscle and the flexor tendon sheaths. Normally it forms a slight ventral concave line and is convexly bowed in a ventral direction or completely absent under pathological conditions such as fractures.

Subluxation or dislocation of the distal radioulnar joint commonly can be recognized adequately on routine PA and lateral views. On the PA radiograph, the distal radioulnar joint should measure approximately 2 mm. Incongruity at this joint may cause widening or narrowing of this joint space, but if it does not, subluxation or dislocation of the distal radioulnar joint may be overlooked. Normally on a true lateral radiograph congruence of the distal radioulnar joint is demonstrated by nearly complete overlap of the ulnar head and the distal radius (Fig. 10.7), and dorsal or ventral dislocation causes loss of this radial and ulnar superimposition. However, as shown in the literature (MINO et al. 1983), slight supination or pronation of the wrist from the neutral position and slight variations of normal will render analysis for distal radioulnar incongruity inaccurate. Therefore in uncertain cases, advanced imaging techniques such as computed tomography (CT) or magnetic resonance imaging (MRI) should be used when there is a question of subluxation of the distal radioulnar joint.

10.1.4.2 Computed Tomography

In the majority of cases the simple radiographic examination is satisfactory for evaluation of distal forearm injuries. However, in selected difficult cases CT may add significant information compared with conventional radiographs. The advantage of CT is its improved contrast resolution and planar representation of the bones without the superimposition inherent in radiography. Another advantage of CT is that primary images in different planes (e.g., axial, coronal, and sagittal) can be obtained. Furthermore, the

Fig. 10.7. a True lateral radiograph of a normal wrist. Congruence of the distal radioulnar joint is demonstrated by nearly complete overlap of the ulnar head and the distal radius. **b** Same patient as in **a**. The radiograph was obtained in slight pronation of the wrist. The ulnar head is projected dorsal to the radius, which may give rise to the misdiagnosis of dorsal subluxation of the distal radioulnar joint

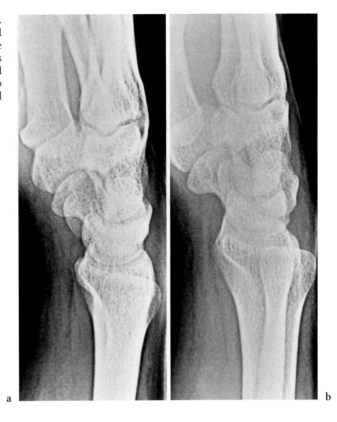

a   b

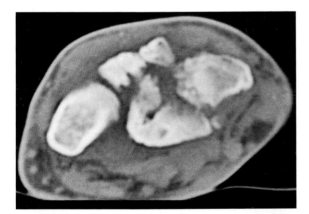

Fig. 10.8. Axial CT through the distal radius and ulna demonstrates a complex intra-articular fracture of the distal radius. CT may be helpful for better evaluation of the degree of diastasis of the fracture fragments

spiral-CT technique allows multiplanar reconstructions in any desired plane and high-quality three-dimensional reconstructions by a single examination.

Indications for CT include complex fractures, especially intra-articular fractures, occult fractures, assessment of fracture healing, and post-surgical evaluation (STEWART and GILULA 1992; YIN et al.

1996a). As suggested in recent studies on CT examination of distal radius fractures, imaging in axial and sagittal or axial and coronal planes with 2-mm continuous sections is usually sufficient. The axial plane is very useful to show the configuration of the fracture patterns involving the distal radial articular surface (Fig. 10.8), and this plane readily shows the degree of diastasis of radioscaphoid and radiolunate fossae fragments, possible incongruity of the distal radioulnar joint, and volar and dorsal cortical comminution of the radius. The sagittal (Fig. 10.9) and coronal planes are useful for demonstration of congruity and angulation of radiocarpal joint surfaces and the degree of dorsal and volar surface comminution, as well as elevation or depression of the distal radial articular surface. Recognition of fracture fragment size and position can have a major influence on whether or not to operate and on which approach may be most suitable. Central pylon type fracture depression may be invisible on plain radiographs.

As discussed earlier in this chapter, distal radioulnar subluxation or dislocation occasionally can be diagnosed on a true lateral radiograph. Sometimes, however, it may be difficult to obtain a true lateral radiograph because pain in an acutely injured wrist, casting, or inconsistent positioning by the

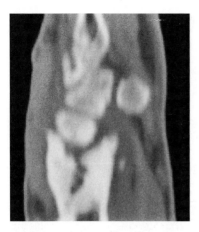

Fig. 10.9. Sagittal multiplanar reconstruction obtained from axial scans of the same patient as in Fig. 10.8 allows more accurate evaluation of the degree of depression of the articular surface of the distal radius

technologist may be a limiting factor. Positioning the wrist as little as 10° off lateral makes the lateral radiograph completely unreliable in the assessment of distal radioulnar joint congruity. In addition, the ulna may show subluxation only in certain positions and the dorsally prominent ulna may be a normal variant. Comparison with the opposite wrist in the lateral position may be helpful. CT is the technique of choice for corroborating distal radioulnar incongruency (Cone et al. 1983; Frahm et al. 1989; Mino et al. 1983; Stewart and Gilula 1992). Mino et al. (1983) described CT criteria for the diagnosis of distal radioulnar subluxation or dislocation. On the axial plane, two lines have to be drawn, one through the dorsal border of the distal radius and the second through the palmar border of the distal radius at the level of the sigmoid notch and Lister's tubercle (Fig. 10.10). Articulation of the distal radioulnar joint is normal if the ulnar head lies between these two lines. Additional axial CT scans should be performed in supination and pronation to avoid picturing a dynamic subluxation that is reduced, and in a position that is painful for the patient in the hope of finding the subluxation in that painful position. Wechsler et al. (1987) cited poor experience with these criteria and introduced the epicentre and congruity methods as being more accurate for the diagnosis of distal radioulnar subluxation/dislocation.

10.1.4.3 Magnetic Resonance Imaging

Although MRI cannot be used as the imaging technique of first choice for evaluating acute distal radius

fractures, it provides a powerful new diagnostic tool to assess bony, ligamentous, and soft tissue abnormalities which sometimes are related to fractures of the distal forearm.

Magnetic resonance imaging can be used for detection of occult fractures (Fig. 10.11), stress fractures, and osteochondral lesions of the distal forearm if plain films are negative and there is a high clinical suspicion of abnormality. These lesions can easily be demonstrated by obtaining T1-weighted images and fat-suppressed sequences (such as the STIR sequence) in a coronal plane. In addition MRI is helpful for evaluation of fracture healing or non-union in selected cases.

Magnetic resonance imaging can be useful for the diagnosis of subluxation or dislocation of the distal radioulnar joint. Compared with CT, MRI has the additional advantage of simultaneous identification of the radioulnar ligaments and the TFCC, MRI allows more accurate characterization of associated effusion in the distal radioulnar joint, which may be a secondary sign of ligament and TFCC pathology.

For injuries of flexor or extensor tendons as well as injuries to the median nerve, which are possible complications in distal radius fractures, MRI can be a very helpful diagnostic imaging modality (Reicher and Kellerhouse 1990). Evaluation of carpal tunnel disease after malunions of distal radius fractures and evaluation and staging of reflex sympathetic dystrophy also can be performed successfully with MRI (Schimmerl et al. 1991).

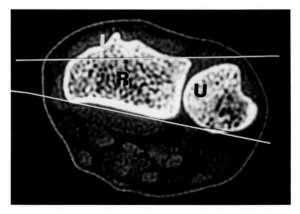

Fig. 10.10. Axial CT of the distal radioulnar joint at the level of Lister's tubercle. Two lines have to be drawn, one through the dorsal border of the distal radius and the second through the palmar border of the distal radius. Articulation of the distal radioulnar joint is normal if the ulnar head lies between these two lines

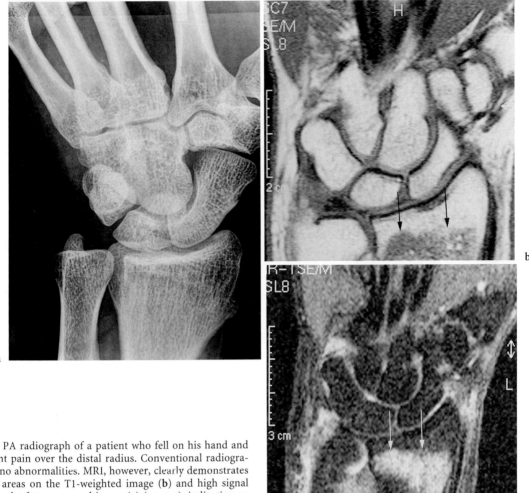

Fig. 10.11. a PA radiograph of a patient who fell on his hand and had persistent pain over the distal radius. Conventional radiography showed no abnormalities. MRI, however, clearly demonstrates hypointense areas on the T1-weighted image (**b**) and high signal intensities on the fat-suppressed image (**c**) (*arrows*), indicating an occult fracture of the distal radius

10.1.5 Special Features in Children

In children less than 12 years old, fractures of the distal forearm account for as many as 35% of all fractures, and in more than 50% of cases the fractures are located in the distal sixth of the radius and ulna (THOMAS et al. 1975). Between the ages of 6 and 10 years, most fractures are located 2–4 cm proximal to the distal growth plate, whereas between the ages of 10 and 16 years, separations of the distal radial epiphysis are more common.

Torus fractures (Fig. 10.12) are the result of a fall on the outstretched hand. In this condition compression forces are created in the posterior cortex, leading to a buckling or folding of the cortex (buckled cortex). The anterior cortex remains intact and is usually slightly angulated.

Greenstick fractures (Fig. 10.13) are the result of a force greater than in Torus fractures, leading to com-

plete disruption of a portion of the cortex with angulation at the fracture site.

Separation of the growth plate of the distal radius accounts for almost 50% of all epiphyseal injuries (PETERSON and PETERSON 1972). It can result from a fall on the outstretched hand resulting in shearing forces within the growth plate, or, as described in the literature (ROWE 1979), from weight lifting. In most cases separation of the growth plate takes the form of either a Salter-Harris type 2 (fracture through the growth plate and metaphysis) or a Salter-Harris type 1 (isolated fracture through the growth plate) lesion. Commonly the epiphyseal center is displaced posteriorly, resulting in a "Colles-like" fracture; however, it also may be displaced in a volar direction (Smith-like fracture). Usually there is an additional fracture of the ulnar styloid process. Radiological diagnosis can easily be done on the lateral view by identifying the dorsal or volar displacement of the ossification

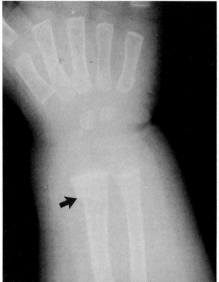

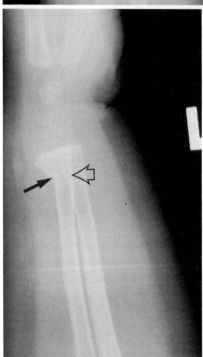

Fig. 10.12a,b. Torus fracture of the distal radius in a 6-year-old boy. On the PA view (**a**) there is buckling of the cortex of the metaphysis of the distal radius (*arrow*). On the lateral view (**b**) there is angulation of the posterior cortex (*closed arrow*); the anterior cortex is intact (*open arrow*)

the corner sign is projected en face and may be obscured by the surrounding bone.

10.1.6 Follow-up and Complications

The goal of fracture treatment is bony union in as close to an anatomic position as is possible and reasonable. Postreduction radiographs in at least two planes should be obtained for evaluation of the adequacy of treatment. Radial length, palmar tilt, radial inclination, and congruity of articular surfaces must be evaluated after reduction to avoid malunion, nonunion, and other complications. Weekly serial PA and lateral radiographs should be obtained for evaluation of fracture healing. Fixation devices such as external fixations and Kirschner wires in cases of open reductions have to be examined by radiography for assessment of proper position.

Complications after fractures of the distal forearm occur in about 30% of cases (COONEY et al. 1980). They include malunion with subsequent develop-

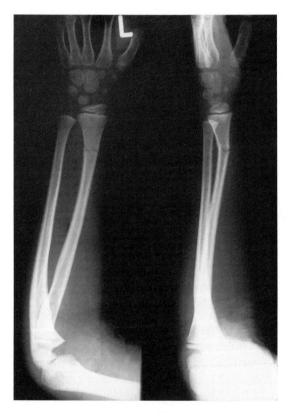

Fig. 10.13. Greenstick fracture of the distal radius. A complete disruption of a portion of the cortex with angulation at the fracture site can be seen

center. The accompanying dorsal metaphyseal fragment, the so-called corner sign, is readily apparent on the lateral view. On the PA view, separation of the growth plate may be overlooked since medial or lateral displacement of the epiphysis is minimal, and

ment of arthrosis, entrapment of the flexor and extensor tendons, compression of the median nerve due to dislocation and malunion of fracture fragments, and reflex sympathetic dystrophy. It is also important to note that distal radius fractures are sometimes accompanied by scaphoid fractures, injuries of the triangular fibrocartilage complex, and tears of the carpal ligaments. Therefore, radiological examination of these structures should routinely be performed for correct diagnosis and to avoid complications.

10.1.7 Diagnostic Algorithm

The imaging technique of first choice is conventional radiography in at least two planes, the lateral and the PA. Additional planes such as the oblique view may be employed for better evaluation of fracture lines and fragments. In most cases routine radiographs allow adequate diagnosis. In cases of complex and comminuted trauma, CT should be performed. This technique allows a more precise evaluation of articular surfaces and evaluation of the location of fracture fragments. As mentioned earlier, CT is the imaging technique of choice in uncertain cases of subluxation or dislocation of the distal radioulnar joint. In selected cases CT is superior to conventional radiography for the evaluation of fracture healing. MRI should be performed if there is clinical suspicion of fracture-associated soft tissue injuries of the tendons, the median nerve, the TFCC, or the ligaments of the wrist. MRI is also a very sensitive and specific imaging technique for evaluation of occult fractures and fracture healing if conventional radiography is inconclusive or negative.

10.2 Carpus

10.2.1 General Considerations

Compared with fractures of the distal forearm, fractures of the carpal bones occur ten times less often. Frequently, fractures of carpal bones involve multiple bones but they may also occur in a single bone. The most common site of a carpal bone fracture is the scaphoid bone, such fractures accounting for 60%–70% of all carpal injuries (DUNN 1972). The second most commonly fractured bone is the triquetral bone, accounting for 10%–20% of cases. Dislocations and fracture dislocations are relatively

rare and account for 10%. In children under the age of 12 years, carpal injuries are rare.

10.2.2 Anatomy and Biomechanics

The carpus is a highly complex joint composed of eight bones which are arranged in a proximal and a distal row (KAUER 1986; KAUER and DE LANDE 1987). The proximal row consists of the scaphoid, the lunate, the triquetrum, and the pisiform. The distal row consists of the trapezium, the trapezoid, the capitate, and the hamate. Though there are separate articulations between each of these bones, functionally the distal and proximal rows form separate units. The scaphoid bone acts as a connecting link between these two rows and therefore is more susceptible to injury than the other carpal bones. There are three distinct articulations: the radiocarpal joint between the radius, the TFCC, and the proximal carpal row; the midcarpal joint between the proximal and distal carpal rows; and the carpometacarpal joint between the distal carpal row and the metacarpals. The radiocarpal joint and the midcarpal joint are each covered by a separate joint capsule and are separated by ligaments. There is normally no communication between these two joints. The range of motion is high in the radiocarpal joint and decreases from proximal to distal. There is nearly no range of motion in the carpometacarpal joint. Dorsiflexion is primarily a function of the midcarpal joint, supported by the radiocarpal joint, whereas volar flexion mainly occurs in the radiocarpal joint, supported by the midcarpal joint.

Numerous extrinsic and intrinsic ligaments (MAYFIELD 1992) connect the carpal joints. By definition, the intrinsic (interosseous) ligaments connect the individual carpal bones. The most important intrinsic ligaments are the scapholunate and lunotriquetral ligaments, as rupture of these ligaments may lead to carpal instability. The extrinsic ligaments arise from the distal radius and ulna and attach at the carpal bones, or they course between the carpal bones. They are divided into a dorsal and a volar group. In general, the volar ligaments are thicker and stronger than the dorsal ligaments and provide more for carpal stability. A strong volar radiocarpal ligament is the radiocapitate (or radioscaphocapitate) ligament. It arises from the radial styloid process, transverses the waist of the scaphoid, and inserts in the volar center of the capitate. This ligament avoids volar displacement of the

262 V.M. Metz

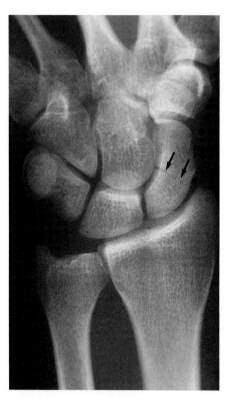

Fig. 10.14. PA radiograph of the wrist with a transverse fracture of the scaphoid located in the waist (*arrows*)

scaphoid. The strongest volar radiocarpal ligament is the radiotriquetral (or radiolunotriquetral) ligament. It arises from the radial styloid process just medial of the radioscapite ligament, crosses the lunate, and terminates at the volar surface of the triquetrum. In dorsiflexion of the wrist an interligamentous space develops between the radiocapite ligament and the radiotriquetral ligament, which is referred to as the space of Poirier. This space is a weak point which explains why the carpus tends to dislocate between the capitate and lunate at the site of the space of Poirier.

The mechanism of carpal injury has been the subject of considerable controversy (MAYFIELD 1992). Most commonly the injury is caused by a fall on the outstretched hand resulting in dorsiflexion and ulnar deviation of the hand combined with supination of the carpus against the fixed pronated forearm. This condition leads to a force which is focused between the radial styloid process and the capitate across the waist of the scaphoid and within the midcarpal joint. Because the proximal carpal row is more tightly fixed to the radius by the radiocarpal ligaments than the distal carpal row, dislocation is more likely to occur between the distal and the proximal carpal row than

between the radius and the proximal carpal row. In general, the resultant injury is dependent upon the severity of the force involved, the degree of extension, ulnar and radial deviation, and the degree of intercarpal supination. JOHNSON (1980) described a vulnerable arc which roughly follows the direction of the volar carpal ligaments and in which most carpal injuries occur. This zone starts at the radial styloid including the waist and proximal pole of the scaphoid and the scapholunate joint. It then courses distally to the body of the capitate, turns toward the hamate and the lunotriquetral joint, and finally ends at the ulnar styloid.

10.2.3 Fractures, Dislocations and Instabilities

10.2.3.1 Fractures

The most frequently fractured carpal bone is the *scaphoid*; as mentioned above, fractures to this bone account for 60%–70% of all carpal injuries (DUNN 1972). Fractures of the scaphoid commonly occur between the ages of 15 and 40 years. They are very rare in young children and relatively rare after the age of 60 years. Seventy percent of fractures are located in the waist (Fig. 10.14), 20% involve the proximal pole, and 10% are located in the distal pole (RUSSE 1960). The fracture line most commonly runs transverse or slightly oblique to the long axis of the

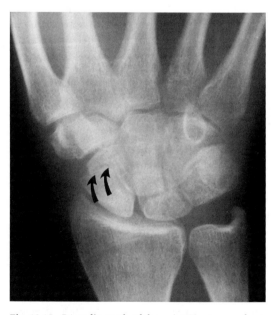

Fig. 10.15. PA radiograph of the wrist. Transverse fracture of the distal pole of the scaphoid (*arrows*) with dislocation of the distal fragment

scaphoid. Vertically oriented fractures are rare. The mechanism of injury is a fall on the dorsiflexed outstretched hand leading to severe stress on the narrow waist of the scaphoid. Fractures of the distal pole (Fig. 10.15) and the tuberosity are the result of compression forces transmitted by the thumb and index finger through the trapezium and trapezoideum. If a fracture of the scaphoid is identified, the distal forearm and the wrist should be examined carefully for associated injuries such as fractures of the radial styloid, capitate and lunate, scapholunate dissociation, perilunate dislocations, and other forms of carpal instability.

The second most commonly fractured carpal bone is the *triquetrum*, with an incidence of 7%–20% (BORGESKOV et al. 1966; BONE and GELBERMAN 1987). Most often the fracture is an avulsion from the dorsal surface at the site of the attachment of the lunotriquetral ligament. Fractures of the body of the triquetrum are rare. These fractures are commonly nondisplaced, and are often comminuted. They are the result of a compression of the triquetrum between the hamate and the ulnar head during extreme dorsiflexion and ulnar deviation of the wrist.

Fractures of the *lunate* are rare and occur in less than 3% of fractures of the carpal bones. As in the case of the triquetral bone, these fractures may be chip fractures of the dorsal or volar surface, or, occasionally, may occur as complete transverse fractures. The latter are due to shearing forces from impaction of the lunate against the rim of the distal radius. Disturbance of the vascular blood supply may occur after apparently trivial trauma or an obvious fracture of lunate. This disturbance may lead to Kienböck's disease (lunatomalacia, avascular necrosis).

Fractures of the *pisiform bone* are rare and account for less than 1%–7% of fractures of carpal bones (BORGESKOV et al. 1966; BONE and GELBERMAN 1987). The pisiform bone may be fractured by a direct blow, or by a fall on the outstretched hand directly impacting on the hypothenar eminence. The fracture may be comminuted or simple.

Fractures of the *trapezium* and *trapezoid* account for 3%–5% and 1%, respectively (BORGESKOV et al. 1966; BONE and GELBERMAN 1987). The mechanism of injury is abduction of the thumb, leading to a vertical shear or compression fracture. Fractures of the trapezium may be associated with dislocation or subluxation of the first carpometacarpal joint.

Although the *capitate* is the largest carpal bone, fractures of the capitate are uncommon (1%–3%). They are rare as isolated fractures and usually occur

in association with fractures of the scaphoid or perilunate dislocations (RAND et al. 1982). Most commonly capitate fractures are transverse fractures of the waist or head. Often the proximal fracture fragment is displaced and rotated 90°, or is completely inverted by 180° and entrapped between the capitate and lunate with or without perilunate dislocation (MONAHAN and GALASKO 1972). In rare cases fractures are located transversely at the head of the capitate. The fractured proximal fragment may or may not be displaced; it may be accompanied by a fracture of the scaphoid waist, and may occur in association with perilunate dislocation.

Fractures of the *hamate* may be located in the body or the hook (BORGESKOV et al. 1966; BONE and GELBERMAN 1987). They are rare and account for 1%–6% of all fractures. Most commonly the hook of hamate is fractured as the result of a direct blow or occurs as an avulsion fracture caused by the pull of the transverse carpal ligament. Usually the fracture occurs at the base of the hook. Fractures of the body of the hamate may occur as isolated fractures or in association with complex perilunate fracture dislocations. Fractures of the distal articular surface may occur in association with dislocation of the fourth and fifth carpometacarpal joints.

10.2.3.2 Dislocations

Carpal dislocations account for approximately 10% of all carpal injuries (DUNN 1972; GILULA 1979, GILULA and WEEKS 1978; JOHNSON 1980). In most cases they are the result of a fall on the outstretched hand that results in extensive dorsiflexion and ulnar deviation of the wrist.

Carpal dislocations can be divided into two major types: lunate and perilunate. They may occur with or without associated fractures of carpal bones. The key to identification of normal anatomic position is the distal radial articular surface, the lunate, and the capitate (Fig. 10.16a). Under normal conditions on the lateral radiograph, the lunate and the capitate are centered over the distal radius. Generally, on the lateral view, whichever bone is centered over the radius, whether it is the lunate or the capitate, will be the bone that is considered in regular anatomic position. In lunate dislocation (Fig. 10.16b) the lunate is displaced ventrally or dorsally away from the radius and the head of the capitate is centered over the radius (ventral or dorsal lunate dislocation). In contrast, in perilunate dislocation (Fig. 10.16c) the lunate stays in anatomic position and the capitate head is

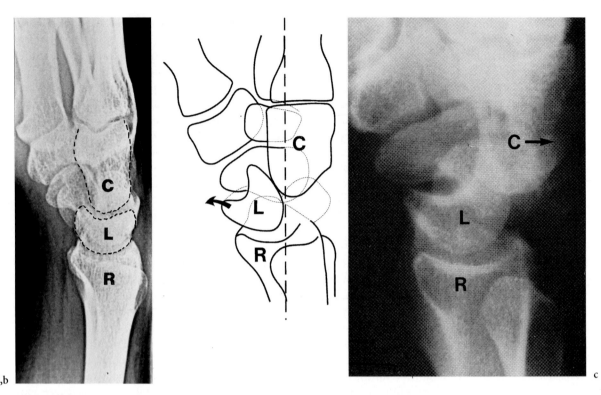

Fig. 10.16. a Lateral view of the wrist in the neutral position. Normally, the capitate (*C*) is centered over the lunate (*L*) and the lunate is centered over the distal radius. In ventral lunate dislocation (**b**) the lunate is displaced ventrally away from the radius but the capitate head is centered over the radius. In dorsal perilunate dislocation (**c**) the lunate stays in the anatomic position and the head of the capitate is displaced dorsally with respect to the radius

displaced ventrally or dorsally with respect to the radius (ventral or dorsal perilunate dislocation). If there is an additional fracture of a carpal bone, the term "trans" indicates which bone is fractured (e.g., transscaphoid perilunate dislocation). When there is a dislocation between the capitate, other carpal bones, and the lunate and neither the lunate nor the capitate centers over the distal radius, the term "midcarpal dislocation" is used. In rare cases a carpal fracture dislocation separates the carpometacarpal axes in the sagittal plane (Fig. 10.17). Again, the fractured bone is named first by using the term "trans," and then the site of carpal joint separation is identified (e.g., transtriquetrum perihamate).

10.2.3.3 Instabilities

"Carpal instability" is a term that describes abnormalities in the alignment of the carpal bones. This condition can occur in association with scaphoid fractures, in association with or as a result of lunate/ perilunate dislocations, or as a result of an

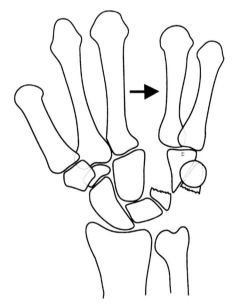

Fig. 10.17. Schematic drawing of transtriquetral perihamate dislocation. Due to a fracture of the triquetrum, indicated by the term "trans," there is separation of the carpometacarpal axes in the sagittal plane (*arrow*)

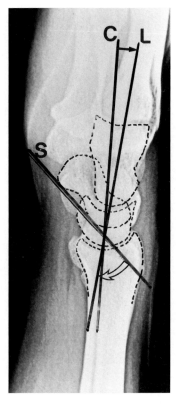

Fig. 10.18. Normal alignment of the carpal bones. Under normal conditions the capitolunate angle (*closed arrow*) is between 0° and 30°, and the scapholunate angle (*open arrow*) is between 30° and 60°. *C*, Axis of the capitate; *L*, axis of the lunate; *S*, axis of the scaphoid

rotatory subluxation of the scaphoid (or so-called scapholunate dissociation).

Understanding of normal carpal anatomy on lateral wrist radiographs is essential for the correct interpretation of carpal alignment. The key to correct identification of normal or abnormal carpal alignment is the capitate, the lunate, the scaphoid, and the radius (Fig. 10.18). The capitate is centered with its head to the distal concavity of the lunate. The lunate is centered in the concavity of the distal radius. The axis of the capitate can be defined by drawing a line from the midportion of the capitate head to the superimposed midportion of the base of the second through fifth metacarpals. The axis of the lunate can be identified by joining the distal volar and dorsal portions of the lunate and drawing a line perpendicular to the line mentioned above. The axis of the scaphoid is identified by drawing a tangential straight line joining the distal and proximal ventral poles of the scaphoid. The axis of the radius is defined by a line which runs through the middle of the diaphysis of the radius. For evaluation of carpal ligament instability two angles have to be measured: the scapholunate and the capitolunate. Normally, the

interruption of the extrinsic and/or intrinsic carpal ligaments (Dunn 1972; Gilula 1979; Gilula and Weeks 1978; Johnson 1980).

Two types of carpal instability can be differentiated: static and dynamic. Static instabilities are constantly present and can be recognized on a (static) routine radiographic examination. Dynamic instabilities are not constantly present on routine radiographs and need stress or motion to produce them. Therefore they may be diagnosed only by using instability series (discussed later in this chapter). Carpal instabilities may be without clinical symptoms, or even may occur as normal variants. Therefore, in any case of suspected instability, radiological examination of both wrists should be performed. In other cases, carpal instability may progress to further disruption, leading to severe loss of wrist function and advanced degenerative joint disease. Five static carpal instabilities have been described: dorsiflexion instability, volar flexion instability, ulnar translocation, dorsal and palmar carpal subluxation, and

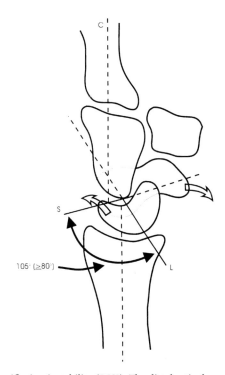

Fig. 10.19. Dorsiflexion instability (DISI). The distal articular surface of the lunate tilts dorsally (*open arrow*). The scaphoid bone remains in its normal position or, as is more common, tilts ventrally (*open arrow*). This leads to an increase in the scapholunate angle of more than 60°. The capitolunate angle remains normal or may be increased to more than 30°. *S*, Axis of the scaphoid; *L*, axis of the lunate; *C*, axis of the capitate

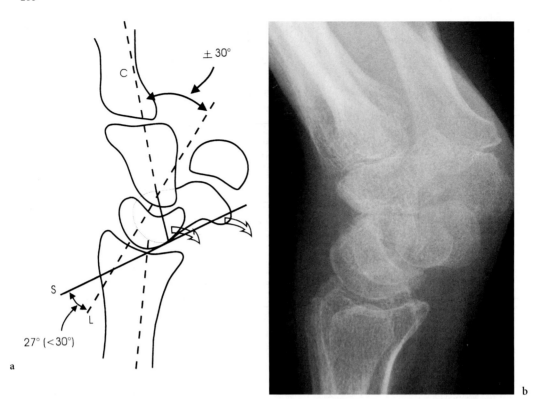

a

b

Fig. 10.20. Schematic drawing (**a**) and lateral radiograph (**b**) of palmar flexion instability (VISI). In VISI the distal articular surface of the lunate displays palmar tilting (*open arrow*). In this condition the lunate and the scaphoid (*open arrow*) show palmar flexion, leading to a scapholunate angle that is 30° or less. The capitolunate angle is increased to more than 30°. *S*, Axis of the scaphoid; *L*, axis of the lunate; *C*, axis of the capitate

scapholunate angle (Fig. 10.18) is between 30° and 60°. Between 60° and 80° the scapholunate angle is questionably abnormal. If it is more than 80° or less than 30°, it is definitely abnormal. However, it is important to note that these measurements are only reliable if the wrist is examined in a true lateral and neutral position without any flexion or extension or ulnar or radial deviation of the wrist. Under normal conditions the capitolunate angle (Fig. 10.18) is between 0° and 30°; it is abnormal when it exceeds 30°.

Dorsiflexion instability (DISI) (Fig. 10.19) is a condition in which the distal articular surface of the lunate tilts dorsally. The scaphoid bone either retains in its normal position or, as is more common, tilts ventrally more than normal. This causes an increase in the scapholunate angle of more than 60°. The capitolunate angle remains normal or may be increased to more than 30°.

In *palmar flexion instability* (VISI) (Fig. 10.20) the distal articular surface of the lunate displays a palmar tilt. In this condition the lunate and the scaphoid

show palmar flexion, leading to a scapholunate angle that is 30° or less. The capitolunate angle is increased to more than 30°.

In cases of a VISI or DISI, two additional lateral views, one with the wrist in maximal extension and the other with the wrist in flexion, should be performed. These views allow evaluation if there is normal or abnormal motion between the carpal bones. Normally, during wrist flexion the axis of the lunate should flex with respect to the radial axis, and the capitate axis should flex with respect to the lunate axis. Similarly, during wrist extension the axis of the lunate should extend with respect to the radial axis, and the capitate axis should extend with respect to the lunate axis. Abnormal intercarpal motion in different directions is consistent with carpal ligament instability and supports the diagnosis of VISI and DISI.

In *ulnar translocation*, a less common form of carpal instability, the carpus merely suffers ulnar subluxation. Two types have been described: Type I can be diagnosed when the space between the radial

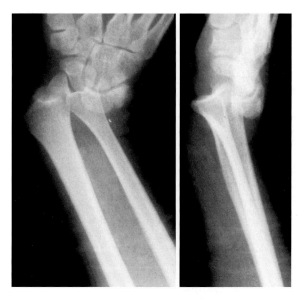

Fig. 10.21. Posttraumatic dorsal carpal luxation. The total carpus is displaced dorsal to the radius

styloid and the scaphoid is wider than the width of other intercarpal joints or when more than one-half of the proximal articular surface of the lunate lies ulnar to the radius. In type II there is a marked scapholunate diastasis; the scaphoid, however, stays in the scaphoid fossa of the distal radius and the remainder of the carpus translocates ulnarly.

In *dorsal or palmar carpal subluxation* (Fig. 10.21) the total carpus is displaced dorsal or palmar to the midplane of the distal radius seen on the lateral view. It usually follows an old Colles' fracture or may be associated with an old impacted fracture of the dorsal rim of the distal radius. Dorsal or palmar subluxation indicates severe injuries of the radiocarpal ligaments.

Rotatory subluxation of the scaphoid (or scapholunate dissociation, or scapholunate instability) is the most common form of carpal instability. This injury occurs when acute dorsiflexion of the wrist causes rotation of the scaphoid on its transverse axis. It can be diagnosed when the scapholunate joint space is abnormally wide (Fig. 10.22). This increase in the width of the scapholunate joint space indicates a rupture of the scapholunate interosseous ligament (= scapholunate dissociation). If there is an additional rupture of ventral radiocarpal ligaments, the scaphoid tilts ventrally and the term "rotatory subluxation" of the scaphoid is applicable. If the scaphoid tilts ventrally, it foreshortens and displays a "signet ring" shape on the

neutral PA radiograph due to overlapping edges of the scaphoid. Abnormal scaphoid foreshortening is supported when the radioscaphoid angle on the lateral view is less than 110°. Rotatory subluxation of the scaphoid may progress to VISI or DISI with time.

10.2.4 Examination Methods

10.2.4.1 Plain Film Radiography

For routine roentgenographic survey of the wrist a minimum of three views should be performed: the PA, lateral, and oblique projections (MANN et al. 1992; YIN et al. 1996b). For the PA view the hand (not the wrist) is placed flat on the cassette in neutral position with the axis of the radius collinear with the axis of the third metacarpal (without *any* ulnar or radial deviation). Neutral position is of importance because under normal conditions the scaphoid foreshortens with radial deviation or palmar flexion (and elongates with ulnar deviation or dorsal flexion) and takes the configuration of a signet ring (Fig. 10.23). A signet ring sign, seen on a true neutral PA view, however, is a pathological feature indicating rotatory subluxation of the scaphoid. In addition, as mentioned earlier, for the PA view, the humerus should be abduced 90° from the chest wall so that the elbow

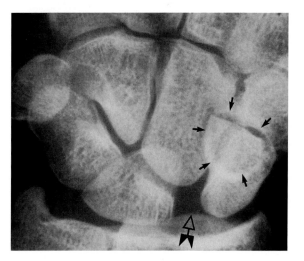

Fig. 10.22. PA radiograph in the neutral position in a patient with rotatory subluxation of the scaphoid. The scapholunate joint space (*open arrow*) is abnormally wide. Due to the ventral tilting of the scaphoid it is foreshortened and attains the shape of a signet ring (*small arrows*)

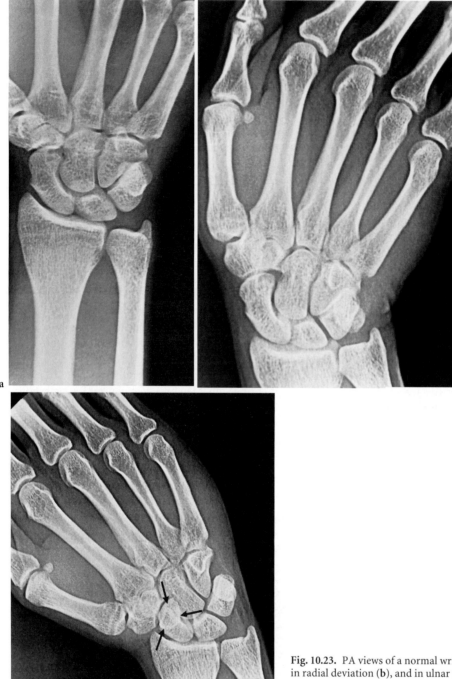

Fig. 10.23. PA views of a normal wrist in the neutral position (**a**), in radial deviation (**b**), and in ulnar deviation (**c**). In radial deviation the scaphoid is foreshortened and attains the shape of a signet ring (*arrows*). In ulnar deviation the scaphoid is elongated. The latter view may be a helpful additional view for evaluation of the scaphoid

is at the same level as the shoulder and flexed 90° (HARDY et al. 1987). For the oblique (semipronation) view (Fig. 10.24), the hand is rotated 45° off the cassette and the fingers held straight. In this view the trapeziotrapezoid and the trapezioscaphoid joints

are profiled and parallel and an additional view of the head of the capitate and the scaphoid is provided. The lateral view is performed by further rotation of the hand into a radioulnar projection. Again, for this view the humerus is adducted against the chest wall with the elbow flexed 90°. It is important to keep the wrist and fingers straight (without any flexion or extension) for optimal evaluation of carpal alignment.

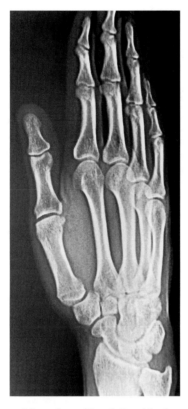

Fig. 10.24. Oblique view of the wrist and hand. For this view the hand is rotated 45° off the cassette and the fingers held straight. This view better profiles the scapho-trapezio-trapezoid joint and is an additional view for the head of the capitate and for the scaphoid

Other views may be necessary to investigate specific problems in various sites of the wrist and hand. To better profile the scaphoid, the wrist is initially placed in the routine PA view and then in ulnar deviation (Fig. 10.23c). The film in this position demonstrates the scaphoid, free of the distortion caused by its normal volar tilt when the wrist is in the neutral position. The carpal tunnel view (Fig. 10.25) demonstrates an axial view of the hook of hamate, the pisiform, and the volar margin of the trapezium. The carpal tunnel view is most easily performed by laying the forearm flat on the cassette, with the hand maximally dorsiflexed by means of the patient's opposite hand or a strap. Another way to achieve optimal depiction of the pisiform bone and to profile the pisotriquetral joint is use of an AP semisupinated oblique view, with the wrist supinated 30° from the lateral position. A fluoroscopic spot film should be employed when detailed carpal views fail to demonstrate an abnormality in a clinically suspicious area. Instability series (TRUONG et al. 1994; YIN et al. 1996b) under frequent spot filming or videotaping should be performed if there is any clinical or plain film suspicion of carpal malalignment. Instability series include PA views in the neutral position and radial and ulnar deviation, a semipronated oblique view, lateral views in the neutral position, full flexion and extension, and radial and ulnar deviation, 30° off-lateral views, and an AP clenched fist view.

As with the distal forearm, soft tissue evaluation is of major importance and may be the key to correct diagnosis in trauma. Several superficial and deep fat planes on the PA and lateral radiographs have been described (CURTIS et al. 1984), and are useful in the

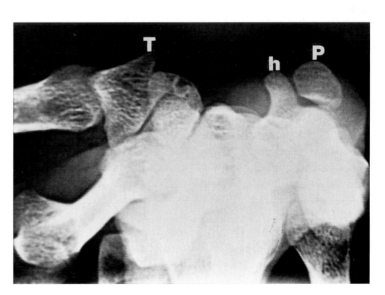

Fig. 10.25. Carpal tunnel view demonstrating an axial view of the tuberculum of the trapezium (*T*), the hook of hamate (*h*), and the pisiform bone (*P*)

evaluation of radiographs of the wrist following trauma. The scaphoid fat stripe, seen on the PA view, lies between the radial collateral ligament and the tendon of the abductor pollicis longus muscle and courses from the ulnar styloid to the trapezium. Fractures of the scaphoid may be extremely subtle and therefore attention should always be directed to the scaphoid fat pad. Swelling, displacement, or obliteration of this fat pad occurs in one-third of all carpal fractures and is usually associated with scaphoid fractures. However, the scaphoid fad pad also may be abnormal in cases of fractures of the radial styloid and of the trapezium.

On the lateral plane the dorsal skin-subcutaneous fat zones of the wrist are superficial fat planes and should be evaluated carefully. Dorsal wrist swelling often occurs in fractures or dislocations of the carpal bones but also may be observed in patients without fractures. However, if significant dorsal wrist swelling is present, a fracture should be searched for diligently. After careful examination of the soft tissues, the osseous elements should be evaluated. Understanding of what is normal and application of some basic principles will lead to correct diagnosis.

Normally, the widths of the radiocarpal, intercarpal, and carpometacarpal joint spaces are 2 mm or less (GILULA 1979; GILULA and WEEKS 1978) (Fig. 10.26). However, accurate measurement of a joint space width is only reliable if the joint space in question is in true profile and measurement is performed at the joint's midportion. If a joint space is not in profile on standard radiographs and there is any clinical or radiological suspicion of an abnormality, fluoroscopic controlled views should be added. When a joint space is 4 mm or more wide, it is considered to be definitely abnormal and indicates ligamentous injury. The concept of parallelism of articulating joint surfaces helps to differentiate normal from abnormal bone alignment. On the exactly performed routine PA view, parallelism exists between the radius, scaphoid, and lunate bones; between the bones of the proximal and distal carpal rows; at the intercarpal joints of the proximal and distal carpal rows; between the distal carpal bones and the metacarpals; and between the metacarpophalangeal and interphalangeal joints. Under normal conditions, on a true PA view the articular surfaces between the aforementioned bones do not overlap each other. Overlapping of articular surfaces between these bones indicates subluxation or dislocation. Under normal conditions there are three

smooth carpal arcs (Fig. 10.26) that can be observed in the PA or AP view (GILULA 1979; GILULA and WEEKS 1978). Break (stepoff) of any of these arcs may indicate ligamentous/bony abnormality at the site of the broken arc.

10.2.4.2 Radionuclide Bone Imaging

Raidionuclide bone imaging (RNBI) is an extremely sensitive imaging technique for evaluation of subtle wrist injury, but displays low specificity. It is very valuable for detection or exclusion of osseous, osteochondral, and soft tissue abnormalities and is used following acute trauma in patients with significant clinical symptoms and in whom standard radiographs fail to demonstrate an abnormality (GANEL et al. 1979; HOLDER 1992). In areas of intense focal tracer uptake, an occult fracture must be excluded by additional, more detailed roentgenograms in differ-

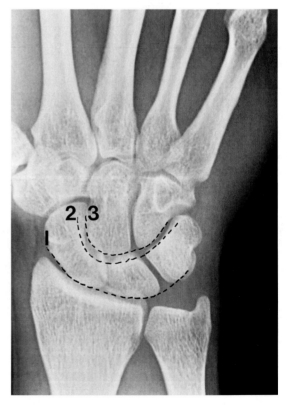

Fig. 10.26. PA view of the wrist in the neutral position. The width of the joint spaces is 2 mm or less and all joint spaces are of symmetrical width. Three smooth arcs can be drawn (*1, 2, 3*). Note also parallelism between the carpal bones

ent planes or by other imaging techniques such as magnification views, CT, or MRI. Mildly increased focal tracer accumulation commonly suggests a ligamentous or cartilagous abnormality. The lack of focal tracer uptake on delayed images is useful in excluding osseous involvement. Three-phase scintigraphy can be used for determination of the age of a fracture as well as fracture healing when radiographs are inconclusive.

Radionuclide bone imaging is also valuable for diagnosis of reflex sympathetic dystrophy (RSD), which is not uncommon after fractures of carpal bones. A specific scintigraphic pattern for RSD has been established with a sensitivity and specificity of 96% and 97%, respectively, on delayed bone images which show diffusely increased activity involving predominantly the juxta-articular zones of bones of the wrist and hand. Three-phase scintigraphy is a most valuable method for the diagnosis of especially the early stages of RSD, which often are not detected on conventional radiographs, and for follow-up, affecting therapeutic regimens.

Another condition in which RNBI can be helpful is evaluation of posttraumatic avascular necrosis (AVN) of carpal bones or carpal bone fracture fragments. Early detection of AVN is of major importance for treatment and prognosis. RNBI is superior to radiography for early detection of AVN, but has a very low sensitivity. However, the sensitivity and specificity of MRI for the detection of AVN is higher and therefore MRI is the imaging technique of choice in these cases (as discussed later in this chapter).

10.2.4.3 Arthrography

When the clinical situation, plain films, and instability series suggest a ligamentous or cartilaginous abnormality, arthrography may be helpful in identifying these defects.

The wrist consists of several synovium-lined major and minor compartments that usually do not communicate. The major compartments are the radiocarpal compartment (RCC), the distal radioulnar compartment (DRUC), and the midcarpal compartment (MCC). Arthrography should be performed by utilizing fluoroscopic control (GILULA et al. 1983) and frequent spot filming. Needle placement should always be away from the symptomatic site in the midcarpal and radiocarpal compartments so that local contrast extravasation

will not be confused with pathology. The wrist should be exercised in several positions; this may open a small communicating defect which may not be apparent on static views. For a "complete" arthrographic study of the wrist designed to show the maximum number of abnormal communicating and noncommunicating defects, all three major compartments should be injected. A ligamentous, cartilaginous, or capsular communicating tear may be complete (through and through) and seen on both adjacent compartments which are injected (bidirectional communication). A communicating defect may also display "one-way valve" behavior (unidirectional communication) and therefore can be overlooked when only one compartment is injected (LEVINSOHN et al. 1991; RESNICK 1980; WILSON et al. 1991). A ligamentous or cartilaginous defect may also occur as an incomplete defect (not through and through or not communicating between two adjacent compartments) and therefore can be detected only by injecting both adjacent wrist compartments. For example, a proximal avulsion of the TFCC from the ulnar styloid can only be seen with DRUC arthrography and not with RCC

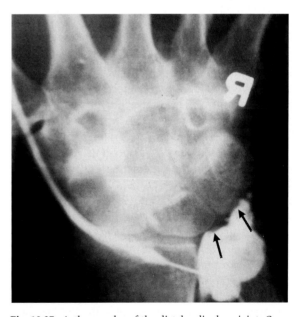

Fig. 10.27. Arthrography of the distal radioulnar joint. Contrast passes around the ulnar styloid into the soft tissues (*arrows*), indicating an avulsion of the TFCC from its insertion to the styloid process. However, there is no communication to the radiocarpal joint (noncommunicating defect). This pathology would be missed by injecting the radiocarpal joint only. There is contrast dye in the midcarpal compartment from earlier injection

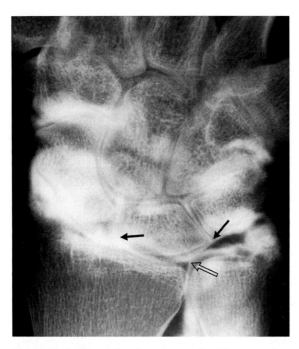

Fig. 10.28. Radiocarpal wrist arthrography. There are clear communications from the radiocarpal compartment into the midcarpal compartment through defects of the scapholunate and the lunotriquetral ligaments (*arrows*). There is also communication to the distal radioulnar joint through a defect of the TFCC (*open arrow*)

10.2.4.4 Computed Tomography

In selected cases CT may add significant information compared to conventional radiography. Indications for wrist CT include evaluation of complex or occult carpal fractures, the assessment of fracture healing (Fig. 10.29) and fracture complications, and postsurgical evaluation (BUSH et al. 1987; HINDMAN et al. 1989; TALEISNIK 1985; WOOD and BERQUIST 1992; YIN et al. 1996a).

Computed tomography should be performed in a tailored manner depending on the clinical question. It is important to obtain CT sections at right angles to the surface to be detailed (e.g., if a fracture line has to be examined, the wrist should be placed on the CT table so that the CT section passes at right angles to the fracture line). Thin sections at close intervals, e.g., 2-mm thin sections at 1- or 2-mm intervals, should be performed. To answer specific problems, such as exact evaluation of the displacement of a fracture fragment or the amount of healing present following a fracture or osteotomy, CT of the wrist should be performed in at least two planes. The coronal plane can be obtained with the patient prone on the CT table, with the arm elevated above the head, the elbow flexed, and the hand placed with its ulnar side on the table. For the sagittal plane the patient

arthrography (Fig. 10.27). Additionally patients may have more than one abnormality in different compartments which would be missed by using single-compartment arthrography alone. The most common sites of abnormal intercompartmental communications due to ligamentous tears are the scapholunate and the lunotriquetral ligaments and the TFCC (Fig. 10.28).

It must be noted that the clinical significance of some arthrographic findings is difficult to assess. As reported in the literature (MANASTER et al. 1989; METZ et al. 1993a), there is often a poor correlation between symptom sites and abnormalities detected on arthrography. The reason for this poor correlation is uncertain. However, ligamentous and triangular fibrocartilage defects increase in number with age. Therefore asymptomatic defects must exist. Abnormalities detected on arthrography must always be carefully correlated with clinical and physical examinations. Perhaps the use of bilateral wrist arthrography to detect asymmetric defects may show these defects and may have a better correlation with symptom sites.

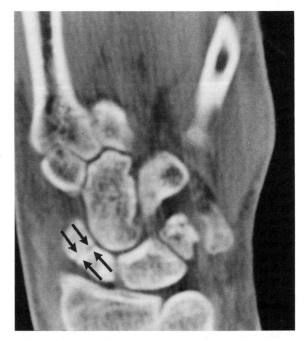

Fig. 10.29. Coronal CT of the wrist in a patient with an old fracture of the scaphoid. Sclerotic margins at the fracture site (*arrows*) can be detected; however, there is no evidence of bony bridging, indicating pseudarthrosis

and his arm are positioned in the same way, but the palm of the hand is flat on the CT table. For the axial plane the patient can be in the prone, supine, or lateral decubitus position with the arm extended straight over the head. Examination of the scaphoid in its long axis can be achieved by placing the wrist obliquely across the table such that the line between Lister's tubercle and the thumb base is parallel to the gantry sections. If there is metal (wires, Herbert screws) within the wrist bones, the wrist should be positioned so that the long axis of the metal is parallel to the gantry sections. Placing the metal object at right angles to the gantry may decrease the metal artifacts.

The advantage of spiral-CT (helical-CT, or volume scanning) is that thin-section overlapping images can be acquired with reduced examination time and radiation exposure for the patient. Due to the overlapping and continuous scanning with current software reconstructions, an infinite number of anatomic planes (Fig. 10.29) as well as 3-D reconstructions can be obtained with excellent quality. Multiplanar reconstructions can be very helpful for the evaluation of complex carpal trauma. 3-D reconstructions allow modeling of fracture fragments and preoperative planning at a clinical as well as a research level.

Fractures of the scaphoid and the hook of hamate are sometimes difficult to diagnose on conventional radiographs and therefore may be overlooked. Consequently, patients with negative radiographs but clinical symptoms should be further investigated by means of CT. Fracture complications can only be avoided by early detection. Fractures of the scaphoid waist are slow healing and often associated with nonunion and/or avascular necrosis of the proximal fracture fragment. It is of major importance to determine as early as possible whether or not a fracture has good potential for healing. CT may be helpful for early detection of these complications.

Evaluation of the wrist following treatment of wrist fractures can be difficult with conventional radiography or even with conventional tomography due to artifacts from casting material or metal implants or inability to obtain proper positioning. CT has advantages over conventional radiography and conventional tomography in assessing fusions because CT avoids the overlapping bone surfaces seen on radiography and the blur seen on conventional tomography. CT is very sensitive in detecting subtle calcification or areas of bone formation. Therefore CT can be superior in evaluating treatment success and fracture healing. CT is a very reliable method for detecting nonunion of carpal fractures, bone graft incorporation, and osseous fusion.

10.2.4.5 Magnetic Resonance Imaging

In recent years MRI has provided an important, noninvasive approach for examination of the traumatized wrist. Indeed, MRI is currently the best method to simultaneously and directly visualize bones, cartilages, and soft tissues without using ionizing radiation.

During the past few years much attention has been paid to evaluation of the TFCC and the extrinsic and intrinsic carpal ligaments of the wrist with MRI (BRODY and STOLLER 1993; GOLIMBU et al. 1989; ROMINGER et al. 1993; TOTTERMAN et al. 1993). It has been shown that MRI, by using special techniques and dedicated surface coils, is able to depict these soft tissues with high quality (Fig. 10.30). It is important to note that MRI is the *only* imaging modality which can allow direct topographic visualization of all these structures.

Magnetic resonance imaging is the most sensitive imaging technique for the detection of osteonecrosis of carpal bones (Fig. 10.31), which may occur after fractures (REINUS et al. 1986; TRUMBLE and IRVING 1990). Compared with plain radiography and even with scintigraphy, MRI is more sensitive and specific in detecting early osteonecrosis. As MR findings depend on death of fat cells, which takes from 2 to 5 days, avascular necrosis may be seen as early as 5 days after trauma. Typically, early stages of avascular necrosis have low signal intensity on T1-weighted images and show an inhomogeneous increase in signal intensity on T2-weighted images. T1-weighted sequences after intravenous administration of gadolinium should be performed as they allow some kind of "staging" of avascular necrosis. It has been reported that patients in whom there is an increase in signal intensity have a better prognosis than those without enhancement. Enhancement after intravenous administration of gadolinium indicates vitality of the avascular fracture fragment and therefore influences therapy and prognosis. It must be noted that differential diagnosis of early stages of osteonecrosis and bone marrow edema ("bone bruise") may be difficult as both conditions show similar signal intensities on MRI (high signal on T2 and low signal on T1). However, it has been reported that the signal changes in cases of osteonecrosis are more inhomogeneous than those of bone bruise.

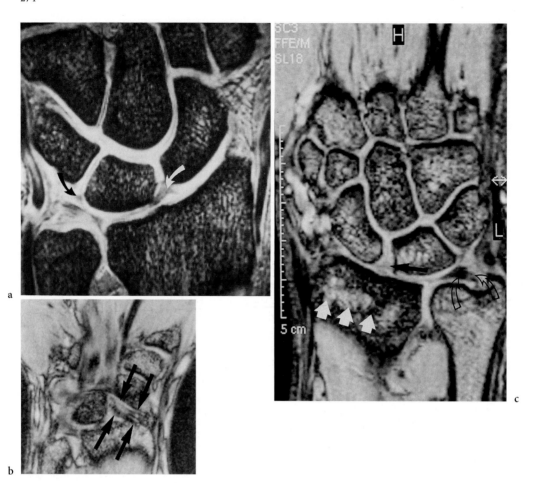

a

b

c

Fig. 10.30a–c. Coronal gradient recalled echo MR images of the wrist. **a** Normally, the scapholunate (*white curved arrow*) and the lunotriquetral interosseous ligaments (*black curved arrow*) are triangular shaped and of low to intermediate signal intensity, and can be depicted with high quality using MRI. **b** With thin sections even the very thin extrinsic ligaments of the wrist, such as the volar radioscaphocapitate ligament (*ar-* *rows*), can be depicted with MRI as alternating bands of low to intermediate signal intensity. **c** In a patient with a fracture of the distal radius (*white arrows*), the scapholunate ligament (*black arrow*) is no longer visible, indicating a tear of this ligament. The scapholunate joint space is of abnormal width. *Curved arrows*, TFCC

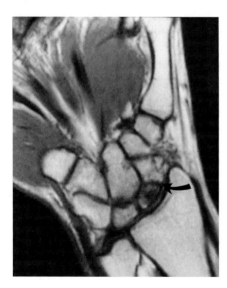

Fig. 10.31. T1-weighted coronal MRI of the wrist in a patient with a scaphoid fracture (*arrow*). The proximal pole of the scaphoid is of very low signal intensity, indicating avascular necrosis of the proximal fracture fragment

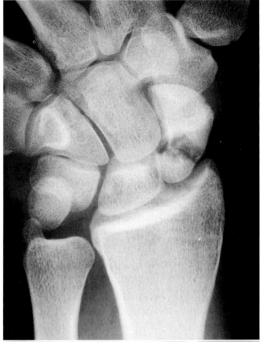

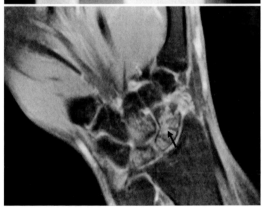

Fig. 10.32. **a** PA radiograph of the wrist with a scaphoid fracture. On the radiograph there is no evidence of bony bridging of the fractured fragments. **b** On the coronal fat-suppressed MR image after i.v. administration of gadolinium (same patient as in **a**), fibrous bridging of the fracture fragments is demonstrated (*arrow*)

Evaluation of occult fractures or fracture healing (Fig. 10.32) and follow-up after bone graft incorporation are other indications for which MRI may be superior to other imaging techniques, thereby allowing the very early diagnosis which is imperative for successful treatment.

As discussed earlier, reflex sympathetic dystrophy (RSD) may occur in association with fractures of the carpal bones. MRI has been reported to be a helpful imaging technique in the diagnosis and follow-up of RSD (SCHWEITZER et al. 1995). A coexistence of signal intensity changes of soft tissue and bone marrow due to edema, which seem to be typical features in patients with RSD, has been described. In addition, MRI potentially allows the detection of the different stages of RSD, which may have consequences for therapeutic procedures.

10.2.5 Special Features in Children

As mentioned above, fractures and dislocations of the carpus are rare in children.

In contrast to scaphoid fractures in adults, fractures of the scaphoid in children most commonly are distal avulsion fractures or transverse fractures of the distal third of the scaphoid (LARSON et al. 1987; MUESSBICHLER 1961). Only 15% of the fractures occur at the waist of the scaphoid. Scaphoid fractures in children are usually the result of a severe direct blow to the wrist and are often associated with other fractures of the distal forearm, wrist, and hand. In young children the fracture may be located through the osteochrondrous junction and therefore may be overlooked. In this case the fracture can be identified subsequently with further progression of the ossification of the scaphoid. If the fracture occurs through the ossific nucleus, it should not be misinterpreted as a fracture of the proximal pole.

10.2.6 Pitfalls

As a frequent normal variant, on the radial margin of the waist of the scaphoid there is a small angular tubercle and the margins of the bony trabeculae within the scaphoid bone arising from this tubercle may be mistaken for the margins of a fracture (Fig. 10.33). To avoid such a misinterpretation, the opposing articular surface of the scaphoid should be examined carefully for evidence of discontinuity. If there is intact cortex, a fracture is very unlikely.

The look of hamate arises from a secondary ossification center and may not be united with the body of the hamate. This condition may lead to the misinterpretation of a fracture. However, differentiation between a fracture and a nonunited secondary ossification center can easily be achieved by watching the margins of the two bones. The margins of a fracture are irregular and have no cortical bone on the opposing margins, as is seen with a secondary ossification center. Similarly, sometimes the pisiform bone may have more than one ossification center and this should not lead to misdiagnosis of a fracture.

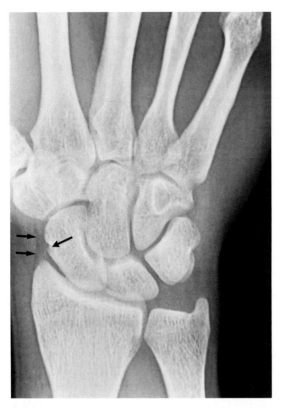

Fig. 10.33. Normal scaphoid with a prominent tubercle as a normal variant which should not be misinterpreted as a fracture. Note the normal appearance of the scaphoid fat stripe (*small arrows*)

Hohl 1963). The main artery of the scaphoid enters the scaphoid in the anterolateral region of the waist. In most individuals it supplies the scaphoid waist, a part of the distal pole, and the entire proximal pole. The distal pole and the tuberosity are invariably supplied by an additional artery that enters the tuberosity. In general, the prognosis is best in fractures of the distal third and is worst in fractures of the proximal third since the latter fractures invariably deprive the proximal fragment of its blood supply. If the fracture runs through the scaphoid waist, the prognosis depends on whether the fracture is situated distal or proximal to the entrance of the main artery. If it is distal, complications are unlikely, whereas if it is proximal, nonunion or delayed union is likely (30%).

Malunited fractures of the scaphoid may lead to radioscaphoid impingement or radioscaphoid arthrosis. In most cases malunion results from a failure to recognize an inadequate reduction. Usually malunion leads to a humpback deformity characterized by a palmar angulation of the distal fracture fragment. This may lead to foreshortening of the carpal height and further, due to an increase in the scapholunate angle, to dorsal carpal instability.

Like fractures of the scaphoid, fractures of the lunate may lead to ischemic necrosis. Posttraumatic avascular necrosis of the capitate is very rare. Necrosis of the proximal pole of the capitate may occur in patients with fractures of the isthmus of the capitate. Because the blood supply of the capitate bone enters the distal pole, a fracture at the site of the isthmus of the capitate may disrupt the blood supply of the proximal pole (Pellegrini 1988).

The most common complication of fractures of the hook of hamate is nonunion as a result of delayed diagnosis. The diagnosis is often difficult to make on routine radiographs. Three signs on the PA radiograph have been reported to suggest fracture of the hook of hamate: (a) absence of the hook, (b) lack of the normal cortical ring, and (c) sclerosis at the region of the hook, indicating reactive bone formation in a nonunited fracture. As a result of nonunion, persistent pain, ulnar nerve neuropathy, and attritional flexor tendon rupture may occur.

As mentioned earlier, the joint space width between the carpal bones should be approximately 2 mm and all joint spaces should be of similar width. When a joint space is widened, it may indicate a tear of an intercarpal ligament. However, as reported in the literature (Metz et al. 1993b), a wide scapholunate joint space may occur in persons with lunotriquetral coalitions as a normal variant and should not be misinterpreted as indicating a tear of the scapholunate ligament.

10.2.7 Follow-up and Complications

Fractures of the scaphoid are frequently associated with complications such as delayed union, nonunion, avascular (ischemic) necrosis, and malunion. Early detection and close radiological follow-up are mandatory to avoid these complications.

The prognosis for union and the tendency for nonunion or delayed union or ischemic necrosis depend on the fracture site (Dobyns and Linscheid 1984; Gelberman and Gross 1986; Mazet and

10.2.8 Diagnostic Algorithm

The imaging technique of first choice in a patient with a history of wrist trauma is the routine three-view (PA, lateral, oblique) plain film examination. In many cases, these three views will allow correct diagnosis. If routine radiographic survey is negative, and the patient's history and clinical symptoms and careful clinical examination are suspicious for a bony or ligamentous injury, special views centered on the site of pain (e.g., scaphoid views, carpal tunnel view, semisupinated off-lateral view) should be performed. If these views still show no abnormality, advanced imaging techniques are required, depending on their availability and the experience of the radiologist. Bone scan is a more sensitive survey tool, but its specificity is low. If there is an increased uptake on bone scan, further investigation depends on where the increased uptake is centered. If bone scan depicts hot to very hot spots, it is more suggestive of a bony lesion. In this condition, CT and/or MRI can be performed to make the correct diagnosis. If bone scan shows only mildly increased tracer uptake, a ligamentous or cartilaginous injury is more likely, and instability series or even arthrography should be performed. However, with a good-quality MR unit and an experienced physician, MRI can be performed instead of arthrography and can be very helpful for the depiction of ligamentous or cartilaginous injuries. As mentioned earlier in this chapter, MRI is also a very sensitive and specific new diagnostic tool for the detection of occult fractures and the evaluation of fracture healing, and it is the imaging technique of choice for the early detection of osteonecrosis of wrist bones. CT should be performed in cases of complex carpal trauma, for evaluation of treatment success and fracture healing, if routine radiographs are inconclusive.

10.3 Hand

10.3.1 General Considerations

The most common sites of injuries in the entire skeletal system are the metacarpals and phalanges (DUNN 1972; GREEN and ROWLAND 1991). In general, fractures of the phalanges are more common than fractures of the metacarpals. Of all phalangeal fractures, the distal phalanges of the first and third digits are the most common sites of fractures, accounting for 50%. The next most common sites (15%) are the proximal phalanges of the first and second fingers. Fractures of the middle phalanx are least common. Fractures of the metacarpals are more commonly located in the little finger and the thumb. In up to 90% of cases a single phalanx or metacarpal is injured; simultaneous fractures of multiple bones are rare. Fractures of the phalanges and metacarpals

are classified as either extra-articular, located in the body or the shaft of the bones, or intra-articular, consisting of avulsion fractures of the proximal and distal margins of the phalanges at the site of the attachments of the tendons and collateral ligaments. Each phalanx and metacarpal bone has its own peculiar trauma pattern; however, description of all these individual injuries would lengthen this chapter excessively.

10.3.2 Anatomy

The collateral ligaments arise from the lateral margin of the head of the metacarpal and phalangeal bones and insert at the lateral margrin of the base of the apposing phalanx. Each metacarpophalangeal and interphalangeal joint is covered by a capsule which has a dense fibrous structure on the volar side, termed the volar plate. This volar plate consists distally of stiff fibrocartilage that is firmly attached to the volar aspect of the base of the phalanx and additionally is fixed on the lateral side of the head of the metacarpal or phalangeal bone by the accessory collateral liagments. Proximally the volar plate becomes thinner and more elastic and is attached on the proximal phalanx/metacarpal by two lateral bands. The central portion of this plate is not attached.

The extensor tendon complex overlying the dorsum of the proximal interphalangeal joint divides proximal to the joint into three parts. The middle part inserts on the base of the middle phalanx, whereas the two lateral parts pass distally on each side of the phalanx and are joined by slips from the lumbrical and interosseous muscles. These structures run laterally of the proximal interphalangeal joint, distally, and then again join and are finally attached over the distal portion of the middle phalanx. The common extensor tendon then attaches on the dorsal aspect of the base of the distal phalanx.

10.3.3 Fractures, Dislocations, and Soft Tissue Injuries

Fractures of the first metacarpal bone most commonly (78%) are located at the base or proximal portion (GEDDA 1954). It is important for orthopedic management to recognize whether these fractures are intra-articular (as is more common) or extra-articular since extra-articular fractures can be treated by closed means. Fractures of the first metac-

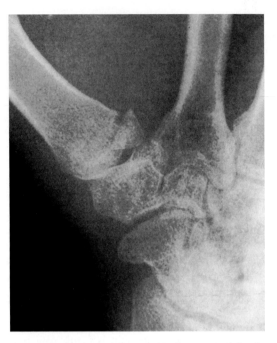

Fig. 10.34. Bennett's fracture. This fracture is defined as an oblique fracture of the base of the first metacarpal that extends into the first carpometacarpal joint

position while the rest of the first metacarpal is dorsally and radially dislocated due to the pull of the abductor pollicis muscle. Therefore the fracture should be defined as a fracture dislocation. Another type of intra-articular fracture of the first metacarpal is *Rolando's fracture* (GREEN and ROWLAND 1991) (Fig. 10.35), which is less common than Bennett's fracture. It is defined as a comminuted Bennett's fracture with a Y, V, or T configuration of the fracture line.

Boxer's fracture (Fig. 10.36) is a transverse fracture of the neck of a metacarpal bone with volar angulation of the distal fracture fragment (GREEN and ROWLAND 1991). It commonly occurs in the fifth metacarpal but may be seen in any of the metacarpal bones. The mechanism of trauma is a blow struck with the fist.

Fractures of the metacarpal base most commonly are located in the fourth and fifth metacarpals. In these fractures the adjacent carpometacarpal joints must be examined carefully for presence of subluxations or dislocations of the joints. *Fractures of*

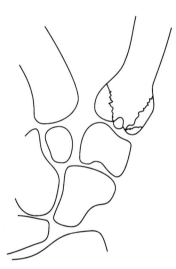

Fig. 10.35. Schematic drawing of Rolando's fracture. It is defined as a comminuted intra-articular fracture of the first metacarpal with a Y, V, or T configuration of the fracture line

arpal are the result of a fall or a blow along the longitudinal axis, or may occur after hyperabduction or hyperextension of the thumb. *Bennett's fracture* (Fig. 10.34) is defined as an oblique fracture of the base of the first metacarpal that extends into the first carpometacarpal joint (PELLEGRINI 1988). Commonly, a small volar fragment of the base remains in

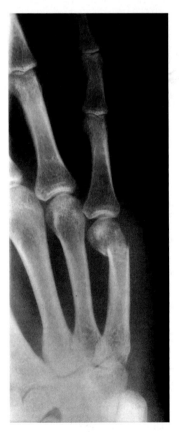

Fig. 10.36. Boxer's fracture of the fifth metacarpal. This is a transverse fracture of the neck of a metacarpal bone with volar angulation of the distal fracture fragment

the shaft of the metacarpals (Fig. 10.37) may be transverse or oblique. Transverse fractures of the shaft frequently are angulated dorsally due to the extension of the proximal fragment by the extensor carpi ulnaris and extensor carpi radialis tendons. Oblique shaft fractures may result in shortening and rotational deformity which often is not evident on radiographs. *Fractures of the head of the metacar-*

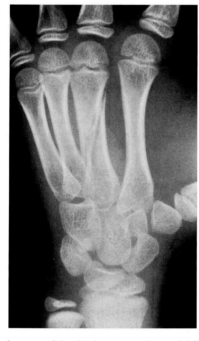

Fig. 10.37. Oblique fracture of the third metacarpal in a child

pals frequently occur at the second metacarpal, followed by the fifth metacarpal. They are rare in the thumb.

Gamekeeper's thumb is defined as a valgus injury of the metacarpophalangeal joint resulting in disruption of the ulnar collateral ligament. Frequently this injury is accompanied by a fracture of the base of the proximal phalanx. In 40% of cases of ulnar collateral ligament disruption the so-called Stener lesion occurs. In this lesion the proximal portion of the torn ulnar collateral ligament is folded back and trapped by the aponeurosis of the adductor pollicis muscle.

The most common sites of *fractures of the proximal phalanx* are the proximal portion and the midportion of the thumb and the index finger as a result of a direct blow or a fall. Intra-articular involvement is rare. Occasionally an avulsion fracture may occur at the lateral margin of the base of the proximal or middle phalanx at the site of the attachment of the collateral ligaments (GREEN and ROWLAND 1991). The fractures may be oblique, with a tendency for shortening and rotation of the digit, or transverse with typical volar angulation.

As mentioned above, *middle phalanx fractures* are rare and are the result of direct blows or crushing injuries. Commonly, the distal shaft of the index and middle finger are involved. Angulation of the fracture fragment depends upon their relation to the insertion of the flexor sublimis tendon. Fractures distal to this insertion lead to volar angulation of the proximal fragment, whereas in fractures located proximal

Fig. 10.38. PA (**a**) and lateral (**b**) view of the fifth finger with a volar plate avulsion fracture. A very small undisplaced fracture (*arrows*) can be seen at the base of the middle phalanx. On the PA view it can be easily overlooked

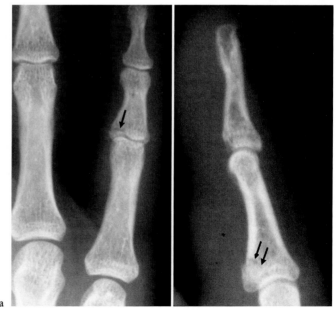

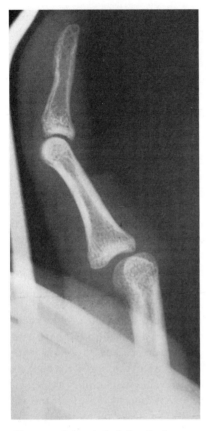

Fig. 10.39. Buttonhole deformity due to a rupture of an extensor tendon from its attachments to the dorsal base of the middle phalanx. In this deformity the finger is typically flexed at the proximal interphalangeal joint and extended at the distal interphalangeal joint

sites of fractures of the hand. The ungual tufts (Fig. 10.40) are most frequently fractured and fractures may vary from a simple marginal chip fracture to severely comminuted fractures. Transverse and longitudinal fractures are less common and may or may not be associated with displacement or angulation.

The "*mallet finger*" deformity or baseball finger is suspected when a distal phalanx is maintained in palmar flexion due to rupture of an extensor tendon at its insertion on the dorsal surface of the base of the distal phalanx (McMinn 1981). It may be associated with an avulsion fracture of the dorsal aspect of the base of the distal phalanx. The trauma mechanism is a blow on the tip of the finger which forcibly flexes the distal phalanx while the extensor tendon is taut.

Dislocations and subluxations of the metacarpophalangeal and interphalangeal joints may occur in the dorsal, the lateral, and the volar direction (Green and Rowland 1991). Dorsal dislocations are the most common types of dislocation whereas volar dislocations are extremely rare. Lateral dislocations more precisely should be termed subluxations because displacement typically is minimal. The trauma mechanism of lateral subluxation involves rotatory, twisting forces leading to disruption of the collateral ligaments (Fig. 10.41) and partial tears of the volar plate. Dorsal dislocations of

to the insertion, the distal fracture fragment shows volar angulation.

A common type of injury is *volar plate avulsion fractures* (Fig. 10.38). They are the result of a hyperextension trauma (ballplayers) leading to an avulsion of the volar plate at its insertion on the base of the middle phalanx. Typically, the avulsed fragment is very small and undisplaced and therefore can be easily overlooked.

Rupture of a extensor tendon leads to a condition which is called the "*buttonhole*" *deformity* (Green and Rowland 1991) (Fig. 10.39). In this injury, the extensor tendon is ruptured from its attachments to the dorsal base of the middle phalanx or there is a rupture of the central slip that keeps the tendon over the dorsal midline of the proximal interphalangeal joint. The finger is flexed at the proximal interphalangeal joint and extended at the distal interphalangeal joint.

Fractures of the *distal phalanges*, especially of the middle finger and the thumb, are the most common

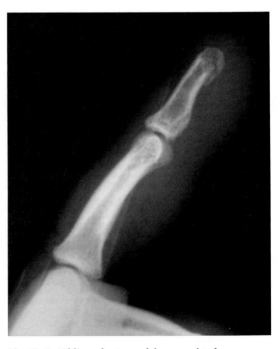

Fig. 10.40. Oblique fracture of the ungual tuft

Fig. 10.41A–D. Tear of the collateral ligament of the proximal interphalangeal joint of the fifth finger. On the PA (**A**) and lateral (**B**) views no abnormalities can be found. On the stress view in ulnar direction (**C**), however, there is clear evidence of a radial collateral ligament tear. On the stress view in radial direction (**D**) there is no abnormal widening of the joint space

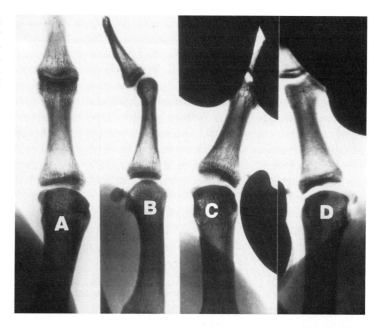

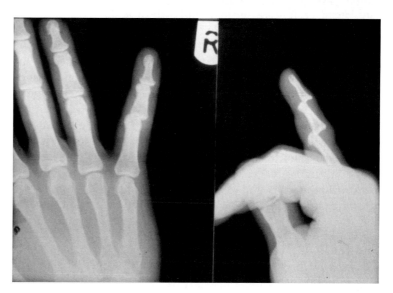

Fig. 10.42. Dorsal dislocation of the proximal and distal interphalangeal joints of the fifth finger

the interphalangeal (Fig. 10.42) and metacarpophalangeal joints are the result of hyperextension forces associated with some longitudinal compression, usually due to a fall on the outstretched hand. Dorsal dislocations are associated with rupture of the volar plate and may be manifested by a small avulsion fracture from the insertion of the volar plate at the base of the phalanx. In general, dislocations are divided into simple and complex types. In complex dislocations, soft tissues such as the volar plate, the collateral ligament, or the joint capsule becomes entrapped within the joint. Therefore this type of dislocation is irreducible and requires open reduction to

remove the soft tissues. The only radiographic sign of a complex dislocation is persistent incongruity of the joint. In simple dislocation no soft tissues are entrapped and therefore reduction by closed means is easy.

10.3.4 Examination Methods

10.3.4.1 Plain Film Radiography

For routine roentgenographic survey of the hand a minimum of three views should be performed (YIN et al. 1996b): the PA, the lateral and the oblique projections. The central beam for examinations of the hand should be at the capitate of the third metacarpal. For the oblique view, the hand is rotated 45° off the cassette and the fingers held straight (positioned on a step sponge) to obtain the interphalangeal and metacarpophalangeal joints in true profile. Other views may be necessary to investigate specific problems in various sites of the hand (Yin et al. 1996b). The second through fifth digits normally are well depicted on the routine PA and oblique views. Anteroposterior (AP) views profile slightly different portions of the carpometacarpal, the metacarpophalangeal, and the interphalangeal joints and may be of additional value for depiction of occult fractures. For the lateral projection of an individual digit, it may be necessary to overpronate the hand and place the second or third finger against the cassette and to keep the other digits out of the field to prevent superimposition. For true frontal and lateral projections of the thumb, which is depicted in an oblique view on routine radiographs, it is necessary to overpronate the forearm and hand and to position the thumb in contact with the cassette surface. The true lateral projection of the thumb can be obtained by overpronating the hand and placing the radial surface of the thumb to the cassette. Fluoroscopic spot film and stress views can be performed when detailed carpal views fail to demonstrate an abnormality in a clinically suspicious area. Abduction stress views of the thumb have to be performed for evaluation of the collateral ligament. An increase to more than 30° in the angle between the first metacarpal and the proximal phalanx is characteristic.

As in any other area of the body, careful evaluation of the soft tissues is of major importance and may be the clue to correct diagnosis (Curtis et al. 1984). The dorsal skin-subcutaneous fat zones of the hand are superficial fat planes and can be evaluated on the lateral plane. Dorsal hand swelling is strongly associated with fractures of metacarpals II–V. Combinations of dorsal wrist and hand swelling after trauma occur in cases of (a) carpometacarpal dislocation, (b) proximal intra-articular fracture of one or more of metacarpals II–V, or (c) combinations of metacarpal and carpal fractures. Swelling of the thenar skin-subcutaneous fat plane are associated with fractures of the first metacarpal and sometimes with fractures of the proximal first phalanx. Hypothenar swelling may occur in cases with fractures of metacarpals II–V. Metacarpophalangeal joint swelling may be indicative of a fracture in that region. Injuries at the metacarpophalangeal joints

lead to a focal swelling over the joint and involve only the more distal parts of the dorsal hand soft tissues. Swelling at the interphalangeal joints also may be an indicator of a fracture. Swelling in this region tends to be more tubular, and eccentric swelling at one side of an interphalangeal joint is most suggestive of a collateral ligament injury.

The concept of parallelism of articulating joint surfaces helps to differentiate normal from abnormal bone alignment. Parallelism exists between the distal carpal bones and the metacarpals, and between the metacarpophalangeal and interphalangeal joints. In addition, under normal conditions, the articular surfaces between the bones mentioned above on a true PA view do not overlap each other. Overlapping of articular surfaces between those bones is most suggestive of subluxation or dislocation.

10.3.4.2 Arthrography

The most common indications for finger arthrography are acute injuries of the capsule and collateral ligaments of the finger, tendon derangements, and defects of the volar plate of the metacarpophalangeal joints. Arthrography should be performed acutely because the joint capsule usually seals spontaneously in less than 1 week. The most frequent finger joint evaluated by arthrography is the metacarpophalangeal joint of the thumb to diagnose disruption of the ulnar collateral ligament in patients in whom the results of clinical examination or stress radiography are equivocal. Another lesion which may be diagnosed with arthrography is the Stener lesion of the thumb (mentioned above). In this lesion the proximal portion of the torn ulnocarpal collateral ligament is folded back and trapped by the aponeurosis of the adductor pollicis muscle and appears on arthrography as a filling defect on the ulnar side of the joint capsule. Injuries of the volar plate can be diagnosed on arthrography as extravasations of contrast material ventrally, occasionally with additional filling of the adjacent tendon sheaths.

10.3.4.3 Ultrasonography and Magnetic Resonance Imaging

Traumatic tendon ruptures and tears of the collateral ligaments of the digits and disruption of the ulnar collateral ligament of the thumb commonly are clinically obvious. However, if the patient cannot cooperate, or if a partial rupture is suspected, or for

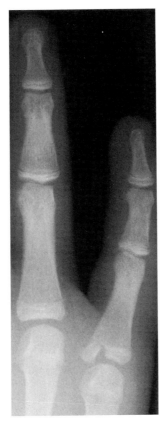

Fig. 10.43. Salter-Harris type 3 fracture of the base of the proximal phalanx of the fifth finger

detection of a Stener lesion, ultrasonography or MRI can be helpful in making the correct diagnosis and planning further treatment (DRAPE et al. 1994; O'CALLAGHAN et al. 1994).

10.3.5 Special Features in Children

The most common sites of fractures in children are the proximal phalanges, and the epiphysis (Fig. 10.43) and metaphysis (WORLOCK and STOWER 1986) are frequently involved. Most epiphyseal fractures are Salter-Harris type 2 lesions. Greenstick and torus fractures are common in children and frequently are located at the base of the proximal phalanges. Often two adjacent bones are involved and therefore when one fracture is identified, the adjacent corresponding bone should be evaluated carefully. Salter-Harris type 1 injuries, located at the distal phalanges, are often associated with severe lacerations of the nail bed and are essentially open injuries. Osteomyelitis may occur as a complication and antibiotic coverage should be performed.

References

Alffram P, Bauer GCH (1962) Epidemiology of fractures of the forearm. J Bone Joint Surg [Am] 44:105–114

Borgeskov S, Christiansen B, Kjaer A, Bladev I (1966) Fractures of the carpal bones. Acta Orthop Scand 37:276–287

Botte MJ, Gelberman RH (1987) Fractures of the carpus, excluding the scaphoid. Hand Clin 3:149–161

Brody GA, Stoller DW (1993) The wrist and the hand. In: Stoller DW (ed) Magnetic resonance imaging in orthopedics and sports medicine, 1st edn. J.B. Lippincott, Philadelphia, p 683

Bush CH, Gillespy T, Dell PC (1987) High-resolution CT of the wrist: initial experience with scaphoid disorders and surgical fusions. AJR 149:757–760

Cone RO, Szabo R, Resnick D, Gelberman R, Taleisnick J, Gilula LA (1983) Computed tomography of the normal radio-ulnar joint. Invest Radiol 18:541–545

Cooney WP, Dobyns JH, Linscheid RL (1980) Complications of Colles' fractures. J Bone Joint Surg [Am] 62:613–619

Curtis DJ, Downey EF, Brower AC et al. (1984) Importance of soft-tissue evaluation in hand and wrist trauma: statistical evaluation. AJR 142:781–788

Dameron TB (1972) Traumatic dislocation of the distal radioulnar joint. Clin Orthop 83:55–63

De Oliveira JC (1973) Barton's fractures. J Bone Joint Surg [Am] 55:586–594

Dobyns JH, Linscheid RL (1984) Fractures and dislocations of the wrist. In: Rockwood CA Jr, Geen DP (eds) Fractures in adults. J.B. Lippincott, Philadelphia, p 411

Drape JL, Dubert T, Silbermann O, Thelen P, Thivet A, Benacerraf R (1994) Acute trauma of the extensor hood of the metacarpophalangeal joint: MR imaging evaluation. Radiology 192:469–476

Dunn AW (1972) Fractures and dislocations of the carpus. Surg Clin North Am 52:1513

Frahm R, Saul O, Drescher E (1989) CT-Diagnostik bei Fehlstellung nach distaler Radiusfraktur. Radiologe 29:68–72

Frykman G (1967) Fractures of the distal radius including sequelae-shoulder-hand-finger syndrome, disturbance in the distal radioulnar joint, and impairment of nerve function. Acta Orthop Scand (Suppl) 108:1–55

Ganel A, Engel J, Oster Z, Farenc I (1979) Bone scanning in the assessment of fractures of the scaphoid. J Hand Surg 4:540–543

Gedda KO (1954) Studies on Bennett's fracture. Anatomy, roentgenology and therapy. Acta Chir Scand 193:1–9

Gelberman RH, Gross MS (1986) The vascularity of the wrist, identifying aterial patterns at risk Clin Orthop 202:40–49

Gilula LA (1979) Capal injuries. Analytic approach and case exercises. AJR 133:503–517

Gilula LA, Weeks PM (1978) Post-traumatic ligamentous instabilities of the wrist. Radiology 129:641–651

Gilula LA, Totty GW, Weeks PM (1983) Wrist arthrography: the value of fluoroscopic spot viewing. Radiology 146:555–556

Golimbu CN, Firooznia H, Melone CP Jr et al. (1989) Tears of the triangular fibroscartilage of the wrist: MR imaging. Radiology 173:731–733

Graham HK, McCoy GF, Mollan RAB (1985) A new injury of the distal radioulnar joint. J Bone Joint Surg [Br] 67:302–304

Green DP, Rowland SA (1991) Fractures and dislocations of the hand. In: Rockwood CA et al. (eds) Fractures, 3rd edn. J.B. Lippincott, Philadelphia, p 441

Hardy TH, Totty WG, Reinus WR, Gilula LA (1987) Posteroanterior wrist radiography: importance of arm positioning. J Hand Surg [Am] 12:504–508

Head RW (1971) Anterior dislocation of the distal ulna without accompanying fracture of the ulna styloid. Br J Radiol 44:468–470

Hindman BW, Kulik WJ, Lee G, Avolio RE (1989) Occult fractures of the carpals and metacarpals: demonstration by CT. AJR 153:529–532

Holder LE (1992) Radionuclide bone imaging in surgical problems of the hand. In: Gilula LA (ed) The traumatized hand and wrist, 1st edn. W.B. Saunders, Philadelphia, p 19

Johnson RP (1980) The acutely injured wrist and its residuals. Clin Orthop 149:33–44

Jupiter JB (1991) Fractures of the distal end of the radius. J Bone Joint Surg [Am] 73:461–469

Kauer JMG (1986) The mechanism of the carpal joint. Clin Orthop 202:16–26

Kauer JMG, de Lande A (1987) The carpal joint. Anatomy and function. Hand Clin 3:23–29

Knirk JL, Jupiter JB (1986) Intraarticular fractures of the distal end of the radius in young adults. J Bone Joint Surg [Am] 68:647–659

Larson B, Light TR, Ogden JA (1987) Fracture and ischemic necrosis of the immature scaphoid. J Hand Surg [Am] 12:122–126

Levinsohn EM, Rosen DI, Palmer AK (1991) Wrist arthrography: value of the three-compartment injection method. Radiology 179:231–239

Manaster BJ, Mann RJ, Rubenstein S (1989) Wrist pain: correlation of clinical and plain film findings with arthrographic results. J Hand Surg [Am] 14:466–473

Mann FA, Wilson AJ, Gilula LA (1992) Radiographic evaluation of the wrist: what does the hand surgeon want to know? Radiology 184:15–19

Mayfield JK (1992) Wrist ligament anatomy and biomechanics. In: Gilula LA et al. (eds) The traumatized hand and wrist. W.B. Saunders, Philadelphia, p 241

Mazet RJR, Hohl M (1963) Fractures of the carpal navicular. J Bone Joint Surg [Am] 45:82–111

McMinn DJW (1981) Mallet finger and fractures. Injury 12:477–481

Metz VM, Mann FA, Gilula LA (1993a) Three-compartment wrist arthrography: correlation of pain site with location of uni- and bidirectional communications. AJR 160:819–822

Metz VM, Schimmerl SM, Gilula LA (1993b) Wide scapholunate joint space in lunotriquetral coalition: a normal variant? Radiology 188:557–559

Mino DE, Palmer AK, Levinsohn EM (1983) Radiography and computerized tomography in the diagnosis of incongruity of the distal radio-ulnar joint. A prospective study. J Bone Joint Surg [Am] 67:247–252

Monahan PRW, Galasko CSB (1972) The scapho-capitate fracture syndrome. A mechanism of injury. J Bone Joint Surg [Br] 54:122–124

Muessbichler H (1961) Injuries of the carpal scaphoid in children. Acta Radiol 56:316–368

O'Callaghan BI, Kohut G, Hoogewoud HM (1994) Gamekeeper thumb: identification of the Stener lesion with US. Radiology 192:477–480

Pellegrini VD (1988) Fractures at the base of the thumb. Hand Clin 4:87–90

Peterson CA, Peterson HA (1972) Analysis of the incidence of injuries of the growth plate. J Trauma 12:275–281

Rand JA, Linscheid RL, Dobyns JH (1982) Capitate fractures. A long-term follow-up. Clin Orthop 165:209–216

Reicher MA, Kellerhouse LE (1990) Carpal tunnel disease, flexor and extensor tendon disorders. In: Reicher MA, Kellerhouse LE (eds) MRI of the wrist and hand. Raven Press, New York, p 49

Reinus WR, Conway WF, Totty WG et al. (1986) Carpal avascular necrosis: MR imaging, Radiology 160:689–693

Resnick D (1980) Arthrography and tenography of the hand and wrist. In: Dalinka MK (ed) Arthrography, 1st edn. Springer, New York Berlin Heidelberg

Rominger MB, Bernreuter WK, Kenney PJ, Lee DH (1993) MR imaging of anatomy and tears of the wrist ligaments. RadioGraphics 13:1233–1246

Rowe TA (1979) Cartilage fracture due to weight lifting. Br J Sports Med 12:130–132

Russe O (1960) Fracture of the carpal navicular. J Bone Joint Surg [Am] 42:759–768

Schimmerl S, Schurawitzky H, Imhof H et al. (1991) Morbus Sudeck – MRT als neues diagnostisches Verfahren. Fortschr Röntgenstr 154:601–604

Schweitzer ME, Mandel S, Schwartzmann RJ, Knobler RL, Thamoush AJ (1995) Reflex sympathetic dystrophy revisited: MR imaging findings before and after infusion of contrast material. Radiology 195:211–214

Short WA, Palmer AK, Werner FW, Murphy DJ (1987) A biomechanical study of distal radial fractures. J Hand Surg [Am] 12:529–534

Snook GA, Chrisman OD, Wilson TC, Wietsma RD (1969) Subluxation of the distal radioulnar joint by hyperpronation. J Bone Joint Surg [Am] 51:1315–1318

Stewart NR, Gilula LA (1992) CT of the wrist: a tailored approach. Radiology 183:13–20

Taleisnik J (1985) Radiographic examination of the wrist. In: Taleisnik J (ed) The wrist. Churchill Livingstone, New York, p 38

Thomas EM, Tuson KW, Brown PS (1975) Fractures of the radius and ulna in children. Injury 7:120–124

Thomas FB (1957) Reduction of Smith fracture. J Bone Joint Surg [Br] 39:463–470

Totterman SM, Miller R, Wasserman B, Blebea JS, Rubens DJ (1993) Intrinsic and extrinsic carpal ligaments: evaluation by three-dimensional Fourier transform MR imaging. AJR 160:117–123

Trumble TE, Irving J (1990) Histologic and magnetic resonance imaging correlations in Kienböck's disease. J Hand Surg [Am] 15:879–885

Truong NP, Mann FA, Gilula LA, Kang SW (1994) Wrist instability series: increased yield with clinical-radiologic sereening criteria. Radiology 192:481–484

Wechsler RJ, Webbe MA, Rifkin MD et al. (1987) Computed tomography diagnosis of distal radioulnar subluxation. Skeletal Radiol 16:1–4

Wilson AJ, Gilula LA, Mann FA (1991) Unidirectional joint communications in wrist arthrography: an evaluation of 250 cases. AJR 157:105–109

Wood MB, Berquist TH (1992) The wrist and hand. In: Berquist TH (ed) Imaging of orthopedic trauma. Raven Press, New York, p 749

Worlock PH, Stower MJ (1986) The incidence and pattern of hand fractures in children. J Hand Surg [Br] 11:198–203

Yin Y, McEnery KW, Gilula LA (1996a) Computed tomography – applications and tailored approach. In: Gilula LA, Yin Y (eds) Imaging of the wrist and hand. W.B. Saunders, Philadelphia, p 411

Yin Y, Mann FA, Gilula LA (1996b) Positions and techniques. In: Gilula LA, Yin Y (eds) Imaging of the wrist and hand. W.B. Saunders, Philadelphia, p 93

11 Pelvis, Hip, and Proximal Femur

J. Brossmann, H. Schwarzenberg, and M. Heller

CONTENTS

11.1 Pelvis

11.1.1 General Considerations

Injuries of the bones and ligaments of the pelvic ring result from severe trauma, most often sustained in motor vehicle and motor bike accidents (60%–70%), followed by work-related accidents, sports-related injuries, attempted suicide, and other causes. A high number of pelvic fractures following minor trauma were reported in osteoporotic patients by Melton et

J. Brossmann, MD, Klinik für Radiologische Diagnostik, Klinikum der Christian-Albrechts-Universität, Arnold-Heller-Straße 9, 24105 Kiel, Germany
H. Schwarzenberg, MD, Klinik für Radiologische Diagnostik, Klinikum der Christian-Albrechts-Universität, Arnold-Heller-Straße 9, 24105 Kiel, Germany
M. Heller, MD, PhD Professor, Direktor der Klinik für Radiologische Diagnostik, Klinikum der Christian-Albrechts-Universität, Arnold-Heller-Straße 9, 24105 Kiel, Germany

al. (1981). Linked with high-energy traumas is a high incidence of soft tissue damage and internal injuries of the pelvic region, featuring internal hemorrhage and injuries to the urinary tract and other viscera (Jungbluth and Sauer 1977). Further, more than 50% of the pelvic fractures are combined with injuries of the extremities, thorax, and head (Peltier 1965). Since physical signs of pelvic injury may not be obvious, it is important to keep the possibility of internal pelvic injuries in mind if patients are unconscious and severely traumatized.

The diagnosis and classification of fractures require a profound knowledge of the anatomy and the trauma mechanics. The incidence of additional injuries (visceral injuries, hemorrhage) and the rate of complications are greater in patients with unstable pelvic fractures (Looser and Crombie 1976; Campbell 1983). Therefore, the correct diagnosis is important for treatment planning and further observation of the patient.

11.1.2 Anatomy and Biomechanics

The pelvis is a ring-like structure, the major function of which is transmission of the body weight to the lower extremities, and protection of the pelvic viscera (Williams et al. 1989). It is formed by the articulation of the two innominate bones and the sacrum. The innominate bones are joined anteriorly at the symphysis pubis and articulate posteriorly with the sacrum, creating the left and right sacroiliac joints (Fig. 11.1). The innominate bone is composed of three elements, the ilium, pubis, and ischium, which join in the region of the acetabulum (Fig. 11.2).

The ilium, which is the largest of the three elements, consists of a body and a wing (ala ilii). The arcuate line and the margin of the acetabulum represent the border of these two parts at the internal and external surfaces, respectively. The body of the ilium forms approximately 40% of the acetabulum. The iliac wing has wide surfaces and forms cranially a

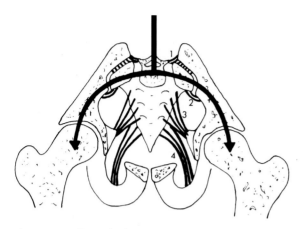

Fig. 11.1. Load transfer from the trunk via the sacroiliac joints and the posterior column of the hip joint to the lower extremities. *1*, Dorsal and interosseous sacroiliac ligaments; *2*, anterior sacroiliac ligament; *3*, sacrospinal ligament; *4*, sacrotuberal ligament. (From HELLER and JEND 1986)

crest, which is anteriorly and posteriorly terminated by the anterior superior and the posterior superior iliac spine.

The ischium is smaller than the ilium and forms the posteroinferior aspect of the innominate bone. It is made up of the body and a descending ramus. The body forms approximately 40% of the posteroinferior aspect of the acetabulum. The ischial tuberosity creates the posteroinferior angle of the ischium. The ischial spine arises on the posteromedial surface of the ischial body. The ramus forms the inferior border of the obturator foramen and joins the inferior pubic ramus medially to complete the obturator foramen.

The pubic bones consist of three parts, a superior and inferior ramus, and a body. The superior rami create the superior and medial borders of the obturator foramen and the anteroinferior 20% of the acetabular surface. The inferior rami extend inferiorly to fuse with the ischial ramus.

The sacrum is composed of the five fused sacral vertebrae. Its ventral surface is concave and displays four pairs of pelvic sacral foramina within the sacral wings. The triangular shaped coccyx articulates with the inferior aspect of the sacrum and consists variably of three to five rudimentary vertebrae, which are fused. Its anterior angulation to the sacrum is highly variable.

The articulations of the pelvic ring are the sacroiliac joints and the pubic symphysis. The sacroiliac joints are held together by the anterior, dorsal, and interosseous sacroiliac ligaments (Fig. 11.1). The dorsal sacroiliac ligament is the strongest ligament of the body. The iliolumbar ligaments reach from the

iliac crest to the transverse processes of the fifth lumbar vertebra. The pubic symphysis is strengthened superiorly by the superior pubic ligament and inferiorly by the arcuate pubic ligament. The fibrocartilaginous interpubic disc connects the adjacent surfaces of the pubic bones, which are covered with hyaline cartilage.

The articular surface of the acetabulum forms an incomplete ring, which is termed the lunate surface (Fig. 11.2). The hemispheric acetabular fossa is directed anterolaterally and is bordered by a bony rim, the acetabular limbus. Ventro-caudally, the acetabular limbus is open (incisura acetabuli). The depth of the acetabulum is increased by the acetabular labrum, which represents a fibrocartilage rim. Biomechanically, the acetabulum can be divided into three different columns (Fig. 11.2): the cranial column, which consists of the ilium and forms the apex of the acetabulum; the posterior column, which creates the posterior rim of the acetabulum and is formed by a vertical portion of the ischium and a dorsal part of the ilium; and the anterior column, which is formed by the pubis and parts of the ilium and creates the anterior border of the acetabulum. The Anglo-American literature describes only two columns, a dorsal (ilioischial) and a ventral (iliopubic) column (JUDET et al. 1964; ROGERS 1992; BURGESS and TILE 1991). The medial face of the posterior column and the inner aspect of the acetabular region are described as the quadrilateral surface (Fig. 11.2).

To describe the functional mechanism, the pelvis can be divided into the anterior and posterior arch. The main function of the posterior arch is to transmit the weight of the body to the lower extremity (Fig. 11.1). It consists essentially of the upper sacrum and strong bony pillars of the ilium, which run from the sacroiliac joint to the cranial and dorsal aspects of the acetabulum. The posterior arch is the most important element for the stability of the pelvic ring. The anterior arch consists of the pubic bones and the superior rami, and acts as a tie-beam to prevent separation of the lateral pillars of the posterior arch. Since the anterior arch is weaker, fractures are more likely to occur there. Additional stabilizers are the sacrospinous, sacrotuberous, iliolumbar, and lateral lumbosacral ligaments.

11.1.3 Classification of Pelvic Fractures

Fractures of the pelvis are usually classified into stable and unstable fractures (PELTIER 1965;

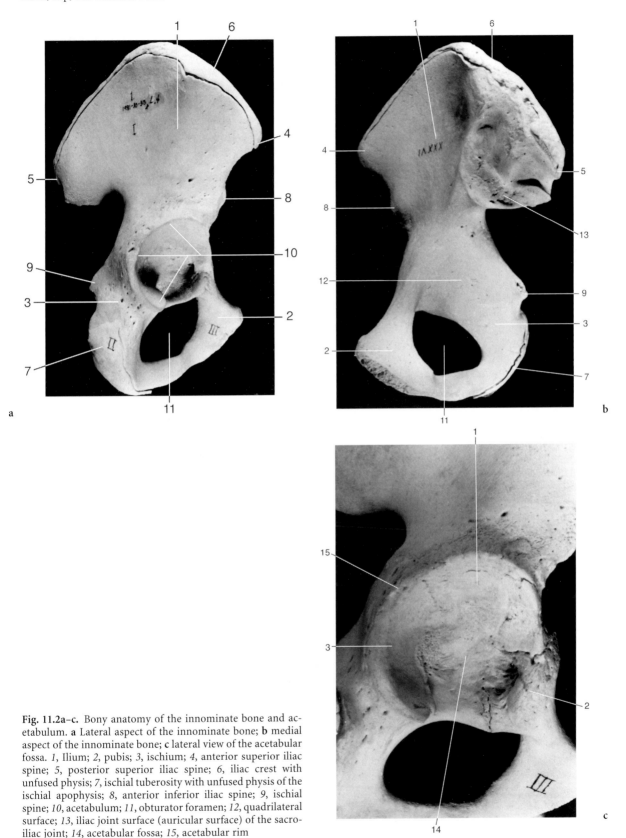

a

b

c

Fig. 11.2a–c. Bony anatomy of the innominate bone and acetabulum. **a** Lateral aspect of the innominate bone; **b** medial aspect of the innominate bone; **c** lateral view of the acetabular fossa. *1*, Ilium; *2*, pubis; *3*, ischium; *4*, anterior superior iliac spine; *5*, posterior superior iliac spine; *6*, iliac crest with unfused physis; *7*, ischial tuberosity with unfused physis of the ischial apophysis; *8*, anterior inferior iliac spine; *9*, ischial spine; *10*, acetabulum; *11*, obturator foramen; *12*, quadrilateral surface; *13*, iliac joint surface (auricular surface) of the sacroiliac joint; *14*, acetabular fossa; *15*, acetabular rim

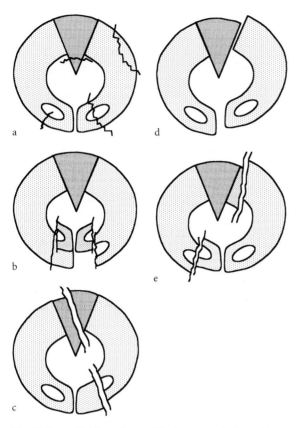

Fig. 11.3a–e. Stable and unstable fractures of the pelvis. **a** Stable fractures: fractures of a single pubic ramus, both pubic rami unilaterally, the iliac wing, and the sacrum and the coccyx horizontally below the sacroiliac joints. **b–e** Unstable fractures: **b** straddle fracture; **c** Malgaigne fracture; **d** dislocation; **e** bucket handle fracture

THAGGARD et al. 1978; ROGERS 1992). Generally, stable fractures of the pelvis are considered those which concern the margins of the pelvis and those which represent single breaks in the anterior pelvic ring without interruption of the dorsal ring structure. About two-thirds of all fractures of the pelvis are stable. In unstable fractures of the pelvic ring, the structures for weight-bearing, the posterior arch and its joints and ligaments, are affected (Fig. 11.3).

Stable fractures comprise avulsion fractures, isolated fractures of the ilium, transverse fractures of the sacrum and coccyx, and single breaks in the anterior pelvic ring without disruption of the public symphysis (fractures of a single public ramus, fractures of both public rami unilaterally, and nondisplaced fractures). More controversial is the classification of displaced unilateral and bilateral fractures of the anterior pelvic arch (Fig. 11.3). Until recently, they were classified as stable, using conventional radiography. However, CT and bone scintigraphy have proved

that these injuries are associated with concurrent osseous and ligamentous injuries about the region of the sacroiliac joint (CHENOWETH et al. 1980; NUTTON et al. 1982; HELLER and JEND 1986). These types of fracture are referred to as extended pubic fractures (ROGERS 1992) or as unstable incomplete fractures of the pelvic ring (KREITNER and WEIGAND 1993). Therefore, bilateral fractures of the anterior pelvic arch (straddle fracture) and disruption of the symphysis pubis are considered unstable.

In unstable fractures and fracture dislocations of the pelvic ring the posterior pelvic ring is disrupted. These lesions are regularly combined with a lesion of the anterior pelvic ring. Disruptions of the sacroiliac joint, vertical and oblique fractures of the sacrum with and without involvement of the sacroiliac joint, fractures of the ilium through the weight-bearing pillars, and involvement of the posterior column of the acetabulum are considered unstable fractures. Isolated fractures of the posterior arch are very rare and have to be regarded as unstable. Injuries of the acetabulum will be discussed separately. In any case, a fracture of either the anterior or the posterior arch demands a search for a second disruption of the pelvic ring.

Another, more complex classification system of pelvic fractures was described by TILE and PENNAL (TILE and PENNAL 1980; PENNAL et al. 1980). Briefly, it is based on clinical, radiographic, and biomechanical observations and reduces the mechanisms of injury to vertical shear forces, lateral, and anterior compression (Fig. 11.4). This classification takes into consideration the integrity of ligaments and whether a fracture is dislocated or impacted.

Anterior-posterior compression leads to diastasis of the symphysis pubis and disruption of the sacroiliac joint uni- or bilaterally (open-book injury, pelvic dislocation). With increasing diastasis, the anterior sacroiliac, sacrotuberous, sacrospinous, and finally the posterior sacroiliac ligaments are disrupted, the latter indicating instability (see also Sect. 11.1.5.3.2). Lateral compression is the most common mechanism of injury. It results in internal rotation of the affected hemipelvis, dislocated and overlapping fractures of the pubic rami and/or disruption of the symphysis pubis, which are combined with impacted fractures of the lateral wing of the sacrum. Disruption of the posterior sacroiliac ligaments is again the benchmark for instability. Vertical shearing injuries (Malgaigne fractures) are always considered unstable. Shearing forces are directed in the caudal-cephalad direction, causing fractures of the inferior and superior pubic rami and

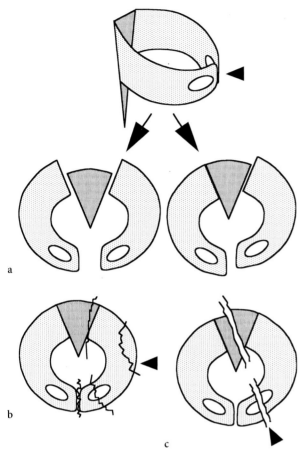

Fig. 11.4a–c. Biomechanical mechanisms of pelvic injuries. **a** Anterior compression; **b** lateral compression; **c** vertical shearing. For details see text

vertical fractures of the ilium or oblique fractures of the lateral sacrum and/or disruptions of the sacroiliac joint. Generally, the affected hemipelvis is displaced posterosuperiorly.

11.1.4 Examination Methods

Although computed tomography is the most important technique for evaluating pelvic trauma and related injuries, plain films are more readily available and are the first diagnostic method to be ordered. One must be familiar with the different projections and must know their limitations.

Most fractures can be detected by *plain radiography*. On the *anteroposterior (a.p.) radiograph of the pelvis*, which should always include both hips, several important landmarks have to be analyzed. The width of the symphysis pubis (normal ≤5 mm) and of the sacroiliac joints (normal 2.5–4 mm) has to be evaluated. The symmetry of the sacroiliac joints and

the iliac wings has to be compared, because asymmetry may be the only sign indicating disruption of the posterior elements. A fracture of the fifth lumbar transverse process might give a clue to underlying disruption of the sacroiliac joints or a vertical fracture of the posterior pelvic arch. The sacral foramina and especially their superior rims have to be scrutinized for disruptions and distortions. The a.p. radiograph of the pelvis is well suited for the diagnosis of injuries to the anterior pelvic arch. Limitations of plain films lie in the evaluation of the posterior elements, which may be obscured by abdominal gas and feces.

If the patient history, the physical examination, or the a.p. radiography of the pelvis suggests an acetabular fracture, coned down *a.p. views of the hip* should be obtained. Oblique radiographs provide additional information (see below). The following important bony contours should be analyzed, which give clues to fractures of the acetabulum (Figs. 11.5, 11.6). The iliopectineal line extends from the foramen ischiadicum to the pubic tubercle. Disruption of this line represents a fracture of the anterior column of the acetabulum. Fractures of the posterior column of the acetabulum lead to disruption of the ilioischial line. Other important landmarks are the line of the anterior and posterior acetabular rim and the teardrop. The medial limb of the teardrop corresponds to the cortical bone of the quadrilateral surface, whereas its lateral portion represents the medial wall of the acetabulum anterior to the acetabular notch.

The 45° rotated *obturator* and *ala views* (Judet views, internal and external oblique views) provide additional projections of the acetabular region. On the ala view (supine patient rotated toward the af-

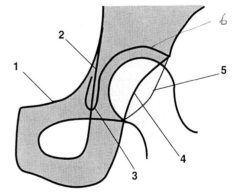

Fig. 11.5. Bony contours in the a.p. radiograph of the hip. *1*, Iliopectineal line; *2*, ilioischial line; *3*, teardrop figure; *4*, anterior acetabular rim; *5*, posterior acetabular rim *6 dome*

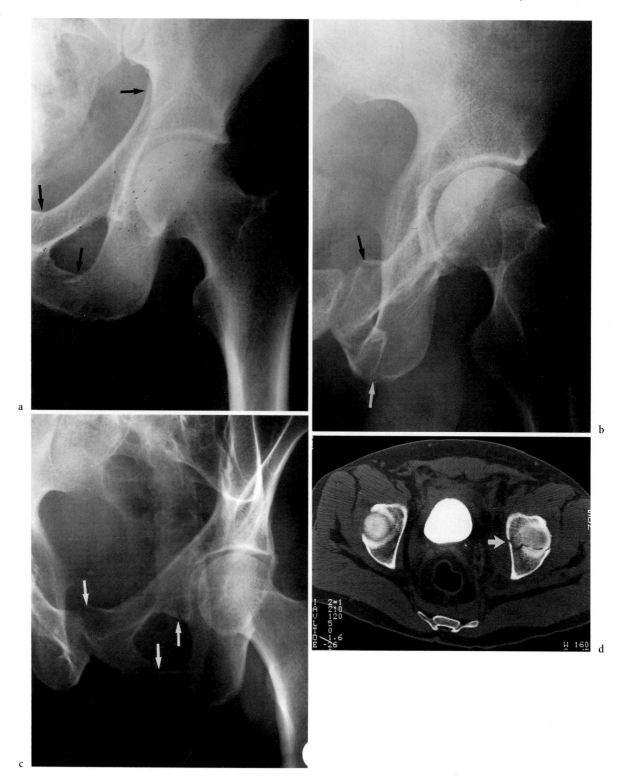

Fig. 11.6a–d. Fractures of the superior and inferior pubic rami, and the anterior column of the acetabulum (*arrows*). **a** Anteroposterior radiograph of the hip. **b** Ala view without evidence of fracture of the posterior column of the acetabulum. **c** Obturator view: an additional fracture of the anterior column reaching the obturator foramen is revealed. **d** Transaxial CT shows fracture of the acetabular dome and the quadrilateral surface, which is not displayed on the plain radiographs

fected side), the quadrilateral surface of the pelvis, the anterior surface of the acetabulum, and the anterior column are better depicted (Fig. 11.6). The obturator view (supine patient rotated toward the unaffected side) allows better judgement of the posterior rim of the acetabulum, the posterior column, and the relationship between the acetabulum and the femoral head (Fig. 11.6). Instead of turning the patient to the affected side for the ala view, the radiograph can also be taken in prone position with the affected side elevated.

Additional views have to be obtained if dislocations in the sagittal and frontal plane are suspected. The *inlet view*, an a.p. projection of the pelvis with a 30–40° cranially angulated tube (craniocaudal beam), allows assessment of the anterior-posterior displacement of the sacrum and ilium, the mediolateral dislocation of the fragments, and rotational distortions of the anterior pelvic arch (Fig. 11.7a). In the *outlet view*, the tube is angulated 30–40° in the

caudal direction (caudocranial beam), thus allowing evaluation for craniocaudal displacement of the pelvic structures. At the same time, the sacrum is projected approximately perpendicular to its long axis, which facilitates its evaluation. *Lateral views of the sacrum and coccyx* may be necessary to evaluate for fractures.

Conventional tomography can be done for the diagnosis of fractures of the posterior elements of the pelvic arch and the acetabulum, but has been widely replaced by computed tomography.

Computed tomography (CT) is the most accurate method to display the anatomy of the traumatized pelvis without superimposed structures (HELLER et al. 1980). For the examination no patient positioning is necessary. Fractures of the pelvic ring, dislocated fragments, and their relation to adjacent pelvic structures can be better appreciated with CT (Fig. 11.7b). CT can demonstrate bowel entrapment (CATSIKIS et al. 1989) and, indirectly, injuries of the lower urinary tract by revealing hematomas of the symphyseal area and by detecting paravesical contrast extravasation as a sign of bladder rupture (CAMPBELL 1983). Indirect signs of fractures like hematomas of the internal obturator muscle and piriformis muscles are easily visualized.

The greatest advantage of CT, however, is the superior delineation of structures of the posterior pelvic ring. Plain radiography has great disadvantages in diagnosing injuries of the posterior arch or the acetabular region. About 29% of sacroiliac disruptions, 57% of acetabular rim fractures, 34% of the vertical fractures of the sacrum and the dorsal ilium, and 30% of the intra-articular and periarticular fragments of acetabular and sacral fractures were missed with plain film radiography (SCHILD et al. 1981; HELLER and JEND 1986; EGUND et al. 1990). CT is the most important method for the diagnosis of disruptions of the sacroiliac joint. On plain radiographs, intra-articular vacuum phenomena as a sign of joint sprains are missed in almost 100% of cases. Likewise, 33% of the disruptions of the anterior and 8% of the disruptions of both the anterior and posterior sacroiliac ligaments are missed on plain radiography. CT is also superior to plain radiography in the diagnosis and staging of fractures of the acetabular dome and the posterior column and in the detection of intra-articular fragments (KAULBACH et al. 1989).

The pelvis should be scanned with a 5–10 mm slice thickness after administration of an intravenous contrast agent, but slice thickness should be reduced at least to 3 mm in the region of the acetabulum. Multiplanar reformation of CT data and 3D recon-

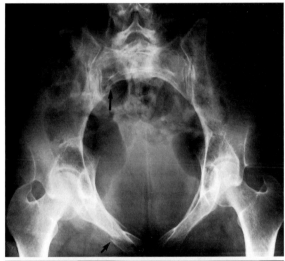

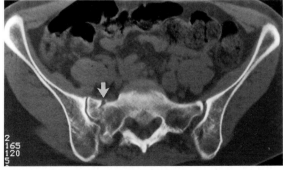

Fig. 11.7a,b. Malgaigne fracture of the pelvis. Fractures of the superior and inferior pubic rami; fracture of the right sacral wing. **a** Inlet view: a slight a.p. offset can be noted. Only subtle signs of the sacral fracture are present. **b** Transaxial CT shows the sacral fracture

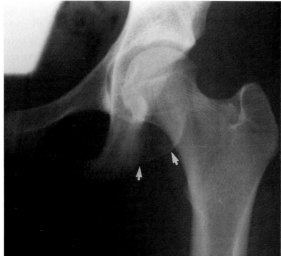

a

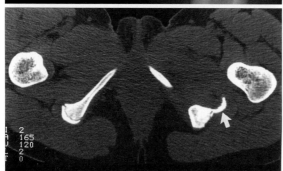

b

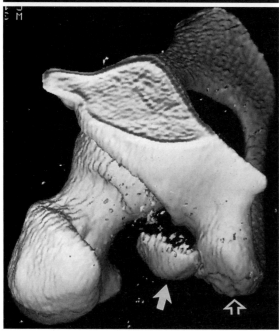

c

Fig. 11.8a–c. Avulsion fracture of the ischial tuberosity. **a** A bony fragment is projected inferomedial to the femoral head (*allows*). **b** Transaxial CT shows avulsion of the left ischial tuberosity (*allow*). **c** 3D display (posterosuperior view) of the avulsed fragment (*allow*) and the donor site (*open arrow*)

structions help to display complex fractures and fragment dislocations, and ease the surgical planning (MARTINEZ et al. 1992; MAGID 1994) (Fig. 11.8). Latest developments in geometric fidelity and possibilities of interactive measurements allow use of CT for preoperative planning, such as determination of the amount and type of bone graft and the selection of the best-fitting prosthesis (MAGID 1994).

Bone scintigraphy in the diagnosis of acute pelvic trauma is limited to instances when CT is not available and injuries of the posterior elements are suspected, but cannot be excluded by conventional radiographic means. It is highly sensitive but not very specific and should be performed at the earliest 4 days after the trauma.

Until recently, *magnetic resonance imaging* (MRI) had no application in the diagnostics of pelvic trauma. More recent reports suggest the application of MRI for the detection of sciatic nerve injury after pelvic trauma (POTTER et al. 1994). In cases with persisting bleeding associated with pelvic trauma, *Angiography* may become necessary to localize the injured vessels. Usually, multiple branches of the internal iliac artery are disrupted and rarely major vessels are lacerated. Since the surgical approach is often ineffective, the most promising treatment is percutaneous selective embolization (PANETTA et al. 1985). *Retrograde urethrography* and *cystography* may be necessary to rule out urethral tears or ruptures of the bladder (CAMPBELL 1983). For more details, see Chap. 7.

11.1.5 Trauma Pattern and Pathomorphology

The description of fractures will follow the functional classification in stable and unstable fractures and differentiates topographically between fractures of the margins of the pelvis and fractures of the anterior and posterior pelvic arch.

11.1.5.1 Marginal Fractures of the Pelvis

11.1.5.1.1 Avulsion Fractures of the Pelvis. Avulsion fractures occur mostly in young athletes at attachment sites of major muscles and are related to abrupt and forceful contractions of the respective muscles. Typical sites in the pelvis are the spina iliaca anterior superior (sartorius muscle), the spina iliaca anterior inferior (rectus femoris muscle), and the ischial tuberosity (adductor muscles) (Fig. 11.8). Avulsion injuries are generally treated conserva-

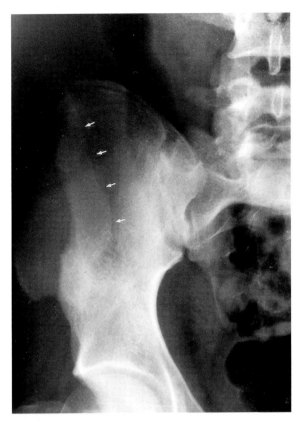

Fig. 11.9. Fracture of the iliac wing (*arrows*) – Duverney fracture

tively. Exuberant callus formation may simulate a bone tumor.

11.1.5.1.2 Fractures of the Iliac Wing. Isolated fractures of the iliac wing – Duverney fractures – account for a small percentage of pelvic fractures. They are caused by direct lateral compression (Figs. 11.4, 11.9). Fracture lines are variable, but regularly involve the anterior part of the ala and the iliac crest. Due to adjacent muscle attachments, gross displacements are rarely observed and therapy is usually conservative (PELTIER 1965). Additional oblique radiographs should exclude involvement of the hip and sacroiliac joint.

11.1.5.1.3 Fractures of the Sacrum and Coccyx. Fractures occur due to direct blows or falls onto the lower back. Diagnosis is difficult on the plain a.p. radiographs because of superimposed gas and feces, and lateral radiographs are necessary. Studies showed that fractures of the sacrum were missed in up to 70% of cases on plain radiographs, and CT evolved as the method of choice (SCHILD et al. 1981; HELLER and JEND 1986). Sacral fractures are usually transverse and caudal to the sacroiliac joint at the level of the third or fourth sacroiliac segment. The caudal fragment is usually angulated anteriorly. Isolated vertical or oblique fractures of the sacrum are extremely rare and one should be suspicious for a fracture elsewhere in the pelvic ring. A pitfall might be the high variability of the angulation of the coccyx in relation to the sacrum, since it may show up to 90° forward angulation as a normal variant.

11.1.5.2 Fractures and Disruptions of the Anterior Pelvic Arch

Fractures and disruptions of the anterior pelvic arch comprise uni- and bilateral fractures of the pubic and ischial rami and contusions or disruptions of the pubic symphysis (Fig. 11.3). Generally, these injuries are sufficiently diagnosed on a plain a.p. radiographs. Displacements in the sagittal plane and fracture extensions into the acetabular region are more reliably seen with CT. CT can also show soft tissue hematomas as indirect signs of injuries of the urethra and the urinary bladder. Single fractures of the ischial rami are considered most common. Since this type of fracture is often associated with an additional fracture of the superior pubic ramus and extension into the ipsilateral acetabulum is possible, a close examination of this region is suggested, possibly with CT. Fractures of the superior pubic ramus are usually easy to diagnose if located medially, but may be difficult to see if found laterally, where they can extend into the acetabular region. Additional oblique views and CT evaluation are helpful (Fig. 11.6).

Simultaneous fractures of the inferior and superior pubic ramus are referred to as unilateral fractures of the anterior pelvic arch and are considered stable if there is no evidence of severe displacement of the fragments or a disruption of the pubic symphysis (Fig. 11.3). With increasing displacement, resulting from a greater force, the probability of concomitant injuries of the posterior arch of the pelvis is higher, particularly about the sacroiliac joint (Fig. 11.7). In subtle cases and in the presence of complaints, CT is the method of choice for the diagnosis of occult injuries (HELLER and JEND 1986; CHENOWETH et al. 1980). Bilateral fractures of the anterior pelvic arch (straddle fracture) and disruptions of the symphysis pubis are considered unstable (Figs. 11.10, 11.11). The normal width of the symphysis is 5 mm.

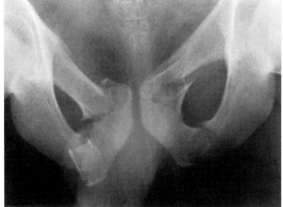

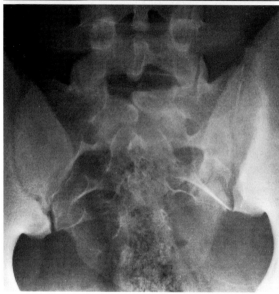

Fig. 11.10. a Bilateral fractures of the superior and inferior pubic rami – straddle fracture. **b** Disruption of the left sacroiliac join in the same patient

11.1.5.3 Fractures and Disruptions of the Posterior Pelvic Arch

Fractures or disruptions of the posterior pelvic ring involve the weight-bearing elements and are therefore considered unstable. They enclose disruptions and fractures of the sacroiliac joint, fractures of the sacrum, fractures of the ilium through the weight-bearing pillars, and involvement of the posterior column of the acetabulum. The latter will be discussed separately.

11.1.5.3.1 Fractures of the Sacrum. As mentioned before, only 30% of the sacral fractures are detected on plain radiographs (SCHILD et al. 1981; HELLER and JEND 1986). Transverse and sagittal fractures are the types of fractures which are described. Transverse

fractures of the sacrum and coccyx are considered as marginal fractures of the pelvic ring if they are below the sacroiliac joints. Sagittal fracture lines are commonly within the sacral wings and involve the sacral foramina (Fig. 11.12). Frequently, the sacroiliac joints are involved. Comminuted fractures of the sacrum are a result of great traumatizing forces. CT allows the functional classification of the trauma pattern, as it can differentiate impacted fractures of the sacrum following pelvic compression from dislocations, which occur in burst fractures.

11.1.5.3.2 Fractures and Disruptions of the Sacroiliac Joints. This kind of injury can follow all three kinds

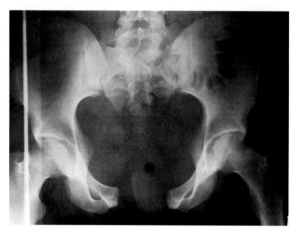

Fig. 11.11. Open book injury. Disruption of the symphysis pubis and of the sacroiliac joints

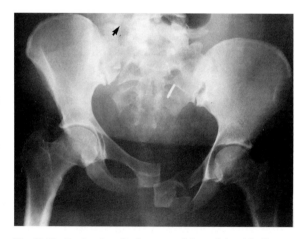

Fig. 11.12. Bucket handle fracture of the pelvis with disruption of the symphysis pubis and fractures of the left inferior and superior pubic rami. Fracture of the right sacral wing and widening of the left sacroiliac joint. Note fracture of the right transverse process of L5 as a sign of disruption of the posterior arch (*arrow*)

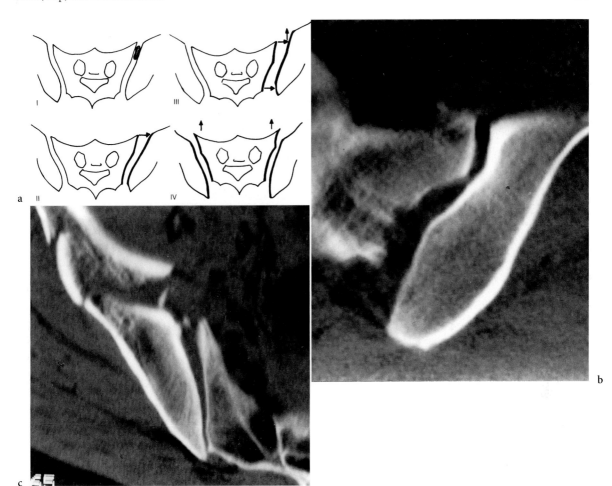

Fig. 11.13a–c. Four grades of lesions of the sacroiliac joints. **a** Schematic representation. *I*, Vacuum phenomenon; *II*, disruption of the anterior sacroiliac ligament; *III*, unilateral disruption of the anterior and posterior sacroiliac ligaments; *IV*, complete bilateral ruptures of the anterior and posterior sacroiliac ligaments with dislocation of the sacrum. (From HELLER and JEND 1986). **b** Transaxial CT of a grade I lesion. **c** Transaxial CT of a grade II lesion

of injury mechanism, anterior compression, lateral compression, and vertical shearing (Fig. 11.4). These forces cause disruption of the anterior sacroiliac, the sacrotuberal, the sacrospinal, and finally the posterior sacroiliac ligaments (Fig. 11.1). The stability of the sacroiliac joint is based on the integrity of the posterior sacroiliac ligaments. Fractures of the ilium are usually oriented vertically and just lateral and parallel to the sacroiliac joint. They may extend into the sacroiliac joint.

On conventional a.p. radiographs, widening of the sacroiliac joints, displacements of the ilium, and asymmetric iliac wings are hints of posterior involvement (Figs. 11.10–11.12). A fracture of the fifth transverse process gives an important clue to a disruption of the posterior arch (attachment of the iliolumbar ligament). CT has proved to be superior to conventional radiography, which is less sensitive for the

detection of subtle injuries of the sacroiliac joint (HELLER and JEND 1986). Based on CT, disruptions of the sacroiliac joints can be classified into four categories (Fig. 11.13).

Class 1: Short-term or persisting alterations of the articular pressure result in intra-articular collection of gas. This effect is known as the vacuum phenomenon. Usually, there are no concurrent disruptions of the sacroiliac ligaments. This pattern can only be recognized with CT and is considered stable.

Class 2: In this pattern, the sacroiliac joint space is widened about the anterior margin of the joint (normal range: 2.5–4 mm). The posterior joint width remains normal. This indicates a disruption of the anterior sacroiliac ligament. Class 2 injuries are also stable, since the posterior sacroiliac ligaments are intact.

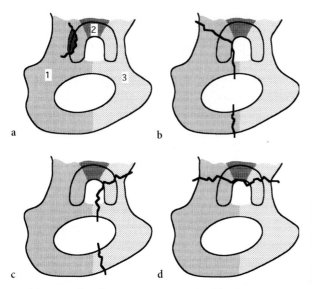

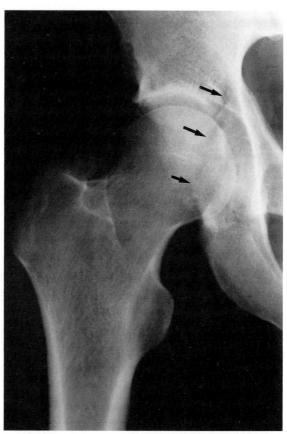

Fig. 11.14a-d. Schematic representation of four basic patterns of acetabular fractures. *1*, Ischium; *2*, ilium; *3*, pubis. **a** Fracture of the acetabular rim; **b** fracture of the posterior column; **c** fracture of the anterior column; **d** transverse fracture with involvement of both the anterior and the posterior column. For details see text

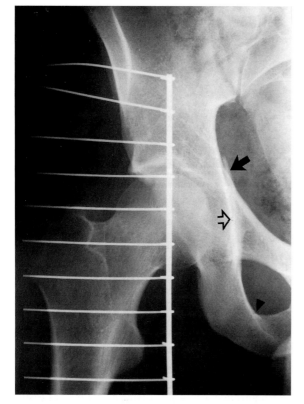

Fig. 11.16. Fracture of the anterior acetabular column. The iliopectineal line is disrupted and there is subtle medial displacement of the anterior column (*arrow*) and the teardrop figure (*open arrow*). Note the subtle fracture of the inferior pubic ramus (*arrowhead*)

Fig. 11.15. Fracture of the posterior acetabular column. The fracture line (*arrows*) extends from the posterior acetabular rim toward the ilioischial line and the sciatic notch. Fracture of the inferior pubic ramus is not displayed

Class 3: Widening of the entire extent of the sacroiliac joint shows disruption of the anterior and posterior sacroiliac ligaments. This injury is therefore classified as unstable. An equivalent finding is posterior bony avulsion of the sacroiliac joint, which serves for attachment of the dorsal sacroiliac ligaments.

Class 4: Dislocation of the sacrum. This group encompasses bilateral complete disruptions of both the anterior and posterior sacroiliac ligaments and dislocation of the sacrum in the anterior and posterior direction. In this type of injury, neurologic injuries are frequent.

11.1.5.4 Fractures of the Acetabulum

Although the acetabulum forms part of the hip joint, fractures involving the acetabulum are considered pelvic fractures. Approximately 20% of all pelvic

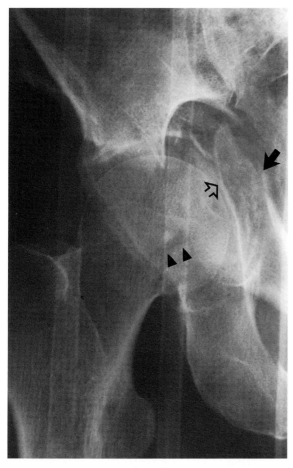

Fig. 11.17. Transverse fracture of the acetabulum with involvement of the acetabular dome. The iliopectineal line (*arrow*) and the ischiopubic line (*open arrow*) are disrupted. There is medial displacement of the femoral head and the anterior and posterior columns. Note the transverse fracture line of the posterior acetabular rim (*arrowheads*)

ent basic types of acetabular fracture can be described. They can occur in various combinations. The classification is oriented along the involvement of the biomechanically important pillars (Figs. 11.14–11.17). With CT, the important structures of this classification can be identified (Figs. 11.18, 11.19).

Type 1 comprises fractures of the anterior, the superior, or the posterior acetabular rim. The fractures of the posterior acetabular rim are most common and are regularly associated with a transient or

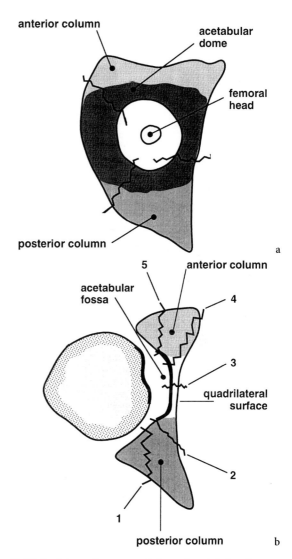

Fig. 11.18a,b. Schematic representation of acetabular fractures on transaxial CT. **a** Fractures of the acetabular dome. **b** Transaxial CT through the acetabular fossa. This section serves as a guide structure to identify the anterior and posterior columns. *1*, Fracture of the posterior acetabular rim; *2*, fracture of the posterior column; *3*, fracture of the quadrilateral surface; *4*, fracture of the anterior column; *5*, fracture of the anterior acetabular rim

fractures in adults involve the acetabulum (LANSINGER 1977). Acetabular fractures are usually caused by a force applied directly to the trochanter major or transmitted to it from a remote site, driving the head of the femur into the acetabulum (dashboard injury). They may also result from fractures of the pelvic ring with direct involvement of the hip joint (JUDET et al. 1964; JUNGBLUTH and SAUER 1977; SCHMITT et al. 1987). The position of the femoral head in relation to the acetabulum at the time of the accident determines the type of acetabular fracture. They can be accompanied by posterior dislocations of the hip. A dislocation or subluxation of the femoral head is present in up to 75% of all acetabular fractures.

According to the most accepted classification of Judet and Letournel (JUDET et al. 1964), four differ-

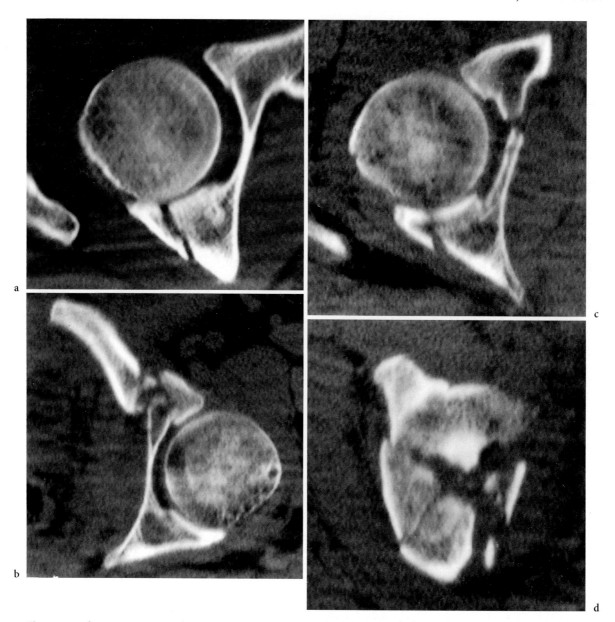

Fig. 11.19a-d. Representation of acetabular fractures on transaxial CT. **a** Fracture of the posterior rim of the acetabulum; **b** fracture of the anterior acetabular rim and the anterior column; **c** fractures of the quadrilateral surface and the posterior acetabular rim; **d** fractures of the acetabular dome

permanent posterior dislocation of the femoral head. About 30% of all acetabular fractures are type 1 fractures. Generally the size of the acetabular fragment increases with the abduction of the femur at the time of the accident. These fractures may be difficult to diagnose on plain films. CT and probably 3D reconstructions are necessary to assess the fracture correctly. On CT, a fracture line is seen which extends from the hip joint through the rim toward the outer aspect of the pelvis (Figs. 11.18, 11.19).

Type 2 represents fractures of the posterior (ilioischial) column. These fractures usually begin above the acetabulum in the region of the sciatic notch, extend through the posterosuperior aspect of the acetabulum and the acetabular notch, and include the inferior pubic ramus. On plain radiographs, the ilioischial line and the dorsal rim of the acetabulum are interrupted and may be displaced while the iliopectineal line and the anterior rim of the acetabulum are intact (Fig. 11.15). On CT, a fracture line is seen which extends from the hip joint medially through the posterior column (Figs. 11.18, 11.19).

Type 3 comprises fractures of the anterior (iliopubic) column. The fracture line starts about the anterior inferior iliac spine, extends through the anterosuperior acetabulum, and ends at the obturator foramen. A second fracture line is seen in the superior pubic ramus, the pubic body, or the inferior ramus about the area of the ischiopubic junction. On plain radiographs, disruptions of the iliopectineal line and the anterior rim of the acetabulum can be detected and the anterior column and the "teardrop" may be medially displaced. Additional fractures of the anterior acetabular margin may be present (Fig. 11.16). On CT examination, the fracture is seen extending from the hip joint anteriorly to the inner aspect of the pelvis, separating the anterior column (Figs. 11.18, 11.19).

Type 4 is described as a transverse acetabular fracture which crosses the acetabular fossa and involves the anterior and posterior columns (Fig. 11.17). The fracture may be in the area of weight bearing (superior location) or below this region (inferior location). The latter has the better prognosis. The obturator foramen is not involved in this fracture type. Radiographically, the iliopectineal and ilioischial lines are disrupted. Coexisting fractures and disruptions about the symphysis pubis and the sacroiliac joints have to be excluded. On CT, purely transversely orientated fracture lines can be missed but type 4 fractures are generally diagnosed because most are orientated obliquely.

In transverse acetabular fractures, an additional fracture line may extend caudally from the acetabular fossa, creating a T-shaped fracture of the acetabulum. This can be best appreciated on CT, where this fracture line can be seen on the quadrilateral surface (Figs. 11.18, 11.19). There may be coexisting fractures of the posterior, and rarely of the anterior and superior acetabular margin. Involvement of the dome, which is referred to as the third column (HELLER and JEND 1986), may cause considerable therapeutic problems. These fractures are often comminuted and coincide with fractures of both the anterior and the posterior column.

11.1.5.5 Miscellaneous

The pelvis is a common location for stress fractures, with a special preference for the pubic rami. They may also appear in the supra-acetabular region and rarely in the sacral wings. Radiographically they

appear as circular or linear sclerotic zones but are more readily apparent on bone scintigraphy (Fig. 11.20). Insufficiency fractures are usually associated with osteoporosis and are generally found in postmenopausal females. Rarely they are related to hyperparathyroidism, radiation osteitis, or steroid medication. Insufficiency fractures are generally located in the sacrum and the pubic body and are less frequent in the acetabular region and the ilium (DE SMET and NEFF 1985). Multiple insufficiency fractures are common. On radiographs, insufficiency fractures appear as poorly defined patchy areas of sclerosis. Bone scintigraphy can be positive before radiographic signs appear (Fig. 11.21).

11.1.6 Complications Associated with Pelvic Fractures

The mortality associated with pelvic fractures is about 10%, most fatalities being caused by hemorrhage and exsanguination. Blood loss associated with pelvic fractures can be as much as 4l and is highly related to disruption of the posterior arch (Fig. 11.22). Positioning of the patient increases hemorrhage and therefore radiographic views that require

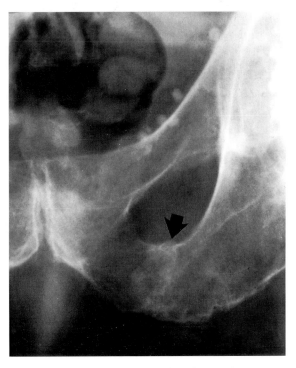

Fig. 11.20. Stress fracture of the left inferior pubic ramus 1 year after total hip replacement

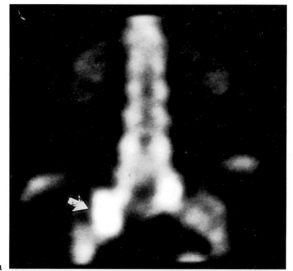

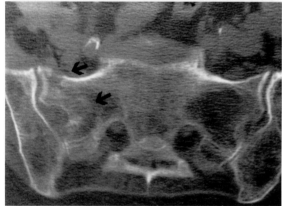

Fig. 11.21a,b. Insufficiency fractures of the sacrum in a female patient with breast cancer. Sacral pain was attributed to metastases. **a** Bone scan shows increased radionuclide uptake in the region of the right iliac wing. **b** CT of the sacrum reveals subtle insufficiency fracture lines (*arrows*)

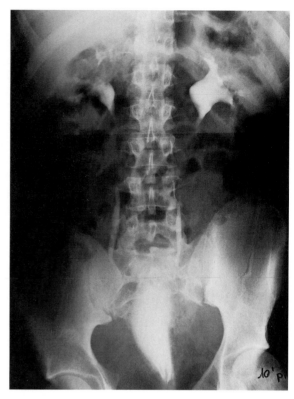

Fig. 11.22. Massive pelvic hematoma with compression of the bladder. The hematoma was caused by disruption of the left sacroiliac joint and fracture of the left iliac wing

movement of the patient should be restricted or replaced by CT.

Injuries of the urinary tract are commonly associated with fractures of the anterior pelvi arch. The urethra is more often injured than the bladder, and males are almost exclusively affected. The most common location for urethral injuries is the membranous portion, which is highly susceptible to shearing forces and resulting transection or laceration (CAMPBELL 1983). Injuries to the bladder occur either by sharp edges of fragments or indirectly by increased intra-abdominal pressure, if the bladder is distended. Ruptures may be intra- or extraperitoneal (Fig. 11.23).

Injuries of the viscera are more frequent in fractures involving the posterior arch, reflecting the different forces involved. In about 20% of pelvic fractures, visceral injuries occur (laceration of the liver

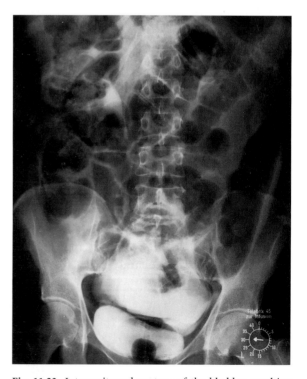

Fig. 11.23. Intraperitoneal rupture of the bladder, resulting from blunt pelvic trauma. Absence of the left kidney on pyelogram

and spleen, rupture of the diaphragm). Bowel may become entrapped in the fracture or can be perforated by fragments (CATSIKIS et al. 1989). In about 12% of the pelvic fractures, neurologic deficits are reported as complications, generally related to fractures of the sacrum and associated injuries of the lumbosacral nerve roots. By far the most frequent complication of acetabular fractures is posttraumatic osteoarthritis, which is due to the lack of congruency of the joint surface.

11.1.7 Special Features of Trauma in Children and Adolescents

Compared with the more osteoporotic bones of adults, the bones of children require higher energies to cause fractures. The only exceptions are fractures of the cartilaginous growth plates and the apophysis of the pelvis and the hip. When diagnosing pelvic fractures in children, therefore, concomitant injuries of nerves, viscera, and the genitourinary system have to be considered. Apparently the frequency of these complicating injuries is not higher in children, compared with adults.

According to CANALE and KING (CANALE and KING 1991), there are several differences between the pelvis of children and that of adults with respect to trauma and trauma pattern. The pelvis of children is more pliable due to the texture of the bone and the higher elasticity of the joints, so that higher energies can be absorbed. The elasticity of the pelvis allows single displaced breaks without second fractures. Based on the weakness of cartilage, a higher frequency of avulsion fractures and fractures of the triradiate cartilage is seen. Fractures of cartilage can cause growth arrests and unequal growth, as in cases of fractures through the triradiate cartilage with resultant bony bridges. This can lead to an insufficient acetabulum.

The primary and secondary ossification centers of the pelvis can give rise to an erroneous diagnosis of a fracture or avulsion. The primary ossification centers of the pelvis are the ilium, the ischium, and the pubis, which join in the acetabular fossa and create the triradiate cartilage (Fig. 11.2). Before bony fusion at the age of 16–18 years (PONSETI 1978), the lucent lines of the triradiate cartilage junction may be mistaken for fractures. The secondary centers of ossification are the iliac crest, the ischial apophysis, the anterior inferior iliac spine, the pubic tubercles, the angle of the pubis, the ischial spine, and the lateral wings of the sacrum. It is important to know the times of their appearance and fusion with the adja-

cent bone since they can be confused with avulsion fractures (Fig. 11.8). The iliac crests, which appear between 13 and 15 years, fuse with the ilium at the age of 15–17 years. The apophyses of the ischium are first seen at the age of 15–17 years and normally fuse at the age of 19 years, but may be delayed until 25 years. The ossification center of the anterior inferior iliac crest appears at 14 years and fuses at the age of about 16 (WATTS 1976; PONSETTI 1978).

Finally, the battered child syndrome can also include pelvic fractures and should be suspected if the history is not consistent with the sustained trauma and multiple hematomas and fractures with different stages of healing are seen.

11.1.8 Diagnostic Algorithm

In patients with suspected osseous and ligamentous injuries of the pelvis, plain a.p. radiographs and angulated views of the pelvis are the first diagnostic step. The patient should not be positioned for different radiographic projections. In cases of diagnosed or suspected fractures of the pelvis or the acetabular region, CT should be the next diagnostic step. The timing and extent of the CT examination depend greatly on the condition of the patient, the availability of CT, and additional clinical questions. Associated injuries of the thorax and abdomen and of the cranium can be ruled out in the same session. In fractures of the pubic rami and the iliac wing, plain radiography is equivalent to CT. CT is superior to plain radiography in the evaluation of fractures of the posterior pelvic arch and the acetabulum. The degree and direction of dislocations, the extent of the fracture lines, the number and location of fragments, and other related injuries of the pelvis can be easily identified. Conventional tomography should be restricted to those cases in which CT is not available. Multiplanar reconstructions and three-dimensional CT are helpful in the display of complex fractures and the preoperative planning in respect of such fractures. Bone scintigraphy and MRI have not yet found indications in the routine diagnosis of pelvic trauma.

11.2 Hip and Proximal Femur

11.2.1 General Considerations

Usually, fractures of the hip refer to those involving the femoral head and neck or the proximal femur. Fractures of the acetabulum are considered pelvic fractures and have been described in Sect. 11.1, although they are often related to dislocations of the femoral head. Due to specific problems in respect of treatment, complications, and healing, fractures of the proximal femur and the hip are classified into three different types. Intracapsular fractures occur within the joint capsule of the hip and relate to fractures of the femoral head and neck. Intertrochanteric fractures involve the region between the greater and lesser trochanter. Fractures occurring within 5 cm below the lesser trochanter are termed subtrochanteric fractures.

11.2.2 Anatomy and Biomechanics

The hip joint is a synovial joint of ball and socket type and consists of the articulation of the femoral head in the cuplike acetabulum (WILLIAMS et al. 1989). About two-thirds of the femoral head lies within the acetabular fossa. In the adult, the neck of the femur and femoral shaft form an angle of approximately 125–130° (caput-collum-diaphysis angle, CCD) and a forward angle of about 12–15°, which is called anteversion. A buttress of bone (calcar femorale) reinforces the inferior aspect of the femoral neck. The intertrochanteric region consists of the greater and lesser trochanters, which are joined anteriorly by the intertrochanteric line and posteriorly by the intertrochanteric crest. The gluteus medius and minimus muscles (hip abductors) and the iliopsoas muscle (hip flexor) insert on the greater and lesser trochanters, respectively.

The anatomy of the fibrous capsule and the blood supply is important for the classification and prognosis of fractures of the proximal femur (TRUETA 1968; KLENERMAN and MARCUSON 1970). The fibrous joint capsule is attached to the rim of the acetabulum, the acetabular labrum, the transverse ligament, and the edge of the obturator foramen (WILLIAMS et al. 1989). It surrounds completely the femoral neck and inserts anteriorly to the intertrochanteric line, superiorly to the base of the femoral neck, and posteriorly about 1 cm above the trochanteric crest, leaving the dorsal and distal one-third of the femoral neck uncovered (Fig. 11.24). The iliofemoral, ischiofemoral, and pubofemoral ligaments reinforce the joint capsule. The synovial membrane covers all parts of the femoral neck within the joint capsule, and the ligament of the head of the femur.

The blood supply of the neck and the head of the femur depends mainly on vessels that travel within the joint capsule, adjacent to the bone (Fig. 11.24). The medial and the lateral circumflex arteries form a vascular ring at the base of the femoral neck. The anterior part of this ring is within the joint capsule, while the posterior portion is extracapsular. About two to six branches of the vascular ring ascend along the femoral neck, predominantly on the posterosuperior aspect, piercing the bone a few millimeters caudal of the articular cartilage of the femoral head. The lateral epiphyseal arteries are the principal arteries, which originate from the ramus profundus of the medial cirumflex artery. They provide about two-thirds of the blood supply to the femoral head (TRUETA 1968; KLENERMAN and MARCUSON 1970; OGDEN 1974). The medial and inferior epiphyseal arteries and the artery of the round ligament play a minor role in the blood supply of the femoral head. Before the age of 4 years, the metaphyseal vessels mainly supply the femoral head. The developing growth plate creates a barrier to these vessels and gradually the epiphyseal arteries take over the blood supply of the femoral head (OGDEN 1974).

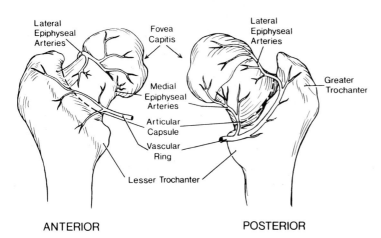

ANTERIOR   POSTERIOR

Fig. 11.24. Vascular supply of the femoral head and insertion of the joint capsule. Note that most parts of the vessels anteriorly are within the joint capsule, opposed to the posterior side. The most important vessel for the supply of the femoral head is the lateral epiphyseal artery. For further details see text. (From ROGERS 1992)

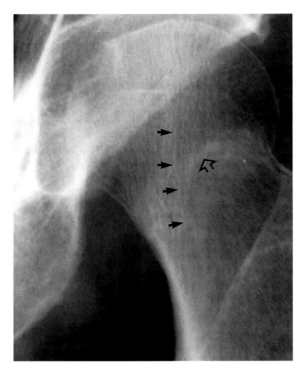

Fig. 11.25. Subtle signs of an incomplete fracture of the femoral neck. Note the slight angulation of the trabeculae (*arrows*) and the zone of increased bone density (*open arrow*)

11.2.3 Examination Methods

Plain radiography is the method of choice for the primary evaluation of fractures of the proximal femur and should be done in two planes. Several important radiographic projections should be known. *Anteroposterior radiographs of the pelvis and hip* have already been discussed above. In patients with suspected fractures of the proximal femur, comparisons to the contralateral side are helpful. For the a.p. view, the feet should be internally rotated, so that the greater trochanter and the femoral neck are seen in profile. With external rotation, the femoral neck is seen shortened, which might be misleading.

Within the femoral neck and head two major groups of trabeculae, the vertically oriented compressive and the tensile trabeculae, can be recognized. They may be distorted in cases of subtle fractures (Fig. 11.25). It is important to study the congruency and continuity of the bony contours of the femoral head and the articulating acetabulum. Dislocations or interposition of soft tissue and fragments may cause only subtle changes. Comparative measurements between the acetabular roof and the femoral head and medially between the femoral head

and the medial line of the teardrop can provide important clues (Waldenström sign). A total distance of more than 11 mm or a difference of more than 2 mm suggests either a large effusion or interposition of soft tissue. Several fat pad signs have been described around the hip, of which only a prominent fat pad of the internal obturator muscle seems reliable, if present asymmetrically.

The second projection to rule out fractures of the proximal femur should be the *groin lateral view* (axial projection) (Fig. 11.26). On this radiograph, the femoral neck, the dorsal cortex, and the anteversion of the neck can be evaluated. It also shows the relation of the femoral head to the neck and the acetabulum. The *frog-leg view* is obtained by external rotation and abduction of the femur with a vertical beam (Fig. 11.27). This projection should not be used in cases with suspected fractures.

Conventional tomography still has a certain application in the proximal femur for the diagnosis of occult fractures and bony defects of the femoral head

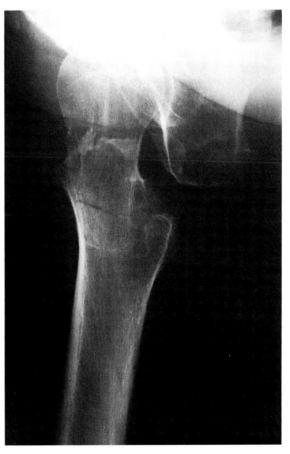

Fig. 11.26. Groin lateral view of a pertrochanteric fracture. Note the diminution of the femoral neck anteversion and the fracture lines

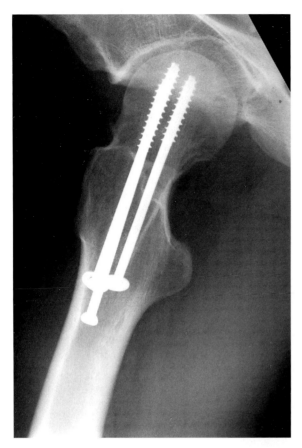

Fig. 11.27. Frog-leg view of the proximal femur after internal fixation of a femoral neck fracture with screws

mur (HOLDER et al. 1990). It has also been used to predict the outcome of femoral neck fractures (ALBERTS et al. 1987).

The application of *magnetic resonance imaging* in the diagnosis of acute trauma of the proximal femur is limited. It has been suggested for the detection of injuries of the femoral head and the sciatic nerve, but its value for diagnosing intra-articular fragments is very limited (POTTER et al. 1994). MRI is very sensitive for bone bruises but it is limited in the detection of cartilaginous injuries. Soft tissue injuries which

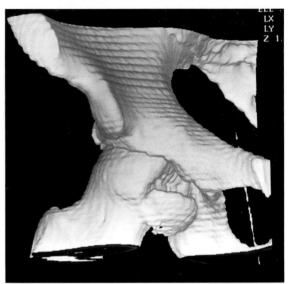

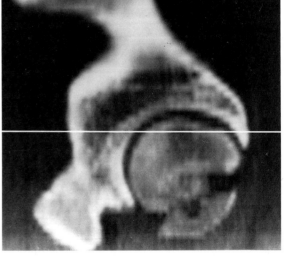

Fig. 11.28a,b. Fracture of the femoral head, Pipkin type 4. **a** 3D reconstruction demonstrating a caudally displaced fragment of the femoral head. **b** Multiplanar reconstruction of the fracture in an oblique sagittal plane, which shows the fracture line directly inferior to the fovea capitis femoris (see also Fig. 11.33).

and intra-articular fragments of the hip joint. Nevertheless, it has been widely replaced by CT.

The superiority of *computed tomography* over other imaging modalities has been discussed for pelvic and acetabular fractures. The extent of fractures of the femoral head and intra-articular fragments can be better evaluated with CT (SCHMITT et al. 1987; KAULBACH et al. 1989). Multiplanar and 3D reconstructions ease the understanding of the complex anatomy and the relationships of fractures and their fragments (Fig. 11.28). Diagnosis of osteonecrosis of the femoral head with CT has been reported (DIHLMANN and HELLER 1985). The application of CT in the diagnosis of acute trauma of the femoral neck and the trochanteric region is limited. Nevertheless, it can be applied for the diagnosis of occult and unusual fractures and is useful in cases with rotational distortions (EGUND et al. 1990).

Bone scintigraphy is highly sensitive for the early detection of osteonecrosis of the femoral head after hip trauma. Bone scintigraphy is also well suited for the detection of occult fractures of the proximal fe-

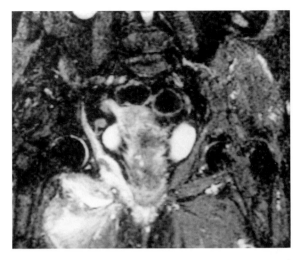

Fig. 11.29. Coronal MRI (short tau inversion recovery, STIR) of a patient with suspected fracture of the right proximal femur proves extensive edema of the iliopsoas muscle and the adductor muscles, consistent with a muscle sprain or partial tear

accompany trauma can be easily detected (Fig. 11.29). MRI is useful in the diagnosis of insufficiency fractures and occult fractures (DEUTSCH et al. 1989; TYRELL and DAVIES 1994). MRI is more sensitive in the diagnosis of occult fractures than bone scintigraphy and may prove the presence of nondisplaced fractures which are missed with CT (POTTER et al. 1994; RIZZO et al. 1993; DEUTSCH et al. 1989) (Fig. 11.30). It is also highly sensitive for the detection of early signs of osteonecrosis, but MRI is considered unsuitable for predicting necrosis of the femoral head following fracture of the femoral neck (SPEER et al. 1990).

11.2.4 Dislocations and Fracture Dislocations of the Hip

11.2.4.1 General Considerations

Dislocations of the hip are infrequent injuries and represent about 5% of all dislocations. Strongest forces are required for dislocations and fracture dislocations of the hip joint, usually occurring during motor vehicle accidents (LARSON 1973; EPSTEIN 1973). Dislocations are mostly produced by indirect forces to the leg which are exerted by the leverarm of the femur: extreme adduction, flexion, and inward rotation of the femur produces a posterior dislocation. Extreme abduction and external rotation of the femur can cause anterior dislocations. Dislocations

of the hip are frequently associated with fractures of both the acetabulum and the femoral head. These injuries may be overlooked in patients with multiple injuries. In such patients, a routine a.p. radiograph of the pelvis and both hips should be obtained. The extent and location of the fracture and the involvement of weight-bearing surfaces of the femoral head and acetabulum must be clarified. Identification of intra-articular fragments is most important for adequate treatment.

11.2.4.2 Classification, Trauma Pattern, and Pathomorphology

The type of dislocation is defined by the position of the femoral head in relation to the acetabulum. Posterior dislocation and fracture dislocation are most common, accounting for about 85% of all hip dislocations (EPSTEIN 1973; JACOB et al. 1987). Anterior dislocations and the extremely rare bilateral dislocations account for the remaining 15% (DAWSON and VAN RIJN 1989; SINHA 1985; STEWART et al. 1975). Sole dislocation of the hip without a fracture is a very rare finding (WEIGAND et al. 1978).

11.2.4.2.1 Posterior Dislocation. Most cases of posterior dislocation are associated with a fracture of the posterior rim of the acetabulum. The size of the fragment is directly related to the degree of adduction at the time of the accident. With increasing adduction it is more likely that the dislocation may occur without an acetabular fracture. Posterosuperior (posterior iliac) dislocation is more common than posteroinferior dislocation (posterior ischial) (Figs. 11.31, 11.32).

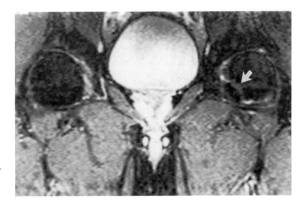

Fig. 11.30. Coronal MRI (T2-weighted spin-echo sequence) shows occult fracture of the femoral head (*arrow*), which could not be diagnosed on plain radiography

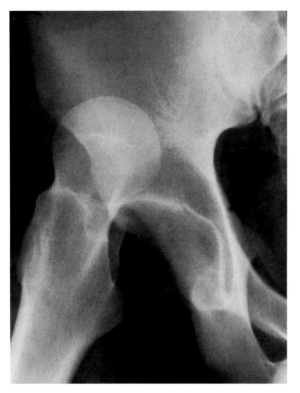

Fig. 11.31. Posterosuperior (posterior iliac) dislocation of the hip

rotated. In obturator dislocations the head of the femur is in the region of the obturator foramen. Pubic dislocation is the least frequent. Anterior dislocations are often associated with fractures of the superolateral portion of the femoral head; they are less often associated with fractures of the acetabular rim and the femoral neck.

11.2.4.2.3 Central Dislocation. A central dislocation occurs when a force is transmitted through the head of the femur towards the acetabular fossa. The result is a marked comminution of the acetabulum with medial displacement of the femoral head into the pelvis. These injuries are often addressed as central dislocations of the hip, but actually represent fracture dislocations (Fig. 11.17).

11.2.4.2.4 Fractures of the Femoral Head. Isolated fractures of the femoral head are rare, because the femoral head is well protected by the acetabulum. Usually, fractures of the femoral head are associated with posterior dislocations of the hip. Fractures occur when the femoral head impacts against the acetabular margin. Severe hyperabduction may cause

Posterosuperior dislocation may be missed on a.p. radiographs of the pelvis because the femoral head may project onto the acetabular fossa. Hints of the presence of a posterior dislocation may be provided by absence of visualization of the lesser trochanter due to posterior rotation and lack of exact congruency of the femoral head with the acetabular fossa. In posteroinferior dislocation the femoral head projects onto the ischial tuberosity. The postreduction radiographs have to be analyzed for intra-articular fragments and interposed tissue (round ligament, acetabular labrum). CT is the method of choice for the evaluation of intra-articular bodies, but it is less sensitive for the diagnosis of nonosseous interponates. In these cases, asymmetric incongruencies of the femoral head with the acetabulum may be the only clues to the diagnosis.

11.2.4.2.2 Anterior Dislocation. Anterior dislocations can be divided into superoanterior (pubic) and inferoanterior (obturator or peroneal) dislocations. In pubic dislocations, the head of the femur is situated over the pubic crest and the femur is externally

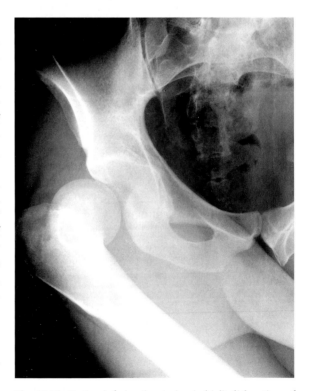

Fig. 11.32. Posteroinferior (posterior ischial) dislocation of the hip

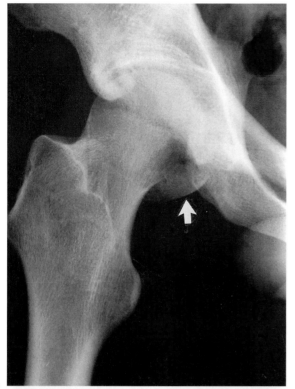
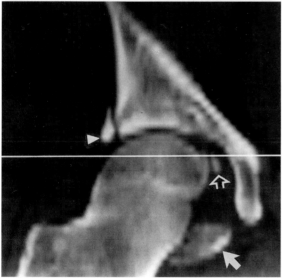

posterior dislocations (ROEDER and DELEE 1980). Fractures of the superolateral femoral head are frequently associated with anterior dislocations of the hip (DELEE 1991). Compression fractures are more common than shearing fractures and may have the appearance of a Hill-Sachs defect. Compression fractures may be difficult to diagnose on a.p. radiographs. CT readily displays the defect as a flattened depression of the femoral head in up to 61% of cases (TEHRANZADEH et al. 1990).

The classification of PIPKIN (1957) is widely accepted in the description of fractures of the femoral head associated with posterior dislocation of the hip. It is based on the relation of the fracture to the fovea capitis femoris and the presence of an associated acetabular and femoral neck fracture. The classification describes four different types of fracture (Figs. 11.33, 11.34). In the AO classification (MÜLLER et al. 1990) the fractures are categorized into three groups, each with three subgroups, according to their morphological and therapeutic complexity and expected outcome (Fig. 11.35).

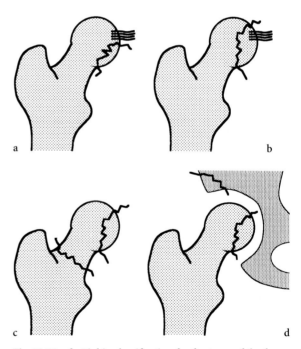

Fig. 11.33a,b. Fracture of the femoral head Pipkin type 4 (see also Fig. 11.28). **a** Anteroposterior radiograph of the hip shows caudal fragment of the femoral head (*arrow*). **b** Multiplanar reconstruction of transaxial CT sections in the frontal plane shows the fracture inferior to the fovea capitis femoris. Note the bony avulsion of the round ligament (*open arrow*) and the fracture of the superior acetabular rim (*arrowhead*)

Fig. 11.34a–d. Pipkin classification for fractures of the femoral head. **a** *Type 1*: fracture of the femoral head below the fovea capitis femoris with the fragment remaining in the acetabular cavity. **b** *Type 2*: fracture of the femoral head above the insertion of the round ligament. This represents the most common fracture type. **c** *Type 3*: fracture type 1 or 2 associated with a fracture of the femoral neck. **d** *Type 4*: fracture type 1 or 2 combined with an acetabular fracture in the posterosuperior region

avulsion of the round ligament (Fig. 11.33). Shear and compression fractures of the anteroinferior aspect of the femoral head result from posterior dislocations. Shear fractures occur in about 10% of

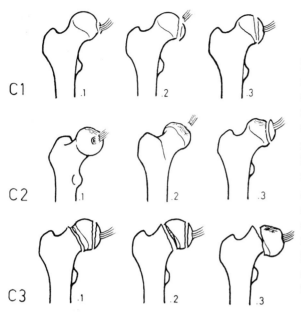

Fig. 11.35. AO classification of fractures of the femoral head. *C1,* Shear fractures of the femoral head: *C1.1,* avulsion of the round ligament; *C1.2,* shear fractures with rupture of the round ligament; *C1.3,* shear fractures with a large fragment of the femoral head. *C2,* Femoral head fractures with depression: *C2.1,* posterior and superior; *C2.2,* anterior and superior; *C2.3,* shear fractures with depression. *C3,* Combination fractures: *C3.1,* shear fractures and transcervical neck fracture; *C3.2,* shear fractures and subcapital neck fracture; *C3.3,* depression fracture and fracture of the femoral neck. (From MÜLLER et al. 1990)

11.2.5 Fractures of the Femoral Neck

11.2.5.1 General Considerations

Fractures of the femoral neck may result from significant injury , but they can occur spontaneously and result from minor trauma, especially in elderly women. They may be the response to cumulative effects of stress in athletes (stress fractures). The incidence of femoral neck fractures is 3–6 times higher in females compared with males and they occur nearly twice as often as intertrochanteric fractures (ALFFRAM 1964; BARNES et al. 1976). Different studies indicate that the severity of osteoporosis is related to fractures of the proximal femur (NILSSON 1970; STEVENS et al. 1962; MUCKLE 1976). An additional predisposing factor is a decreased CCD angle in the elderly. Pathologic fractures may be related to bone tumor, metastasis, osteonecrosis, and other diseases affecting the bone (CALMERS and IRVINE 1988; BILDNER and FINNEGAN 1989).

11.2.5.2 Classification, Trauma Pattern, and Pathomorphology

Fractures of the femoral neck can be classified by the region in which they occur. By far the most frequent and most important fractures occur just distal to the junction of the femoral head with the neck (subcapital fracture). This is the region where the nutrient vessels pierce the bone and can be severed by shearing of fragments. The two other locations for fractures are the midcervical and the basocervical areas of the femoral neck (Fig. 11.36). These fractures are rare and occur in children and adolescents due to severe trauma. Stress fractures, insufficiency fractures, and pathologic fractures have to be considered if the basocervical region is affected in adults. Renal osteodystrophy, steroid therapy, and metastasis have to be excluded.

Subcapital fractures can be incomplete or complete and be displaced or impacted. In incomplete

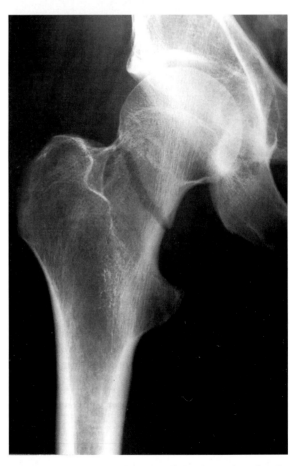

Fig. 11.36. Midcervical fracture of the femoral neck. The femoral head is in a slight valgus position and the femur is externally rotated. AO classification: B2.2

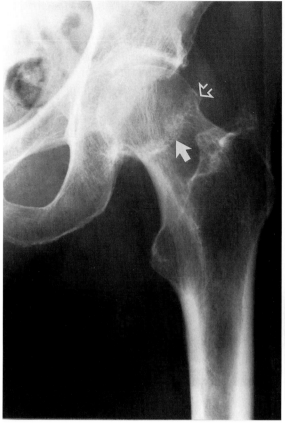
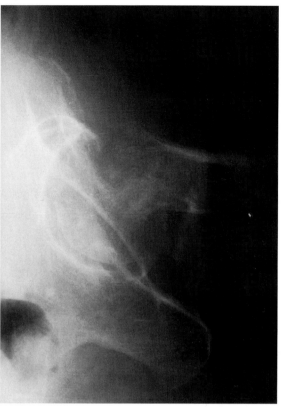

a

b

Fig. 11.37a,b. Subcapital, impacted fracture of the femoral neck. Classification: Garden 1, Pauwels 2, AO B1.2. **a** Impacted fractures in subtle valgus position. The dense sclerotic rim simulates marginal osteophytes and should not be mistaken for a pseudofracture (*arrow*). Note the discrete disruption of the superior cortex of the femoral neck (*open arrow*). **b** The axial radiograph shows the amount of displacement and posterior rotation of the femoral head

fractures, the findings may be limited to subtle irregularities of the cortex, a sclerosed line laterally, and breaks of the trabecular pattern (Fig. 11.25). Complete fractures show a break of the medial cortex of the femoral neck. The femoral head is usually in a valgus position and posterior rotation is best seen on groin lateral views (Fig. 11.37). In displaced fractures, the greater trochanter is externally rotated and displaced superiorly. Varus displacement of subcapital fractures is rare and may be difficult to diagnose. The line of impaction is seen medially and the break in the cortex occurs superiorly. Impacted fracture can produce sclerotic areas in the subcapital area which may be mistaken for marginal osteophytes in osteoarthritis of the hip (Fig. 11.37). Vice versa, osteoarthritis of the hip can produce faint lines of sclerosis that can be misinterpreted as impacted fractures (pseudofracture).

The classifications proposed by Garden and Pauwels are commonly used to stage subcapital frac-

tures (Pauwels 1973; Garden 1961, 1974) (Figs. 11.38, 11.39). The AO classification gives a more compehensive classification of fractures of the femoral neck, however (Müller et al. 1990). In this classification, the fractures of the femoral neck are organized according to their morphological severity, the difficulty of treatment, and their prognosis (Fig. 11.40).

The Garden classification defines four stages. It is based upon whether stable reduction of the fracture can be achieved. *Type 1* represents an incomplete impacted fracture of the femoral neck with disruption of the lateral cortex and valgus position of the femoral head (Fig. 37). In *type 2*, the subcapital fracture is complete, but without rotation and displacement of the femoral head (Fig. 11.41). Types 3 and 4 represent displaced fractures. In *type 3* the complete fracture is partially displaced (Fig. 11.42). The femur is externally rotated and the femoral head is in the varus position, resulting in medially angulated trabe-

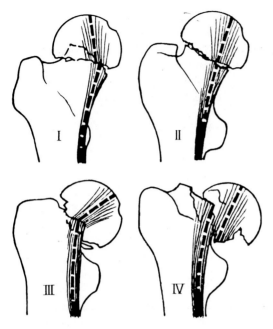

Fig. 11.38. Garden classification for subcapital fractures of the femoral neck, types 1–4. For details see text. (From MÜLLER et al. 1990)

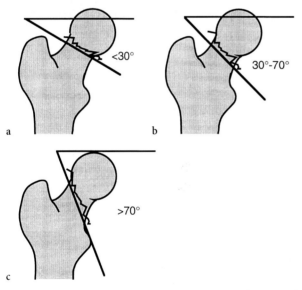

Fig. 11.39a–c. Pauwels classification of subcapital fractures of the femoral neck

culae. The fracture surfaces have maintained partial contact with one another. *Type 4* fractures are completely separated and there is no residual contact of the fracture surfaces (Fig. 11.43). The femoral head has returned to its normal position in the acetabulum and there is no angulation of the trabeculae.

In the classification of Pauwels, the angulation of the fracture line is related to the prognosis. The best prognosis is supposed for *Pauwels 1* fractures, with a fracture line that is horizontal or angulated less than 30° to a horizontal plane (Fig. 11.41) and the worst prognosis is assumed for *Pauwels 3* fractures, which have a fracture line at an angle of more than 70° with the horizontal plane. This classification system has been questioned, because the subcapital fractures are relatively constant in position and direction (GARDEN 1974). They extend as a short spiral from posterosuperiorly to the anteromedial aspect of the femoral neck. The projection of this line depends on the rotation of the femur and can cause the impression of either a horizontal or a rather vertical fracture line (GARDEN 1974).

11.2.6 Fractures of the Trochanteric Region

11.2.6.1 General Considerations

As compared with fractures of the femoral neck, trochanteric fractures are associated with higher forces.

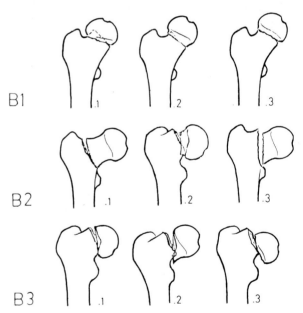

Fig. 11.40. AO classification of fractures of the femoral neck. *B1,* Subcapital fractures impacted in valgus ≥15° (*B1.1*), in valgus <15° (*B1.2*), or without impaction (*B1.3*). *B2,* Transcervical fractures of the femoral neck: basocervical (*B2.1*), midcervical with adduction (*B2.2*), and midcervical shear fractures (*B2.3*). *B3,* Displaced and nonimpacted subcapital fractures: subcapital fractures with moderate displacement in varus and external rotation (*B3.1*), with moderate displacement with vertical translation and external rotation (*B3.2*), and with marked displacement of the femoral head (*B3.3*). (From MÜLLER et al. 1990)

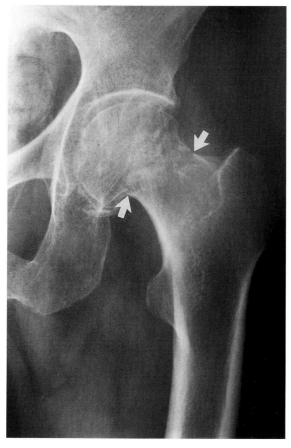

Fig. 11.41. Subcapital fracture of the femoral neck. Classification: Garden 2, Pauwels 1, AO B1.3. Note the subtle breaks of the superior and inferior cortex of the femoral neck (*arrows*)

Elderly patients are more often affected and the incidence is the same in males and females (ALFFRAM 1964; GANZ et al. 1979). Trochanteric fractures are more extensive than fractures of the femoral neck, and cause larger hematomas. Nevertheless, due to better intra-osseous blood supply and the extracapsular location, avascular necrosis and nonunions are infrequent complications. Trochanteric fractures are subdivided into intertrochanteric, subtrochanteric, and avulsion fractures.

11.2.6.2 Classification, Trauma Pattern, and Pathomorphology

11.2.6.2.1 Intertrochanteric Fractures. In intertrochanteric fractures, fracture lines extend between the greater and lesser trochanters and basically four different types can be described (Fig. 11.44). The fracture line of the simple two-part fracture runs between the greater and lesser trochanters. Such fractures may be difficult to differentiate from basocervical fractures of the femoral neck. The greater and lesser trochanters may be separated (three- and four-part fractures) and they may consist of several fragments. Less often, fracture lines extend into the subtrochanteric region and, rarely, reverse fracture lines can be seen. The degree of comminution may be difficult to assess on a.p. radiographs and additional views should be obtained routinely (ANDERSEN et al. 1990).

Trochanteric fractures are usually described according to Evans as stable or unstable (EVANS 1949) or by the AO classification (Figs. 11.45, 11.46a–d). Nevertheless, the terms "stable" and "unstable" only relate to the fact that some fractures are easier to stabilize than others, and none of them is stable without surgery (MÜLLER et al. 1990). Two-part fractures consist of the femoral head and neck proximally and the femoral shaft distally, and are generally stable. In three- and four-part fractures, instability increases

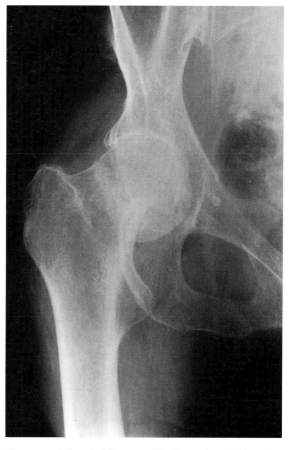

Fig. 11.42. Subcapital fracture of the femoral neck. Classification: Garden 3, Pauwels 2, AO B3.1

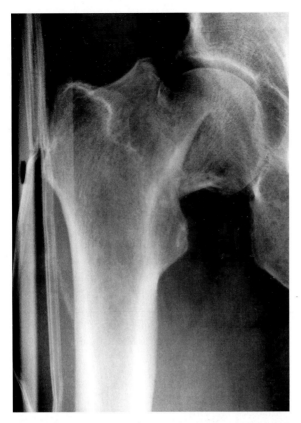

Fig. 11.43. Subcapital fracture of the femoral neck. Classification: Garden 4, Pauwels 2, AO B3.3

lesser trochanter (ROGERS 1992). Subtrochanteric fractures are discussed separately from fractures of the femoral shaft because they are unstable and require specific treatment. They mainly occur in the elderly and are less common than fractures of the femoral neck and intertrochanteric fractures (Fig. 11.47). In young patients they result from severe trauma or represent pathologic fractures (BILDNER and FINNEGAN 1989). Especially in transverse subtrochanteric fractures, pathologic processes have to be excluded.

11.2.6.2.3 Avulsion Fractures of the Trochanters. In juveniles and children, avulsions of the greater trochanter result from abrupt and forceful contractions of the abductors and external rotators of the hip. In adults, localized fractures of the greater trochanters are generally caused by direct trauma. Separation and distraction are usually secondary to avulsion. Avulsion fractures of the lesser trochanter are also more common in children and juveniles. They result from sudden contractions of the iliopsoas muscle. In adults they may be caused by underlying disease and local pathology has to be excluded.

with the degree of comminution, especially if the areas of the calcar femorale and the lesser trochanter are fractured. The highest degree of instability is found in cases in which the fractures extend into the subtrochanteric region and the fracture line runs reversely from medial to lateral in a caudal direction.

The AO classification describes the intertrochanteric fractures according to morphological criteria, the complexity of their treatment, and their prognosis. Type A1 fractures are simple two-fragment fractures with a single disruption of the medial cortex. Type A2 fractures present at least two fracture lines medially and are subdivided by the number of fragments and the dorsal destruction of the cortex. In both type 1 and type 2 fractures the lateral cortex of the femur remains intact. In type A3 fractures, fracture lines extend from the region above the lesser trochanter to the lateral cortex.

11.2.6.2.2 Subtrochanteric Fractures. The definition of subtrochanteric fractures remains controversial, but they are considered to be within 5 cm below the

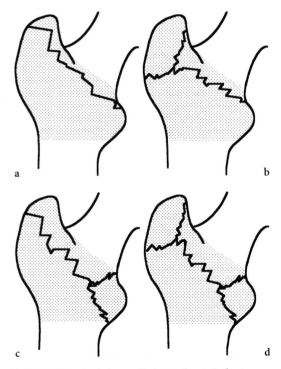

Fig. 11.44a–d. Four basic types of intertrochanteric fracture: **a** simple two-part fractures; **b,c** comminuted fractures with separation of the greater (**b**) and lesser (**c**) trochanter (three-part fractures); **d** comminuted fractures with separation of both trochanters (four-part fracture)

Fig. 11.45. AO classification of trochanteric fractures. *A1*, Simple petrochanteric fractures with single breaks of the medial cortex: *A1.1*, fractures along the intertrochanteric line; *A1.2*, fractures involving the greater trochanter with or without impaction; *A1.3*, fractures extending into the medial cortex below the lesser trochanter. *A2*, Multifragmentary petrochanteric fractures with multiple discruptions of the medial cortex: *A2.1*, with an additional posteromedial fragment; *A2.2*, with several intermediate fragments; *A2.3*, with several intermediate fragments and fracture of the medial cortex below the lesser trochanter. *A3*, Intertrochanteric fractures: *A3.1*, simple reversed fractures, which start about the lesser trochanter, with or without additional fragment of the greater trochanter; *A3.2*, simple transverse fractures with or without involvement of the greater trochanter; *A.3.3*, multifragmentary reversed fractures with separation of the lesser trochanter. (From MÜLLER et al. 1990)

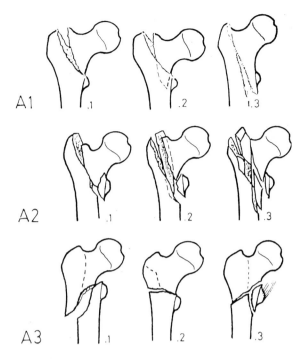

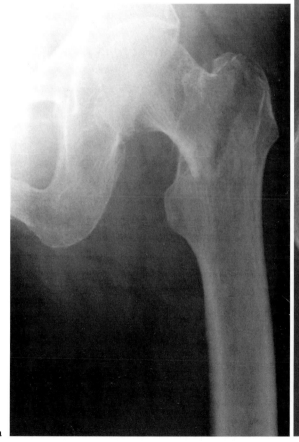

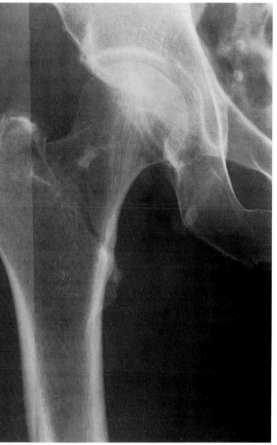

Fig. 11.46a–d. Intertrochanteric fractures. **a** Two-part fracture with fracture extending along the intertrochanteric line. External rotation and cranial migration of the femur. Valgus position of the femoral neck. AO classification A1.1. **b** Three-part fracture with a fragment of the greater trochanter. Fracture line extending through the greater trochanter to the medial cortex above the lesser trochanter. AO classification A1.2. **c** Three-part fracture with separation of the lesser trochanter. AO classification A2.1. **d** Four-part fracture, extending into the subtrochanteric area. The fracture line disrupting the lateral cortex extends from medial to lateral in a caudal direction. AO classification A3.3

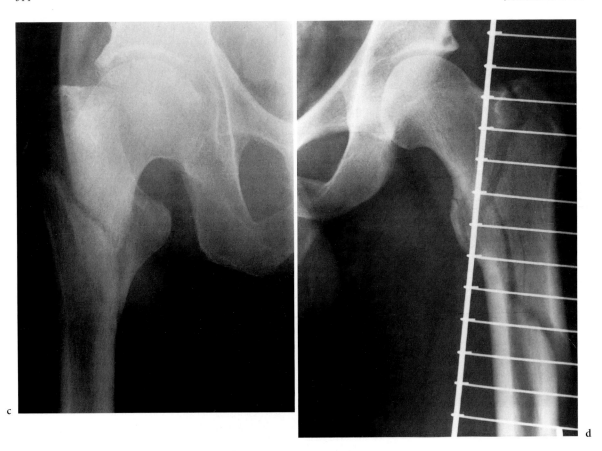

c   d

Fig. 11.46c–d

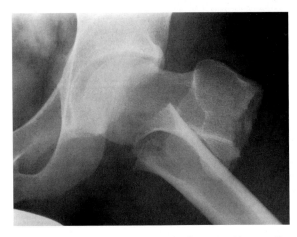

Fig. 11.47. Subtrochanteric transverse fracture with gross displacement following a motor vehicle accident

11.2.7 Miscellaneous

The proximal femur is a common site for pathologic fractures. These fractures usually result from local disease, such as bone tumors and metastasis. They may also be caused by radiation therapy. Nevertheless, subcapital fractures can have a pathologic appearance in osteoporotic patients (SCHWAPPACH et al. 1993). Stress fractures of the femoral neck occur in a physically active population, whereas insufficiency fractures present in bones with underlying disease, such as rheumatoid arthritis, Paget's disease, and renal osteodystrophy (Fig. 11.48). Insufficiency fractures may also be related to steroid therapy (BILDNER and FINNEGAN 1989; HA et al. 1991; TATEISHI et al. 1992; BOGOCH et al. 1993). Both types of fracture can progress to incomplete, complete, and displaced fractures and adequate trauma is generally missing. The most common locations for these types of fracture are the subcapital regions of the femoral neck superolaterally and the base of the femoral neck inferiorly. The radiographic features are ill-defined lines of sclerosis and a focal cortical lucency surrounded by sclerotic bone formation (Fig. 11.48). About 40% of stress and insufficiency fractures are missed on early radiographs, and therefore patients with adequate clinical findings and negative plain film should undergo MRI or bone

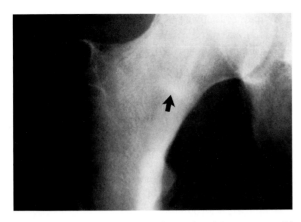

Fig. 11.48. Stress fracture of the femoral neck in a 20-year-old male. Note the circumscribed area of sclerosis (*arrow*)

scintigraphy (ROGERS 1992; HOLDER et al. 1990; DEUTSCH et al. 1989; TYRELL and DAVIES 1994).

11.2.8 Complications

Complications of fractures of the hip and the proximal femur depend greatly on the intra- or extracapsular location and the degree of comminution. Common complications of dislocations and fracture dislocations of the hip are osteoarthritis, avascular necrosis of the femoral head, and sciatic nerve injuries. Less common complications are infections, myositis ossificans, redislocations, and refractures.

Posttraumatic osteoarthritis is the most common complication (EPSTEIN 1973; DELEE 1991) after fractures of the femoral head, but it is less frequent than following acetabular fractures. Avascular necrosis of the femoral head after dislocation of the hip is related to delayed reduction and the type of associated femoral head fracture (Fig. 11.49). Pipkin type 3 fractures have the worst prognosis. In 10%–20% of the dislocations sciatic nerve palsy can be observed, with a preference for the peroneal portion (DELEE 1991). The high frequency of associated injuries of the lower extremity, i.e., fractures of the femur, may cause dislocations of the hip to be missed initially.

Following fractures of the femoral neck, avascular necrosis of the femoral head is the most important complication. The highest incidence of avascular necrosis is found following subcapital fractures. The risk of ischemic complications decreases with a more lateral location of the fracture. Avascular necrosis may occur between 5 months and 3 years after the initial injury (BARNES et al. 1976). The highest risk

for avascular necrosis of the femoral head is reported with Garden type 3 and type 4 fractures and with Pauwels type 2 and type 3 fractures (BARNES et al. 1976; GARDEN 1961; IVERSEN 1986). Nonunion of the fracture results from insufficient reduction and inadequate immobilization and is related to poor blood supply. Nonunions occur in about 25% of femoral neck fractures (BARNES et al. 1976).

11.2.9 Special Features of Trauma in Children and Adolescents

In children, fractures of the hip and the proximal femur are very rare. Except for the epiphyseal growth plate, the proximal femur of children is extremely strong. Pathologic fractures and child abuse have to be anticipated if only minor trauma is reported with these injuries. Simultaneous fractures of the pelvis are frequent and, therefore, should be excluded.

In children, traumatic dislocations of the hip are more frequent than fractures. Dislocations of the hip may be caused by minor trauma and usually occur without additional fractures of the acetabular rim. With increasing rigidity of the bones, greater forces are necessary to dislocate the hip. Posterior dislocations are 7–10 times more common in children than in adults (CANALE and KING 1991). The clinical outcome depends on several factors, including severity of the original trauma, the time between injury and reduction, the success of reduction, and avascular necrosis. A wide joint space after reduction indicates possible entrapment of soft tissue, i.e., joint capsule

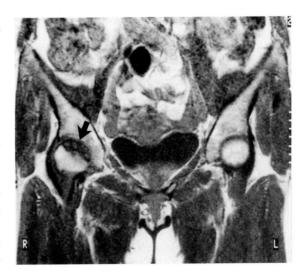

Fig. 11.49. Avascular necrosis of the right femoral head (*arrow*) following depression fracture (T1-weighted coronal MRI)

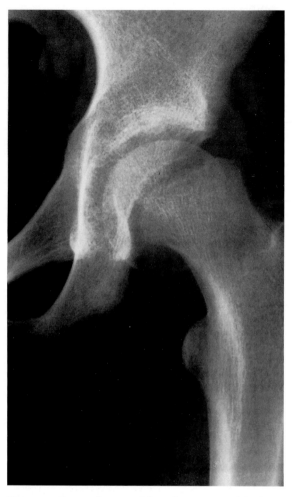

Fig. 11.50. Traumatic transepiphyseal separation of the femoral head

and open reduction with pin fixation in more severe dislocations of the epiphysis.

Unlike in adults, fractures of the femoral neck in children occur in the midcervical and, more frequently, in the basocervical region. Intertrochanteric and subtrochanteric fractures are less frequent than femoral neck fractures. Impacted fractures are rare in children, due to the rigidity of the bones. Cases of nondisplaced fractures and correctly reduced fractures are treated conservatively, while grossly displaced and incorrectly reduced fractures have to be operated on. The initial degree of displacement is crucial for the prognosis.

Avascular necrosis is the most common and most severe complication following injuries to the hip and the proximal femur. The incidence ranges from 100% for dislocated traumatic transepiphyseal fractures to 14% for intertrochanteric fractures (CANALE and KING 1991). Depending on the degree of displacement of fractures of the femoral neck, the frequency of avascular necrosis of the femoral head ranges from 50% in displaced cases to less than 10% in cases without displacement. Premature closure of the epiphysis is found in 9%–61% and may be caused by avascular necrosis and pins crossing the epiphyseal plate. Varus deformity of the hip can result from incorrect reduction, secondary displacement, and premature closure of the epiphysis of the femoral head. Premature closure of the epiphysis of the greater trochanter can lead to coxa valga deformities. Nonunions of fractures occur in 6.5%–13% (CANALE and KING 1991).

and labrum, which has to be excluded. Entrapped soft tissues may not be visible on CT, and MRI and CT-arthrography may be necessary for the diagnosis.

In children, fractures of the proximal femur consist of transepiphyseal separations, transcervical fractures, and basocervical and intertrochanteric fractures (CANALE and KING 1991). Transepiphyseal separations are traumatic epiphyseolysis, which are extremely rare and can be classified as Salter-Harris type 1 fractures (Fig. 11.50). Usually the epiphysis has slipped in a posterior and medial direction. Transepiphyseal fractures can occur with and without dislocation of the femoral head. They have the worst prognosis if the epiphysis is dislocated out of the acetabulum. Since transepiphyseal separation is difficult to detect on a.p. radiographs, additional oblique views are necessary. Treatment consists in closed reduction in patients with mild dislocation

11.2.10 Diagnostic Algorithm

Overall, plain radiography is sufficient to evaluate trauma of the hip and the proximal femur. The initial evaluation should include a.p. radiographs of the pelvis and, if necessary, coned down views of the hip. All fractures should be documented in at least two projections. Additional oblique views help to rule out involvement of the acetabulum. Conventional tomography may be applied for the diagnosis of occult and complex fractures and to document the healing. CT should be performed in all cases with suspected and proven involvement of the femoral head and the acetabulum. CT provides superior demonstration of fractures of the femoral head and acetabulum and of entrapped fragments in the joint space; it is also helpful for the detection of occult fractures. Although CT can be used for the diagnosis of osteonecrosis, this complication of fractures and dislocations is generally better diagnosed with bone scintigraphy and MRI. MRI is the most sensitive imaging modality for the diagnosis of osteonecrosis and for the analysis of viability of the femoral head. It is exquisitely suited to proving occult fractures and associated soft tissue injuries.

References

Alberts KA, Dahlborn M, Ringertz H (1987) Sequential scintimetry in prediction of healing rates after femoral neck fracture. Arch Orthop Trauma Surg 106:168–172

Alffram PA (1964) An epidemiologic study of cervical and trochanteric fractures of the femur in an urban population. Analysis of 1664 cases with special reference to etiologic factors. Acta Orthop Scand 65 (Suppl):1–109

Andersen E, Jørgensen LG, Hededam LT (1990) Evans' classification of trochanteric fractures: an assessment of the interobserver and intraobserver reliability. Injury 21:377–378

Barnes R, Brown JT, Garden RS et al. (1976) Subcapital fractures of the femur. A prospective review. J Bone Joint Surg (Br) 58:2–24

Bildner S, Finnegan M (1989) Femoral fractures in Paget's disease. J Orthop Trauma 3:317–322

Bogoch ER, Oullette G, Hastings DE (1993) Intertrochanteric fractures of the femur in rheumatoid arthritis patients. Clin Orthop 294:181–186

Burgess AR, Tile M (1991) Fractures of the pelvis. In: Rockwood CA Jr, Green DP, Buchholz RW (eds) Rockwood and Green's fractures in adults, vol 2, 3rd edn. Lippincott, Philadelphia, pp 1399–1479

Calmers J, Irvine GB (1988) Fractures of the femoral neck in elderly patients with hyperparathyroidism. Clin Orthop 229:125–130

Campbell JE (1983) Urinary tract trauma. J Can Assoc Radiol 34:237–248

Canale ST, King RE (1991) Pelvic and hip fractures. In: Rockwood CA Jr, Wilkins KE, King RE (eds) Rockwood and Green's fractures in children, vol 3, 3rd edn. Lippincott, Philadelphia, pp 991–1120

Catsikis BD, French WM, Norcus G, Brotman S, Smith JL, Harris RD (1989) CT diagnosis of bowel herniation at pelvic fracture site. J Comput Assist Tomogr 13:148–149

Chenoweth DR, Cruickshank B, Gertzbein SD, Goldfarb P, Janosick J (1980) A clinical and experimental investigation of occult injuries of the pelvic ring. Injury 12:59–65

Dawson I, van Rijn AB (1989) Traumatic anterior dislocation of the hip. Arch Orthop Trauma Surg 108:55–57

De Smet AA, Neff JR (1985) Pubic and sacral insufficiency fractures: clinical course and radiological findings. AJR 145:601–606

DeLee JC (1991) Fractures and dislocations of the hip. In: Rockwoood CA, Green DP, Buchholz RW (eds) Rockwood and Green's fractures in adults, vol 2, 3rd edn. Lippincott, Philadelphia, pp 1481–1651

Deutsch AL, Mink JH, Waxman AD (1989) Occult fractures of the proximal femur: MR imaging. Radiology 170:113–116

Dihlmann W, Heller M (1985) Asterisk-Zeichen und adulte ischämische Femurkopfnekrose. Fortschr Röntgenstr 142:430–435

Egund N, Nilsson LT, wingstrand H, Strömquist B, Pettersson H (1990) CT scans and lipohaemarthrosis in hip fractures. J Bone Joint Surg (Br) 72:379–382

Epstein HC (1973) Traumatic dislocations of the hip. Clin Orthop 92:116–142

Evans EM (1949) The treatment of trochanteric fractures of the femur. J Bone Joint Surg (Br) 31:190–203

Ganz R, Thomas RJ, Hammerle CP (1979) Trochanteric fractures of the femur. Treatment and results. Clin Orthop 138:30–40

Garden RS (1961) Low-angle fixation in fractures of the femoral neck. J Bone Joint Surg (Br) 43:647–663

Garden RS (1974) Reduction and fixation of subcapital fractures of the femur. Orthop Clin North Am 5:683–712

Ha KI, Hahn SH, Chung MY, Yang BK, Yi SR (1991) A clinical study of stress fractures in sports activities. Orthopedics 14:1089–1095

Heller M, Jend HH (1986) Pelvic injuries. In: Heller M, Jend HH, Genant HK (eds) Computed tomography of trauma. Thieme, Stuttgart, pp 89–102

Heller M, Kötter D, Wenzel E (1980) Computer-tomographische Diagnostik des traumatisierten Beckens. Fortschr Röntgenstr 132:386–391

Holder LE, Schwarz C, Wernicke PG, Michael RH (1990) Radionuclide bone imaging in the early detection of fractures of the proximal femur (hip): multifactorial analysis. Radiology 174:509–515

Iversen BJ, Aalberg JR, Naver LS (1986) Complications of fractures of the femoral neck. Ann Chir Gynaecol 75:341–344

Jacob JR, Rao JP, Ciccarelli C (1987) Traumatic dislocation and fracture dislocation of the hip. A long-term follow-up study. Clin Orthop 214:249–263

Judet R, Judet J, Letournel E (1964) Fractures of the acetabulum: classification and surgical approaches for open reduction. J Bone Joint Surg (Am) 46:1615–1648

Jungbluth KH, Sauer HD (1977) Ergebnisse operativ versorgter schwerer Hüftverrenkungsbrüche. Chirurg 48:786–792

Kaulbach C, Heller M, Triebel HJ, Spielmann RP, Richartz-Heller M (1989) Radiologische Diagnostik der Azetabulumfrakturen. Radiologe 29:501–507

Klenerman L, Marcuson RW (1970) Intracapsular fractures of the neck of the femur. J Bone Joint Surg (Br) 52:514–517

Kreitner KF, Weigand H (1993) Becken, Hüftgelenk und proximales Femurende. In: Thelen M, Ritter G, Bücheler E (eds) Radiologische Diagnostik der Verletzungen von Knochen und Gelenken. Thieme, Stuttgart, pp 381–449

Lansinger O (1977) Fractures of the acetabulum. A clinical, radiological and experimental study. Acta Orthop Scand 165 (Suppl):1–125

Larson CB (1973) Fracture dislocations of the hip. Clin Orthop 92:147–154

Looser KG, Crombie HD Jr (1976) Pelvic fractures: an anatomic guide to severity of injury. Review of 100 cases. Am J Surg 132:638–642

Magid D (1994) Computed tomographic imaging of the musculoskeletal system. Current status. Radiol Clin North Am 32:255–274

Martinez CR, DiPasquale TG, Helfet DL, Graham AW, Sanders RW, Ray LD (1992) Evaluation of acetabular fractures with two- and three-dimensional CT. Radiographics 12:227–242

Melton LJ, Sampson JM, Morrey BF, Ilstrup DM (1981) Epidemiologic features of pelvic fractures. Clin Orthop 155:43–47

Muckle DS (1976) Iatrogenic factors in femoral neck fractures. Injury 8:98–101

Müller ME, Nazarian S, Koch P, Schatzker J (1990) The comprehensive classification of fractures of the long bones. Springer, Berlin Heidelberg New York

Nilsson BE (1970) Spinal osteoporosis and femoral neck fracture. Clin Orthop 68:93–95

Nutton RW, Pinder IM, Williams D (1982) Detection of sacroiliac injury by bone scanning in fractures of the pelvis and its clinical significance. Injury 13:473–477

Ogden JA (1974) Changing patterns of proximal femoral vascularity. J Bone Joint Surg (Am) 56:941–950

Panetta T, Sclafani SJA, Golstein AS, Phillips TF, Shaftan GW (1985) Percutaneous transcatheter embolization for massive bleeding from pelvic fractures. J Trauma 25:1021–1029

Pauwels F (1973) Atlas zur Biomechanik der gesunden und kranken Hüfte. Springer, Berlin Heidelberg New York

Peltier LF (1965) Complications associated with fractures of the pelvis. J Bone Joint Surg (Am) 47:1060–1069

Pennal GF, Tile M, Waddel JP, Garside H (1980) Pelvic disruption: assessment and classification. Clin Orthop 151:12–21

Pipkin G (1957) Treatment of grade IV fracture-dislocation of the hip. J Bone Joint Surg (Am) 39:1027–1042

Ponseti IV (1978) Growth and development of the acetabulum in the normal child. J Bone Joint Surg (Am) 60:575–585

Potter HG, Montgomery KD, Heise CW, Helfet DL (1994) MR imaging of acetabular fractures: value in detecting femoral head injury, intraarticular fragments, and sciatic nerve injury. AJR 163:881–886

Rizzo PF, Gould ES, Lyden JP, Asnis SE (1993) Diagnosis of occult fractures about the hip. J Bone Joint Surg (Am) 75:395–401

Roeder L Jr, DeLee JC (1980) Femoral head fractures associated with posterior hip dislocations. Clin Orthop 147:121–130

Rogers LF (1992) Radiology of skeletal trauma. Churchill Livingstone, New York, pp 991–1197

Schild H, Müller HA, Klose K, Ahlers J, Hüwel N (1981) Anatomie, Röntgenologie und Klinik der Sakrumfrakturen. Fortschr Röntgenstr 134:522–527

Schmitt R, Schindler G, Gay B, Brendel H, Riemenschneider J (1987) Computertomographische Diagnostik bei Acetabulumfrakturen. RÖFO 146:628–635

Schwappach JR, Murphey MD, Kokmeyer SF, Rosenthal HG, Simmons MS, Huntrakoon M (1993) Subcapital fractures of the femoral neck: prevalence and cause of radiographic appearance simulating pathologic fracture. AJR 162:651–654

Sinha SN (1985) Simultaneous anterior and posterior dislocation of the hip joints. J Trauma 25:269–270

Speer KP, Spritzer CE, Harrelson JM, Nunley JA (1990) Magnetic resonance imaging of the femoral head after acute intracapsular fracture of the femoral neck. J Bone Joint Surg (Am) 72:98–103

Stevens J, Freeman PA, Nordin BEC et al. (1962) The incidence of osteoporosis in patients with femoral neck fracture. J Bone Joint Surg (Br) 44:520–527

Stewart MJ, McCarroll HR, Mulhollan JS (1975) Fracture-dislocation of the hip. Acta Orthop Scand 46:507–525

Tateishi H, Maeda M, Yoh K, Nakano T, Nakano K (1992) Pathologic fracture associated with amyloid deposition in the bone of a chronic hemodialysis patient. A case report. Clin Orthop 274:300–304

Tehranzadeh J, Vanarthos W, Pais MJ (1990) Osteochondral impaction of the femoral head associated with hip dislocation: CT study in 35 patients. AJR 155:1049–1052

Thaggard A, Harle TS, Carlson V (1978) Fractures and dislocations of bony pelvis and hip. Semin Roentgenol 13:117–134

Tile M, Pennal GF (1980) Pelvic disruption: principles of management. Clin Orthop 151:56–64

Trueta J (1968) Die Anatomie der Gefässe des Oberschenkelkopfes und ihre Empfindlichkeit gegenüber traumatischer Schädigung. H Unfallheilk 97:18–28

Tyrell PN, Davies AM (1994) Magnetic resonance imaging appearance of fatigue fractures of the long bones of the lower limb. Br J Radiol 67:332–338

Watts HG (1976) Fractures of the pelvis in children. Orthop Clin North Am 7:615–624

Weigand H, Sarfert D, Schweikert CH, Walde HJ (1978) Die reine traumatische Hüftluxation des Erwachsenen. Unfallheilk 81:20–27

Williams PC, Warwick R, Dyson M, Bannister LH (1989) Gray's anatomy, 37th edn. Churchill Livingstone, New York, pp 516–526

12 Knee, Including Distal Femur, Proximal Tibia, and Fibula

C. Muhle, M. Reuter, and M. Heller

CONTENTS

C. Muhle, MD, Klinik für Radiologische Diagnostik,
Klinikum der Christian-Albrechts-Universität, Arnold-Heller-
Straße 9, 24105 Kiel, Germany
M. Reuter, MD, Klinik für Radiologische Diagnostik,
Klinikum der Christian-Albrechts-Universität, Arnold-Heller-
Straße 9, 24105 Kiel, Germany
M. Heller, MD, Professor and Direktor, Klinik für
Radiologische Diagnostik, Klinikum der Christian-Albrechts-
Universität, Arnold-Heller-Straße 9, 24105 Kiel, Germany

12.1 Radiographic Techniques

For evaluation of injuries to the knee, the minimum standard radiographic views include anteroposterior and lateral radiographs.

12.1.1 Anteroposterior View

The anteroposterior (AP) view is obtained with the patient supine, the leg extended, and the patella positioned anteriorly. On this view the plateaus slope 15° posteriorly and are not visualized tangentially. The patella overlies the patellofemoral groove and the medial femoral condyle. Its distal portion lies at the level of the intercondylar notch. The head of the fibula is overlapped by the lateral margin of the tibia on the frontal projection. The AP view demonstrates the medial and lateral compartments, as well as the opposing margins of the femoral condyles and the tibial plateaus.

12.1.2 Lateral View

The lateral view is obtained by positioning the patient on the side with the involved knee adjacent to the table top. In this position the knee should be flexed about 15–30°. On the lateral view, the plateaus are manifested by a sharp, well-defined cortical line projected beneath the tibial spine. The medial and lateral plateaus are projected independently. The femoral condyles are rarely perfectly superimposed since the medial condyle is larger and there is invariably a small degree of rotation. The quadriceps tendon is visualized at the superior border of the patella and is separated from the anterior surface of the femur by a layer of fat (prefemoral fat pad). The infrapatellar tendon extends from the inferior margin of the patella to the anterior tibial tubercle and is accentuated by the presence of the infrapatellar fat pad lying between the tendon and the femoral condyles. The lateral view allows assessment of injuries of the patella, the patellofemoral joint, the tibial plateau, and the upper fibula.

12.1.3 Oblique Views

The oblique views are obtained with the patient supine. For the internal oblique view, the leg is internally rotated about 45°. This view provides good detail of the upper fibula and tibiofibular articulation and the medial portion of the patella (Fig. 12.14c).

The external oblique view is obtained using the same parameters but with the leg rotated externally 45°. The fibula is projected behind the upper tibia. It displays the lateral margin of the patella, the medial tibial plateau, and the medial femoral condyle (Fig. 12.7).

12.1.4 Special Projections

12.1.4.1 Notch View

The notch view is specially designed to visualize the intercondylar notch. It is obtained in the posteroanterior projection with the knee flexed. This is helpful in evaluating patients with osteochondrosis dissecans, in visualizing avulsions of the femoral margins of the cruciate ligaments and in detecting osteochondral fragments in the joint space.

12.1.4.2 Patellar Views

Patellar views can be obtained with the patient in either the supine or the prone position. Numerous techniques have been described for evaluation of the patella (BAUMGARTL 1964; LAURIN et al. 1978; MERCHANT et al. 1974; SETTEGAST 1921; WIBERG 1941). In these views the configuration of the patella and femoral condyles and their relative positions are demonstrated. The axial view visualizes the joint surface of the patella, its medial and lateral facets, and the patellofemoral groove. The axial views of the patella are required to evaluate the position of the patella, fractures of the patella, and the patellofemoral joint space (Figs. 12.33, 12.34).

12.1.4.3 Stress Views

For the assessment of suspected ligament injury stress views are difficult to perform in the injured knee. In this situation accompanying pain and swelling cause muscular tension, which hampers this technique. To overcome this limitation anesthetic injection, general anesthesia, or spinal anesthesia is required. The primary benefit of this technique lies in the evaluation of chronic injuries and follow-up of ligamentous reconstructions. The examination can be performed manually by fixing the extremity with a bolster or strap and applying force in the opposite direction or inside commercial devices (Fig. 12.1).

12.1.4.4 Tomography

Tomography is indicated to clarify any suspicious site of fracture irrespective of its location and in the detection of occult fractures (APPLE et al. 1983). It is of particular value in examination of tibial plateau fractures (Figs. 12.11, 12.14). In these cases, tomography has been recommended to evaluate the amount of particular surface depression or displacement, the site of the fracture, and the extent of comminution. Tomography is especially useful in differentiating split-depression fractures from fractures in which depression of the articular surface alone is present.

12.1.5 Ultrasound

Ultrasound is a noninvasive technique and a useful method in the evaluation of joint effusion and

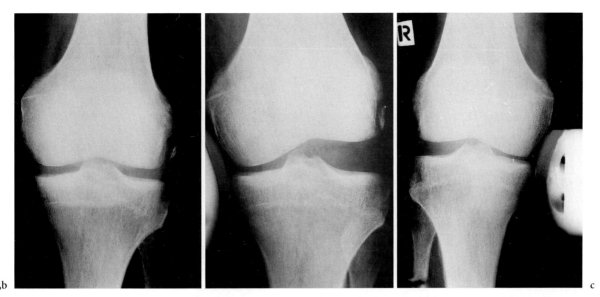

a,b   c

Fig. 12.1a–c. Left knee of a 20-year-old basketball player. **a** Lateral collateral ligament tear with a thin cortical fragment avulsed from the lateral femoral condyle. **b** Stress view (15 kp) demonstrates a lateral joint space opening of 22 mm on the left side compared with 13 mm on the uninjured right side **c**, suggesting a left-sided lateral collateral ligament tear

meniscal, capsular, and synovial cysts and in the detection of patellar tendon or quadriceps tendon ruptures. It also can be helpful in the diagnosis of intra-articular fragments in osteochondral fractures. Compared with magnetic resonance imaging (MRI), ultrasound has been proved to be less sensitive and specific in the detection of meniscal and cruciate ligament tears.

12.1.6 Arthrography

Because of the invasive nature and the very good results of MRI in the detection of meniscal and cruciate ligament tears, MRI has replaced arthrography in the evaluation of meniscal and cruciate ligament injuries (ROGERS 1992).

12.1.7 Angiography

Angiography of the popliteal artery is required in the presence of a supracondylar fracture of the femur, dislocation of the knee, and widely displaced fractures of the proximal tibia or distal femur. The indication for angiography is based on the clinical examination of the leg. When there is a question of diminution of the pulse, coolness of the extremity, or both, angiography may be necessary.

12.1.8 Computed Tomography

Computed tomography (CT) is helpful in evaluating tibial plateaus, the patellofemoral joint, the proximal tibiofibular joint, and the femoral condyles (Figs. 12.9, 12.13). CT better visualizes the degree of comminution of a tibial fracture than does plain film radiography or tomography, and fractures involving the margins of the plateau may be better demonstrated. An added advantage is the ability to perform examinations through casts. Additionally with CT it is possible to obtain reconstruction images in the sagittal, coronal, or oblique plane (Figs. 12.13, 12.21).

12.1.9 Magnetic Resonance Imaging

Magnetic resonance imaging demonstrates excellent visualization of bone and soft tissue structures (CRUES et al. 1987; CRUES and STOLLER 1993; DE SMET et al. 1993; LEE et al. 1988; MINK 1993; ZEISS et al. 1992). The continuity of the menisci, cruciate ligaments and quadriceps and patellar tendons is easily demonstrated. MRI has the added advantage of being noninvasive compared with arthrography and arthroscopy. MRI has become the method of choice in the radiological diagnosis of meniscal tears, collateral ligament tears, cruciate ligament tears, and occult osseous injuries (Figs. 12.15, 12.16; for more details see Sects. 12.3.1.5.1 and 12.3.1.5.2).

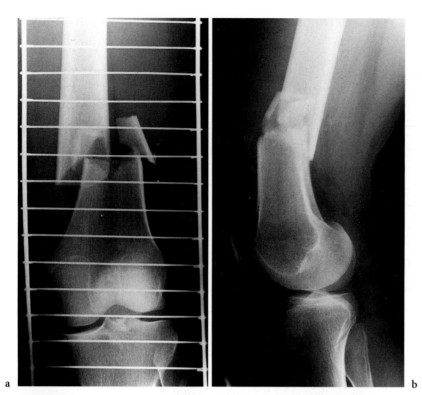

Fig. 12.2a,b. Displaced distal femur fracture with a fragment at the lateral margin of the femur in a 32-year-old man. **a** AP and **b** lateral projections

a

b

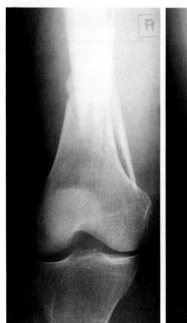
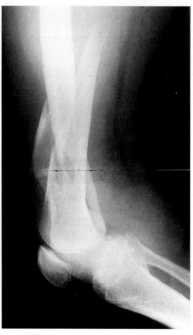

Fig. 12.3a,b. Displaced fracture of the distal femur without involvement of the supracondylar and condylar regions. **a** AP and **b** lateral projections

a

b

12.2 Fractures of the Distal Femur

12.2.1 General Considerations

The average age of patients affected by distal femur fractures is variable but has been taken to be between 40 and 50 years, with no sex predominance

(BERQUIST 1992). Fractures of the distal femur are most often sustained in motor vehicle accidents or falls from heights (Figs. 12.2, 12.3; KUNER 1975). These injuries often result from axial loading combined with varus and valgus stress and rotation. They may occur in association with other injuries, including ligamentous disruption of the knee, patel-

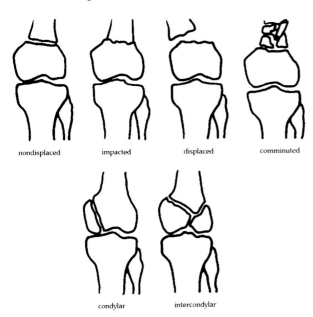

Fig. 12.4. Fractures of the distal femur are classified according to the site and extension of the injury as supracondylar (nondisplaced, impacted, displaced, comminuted), condylar, and intercondylar

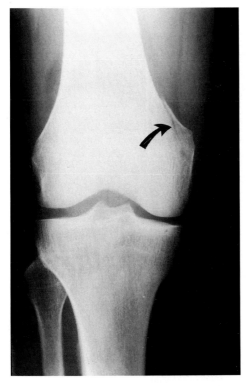

Fig. 12.5. Nondisplaced supracondylar fracture (AP projection). Note the vertical fracture at the medial femoral metaphysis (*arrow*)

lar fractures, fracture-dislocations of the hip, and fractures of the tibial shaft (KIMBROUGH 1961; RESNICK 1995).

12.2.2 Classification, Trauma Pattern, and Pathomorphology

Fractures of the distal femur are classified according to the site and the extension of the fracture line as supracondylar, condylar, or intercondylar (Fig. 12.4).

12.2.2.1 Supracondylar Fractures

Supracondylar fractures are frequently transverse or slightly oblique, with varying degrees of displacement and comminution of the fracture fragments (Fig. 12.5). Because the extension of a fracture into the joint has important therapeutic implications, every supracondylar fracture should be carefully examined to identify or exclude this possibility.

12.2.2.2 Condylar and Intercondylar Fractures

Fractures of the femoral condyles are intra-articular fractures confined to one or both condyles (ROGERS 1992). These fractures, in which sagittal and coronal fracture lines are isolated to the region of a condyle (Fig. 12.6), are more difficult to detect on radiographic examination and may require conventional or computed tomography (COCKSHOTT et al. 1985; DAFFNER and TABAS 1987). Often the femoral condylar fractures are Y or T shaped, with the sagittal component extending into the intercondylar notch. They may then be described as intercondylar fractures (Fig. 12.7).

12.2.3 Examination Methods

Distal femur fractures are normally well demonstrated on anteroposterior and lateral radiographs, but if there is any question of extension into the joint, oblique views are needed (Fig. 12.7; COCKSHOTT 1985; DAFFNER and TABAS 1987). In some cases special projections such as notch views or tomography and CT may be required for full evaluation of the fracture lines and localization of the fragments.

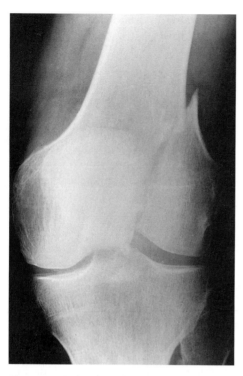

Fig. 12.6. Displaced condylar fracture of the lateral femoral condyle in a 65-year-old man. AP projection

12.2.4 Complications

Complications of dislocated distal femur fractures can result in associated injuries, mainly of the popliteal artery or with fracture-dislocation of the hip (KIMBROUGH 1961). As a result of high-impaction forces, as are encountered in automobile and motorcycle accidents, distal femur fractures also can be associated with fractures of the tibial shaft. The knee is then isolated from the remainder of the extremity, which is described as "floating knee" (LETTS et al. 1986).

12.3 Fractures of the Proximal Tibia

12.3.1 Tibial Plateau Fractures

12.3.1.1 General Considerations

The tibial plateau is the most common site of fractures of the proximal tibia (DOVEY and HERFORDT 1971; HOHL 1967; NEWBERG and GREENSTEIN 1978). The etiology of these injuries is variable. In only 25% of cases are tibial plateau

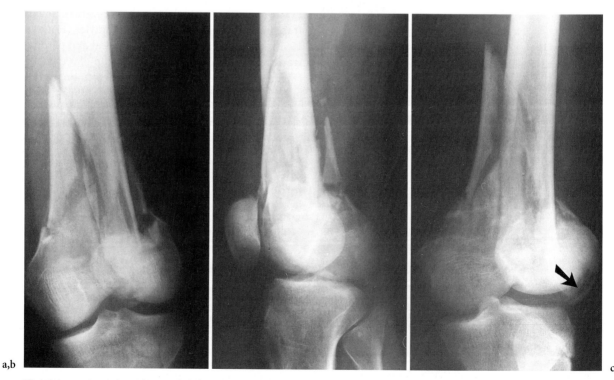

a,b　　　c

Fig. 12.7a–c. Comminuted intercondylar fracture. On the external oblique view (**c**) an avulsed fracture (*arrow*) of the inferior margin of the patella is recognized, which is not well seen on the AP (**a**) and lateral (**b**) projections

Fig. 12.8a–f. Hohl's classification of tibial plateau fractures. **a** Nondisplaced split fracture; **b** central depression fracture; **c** split-depression fracture; **d** displaced depression fracture; **e** local split fracture of the anterior or posterior condylar margin; **f** displaced, comminuted fracture of both tibial condyles. (From Hohl 1967)

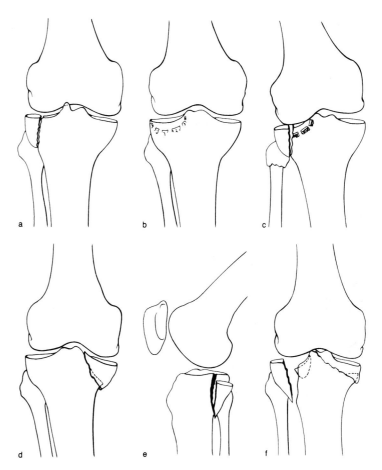

fractures related to motor vehicle accidents ("fender" or "bumper" fractures). Most are the result of twisting falls, and a small number follow blows to the lateral surface of the knee. Although tibial plateau fractures may occur in young persons, tibial plateau fractures predominate in middle-aged and elderly people.

12.3.1.2 Anatomy and Biomechanics

Some anatomic aspects are of interest for the interpretation of tibial plateau fractures. In a knee with normal alignment the greater portion of the weight is transmitted through the medial femoral condyle to the medial tibial plateau. This is evidenced by a greater number of trabeculae within the medial femoral condyle and beneath the medial plateau. The lateral tibial plateau is weaker and less capable of supporting weight because of fewer and finer trabeculae within the lateral tibial condyle. For this reason and because valgus stress is far

more common than varus stress, isolated lateral plateau fractures are seen in 70%–80% of all tibial plateau fractures (Porter 1970). Combined lateral and medial tibial plateau fractures are even more frequent (10%–15%) than isolated medial plateau fractures (5%–10%), fractures of the posterior margin (about 3%), or comminuted bicondylar fractures (10%).

12.3.1.3 Classification, Trauma Pattern, and Pathomorphology

Different classification systems have been suggested for tibial plateau fractures. The most widely utilized classification, however, is that of Hohl, which gives an overview of six different types of tibial plateau fracture (Fig. 12.8; Hohl 1967).

The *nondisplaced split fracture* shows minimal fracture impaction or displacement of less than 3 mm and little disruption of the articular surface (Figs. 12.9, 12.10).

Displaced fractures are graded according to the degree and character of the damage to the tibial plateau. The *central depression fracture* is characterized by mosaic-like depressed fragments (Fig. 12.11). In a *split-depression fracture* an outer portion of the tibial condyle is split off with greater or lesser depression of the more central articular surface (Fig. 12.12). The *displaced depression fracture* is characterized by lack of comminution of the articular surface (Fig. 12.13). However, the entire condyle is impacted or displaced distally and laterally, with resultant angular deformity of the knee. The *local split fracture* is infrequent, but usually involves the anterior or posterior condylar margin without significant central depression of the condyle. The *displaced, comminuted tibial fracture* has been described as the T- or Y-fracture because both condyles are disrupted (Fig. 12.14). Considerable damage to the articular surfaces and menisci is the rule (HOHL 1967).

Although tibial plateau fractures are related to a variety of mechanisms, which include vertical compression, varus and valgus forces, and twisting, lateral tibial plateau fractures are created by a combination of valgus force on the knee caused by abduction of the tibia and compression forces generated by impaction of the femoral condyles against

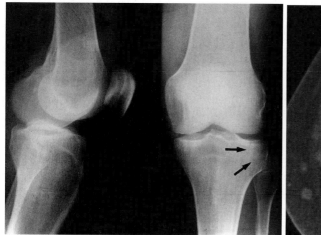
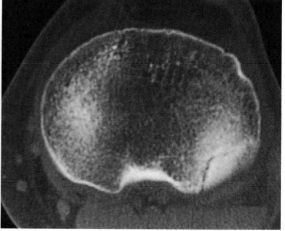

a   b

Fig. 12.9. a AP and lateral views of a nondisplaced split fracture (*arrows*) with minimum depression (3 mm) of the lateral tibial plateau. **b** No displacement of the fracture is seen on the axial CT scan

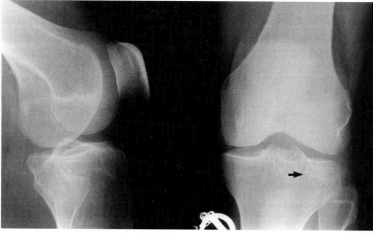
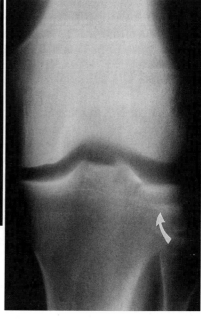

a

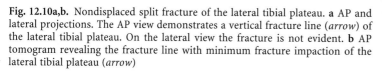

Fig. 12.10a,b. Nondisplaced split fracture of the lateral tibial plateau. **a** AP and lateral projections. The AP view demonstrates a vertical fracture line (*arrow*) of the lateral tibial plateau. On the lateral view the fracture is not evident. **b** AP tomogram revealing the fracture line with minimum fracture impaction of the lateral tibial plateau (*arrow*)

b

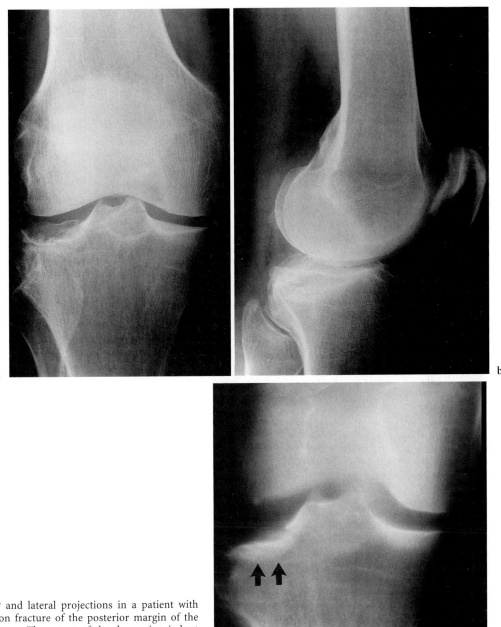

Fig. 12.11 a,b. AP and lateral projections in a patient with a central depression fracture of the posterior margin of the lateral tibial plateau. c The extent of the depression is best visualized on AP tomography (*arrows*)

the tibial plateau. Medial tibial plateau fractures are mainly caused by varus stress and adduction of the tibia, which occur less frequently than valgus stress. Comminuted fractures of the plateaus of both condyles are usually related to vertical compression.

12.3.1.4 Examination Methods

Fractures of the tibial plateau may not be obvious on the routine radiographic examination of the knee, particularly if there is no depression. One of the reasons is the anatomic configuration of the tibial plateau. It is sloped posteriorly from the horizontal axis between 10° and 20°, with an average of 15°. The usual anteroposterior radiograph of the knee is, therefore, not obtained tangential to the tibial joint surface. The anterior margin of the joint is projected superior to the posterior margin because of this angulation. Because of this oblique orientation, depression fragments involving the anterior portion of the plateaus can be overlooked, and depression of

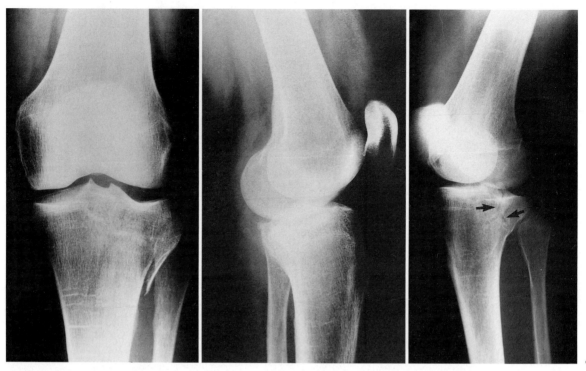

a,b   c

Fig. 12.12. a AP view of a split-depression fracture of the lateral tibial plateau without considerable displacement in a 21-year-old man. **b** The fracture is not visualized on the lateral projection. **c** On the internal oblique view the split fracture (*arrows*) is well seen

fragments involving the posterior portion of the plateau can be overestimated. Therefore oblique projections and conventional or computed tomography with reconstructions are frequently required for accurate assessment of these injuries (Figs. 12.9–12.14; BUTT et al. 1983; COCKSHOTT et al. 1985; DAFFNER and TABAS 1987; ELSTROM et al. 1976; MOORE and HARVEY 1974; NEWBERG and GREENSTEIN 1978; RAFII et al. 1984; SCHILD et al. 1983).

12.3.1.5 Injuries
Associated with Tibial Plateau Fractures

An important feature of tibial plateau fractures is their association with soft tissues injuries of the knee (NICOLET 1965; STALLENBERG et al. 1993).

12.3.1.5.1 Ligamentous Injuries. The incidence of injuries to the collateral ligaments of the knee in association with tibial condylar fractures has been reported to be as high as 12% in operatively and radiographically verified cases. In these patients, tears of the medial collateral ligament and the anterior cruciate ligament are most frequent and usually occur in conjunction with fractures of the lateral

tibial plateau (KUNER 1975; STALLENBERG et al. 1993; WILPPULA and BAKALIM 1972).

MRI of Collateral Ligament Tears. The collateral ligaments are visualized as thin, linear, dark bands of low signal intensity on both T1- and T2-weighted images.

The medial collateral ligament consists of a superficial and a deep portion. The superficial portion of the ligament typically arises from the medial femoral condyle and passes distally to insert approximately 5 cm below the joint line. Superficial fibers are sepa-

Fig. 12.13a–e. Displaced depression fracture of the lateral tibial plateau in a 36-year-old man. **a** On the AP view the fracture is seen as a vertical-oblique line extending from the articular surface to the lateral margin of the tibial plateau. **b** The lateral view demonstrates the depressed fragment of the lateral tibial plateau as a hazy increase in density (*arrows*) at the lateral tibial condyle due to depression and impaction of fracture fragments. **c** Axial CT scan demonstrates a comminuted fracture with a deep central spongiosa defect (*arrow*). **d** Sagittal and **e** coronal CT reconstructions demonstrate the displaced lateral condyle. The fracture line extends to the intercondylar eminence. The articular surface is depressed less than 5 mm

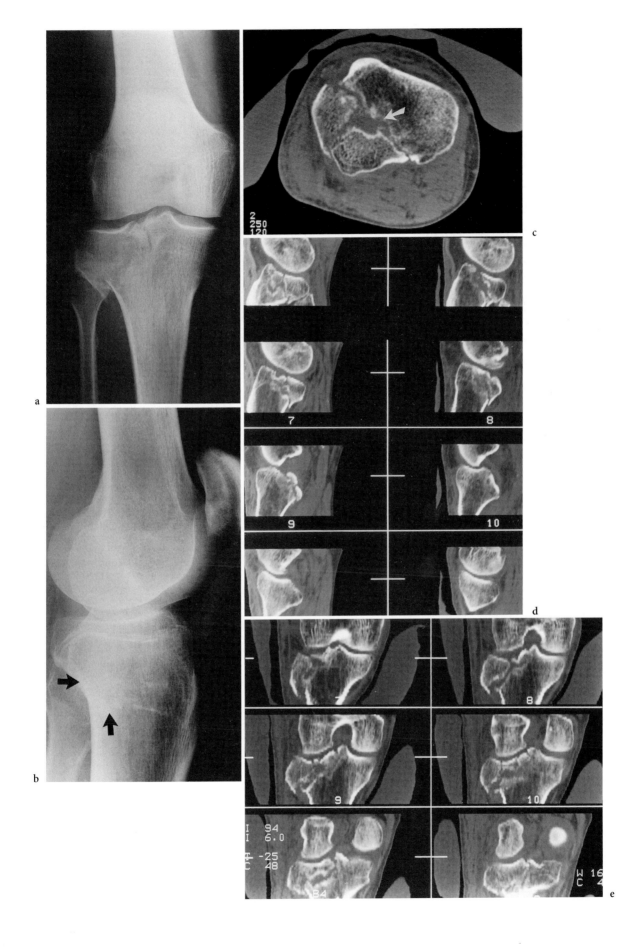

a

b

c

d

e

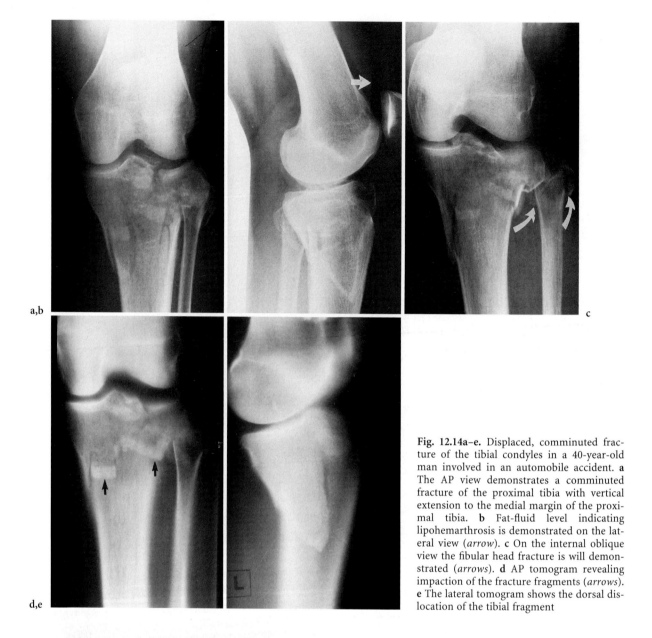

a,b

c

d,e

Fig. 12.14a–e. Displaced, comminuted fracture of the tibial condyles in a 40-year-old man involved in an automobile accident. **a** The AP view demonstrates a comminuted fracture of the proximal tibia with vertical extension to the medial margin of the proximal tibia. **b** Fat-fluid level indicating lipohemarthrosis is demonstrated on the lateral view (*arrow*). **c** On the internal oblique view the fibular head fracture is will demonstrated (*arrows*). **d** AP tomogram revealing impaction of the fracture fragments (*arrows*). **e** The lateral tomogram shows the dorsal dislocation of the tibial fragment

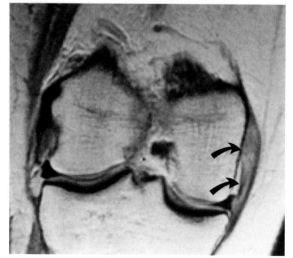

Fig. 12.15. Partial tear of the medial collateral ligament (*curved arrows*) on a coronal T1-weighted spin-echo image (TR 450 ms, TE 20 ms). There is still continuity of the superficial layers; subligamentous hemorrhage of the medial collateral ligament is evident

rated from the deep fibers by a bursa. The deep ligament is firmly attached to the capsule and midportion of the medial meniscus and attaches to the femur and tibia more nearly adjacent to the joint (MINK et al. 1988; MINK 1993).

With complete tears both the tibial collateral and the capsular ligaments are disrupted. This is depicted as discontinuity and serpiginous irregularity of the ligament (Figs. 12.15, 12.25). There is accompanying surrounding hemorrhage and edema of intermediate signal intensity on T1-weighted images that increase in intensity on T2-weighted images.

The lateral collateral ligament is less commonly injured. It is a thin, linear dark band similar in signal intensity to that of the anterior cruciate ligament. The lateral collateral ligament extends from the lateral surface of the femoral condyle to insert on the head of the fibula. The course is oblique from anterosuperior to posteroinferior, and therefore the entire ligament is usually not seen on a single image, like the medial collateral ligament. The appearance of sprains and tears is similar to that of the medial collateral ligament (MINK 1993; ROGERS 1992).

MRI of Cruciate Ligament Tears. On MRI the anterior and posterior cruciate ligaments are distinctive not only in their location and course, but also in the difference in their normal signal. The anterior cruciate ligament is best seen in the sagittal plane with 10–20° of external rotation of the knee. Without such rotation the entire length of the ligament is not captured on one image. The normal anterior cruciate ligament is depicted as a low-signal intensity band, commonly with two or three separate fiber bundles, extending from the anterior tibial plateau to the medial surface of the lateral femoral condyle (LEE et al. 1988; MINK et al. 1988; MINK 1993; VAHEY et al. 1991). The anterior cruciate ligament is the most frequently torn ligament. In an acute tear as depicted on MRI, either the anterior cruciate ligament is obviously disrupted or its anterior margin is wavy or concave and not straight as when the ligament is intact (Figs. 12.16, 12.25). In acute tears fluid or edema is shown with high signal intensity on T2-weighted images. Tears usually appear as foci of increased signal intensity, often accompanied by widening of the ligament (Figs. 12.16, 12.25; MINK et al. 1988; MINK 1993; LEE et al. 1988; ROGERS 1992). In complete tears of the anterior cruciate ligament, discontinuity is present in a low signal intensity band with or without loss of normally parallel margins. Partial or complete ligamentous disruptions may be associated with blurring of the cruciate fascicles due

to edema or hemorrhage. Accurate assessment of partial ligamentous tears is more difficult than the detection of complete disruptions. Posterior bowing of the anterior cruciate ligament or buckling of the posterior cruciate ligament may be associated with increased laxity from a partial or chronic tear of the anterior cruciate ligament. Anterior displacement of the tibia on lateral sagittal images is a secondary sign of anterolateral instability. This anterior drawer sign is dependent on the degree of knee flexion, position-

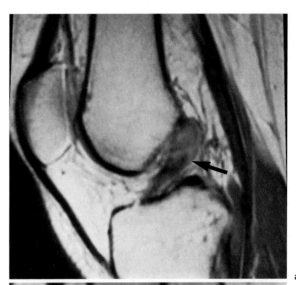

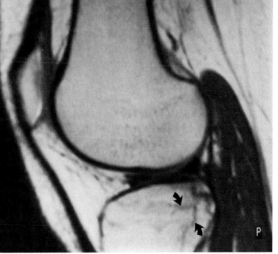

Fig. 12.16a,b. Twenty-seven-year-old soccer player with an anterior cruciate ligament tear and bone bruise of the posterior margin of the tibial condyle. **a** Sagittal T1-weighted image (TR 450 ms, TE 20 ms) revealing fullness in the region of the anterior cruciate ligament tear (*arrow*). The remainder of the ligament is poorly defined and there is no area of distinctly low signal intensity. **b** Note also the branching linear manifestation of a bone bruise (*arrows*) of the posterior margin of the tibial condyle on the sagittal T1-weighted spin-echo image (TR 500 ms, TE 15 ms)

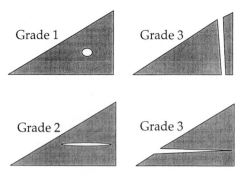

Fig. 12.17. Grading of intrameniscal signal as seen on MRI. In those menisci with punctate areas of increased signal or linear areas of increased signal (grades 1 and 2), focal regions of mucoid degeneration are found. It is likely that some patients with grade 2 increased signal have symptoms associated with mucoid degeneration. Patients with increased signal extending to the articular surface (grade 3) histologically demonstrate meniscal tears

ing, and design of the extremity coil, and its usefulness is limited by lack of comparison with the contralateral knee (MINK et al. 1988; MINK 1993; TUNG et al. 1993; VAHEY et al. 1991).

MRI has demonstrated excellent results in allowing identification of posterior cruciate ligament tears, as confirmed by arthroscopy or arthrotomy (SONIN et al. 1994). The posterior cruciate ligament is usually identified by MRI as a solid black band of low signal intensity that extends in a smooth convex arc from the posterior intercondylar surface of the tibia (ROGERS 1992). Any increase in signal, on either T1- or T2-weighted images, within this normally low signal intensity band can be interpreted as abnormal. Complete disruption of the posterior cruciate ligament demonstrates a loss or gap in ligamentous continuity, whereas partial tears may be more difficult to assess. In some instances an avulsion tear of the tibial plateau may be associated with high-signal ligamentous hemorrhage and a bone marrow fragment (SONIN et al. 1994; STOLLER 1993).

12.3.1.5.2 Meniscal Injuries.
The angular, torsional, and shearing forces which produce disruptions of the tibial condyles also may avulse the corresponding meniscus form its peripheral attachments and it is infrequently found embedded among the fracture fragments. Lateral meniscal injuries are found in 90% of lateral tibial plateau fractures, whereas the medial meniscus is found to be torn in 20% of bicondylar tibial plateau fractures (NICOLET 1965). Acute tears are usually due to athletic injuries with crushing of the meniscus between the tibial and femoral condyles. Chronic repetitive trauma is more

common in the nonathlete and with aging. In this setting, chondrocyte necrosis and increase in mucoid ground substance lead to meniscal tears.

MRI of Meniscal Tears. The menisci are slightly elongated triangles in profile and uniformly black or of low signal intensity. With aging a variable degree of signal often appears within the meniscus (CRUES et al. 1987; CRUES and STOLLER 1993). This initially led to considerable overreading because such signals were misinterpreted as tears of the menisci. It is now recognized that most intrameniscal signal arises from degenerative changes within the meniscus and that only those signals extending to and through the surface of the menisci represent tears (CRUES et al. 1987; CRUES and STOLLER 1993; DE SMET et al. 1993; STOLLER et al. 1987).

Intrameniscal signals are divided into three grades according to the MRI appearance (Fig. 12.17; CRUES et al. 1987; STOLLER et al. 1987):

Grade 1: Globular signal that does not extend to either the superior or the inferior joint surface. Histologically this finding represents a focus of mucinous or myxoid degeneration and is frequently seen

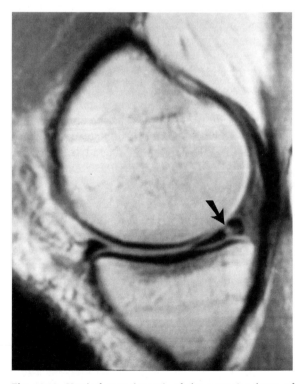

Fig. 12.18. Vertical tear (*arrow*) of the posterior horn of the medial meniscus (grade 3) on a sagittal T1-weighted spin-echo image (TR 450 ms, TE 20 ms) in a 24-year-old soccer player

in asymptomatic individuals. It is considered to be due to mechanical stress.

Grade 2: Linear signal, extending from the periphery on the meniscus at the meniscosynovial junction but confined to the substance of the meniscus without extending to its superior or inferior surface. There should be no vertical component of the signal. It represents further progression of the degenerative process. Patients may be symptomatic but there is no identifiable tear at arthroscopy.

Grade 3: Intrameniscal signal that extends to the articular surface of the meniscus. The articular surface is the superior or inferior surface or free edge of the meniscus, without the meniscus at the meniscosynovial junction or attachment to the joint capsule (Fig. 12.18). Only grade 3 signal alterations represent a tear of the meniscus. Changes in the profile or shape of the menisci are also of importance in the recognition of tears.

12.3.1.5.3 Nerves and Vessel Injuries. Vascular injuries of the popliteal and femoral arteries and nerve damage are comparatively rare, and are found in only approximately 2% of tibial plateau fractures.

12.3.2 Avulsion Fractures

12.3.2.1 General Considerations

Avulsion fractures of the intercondylar eminence occur at the site of origin of the anterior cruciate ligament (Fig. 12.19). These injuries are more common in children and adolescents and often result from a fall from a bicycle (HENARD and BOBO 1983). Such fractures in adults typically are accompanied by ligamentous and meniscal injury, whereas in children they may appear as an isolated phenomenon (MOLANDER et al. 1981).

12.3.2.2 Classification, Trauma Pattern, Pathomorphology, and Methods of Examination of Avulsion Fractures of the Intercondylar Eminence

Avulsion fractures of the intercondylar eminence result from violent twisting, abduction–adduction injuries, or direct contact with the adjacent femoral condyle and are indicative of possible damage to the cruciate ligaments of the knee. Either the anterior tibial spine or, less commonly, the posterior tibial spine is affected, and rarely both are involved. Rou-

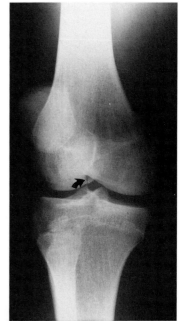

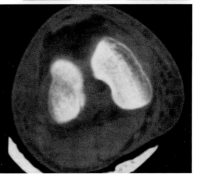

Fig. 12.19a,b. Nondisplaced fracture of the proximal insertion of the anterior cruciate ligament. **a** On the oblique view a small fragment at the proximal insertion of the anterior cruciate ligament is seen (*arrow*). **b** On the axial CT scan a thin fracture line at the medial margin of the lateral femoral condyle is demonstrated

tine radiography supplemented with tunnel projections, radiographs obtained during the application of stress and MRI are important in the assessment of these injuries.

The radiographic appearance of the fracture varies with the degree of displacement (Fig. 12.20). Nondisplaced or minimal displaced fractures (type A; Fig. 12.21) consist of a horizontal fracture line at the base of the anterior portion of the tibial spine (MEYERS and McKEEVER 1959). These are difficult to visualize but are best demonstrated on the lateral view. In more severe injuries the fragment may be lifted upward as a hinge with a gap anteriorly and the fulcrum posteriorly (type B; Fig. 12.22). The frag-

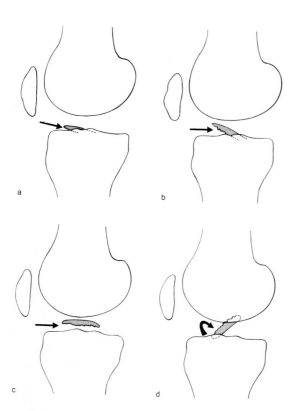

Fig. 12.20a–d. Types of avulsion fracture of the intercondylar eminence. **a** Type A: nondisplaced or minimally displaced avulsion fracture. **b** Type B: displacement of the anterior third to half of the avulsed fragment from the intercondylar eminence produces a beaklike deformity in the lateral projection. **c** Type C: the fragment is completely separated from its bone bed in the intercondylar eminence. **d** Type D: the avulsed fragment is completely lifted from its bone bed of origin in the intercondylar eminence and rotated so that the cartilaginous surface of the fragment faces the bone bed, making union impossible. (From Meyers and McKeever 1959)

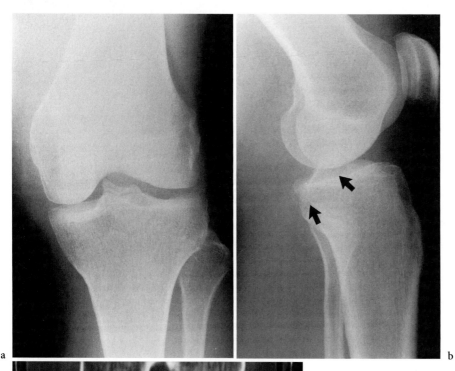

Fig. 12.21a–c. Nondisplaced avulsion fracture (type A) of the intercondylar eminence in a 28-year-old man. **a** AP view. A horizontal fracture line is identified in the intercondylar eminence. **b** On the lateral view the fracture extends to the posterior margin of the intercondylar eminence (*arrows*). **c** On a coronal reconstruction CT scan the fracture extends from the medial to the lateral margin of the intercondylar eminence (*arrows*)

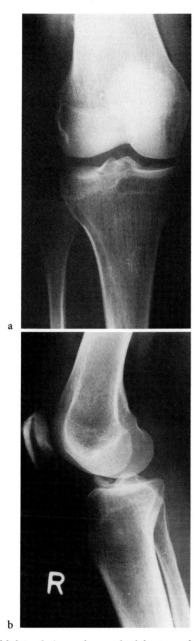

Fig. 12.22. a AP and b lateral views of an avulsed fracture of
the anterior cruciate ligament (type B)

ment may also be completely detached (type C; Fig.
12.23) and even inverted (type D) so that the surface
of the fracture fragment lies superiorly.

Avulsion fractures of the posterior tibial eminence at the site of attachment of the posterior
cruciate ligament are rare (Fig. 12.24). It is unlikely
that such cases represent isolated injuries and
therefore associated injuries of the cruciate
ligament, collateral ligament, and menisci should be
excluded.

12.3.2.3 Trauma Pattern and Pathomorphology of Segond Fracture

Other avulsion fractures may involve the proximal
portion of the tibia. Although, rarely, an avulsion
injury involves the tibial (or femoral) site of attachment of the medial collateral ligament of the knee,
more commonly tibial avulsion occurs at the site of

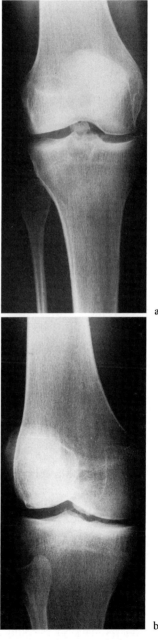

Fig. 12.23. a AP and b external oblique views of an avulsion
fracture of the intercondylar eminence of the tibia. The
avulsed fragment is lifted and completely separated from the
intercondylar eminence (type C)

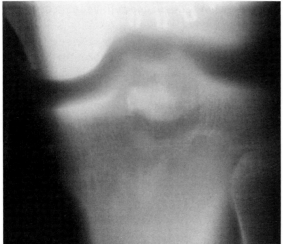

a

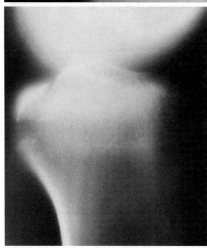

b

Fig. 12.24. a AP and **b** lateral tomograms of the left knee in a 26-year-old football player. Isolated avulsion fracture of the insertion of the posterior cruciate ligament at the posterior margin of the tibial spine

meniscal injuries MRI is often indicated to evaluate fully the bone and soft tissue injury.

12.3.2.4 Trauma Pattern, Pathomorphology, and Methods of Examination of Avulsion Fracture of Gerdy's Tubercle

Avulsion fractures of Gerdy's tubercle of the tibia relate to the tibial band. The bone fragment arising from Gerdy's tubercle lies more anteriorly and slightly more distally compared to the Segond fracture and is best seen on a 45° external rotation view.

12.3.3 Trauma Pattern, Pathomorphology, and Methods of Examination of Subcondylar and Intercondylar Fractures

Subcondylar and intertrochanteric fractures in the condylar portion of the proximal tibia are defined by transverse or obliquely orientated fractures with or without associated fracture of the fibular head (REUTER et al. 1993). They are often comminuted, with one or more fracture lines extending vertically either into the plateaus or into the intercondylar region. These fracture lines may not be immediately obvious on anteroposterior and lateral radiographs, and oblique views may be required for diagnosis.

12.3.4 Trauma Pattern, Pathomorphology, and Methods of Examination of Stress and Insufficiency Fractures of the Tibial Plateau

Stress fractures are commonly seen in military personnel, athletes, and ballet dancers and are localized beneath the medial tibial plateau (ENGBER 1977). Stress fractures are self-limited lesions which respond to limited activity, with resolution of symptoms in approximately 4 weeks. Initial radiographs are frequently normal. In 3–7 weeks a plate-like, 2- to 3-mm-wide band of endosteal callus or sclerosis appears beneath the medial tibial plateau. Periosteal callus is rarely observed, and complete fractures are not encountered.

Elderly people may sustain an insufficiency fracture of the tibial plateau or condyle due to osteoporosis (BAUER et al. 1981; SATKU et al. 1990). These injuries are quite similar to stress fractures in radiographic appearance. Routine radiographs and bone scans may not be as specific in this setting.

insertion of the lateral capsular ligament. This injury, called Segond fracture, occurs with the knee in flexion owing to internal rotation of the tibia (DIETZ et al. 1986). The resulting fracture fragment is located laterally, just distal to the joint line. In 70% to almost 100% of patients with a Segond fracture a disruption of the anterior cruciate ligament is found combined in some patients with medial ligamentous damage. The fracture fragment eventually may merge with the lateral margin of the tibia, producing an outgrowth that simulates an osteophyte. Detection of the fracture can usually be accomplished with routine AP, oblique, or tunnel views. Because of the high incidence of associated anterior cruciate ligament and

MRI usually is more accurate both in diagnosing fractures and in differentiating stress or insufficiency fractures from early osteonecrosis and other knee disorders.

12.3.5 Proximal Fibular and Tibiofibular Joint Injuries

12.3.5.1 General Considerations

Isolated fractures of the head or neck of the fibula are uncommon, but frequently they are combined with ligamentous injuries of the knee or fractures of the lateral tibial plateau or ankle (ROGERS 1992).

12.3.5.2 Classification, Trauma Pattern, Pathomorphology, and Methods of Examination of Proximal Fibular and Tibiofibular Joint Injuries

Fibular head fractures (Fig. 12.14) may result from a direct blow, a varus force (in which an avulsion fracture of the proximal pole or styloid process of the fibula occurs), a valgus force (which is accompanied by a fracture of the lateral tibial plateau and a injury of the medial ligament), or a twisting force of the ankle (in which pronation and external rotation may lead to a fracture in the fibular neck). The combination of adduction stress to the knee, rupture of the lateral capsular and ligamentous structures, injury of the peroneal nerve, and, possibly, an avulsion fracture of the fibula is termed the ligamentous peroneal nerve syndrome.

Dislocations of the tibiofibular joint are uncommon (OGDEN 1974). They may be seen in parachuting, hang-gliding, sky-diving, and horseback riding injuries. They are classified according to whether the displacement of the fibular head is in an anterolateral (which is by far the most common), posteromedial, or superior direction. Superior dislocation is invariably associated with fracture-dislocations of the ankle or fractures of the distal tibia. They may be overlooked if the entire length of the tibia and fibula is not radiographed at the time of the initial examination. Radiographic findings associated with dislocation of the proximal tibiofibular joint may be subtle. As the fibular head is displaced anteriorly, it also moves laterally. This anterolateral movement can be better appreciated upon comparison with radiographs of the uninvolved side or when the relationship of the fibular head to the osseous groove on the posterolateral aspect of the tibia is analyzed carefully. In some instances oblique radiographs may reveal complete separation of the tibia and fibula.

12.4 Knee Dislocations

12.4.1 General Considerations

Knee dislocation is a rare but serious occurrence that has been recorded at the Mayo Clinic only 14 times among 2 million admissions (ROCKWOOD et al. 1991).

12.4.2 Classification, Trauma Pattern, and Pathomorphology

Dislocations of the knee require major force; typical causes include high-energy trauma resulting from motor vehicle accidents, industrial injury, or falls from a great height (Fig. 12.25; HOHL 1975; RESNICK 1995). There are five types of knee dislocation: anterior, posterior, lateral, medial, and rotatory (posterolateral). Anterior dislocation is the most common type, accounting for 30%–50% of knee dislocations; it apparently results from hyperextension of the knee with tearing of the posterior capsule and posterior cruciate ligament. Posterior dislocations are the next most common type and may result from crushing blows to the leg with force applied to the anterior surface of the proximal tibia. Medial, lateral, and rotatory (posterolateral) dislocations of the knee are uncommon, but are often associated with collateral ligament injuries (Fig. 12.25). Although the precise number of ligaments that are torn, stretched, or avulsed during a knee dislocation is variable, involvement of both cruciate ligaments and one or both collateral ligaments is common.

Especially in rotatory (posterolateral) dislocations of the knee, irreducible intra-articular invagination of the medial capsule and medial collateral ligament can be detected.

12.4.3 Examination Methods

In most knee dislocations radiographic diagnosis is not difficult, although different views are required to detect associated osteochondral fractures, fibular head fractures, and avulsion injuries of the tibial spine. Arteriography is required to delineate the status of the popliteal artery in patients with vascular

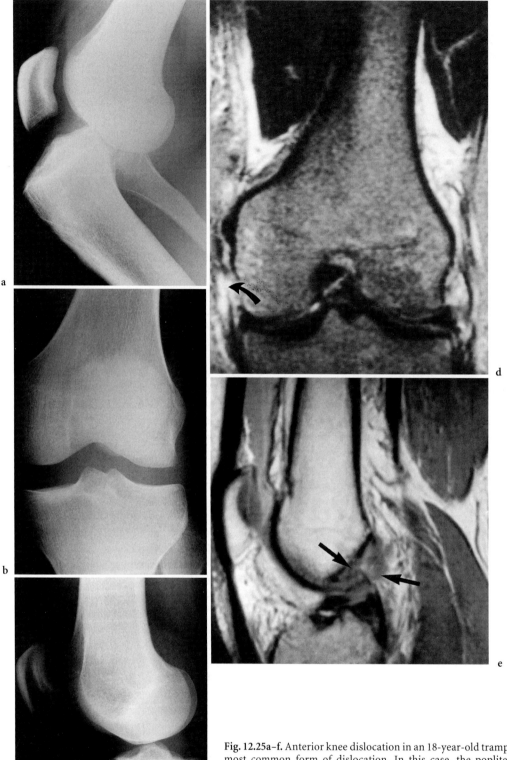

Fig. 12.25a–f. Anterior knee dislocation in an 18-year-old trampolinist. This is the most common form of dislocation. In this case, the popliteal artery was not injured. **a** Anterior knee dislocation. **b,c** After relocation, AP and lateral views demonstrate no evidence of a fracture. **d** Coronal MR image (T2-weighted spin-echo sequence, TR 2400 ms, TE 120 ms) showing a disruption of the medial collateral ligament (*arrow*). **e** On the sagittal T1-weighted spin-echo image (TR 450 ms, TE 20 ms) a tear and discontinuity of the anterior cruciate ligament are seen (*arrows*). **f** Bone contusion (*arrows*) of high signal intensity at the anterior femoral condyle (sagittal T2-weighted spin-echo sequence, TR 2400 ms, TE 120 ms)

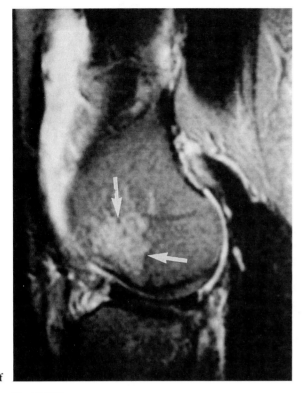

f

Fig. 12.25f

symptoms and signs. For the detection of associated soft tissue injuries, MRI has been recommended as the method of choice (Fig. 12.25).

12.4.4 Complications

Associated injuries may include tibial and fibular fractures in the injured extremity as well as visceral injuries and fractures of the skull. Neighboring structures such as the popliteal vein and tibial and peroneal nerve also may be injured during knee dislocations; popliteal artery injuries occur in 25%–50% of knee dislocations (GREEN and ALLEN 1977).

12.5 Fractures of the Patella

12.5.1 General Considerations

Fractures of the patella are frequent injuries, accounting for 1% of all fractures.

The subcutaneous position of the patella at the anterior aspect of the knee places it in a vulnerable position for direct trauma. Fractures of the patella occur by direct trauma due to motor vehicle accidents, or indirectly from tension forces generated by the quadriceps muscle during falls when severe contraction of the quadriceps muscle occurs with the knee in flexion (Fig. 12.26; MAGERL 1975; FREIBERGER and KOTZEN 1967). Unilateral injuries predominate, although bilateral fractures also are encountered.

12.5.2 Classification, Trauma Pattern, and Pathomorphology

Transverse fractures are typical, representing approximately 50%–80% of all patellar fractures (Figs. 12.27, 12.28). They may divide the patella into equal-sized components or involve the superior or, more commonly, the inferior pole (Fig. 12.29). Longitudi-

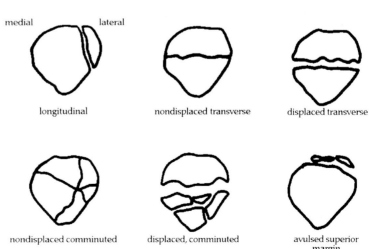

Fig. 12.26. Classification of patellar fractures (adapted from HOHL and LARSON 1975)

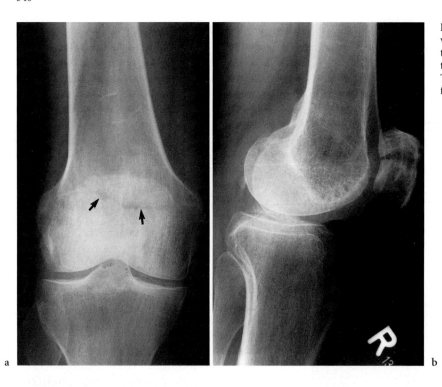

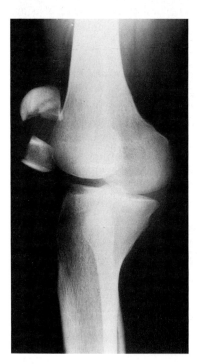

Fig. 12.28. Widely displaced transverse fracture of the patella in a 31-year-old man. On the lateral view the proximal fragment is retracted superiorly by the quadriceps tendon. The distal fragment is angulated anteriorly

nal (Fig. 12.30) and comminuted (Fig. 12.31) or stellate fractures are less frequent and usually result from direct trauma, such as striking the dashboard of an automobile.

12.5.3 Examination Methods

Radiographic diagnosis is easy in most patellar fractures. Comminuted or transverse fracture lines are readily apparent on frontal, oblique, and lateral projections (Figs. 12.27–12.29, 12.31), while longitudinal fractures are best demonstrated on axial radiographs (Fig. 12.30). Fractures of the patella should be differentiated from bipartite or multipartite patella. This anomaly represents a developmental variant of the accessory ossification center and is localized at the superolateral aspect of the bone.

12.5.4 Complications

Complications of fractures of the patella include displacement of osseous fragments, particularly in comminuted fractures, and osteonecrosis appearing 1–3 months after the injury (FREIBERGER and KOTZEN 1967; GILLEY et al. 1981).

Fig. 12.29. **a** AP and **b** lateral views of an avulsion fracture of the inferior pole of the patella (*arrow*)

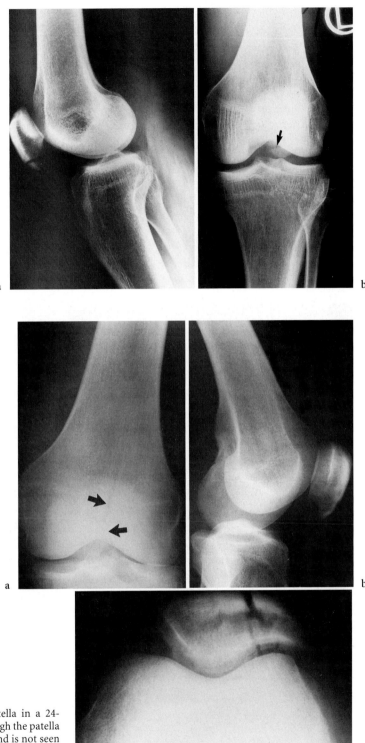

a

b

a

b

c

Fig. 12.30a–c. Longitudinal fracture of the patella in a 24-year-old woman. The longitudinal fracture through the patella is barely visualized on the AP view (**a**; *arrows*) and is not seen on the lateral projection (**b**). **c** On the axial view the fracture is clearly visualized

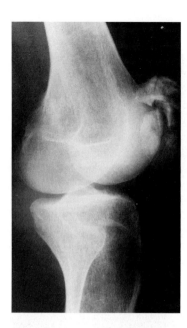

Fig. 12.31. Displaced comminuted fracture of the patella

Fig. 12.32a–d. Osteochondral fracture of the lateral femoral condyle after lateral patellar dislocation in a 27-year-old squash player. **a** On the AP view a small fragment is seen in the intercondylar notch (*arrow*). **b** On the lateral projection the fragment is placed anterior to the femoral condyles (*white arrow*). Note the bone defect at the lateral femoral condyle (*black arrow*). **c** No fracture of the patella is seen on the axial view. Beware of the hypoplastic medial patellar facet representing a predisposing factor for chronic patellar instability. **d** Intraoperative finding of the osteochondral fragment located at the lateral femoral condyle

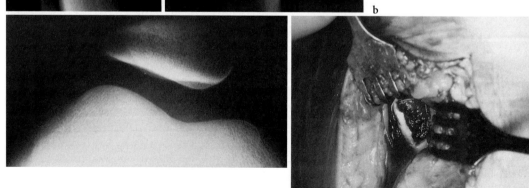

a

b

c

d

12.6 Chondral and Osteochondral Injuries

12.6.1 General Considerations

Chondral and osteochondral lesions involve the articular surface of the knee and have to be rated as severe internal injuries of the joint, since the cartilage lesions will eventually provoke a prearthrosis (MILGRAM et al. 1978). Chondral and osteochondral fractures often occur in adolescents and young adults with no pre-existing knee deformity.

12.6.2 Classification, Trauma Pattern, and Pathomorphology

The lateral femoral condyle and medial surface of the patella are the most common sites of chondral and osteochondral fractures (Fig. 12.32), and the mechanism of injury is usually related to dislocation or relocation of the patella. Osteochondral fractures of the medial femoral condyle may also occur as a result of either rotatory forces applied to a weight-bearing knee or a direct anterior blow to the patella in a flexed knee (GILLEY et al. 1981; FRANGAKIS 1974; FREIBERGER and KOTZEN 1967).

Rotatory or shearing forces generated by acute trauma or impaction forces occurring during a joint dislocation can lead to injury of the articular surface in which a portion of the surface is avulsed (Figs. 12.33, 12.34; JOHNSON-NURSE and DANDY 1985). These injuries may be purely chondral, may include a tiny or large fragment of bone and the entire overlying cartilage (Figs. 12.32–12.34), or rarely may involve bone alone if the overlying cartilage has already been eroded by an unrelated joint process. The resulting fragment may remain in situ or may become a free body in the joint, sometimes lodging and becoming embedded in a distinct portion of the synovial membrane (Figs. 12.32–12.34).

In adolescents and young adults, these fractures usually occur in the subchondral bone due to the lack of calcified cartilage and the elasticity of the articular cartilage, but in adults they often occur at the junction of the calcified and uncalcified cartilage, the so-called tide mark (JOHNSON-NURSE and DANDY 1985; GILLEY et al. 1981).

The pathologic characteristics of chondral and osteochondral fractures are more complex than those of a simple fracture line, consisting of comminution and crushing of cartilage tissue. Beneath the disrupted chondral fragment, the remaining cartilage may appear relatively normal or may demon-strate a blister-like effect. Acutely, any bone that has been separated along with the overlying cartilage appears normal histologically and, at its base, local hemorrhage and crushing of exposed trabeculae may be observed. In more chronic cases, the osteochondral fragment may be attached by a soft tissue pedicle to its site of origin. The composition of this pedicle varies: it may be secure or loose, cartilaginous or fibrous, long or short, and avascular or vascular. In the knee, osteochondral fractures of the femoral condyles commonly result in a mobile lesion containing considerable portions of overlying, intact cartilage and fibrous pedicles. At any site, repair at the base of an osteochondral lesion is associated with

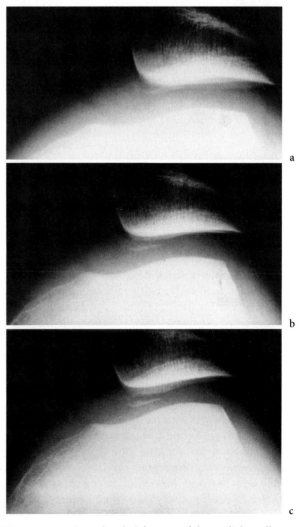

Fig. 12.33a–c. Osteochondral fracture of the medial patellar facet after patellar dislocation. Compared with the axial view at 30° of knee flexion (**a**), the osteochondral fragment and patellar defect are better visualized on the 60° (**b**) and 90° (**c**) axial views. Note the dysplastic patella and the pathologic sulcus angle of the intercondylar groove

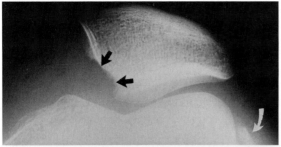

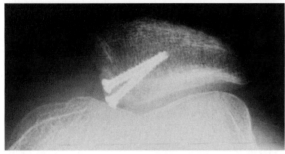

Fig. 12.34a,b. Osteochondral fracture and circumscribed bone defect (*black arrows*) at the medial edge of the patella after patellar dislocation. **a** The fragment (*white arrow*) is displaced at the margin of the lateral femoral condyle. **b** Refixation of the fragment with two screws

fibrocartilaginous proliferative tissue derived from subchondral bone.

12.6.3 Examination Methods

The detection of an osteochondral fragment containing a sizeable piece of bone can be accomplished reasonably well with routine radiography (including anteroposterior, lateral, tunnel, and axial views). In other cases diagnosis may not be possible by radiographic means alone. The fracture fragment may contain only a small segment of bone, not necessarily related to the site of origin (Figs. 12.32, 12.34). It may be located in the suprapatellar bursa, behind the patella, within the intercondylar notch, or beside the femoral condyles within the joint space. Often, when one or two osteochondral fragments are seen, additional chondral fragments may be found at operation. Even when the segment of bone is significant, the actual size of the entire fragment as demonstrated intraoperatively is often much larger than is suggested by radiographs because of the attached but radiographically invisible articular cartilage. Therefore for the depiction of the entire fragment, conventional radiography often has to be supplemented by conventional tomography, CT, or MRI (COCKSHOTT et al. 1985; DAFFNER and TABAS 1987).

In the evaluation of chondral and osteochondral fractures MRI has received considerable attention, including for analysis of the site and size of the lesions and the integrity of the overlying cartilage. On MRI osteochondral fractures may be seen as distinct breaks in the continuity of the low signal intensity of subchondral bone, occasionally with subduction or inward displacement of one or both ends of the fragment, which may be surrounded by a poorly defined region of low signal intensity on T1-weighted images, representing bone contusions. Often the articular bone is simply dented or dimpled inward without a distinct break in the continuity of the cortex. These dents are usually surrounded by an underlying broad-based bone contusion. Although MRI has advantages in the detection of chondral and osteochondral fractures, it is limited in some instances by the inadequacies of standard sequences in accurately delineating articular cartilage. The value of newly developed sequences aimed at the evaluation of chondral lesions remains to be established. Therefore, arthroscopy remains the most accurate method of detailing the chondral defect, whether it be traumatic or osteochondritic in nature. The invasive nature of arthroscopy, however, must be borne in mind.

12.7 Patellar Dislocations

12.7.1 Acute Dislocations of the Patella

12.7.1.1 General Considerations

Patellofemoral instability is a frequent and complex problem that has been studied extensively. Although the incidence of acute patellar dislocations is low, acute patellar dislocation is common among young people, the average age of presentation being approximately 20 years. An acute patellar dislocation may be described as a primary disruption of the patellofemoral relationship where the patella is displaced out of the sulcus.

12.7.1.2 Classification, Trauma Pattern, and Pathomorphology

Acute or traumatic dislocation of the patella is caused by considerable forces produced by a direct blow or an exaggerated contraction of the quadriceps mechanism (SCHARF et al. 1983). The direction of patellar dislocation is most commonly lateral

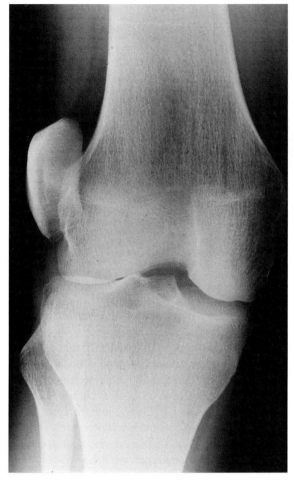

Fig. 12.35. Lateral patellar dislocation of the right knee. AP view

facet or the lateral femoral condyle (Figs. 12.33, 12.34; FREIBERGER and KOTZEN 1967).

12.7.1.4 Complications

Osteochondral fractures occur frequently with dislocation of the patella and may be easily missed on plain x-ray. This had led some clinicians to recommend arthroscopy of all acute patellar dislocations. CT and MRI may be helpful in detecting the cartilage lesions.

12.7.2 Chronic Patellar Instability: Subluxation and Luxation

12.7.2.1 General Considerations

The clinical diagnosis of chronic patellar instability is often difficult, as the resulting symptoms and signs may simulate those of other disorders of the knee. Although observation of the manner in which the patella moves with respect to the femur during flexion and extension of the knee can be accomplished during physical examination, alterations in patellar motion may be subtle.

12.7.2.2 Classification, Trauma Pattern, and Pathomorphology

Recurrent dislocation or subluxation of the patella is a common problem that may result either from an initial acute traumatic dislocation or, more often, from developmental abnormalities. These abnormalities may include the configuration and height of the patella (patella alta, dysplastic patella), the trochlear configuration (deficient height of the lateral femoral condyle, shallowness of the patellofemoral groove), the quadriceps mechanism (lateral insertion of the patellar tendon, muscular weakness, ligament and tendon laxity), genu valgum or recurvatum, or excessive tibial torsion (LANCOURT and CRISTINI 1975; SCHARF et al. 1983).

Lateral dislocation (or subluxation) of the patella is often a transient phenomenon, with spontaneous reduction. Patellar dislocations usually result from a twisting with the knee in flexion and rotated internally on a fixed foot. The patella is pulled laterally from the trochlea and across the lateral femoral condyle, leading to osteochondral injuries of the medial patellar facet, the lateral femoral condyle, or

(Fig. 12.35), although rare patterns of displacement include superior or rotational dislocations, along either the vertical or the horizontal axis of the bone. Medial dislocation of the patella may follow surgical release of the lateral patellar retinaculum.

12.7.1.3 Examination Methods

The diagnosis of acute dislocations of the patella is not difficult if the patella is actually dislocated at the time of presentation. If the patella spontaneously reduces, the diagnosis can be difficult. The patient will usually present with a large hemarthrosis and will have tenderness over the medial retinaculum and under the medial facet of the patella. Often, however, the pain is diffuse, and the diagnosis will remain uncertain.

Radiographs may be helpful if they reveal osteochondral fragments from the medial patella

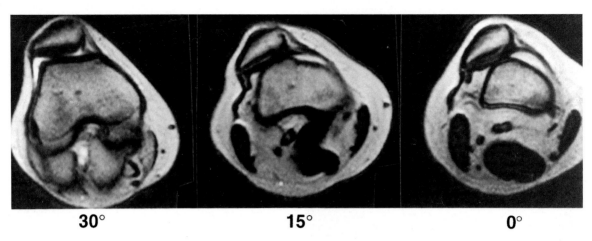

30°   **15°**   **0°**

Fig. 12.36. Eighteen-year-old girl with recurrent patellar dislocation. On this kinematic MRI (TR 10 ms, TE 4 ms) study of the patellofemoral joint, severe lateral patellar subluxation is evident, which was missed on the axial x-ray view at 30° of knee flexion

both structures. The medial retinaculum is injured as a result of dislocation, or a small avulsion fracture at the patellar site of attachment occurs.

12.7.2.3 Examination Methods

Radiographs of the patellofemoral joint must include anteroposterior, lateral, and axial patellar views (BAUMGARTL 1964; DOWD and BENTLEY 1986; WIBERG 1941). A number of different methods based upon the patellar position on the lateral radiograph have been described to confirm the presence of patella alta or baja, i.e., the Blumensaat, Brattstrom, and Insall-Salvati methods (INSALL and SALVATI 1971; LANCOURT and CRISTINI 1975). The advantage of the Insall-Salvati method relates to its lack of dependency on the degree of flexion of the joint. The Insall-Salvati index is determined by the ratio of the length of the patellar tendon to the length of the patella. The value of this ratio is about 1. Any deviation of more than 20% is abnormal.

Axial or tangential (e.g., "sunrise") views of the patella are used in different angle positions (90°, 60°, 45°, 30°) to access the configuration of the trochlea, the patellar shape, and the relationship of the patella to the femur. A variety of techniques for axial patellar radiography have been proposed by different investigators; from these, innumerable indices (such as the congruence angle and the lateral patellofemoral angle) have been developed in an attempt to define the normal patellar position between 30° and 90° of knee flexion (WIBERG 1941; BAUMGARTL 1964; LAURIN et al. 1978; MERCHANT et al. 1974). These methods have proved to be inadequate in assessing

the patellar position at lesser degrees of knee flexion, during which patellar instability is considered to be a greater problem.

Transaxial images provided by CT and MRI allow assessment of the patellar position with the knee in minor degrees of flexion and extension (BROSSMANN et al. 1993; MUHLE et al. 1995; SHELLOCK et al. 1991, 1993; STANFORD et al. 1988). Both imaging techniques allow investigation of patellofemoral relationships during various stages of flexion and extension of the knee; this is usually accomplished by obtaining multiple static images that are viewed in a movie format. Kinematic MRI of the patellofemoral joint under active joint motion demonstrates the influence of quadriceps contraction on the sliding behavior of the patella and provides more information on early patellar subluxation and luxation in the early degree of knee flexion (Fig. 12.36).

12.8 Extensor Mechanism Injuries

12.8.1 General Considerations

The extensor mechanism of the knee consists of the quadriceps and infrapatellar tendons, the patella, and the anterior tibial tubercle. Injuries can be sustained to any of these structures through sudden and severe contraction of the quadriceps muscles while the knee is flexed (NANCE and KAYE 1982). These injuries are often accompanied by small avulsion fractures at either the proximal or distal pole of the patella, avulsion of the anterior tibial tubercle at the insertion of the infrapatellar tendon, or transverse fracture of the proximal or distal pole of the patella.

12.8.2 Classification, Trauma Pattern, and Pathomorphology

12.8.2.1 Quadriceps Tendon Rupture

Rupture of the quadriceps tendon is more likely in the sixth or seventh decade of life and is probably due to a decreased vasculature. Ruptures of the quadriceps tendon are most likely to occur in patients with a previous history of multiple cortisone injections, diabetes mellitus, renal failure, gout, or

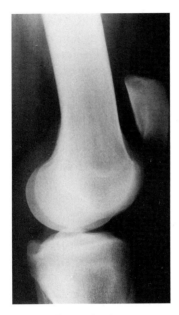

Fig. 12.37. Rupture of the infrapatellar tendon in a 28-year-old volleyball player. On the lateral view the patella is markedly elevated without associated fracture. This finding is typical of rupture of the infrapatellar tendon

hyperparathyroidism. Rarely, spontaneous rupture of the quadriceps tendon is seen in healthy persons (RESNICK 1995). Although the clinical diagnosis of a complete quadriceps tendon rupture should be obvious (based on the patient's history, the inability to extend the knee, a hemarthrosis or soft tissue hematoma and a palpable gap above the patella), it can be delayed or missed (ROCKWOOD et al. 1991).

12.8.2.2 Patellar Tendon Rupture

Patellar tendon ruptures are more likely in patients with chronic patellar tendinitis, and they may occur spontaneously or after sports activity or play in children and adolescents (Fig. 12.37). Failure of the patellar tendon usually occurs at its junction with the inferior pole of the patella or, less commonly, with an avulsion fracture of the tibial tubercle. The superior displacement of the patella is usually obvious, indicating a patella alta, and in most cases is associated with a soft tissue mass, with hemorrhage and hematoma in the region of the patellar tendon. Incomplete tears are not associated with the change in patellar position.

12.8.2.3 Fractures of the Anterior Tibial Tubercle

Fractures of the anterior tibial tubercle are particularly common as a result of jumping activities in adolescents. They are commonly classified into three types (Figs. 12.38, 12.39). When the fracture is fragmented the findings might be confused with those of Osgood-Schlatter's disease. Characteristically, in the

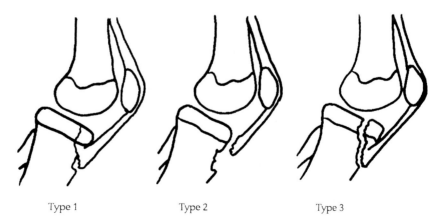

Type 1	Type 2	Type 3

Fig. 12.38. Avulsion fractures of the anterior tibial tubercle. Three types of fractures are described (WATSON-JONES 1955): In type 1 injuries, the tubercle is hinged upward without displacement of the proximal base. The type 2 injury has a smaller portion of the tubercle avulsed, but is retracted proximally. The articular surface is not involved. Type 3 injuries are more severe and extend across the articular surface. There is displacement of the fragment and often comminution

latter all of the separate ossicles are rounded and completely marginated by bone, in contrast to the sharp, angular margins of fracture fragments.

12.8.3 Examination Methods

Radiographic findings associated with complete tears of the quadriceps or patellar tendon reveal soft tissue swelling, distortion of the soft tissue planes above or below the patella, and an inferior (patella

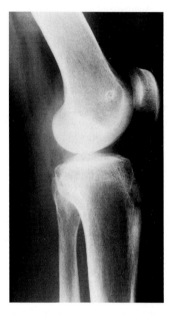

Fig. 12.39. Avulsion fracture of the tibial tubercle in a 24-year-old jumper (type 1). The fracture does not separate the entire tubercle and does not extend into the articular surface

infera) or superior patellar position (patella alta). In quadriceps tendon rupture, additional calcification or ossification within the portions of an avulsed patellar fragment can be seen. Standard arthrography in cases of partial or complete disruption of the quadriceps tendon may be diagnostic. Contrast material introduced into the knee joint will extend outside the quadriceps tendon and, in some cases, into the deep infrapatellar or prepatellar bursa. Owing to the superficial location of the quadriceps and patellar tendons, ultrasonography also may be used in their assessment.

Optimal delineation of the extensor mechanism is obtained by MRI. The latter often distinguishes between a partial and a complete rupture, which has a profound influence on treatment. Normally the quadriceps and patellar tendons are similar in signal intensity to the posterior cruciate and medial and lateral collateral ligaments. Complete tears are manifested by retraction and wavy contours of the separated margins and a mass surrounding the site of the tear that is of intermediate signal intensity on T1- and T2-weighted images. Complications that occur later include angular deformity, leg-length discrepancy, and knee stiffness.

12.9 Special Features of Knee Trauma in Children and Adolescents

12.9.1 General Considerations

Injuries involving the distal femoral and proximal tibial epiphyseal centers are relatively rare. Most are

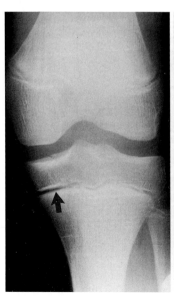
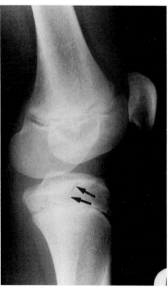

a   b

Fig. 12.40a,b. Salter-Harris type 3 fracture. **a** The AP view demonstrates a vertical fracture of the proximal epiphysis of the tibia and widening (*arrow*) of the medial growth plate. **b** The fracture is clearly demonstrated on the oblique projection (*arrows*)

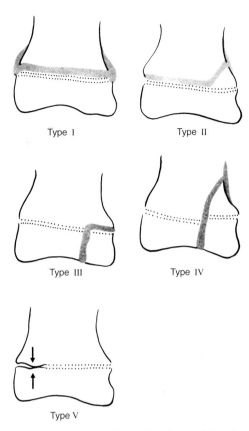

Fig. 12.41. Salter-Harris classification of injuries involving the growth plate. Type I is a separation of the distal femoral growth plate, without fracture through the adjacent epiphysis or metaphysis. Often the diagnosis is made in retrospect when subperiosteal new bone formation occurs along the adjacent metaphysis. The type II injury is characterized by an oblique fracture across one corner of the adjacent metaphysis. It is the most common type of separation seen at the distal femur. Type III injury consists of partial separation of the growth plate, with a vertical fracture line extending from the physis downward to the articular surface of the epiphysis. Type IV injury is uncommon. A vertical fracture line extends from the metaphyseal cortex downward across the growth plate and out through the articular surface of the epiphysis. Type V is defined as a compression through the growth plate. Type IV and type V may lead to growth disturbance with consequent limb-length discrepancy

encountered between the ages of 10 and 17 years as a result of a valgus or hyperextension force at the knee (Aitken et al. 1943; Aitken and Magill 1952). Injuries of the distal femoral epiphysis account for only 1%–2% of all epiphyseal injuries, and proximal tibial epiphyseal separations are even less common. The relative infrequency of proximal tibial epiphyseal injuries (Fig. 12.40) is most likely related to the absence of ligamentous attachments. The collateral ligaments arise on and are firmly attached to the distal femoral epiphyses; the lateral collateral liga-

ment is attached to the fibula, and the medial collateral ligament inserts broadly on the tibial metaphysis with little or no attachment to the margin of the tibial epiphysis.

12.9.2 Classification, Trauma Pattern, and Pathomorphology

Epiphyseal injuries are classified according to Salter and Harris (Fig. 12.41; Salter and Harris 1963). Salter-Harris type II injury accounts for 70% of all epiphyseal separations involving the distal femoral epiphysis (Salter and Harris 1963). The fracture is usually displaced laterally as the result of a valgus force or anteriorly as the result of a hyperextension force. Salter-Harris type III injury limited to one of the condyles, usually the medial condyle, accounts for 15%. These are often undisplaced and relatively obscure and may be difficult to appreciate on the initial radiographs. Salter-Harris type IV fractures account for approximately 10% of injuries. These are condylar fractures with the fracture line extending from the intercondylar notch, usually into the lateral metaphysis, thereby separating off the lateral femoral condyle. Only 3% are Salter-Harris type I injuries without metaphyseal fragments, and a similar percentage are Salter-Harris type V injuries resulting from severe impaction forces and often occurring in association with fractures of the proximal tibia.

The incidence of fractures of the anterior tibial tubercle is low (Baxter and Wiley 1988; Ogden et al. 1980). As mentioned before, acute, traumatic avulsions of the tibial tubercle happen most often during sports or play activities when the patellar ligament pulls hard enough to exceed the combined strength of the growth plate underlying the tubercle, the surrounding perichondrium, and the adjacent periosteum. This can occur upon violent contraction of the quadriceps muscle against a fixed tibia or upon acute passive flexion of the knee strong enough to override the contracted quadriceps. Fractures of the anterior tubercle are classified into three types (Fig. 12.38; see also Sect. 12.8.2.3) (Watson-Jones 1955). In type 1, a small fragment of the distal tubercle is avulsed and displaced upwards. Type 2 is described as a fracture of the entire tubercle and type 3 is classified as a fracture of the entire tubercle extending vertically through the primary ossification center of the proximal tibial epiphysis into the knee joint.

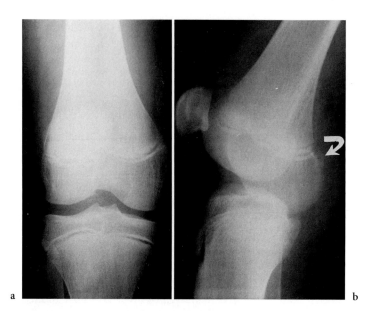

Fig. 12.42a,b. Tear of the lateral capsular ligament in a 15-year-old boy. a No fracture is seen on the AP view. b The lateral view shows an avulsion fracture and a thin cortical fragment at the peripheral margin of the lateral epiphysis (*arrow*)

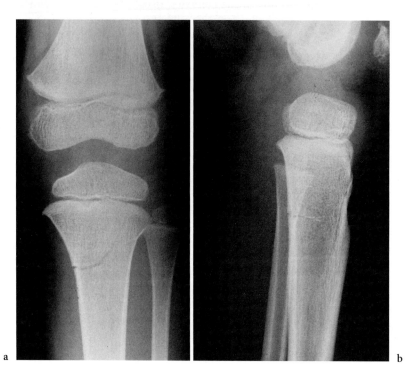

Fig. 12.43a,b. Nondisplaced metaphyseal fracture of the proximal tibia. On the AP (a) and lateral (b) views the fracture line does not extend into the tibial growth plate

12.9.3 Examination Methods

Most epiphyseal injuries are clinically and radiographically apparent. Undisplaced epiphyseal separations are difficult to recognize on radiographic evaluation because the opposing margins of an epiphyseal fracture consist of cartilage and are relatively smooth; therefore the separated epiphysis may glide easily over the opposed metaphysis. This is aided by the pull of tendons and ligaments about the joint. The epiphyseal separation may then reduce spontaneously. Diagnosis is made by identification of a widened growth plate (Fig. 12.40) or by comparative views of the opposite uninjured knee. MRI may further delineate the cartilaginous epiphysis (Rogers 1992).

Anteroposterior and lateral projections have also been helpful in identifying fractures through the epi-

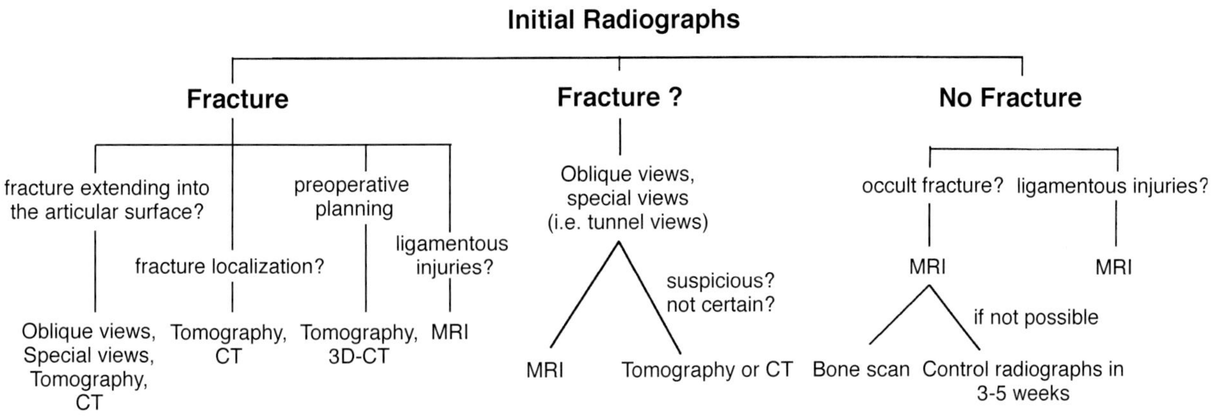

Initial Radiographs

Fig. 12.44. Diagnostic algorithm in knee trauma

physis or metaphysis (Figs. 12.42, 12.43; COCKSHOTT et al. 1985). MRI is recommended as a noninvasive method to evaluate the status of the ligaments in a patient presenting with an epiphyseal injury about the knee. Orthogonal tomograms and CT scans can be helpful in further analysis of Salter-Harris type III and IV fracture-separations before the choice of treatment is made.

12.9.4 Complications

Complications of epiphyseal and apophyseal injuries include popliteal artery injuries, peroneal nerve injuries, premature growth arrest with leg-length discrepancy and angular deformity of the knee.

12.10 Diagnostic Algorithm in Knee Trauma

A diagnostic algorithm in knee trauma is shown in Fig. 12.44.

References

Aitken AP, Magill HK (1952) Fractures involving the distal femoral epiphyseal cartilage. J. Bone Jt Surg [Am] 34:96–108

Aitken AP, Smith L, Blackett CW (1943) Supracondylar fractures in children. Am J Surg 59:161–171

Apple JS, Martinez S, Allen NB, Caldwell DS, Rice JR (1983) Occult fractures of the knee: tomographic evaluation. Radiology 148:383–387

Bauer G, Gustafsson M, Mortensson W, Norman O (1981) Insufficiency fractures in the tibial condyles in elderly individuals. Acta Radiol Diagn 22:619–622

Baumgartl F (1964) Das Kniegelenk: Erkrankungen, Verletzungen und ihre Behandlung mit Hinweisen auf die Begutachtung, Springer, Berlin Heidelberg New York

Baxter MP, Wiley JJ (1988) Fractures of the tibial spine in children. J Bone Joint Surg [Br] 70:228

Berquist TH (1992) Imaging of orthopedic trauma, 2nd edn. Raven Press, New York

Brossmann J, Muhle C, Schröder C, Melchert UH, Spielmann RP, Heller M (1993) Motion-triggered cine MR imaging: evaluation of patellar tracking patterns during active and passive knee extension. Radiology 187:205–212

Butt WP, Lederman H, Chuang S (1983) Radiology of the suprapatellar region. Clin Radiol 34:511–522

Cockshott WP, Racoveanu NT, Burrows DA, Ferrier M (1985) Use of radiographic projections of knee. Skeletal Radiol 13:131–133

Crues JV, Stoller DW (1993) The menisci. In: Mink JH, Reicher MA, Crues JV, Deutsch AL (eds) MRI of the knee. Raven Press, New York, pp 91–140

Crues JV IIIrd, Mink J, Levy TL et al. (1987) Meniscal tears of the knee: accuracy of MR imaging. Radiology 164:445–448

Daffner RH, Tabas JH (1987) Trauma oblique radiographs of the knee. J Bone Jt Surg [Am] 69:568–572

De Smet AA, Norris MA, Yandow DR (1993) MR diagnosis of meniscal tears of the knee: importance of high signal in the meniscus that extends to the surface. AJR 161:101–107

Dietz GW, Wilcox DM, Montgomery JB (1986) Segond tibial condyle fracture. Lateral capsular ligament avulsion. Radiology 159:467–469

Dovey H, Herfordt J (1971) Tibial condyle fractures. Acta Chir Scand 137:521–531

Dowd GSE, Bentley G (1986) Radiographic assessment in patellar instability and chondromalacia patellae. J Bone Jt Surg [Br] 68:297–300

Elstrom J, Pankovich AM, Sassoon H, Rodriquez J (1976) The use of tomography in the assessment of fractures of the tibial plateau. J Bone Jt Surg [Am] 58:551–555

Engber W (1977) Stress fractures of the medial tibial plateau. J Bone Jt Surg [Am] 59:767–769

Frangakis EK (1974) Intra-articular dislocation of the patella. J Bone Jt Surg [Am] 56:423–424

Freiberger RH, Kotzen LM (1967) Fracture of the medial margin of the patella, a finding diagnostic of lateral dislocation. Radiology 88:902–904

Gilley JS, Gelman MI, Edson DM, Metcalf RW (1981) Chondral fractures of the knee. Radiology 138:51–54

Green NE, Allen BL (1977) Vascular injuries associated with dislocation of the knee. J Bone Jt Surg [Am] 59:236–239

Henard DC, Bobo RT (1983) Avulsion fractures of the tibial tubercle in adolescents. Clin Orthop 177:182–187

Hohl M (1967) Tibial condylar fractures. J Bone Jt Surg [Am] 49:1455–1467

Hohl M, Larson RL (1975) Fractures and dislocations of the knee. In: Rockwood CA, Green DP (eds) Fractures. Lippincott, Philadelphia, p 1131

Insall J, Salvati E (1971) Patella position in the normal knee joint. Radiology 101:101–104

Jacobsen K (1976) Stress radiographical measurement of the anteroposterior, medial and lateral stability of the knee joint. Acta Orthop Scand 47:335–344

Johnson-Nurse C, Dandy DJ (1985) Fracture-separation of articular cartilage in the adult knee. J Bone Jt Surg [Br] 67:42–43

Kimbrough EE (1961) Concomitant unilateral hip and femoral-shaft fractures – a too frequently unrecognized syndrome. J Bone Jt Surg [Am] 43:443–449

Kuner EH (1975) Die distale Oberschenkelfraktur: Ursachen, Formen und Begleitverletzungen der distalen Oberschenkelfraktur. H Unfallheilkd 120:1–8

Lancourt JE, Cristini JA (1975) Patella alta und patella infera. Their etiological role in patellar dislocation, chondromalacia, and apophysitis of the tibial tubercle. J Bone Jt Surg [Am] 57:1112–1115

Laurin CL, Levesque HP, Dussault R, Labell H, Peide JP (1978) The abnormal lateral patellofemoral angle. A diagnostic roentgenographic sign of recurrent patellar subluxation. J Bone Jt Surg [Am] 60:55–60

Lee JK, Yao L, Phelps CT (1988) Anterior cruciate ligaments tears: MR imaging compared with arthroscopy and clinical tests. Radiology 166:861–864

Letts M, Vincent N, Gouw G (1986) The "floating knee" in children. J Bone Jt Surg [Br] 68:442–446

Magerl F (1975) II. Die Patellafraktur: Das patellofemorale Gelenk. Ursachen, Formen und Begleitverletzungen der Patellafraktur. H Unfallheilkd 120:45–60

Merchant AC, Mercer RL, Jacobsen RH, Cool CR (1974) Roentgenographic analysis of patellofemoral congruence. J Bone Joint Surg [Am] 56:1391–1396

Meyers MH, McKeever FM (1959) Fracture of the intercondylar eminence of the tibia. J Bone Jt Surg [Am] 41:209–220

Milgram JW, Rogers LF, Miller JW (1978) Osteochondral fractures: mechanisms of injury and fate of fragments. Am J Roentgenol 130:651–658

Mink JH (1993) The cruciate and collateral ligaments. In: Mink JH, Reicher MA, Crues JV, Deutsch AL (eds) MRI of the knee. Raven Press, New York, pp 141–188

Mink JH, Levy T, Crues JV IIIrd (1988) Tears of the anterior cruciate ligament and menisci of the knee: MR imaging evaluation. Radiology 167:769–774

Molander ML, Wallin G, Wilkstad I (1981) Fracture of the intercondylar eminence of the tibia. A review of 35 patients. J Bone Joint Surg [Br] 63:89–91

Moore TM, Harvey JP (1974) Roentgenographic measurement of tibial-plateau depression due to fracture. J Bone Jt Surg [Am] 56:155–160

Muhle C, Brossmann J, Heller M (1995) Funktionelle MRT des Femoropatellargelenkes. Radiologe 35:117–124

Nance EP, Kaye JJ (1982) Injuries of the quadriceps mechanism. Radiology 142:301–307

Newberg AH, Greenstein R (1978) Radiographic evaluation of tibial plateau fractures. Radiology 126:319–323

Nicolet A (1965) Die Meniskusverletzung bei Tibiakopffrakturen. Langenbecks Arch Klin Chir 313:544–545

Ogden JA (1974) Subluxation and dislocation of the proximal tibiofibular joint. J Bone Joint Surg [Am] 56:145–154

Ogden JA, Tross RB, Murphy MJ (1980) Fractures of the tibial tuberosity in adolescents. J Bone Jt Surg [Am] 62:205–215

Porter BB (1970) Crush fractures of the lateral tibial table. J Bone Jt Surg [Br] 52:676–687

Rafii M, Firooznia H, Golimbu C, Bonamo J (1984) Computed tomography of tibial plateau fractures. Am J Roentgenol 142:1181–1186

Resnick D (1995) Diagnosis of bone and joint disorders, 3rd edn. Saunders, Philadelphia

Reuter M, Heller M, Ahlers J (1993) Kniegelenk, distales Femur und proximale Tibia. In: Thelen M, Ritter G, Bücheler E (eds) Radiologische Diagnostik der Verletzungen von Knochen und Gelenken. Thieme, Stuttgart

Rockwood CA, Wilkens KE, King RE (1991) Fractures in children, 3rd edn. Lippincott, Philadelphia

Rogers LF (1992) Radiology of skeletal trauma. Churchill Livingstone, New York

Salter RB, Harris WR (1963) Injuries involving the epiphyseal plate. J Bone Jt Surg [Am] 45:587–622

Satku K, Kumar VP, Chacha PB (1990) Stress fractures around the knee in elderly patients. J Bone Joint Surg [Am] 72:918–922

Scharf W, Wagner M, Schabus R (1983) Zur Entstehung, Diagnostik und Behandlung der Kniescheibenverrenkung. Unfallheilkunde 86:16–21

Schild H, Müller HA, Menke W (1983) Die Tibiakopffraktur – eine CT-Indikation? Fortschr Röntgenstr 139:135–142

Settegast H (1921) Typische Röntgenbilder von normalen Menschen. Lehmanns Med Atlanton 5:211

Shellock FG, Foo THF, Deutsch AL, Mink JH (1991) Patellofemoral joint: evaluation during active flexion with ultrafast spoiled GRASS MR imaging. Radiology 180:581–585

Shellock FG, Mink JH, Fox JM (1993) Patellofemoral joint: kinematic MR imaging to assess patellar tracking abnormalities. Radiology 168:551–553

Sonin AH, Fitzgerald SW, Friedman H (1994) Posterior cruciate ligament injury: MR imaging diagnosis and patters of injury. Radiology 2:445–458

Spritzer CE, Vogler JB, Martinez S, Garret WE, Johnson GA, McNamara MJ, Lohnes J, Herfkens RF (1988) MR imaging of the knee: Preliminary results with a 3 DFT GRASS pulse sequence. Am J Roentgenol 150:597–603

Stallenberg B, Genenois PA, Sintzhoff SA et al. (1993) Fracture of the posterior aspect of the lateral tibial plateau: radiographic sign of anterior cruciate ligament tear. Radiology 187:821–825

Stanford W, Phelan J, Kathol MH, Rooholamini SA, El-Koury GY, Palutsis GR, Albright JP (1988) Patellofemoral joint motion: evaluation by ultrafast computed tomography. Skeletal Radiol 17:487–492

Stoller DW (1993) The knee. In: Stoller DW (ed) Magnetic resonance imaging in orthopaedics and sports medicine. Lippincott, Philadelphia

Stoller DW, Martin C, Crues JV III (1987) Meniscal tears, pathologic correlation with MRI Radiology 163:731–735

Tung GA, Davis LM, Wiggins ME (1993) Tears of the anterior cruciate ligament: primary and secondary signs at MR imaging. Radiology 188:661–667

Vahey TN, Broome DR, Kayes KJ (1991) Acute and chronic

tears of the anterior cruciate ligament: differential features at MR imaging. Radiology 181:251–253

Watson-Jones R (1955) Fractures and joint injuries, 4th edn, vol 2. Williams & Wilkins, Baltimore

Wiberg G (1941) Roentgenographic and anatomic studies on the femoropatellar joint. Acta Orthop Scand 12:319–410

Wilppula E, Bakalim G (1972) Ligamentous tear concomitant with tibial condylar fracture. Acta Orthop Scand 43;292–300

Zeiss J, Saddemi SR, Ebraheim NA (1992) MR imaging of the quadriceps tendon: normal layered configuration and its importance in cases of tendon rupture. Am J Roentgenol 159:1031–1034

13 Ankle

A. Fink, F. Häckl, and M. Heller

CONTENTS

13.1 General Considerations

Traumatic injuries of the ankle joint are very common and usually result from "taking a wrong step" either in sport or in everyday life. The body's reaction is standard: pain, swelling, and impaired function. Unfortunately, these reactions may not tell the whole story; in fact, they can even be misleading. A complete rupture of the joint capsule and one or more of the ligaments may result in less pain than a distortion because the intra-articular effusion or bleeding is not contained in the joint but has ways to diffuse into the surrounding soft tissue, thus placing less stress on the joint capsule. On the other hand,

A. Fink, MD, PhD, Klinik für Radiologische Diagnostik, Klinikum der Christian-Albrechts-Universität zu Kiel, Arnold-Heller-Straße 9, 24105 Kiel, Germany
F. Häckl, MD, Department of Radiology, University of California, San Francisco, CA 94143, USA
M. Heller, MD, PhD, Professor and Direktor der Klinik für Radiologische Diagnostik, Klinikum der Christian-Albrechts-Universität zu Kiel, Arnold-Heller-Straße 9, 24105 Kiel, Germany

the rupture of a small capsular artery may produce a large swelling despite only minor trauma. Since the clinical appearance does not allow a diagnosis to be established with sufficient certainty, the imaging techniques are very important. While there is considerable debate among orthopedic and trauma surgeons over when to operate on ligamental and capsular injuries and when to employ conservative treatment, there is little disagreement that most bone lesions require a surgical approach. The goals of the radiological examination can, therefore, be defined as follows:

1. To prove the existence or absence of osseous lesions, i.e., the "visible joint"
2. To determine the degree of ligamental injury, i.e., the "invisible joint"

The visible joint is for the most part accurately displayed by radiographs in two or three projections and, if necessary, by conventional or computed tomography. The invisible joint is depicted by arthrography and/or magnetic resonance imaging (MRI), while stress examinations give a good idea of the clinically important function of the invisible joint.

13.2 Anatomy

The ankle joint is formed by three bones – the tibia, fibula, and talus – which together make up the "visible joint." The distal ends of the tibia and fibula, i.e., the medial and lateral malleolus, respectively, together form a mortise for the talus, the so-called malleolar fork. The talus is somewhat wedge-shaped (Töndury 1981), i.e., it is wider ventrally than dorsally. This wedge is pressed tightly into the mortise in dorsal flexion of the foot and is only held loosely in plantar flexion, e.g., when wearing high-heels. The talus, being the only bone of the human skeleton on which no muscles attach, is held in the ankle mortise only by the below-mentioned ligaments and by surrounding muscles and tendons.

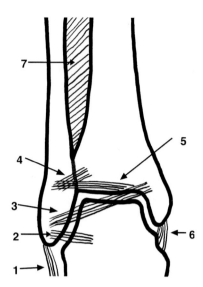

Fig. 13.1. Normal anatomy, posteroanterior view: *1*, calcaneofibular ligament; *2*, posterior fibulotalar ligament; *3*, intermalleolar ligament (see text); *4*, posterior tibiofibular ligament; *5*, transverse ligament (see text); *6*, deltoid ligament; *7*, interosseous membrane

The syndesmosis of the mortise consists of four ligaments and the interosseous membrane: the posterior and anterior tibiofibular ligaments, the interosseous ligament, and the inferior transverse ligament (Figs. 13.1, 13.2). The lower portion of the interosseous membrane strengthens distally to form the interosseous ligament, which, like the interosseous membrane, is angulated downward from medial to lateral. The anterior tibiofibular ligament originates at the anterior tubercle of the tibia and runs downward to attach to the anterior surface of the fibula at the level of the ankle joint. The posterior tibiofibular ligament runs nearly horizontally and has a slightly more medial insertion than its counterpart, the anterior tibiofibular ligament. This insertion point still lies in the lateral to medial third of the tibia. However, the lowest part can reach further to the medial third and is then called the inferior transverse ligament (ROSENBERG et al. 1995). Together, these strong ligaments allow for only very little movement of the fibula. The stability of the syndesmosis is of crucial importance for the proper function of the ankle joint. If, after a rupture of the syndesmosis, the distance is widened by only 1 mm, the articulating surface area is decreased by 30%–53% (quoted after KARL and WRAZIDLO 1987). This reduces the "shock-absorbing" function of the ankle joint by a significant amount.

Between the posterior tibiofibular ligament and the posterior fibulotalar ligament, 56% of the popu-

lation have an additional posterior intermalleolar ligament (PATURET 1951, as quoted in ROSENBERG et al. 1995). Its tibial origin usually lies more medially than that of the posterior tibiofibular ligament (Fig. 13.1). Some of the fibers may blend with the most medial part of the posterior tibiofibular ligament, forming the inferior transverse ligament. It then courses downward and inserts into the fibula slightly superior to the insertion of the posterior fibulotalar ligament. The inferior transverse ligament is sometimes referred to as "marsupial meniscus," since a similar ligament has been found in the ankles of primitive primates. It can have a meniscus-like shape or a meniscus-like appendix and may herniate without an obvious injury into the posterior part of the joint and cause a posterior impingement syndrome (HAMILTON 1993).

Medially, the tip of the tibia is fixed to the talus, navicular bone and calcaneus by the deltoid ligament, a somewhat triangular-shaped complex of four ligaments (from front to back: tibionavicular, anterior tibiotalar, tibiocalcanear, and posterior tibiotalar).

From the distal tip of the fibula three ligaments extend: the anterior fibulotalar, the posterior fibulotalar, and the fibulocalcanear. The lateral ligaments are not as strong as their medial counterparts; hence, the ankle is less well protected laterally. Here

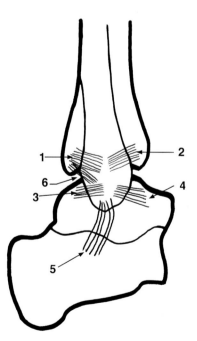

Fig. 13.2. Normal anatomy, lateral view: *1*, posterior tibiofibular ligament; *2*, anterior tibiofibular ligament; *3*, posterior fibulotalar ligament; *4*, anterior fibulotalar ligament; *5*, fibulocalcanear ligament; *6*, intermalleolar ligament

the ligaments are closely related to the tendon sheaths. Thus lateral ligamental tears are often combined injuries. Due to its anatomical position, the fibulocalcanear ligament is not very well connected with the capsule. In cases of a complete tear it may flip into the joint space, either locking the joint or resulting in a posterior impingement syndrome.

13.3 Biomechanics and Classifications of Ankle Trauma

Ankle fractures are often described as:

1. Unimalleolar, when the fracture involves the medial (tibial) or lateral (fibular) malleolus
2. Bimalleolar, when both malleoli are fractured
3. Trimalleolar, when fractures involve the medial and lateral malleoli as well as the posterior lip (the so-called third malleolus or Volkmann triangle) of the distal tibia
4. Complex fractures, when comminuted fractures of the distal tibia and fibula occur (ROGERS 1992)

Although these descriptions might be correct, the diagnosis could be more informative if it were also to consider the underlying pathogenetic mechanism of the trauma.

Between 1948 and 1954, LAUGE-HANSEN, a Swedish radiologist, used cadaver feet to experiment with different injury mechanisms. Based on these experiments and clinical observations, he developed a comprehensive classification of ankle injuries in which he combined the position of the foot and the deforming stress at the time of trauma. His efforts to detect the movement that led to a certain injury were important for the usually conservative approach to treatment in the late 1940s, when good repositioning required reversal of the injury mechanism. Lauge-Hansen's classification has, of course, declined in importance with the advances in osteosynthesis, but it nevertheless serves to offer a basic understanding of the biomechanics of ankle trauma. For the clinical purposes of today, Weber's classification is more commonly used (THELEN et al. 1993; ZWIPP 1991).

13.3.1 Lauge-Hansen's Classification

LAUGE-HANSEN (1953, 1954) described the occurrence of defects that can be expected with the exertion of increasing force on the foot. The shape of the osseous damage allows one to deduce the type of

deforming force responsible for the injury (ARIMOTO and FORRESTER 1980). This in turn provides valuable clues as to the damage that is likely to have occurred before the bone fractured and which ligaments are most likely to have ruptured. An understanding of the mechanisms enables the investigator to focus on less obvious injuries that may be present. LAUGE-HANSEN named four basic categories of ankle trauma according to their *position* and *movement* and described a predictable sequence of injuries to bones and ligaments. A fundamental criticism and possible obstacle in understanding stems from the setup of the experiments: Lauge-Hansen described the movement of the foot relative to the limb while in most injuries the foot is fixed and the leg represents the moving part.

13.3.1.1 Supination-External Rotation (Fig. 13.3)

Stage 1 (SE-1): Rupture of the inferior anterior tibiofibular ligament
Stage 2 (SE-2): + oblique or spiral fracture of the *lateral* malleolus
Stage 3 (SE-3): + rupture of the posterior inferior tibiofibular ligament or fracture of the posterior lip of the tibia (the so-called dorsal Volkmann triangle in the German literature)
Stage 4 (SE-4): + transverse or oblique fracture of the medial malleolus or rupture of the deltoid ligament

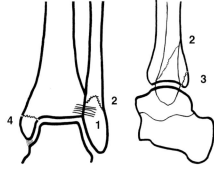

Fig. 13.3. Supination-external rotation: Internal rotation of the leg more often than external rotation of the supinated foot leads firstly to a rupture of the anterior tibiofibular ligament (SE-1) Further rotation results in a spiral or oblique fracture of the fibula (SE-2), often with only minimal displacement. Its inferior margin usually lies at the level of the ankle mortise. Thereafter, the posterior malleolus is fractured or the posterior tibiofibular ligament is torn (SE-3). If the force continues, the initially relaxed medial structures are placed under tension so that a transverse fracture of the medial malleolus or a rupture of the deltoid ligament occurs (SE-4)

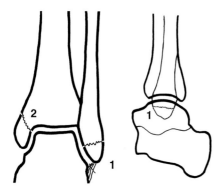

Fig. 13.4. Supination-adduction: The most common type of ankle sprain is a rupture of the anterior talofibular ligament. In about 30% of the cases the calcaneofibular ligament is also disrupted (ROGERS 1992). Its equivalent is a transverse fracture of the lateral malleolus (SA-1). Stage 2 (SA-2) is characterized by an oblique fracture of the medial malleolus

13.3.1.2 Supination-Adduction (Figs. 13.4–13.6)

Stage 1 (SA-1): Transverse fracture of the *lateral* malleolus or tear of the anterior fibulotalar ligament (see Fig. 13.24b)
Stage 2 (SA-2): + vertical or oblique fracture of the medial malleolus

Adduction of the supinated foot usually means varus stress to the ankle by bearing weight on the outside of the foot. At first, a rupture of the fibulotalar ligament or a transverse fracture of the lateral malleolus occurs. Clinically this is suspected on the basis of soft tissue swelling and pain near the lateral malleolus. The radiograph shows either a fracture of the lateral malleolus or an increased talus tilt (see Fig. 13.21) in stress examinations with adduction of the hind foot. If further force is exerted to the foot, the medial malleolus fractures vertically or steeply oblique.

13.3.1.3 Pronation-Abduction (Figs. 13.7–13.9)

Stage 1 (PA-1): Transverse fracture of the medial malleolus or tear of the deltoid ligament (see Fig. 13.25b; same as PE-1)

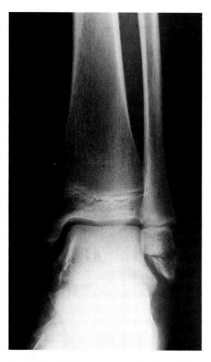

Fig. 13.5. Weber A or supination-adduction injury with a transverse fracture of the distal fibula well below the joint space

It is probably easier to imagine this injury as an inward rotation of the leg on a supinated foot. Then, the lateral structures are injured in sequence from front to back, i.e., anterior tibiofibular ligament, lateral malleolus, posterior tibiofibular ligament, and posterior malleolus. The medial structures – deltoid ligament and medial malleolus – which are initially relaxed because of the supinated position of the foot, are subject to injury only after the lateral structures have lost their stability.

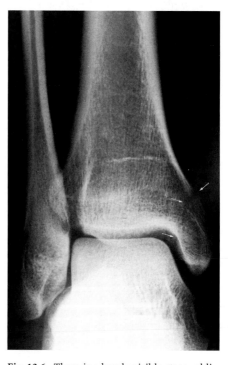

Fig. 13.6. There is a barely visible steep, oblique fracture (*arrows*) of the medial malleolus; this indicates a supination-adduction fracture (SA-2) and makes a tear of the lateral collateral ligament very likely, since no fibular fracture is visible

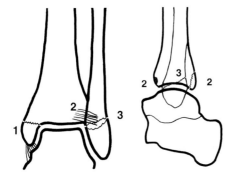

Fig. 13.7. Pronation-adduction: Just as in pronation-external rotation, the initial stage is a transverse fracture of the medial malleolus or a rupture of the deltoid ligament (PA-1). Then, the anterior and posterior tibiofibular ligaments rupture while the interosseous ligament and membrane remain intact (PA-2). The last stage is a short oblique fibular fracture, slightly above the tibial plafond (PA-3). Equivalent to the ligamental tear is an avulsion fracture of the tibial insertion of the anterior tibiofibular ligament or a fracture of the "third malleolus," where the posterior tibiofibular ligament originates

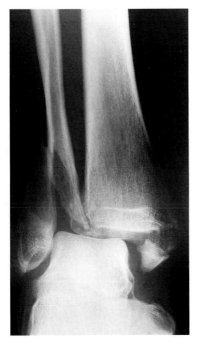

Fig. 13.8. Weber B or pronation-abduction injury: From the initial transverse fracture of the medial malleolus (PA-1) the injury has progressed to stage PA-3, as shown by the steeply oblique fracture of the fibula. The likely rupture of the anterior and posterior tibiofibular ligaments is not as convincingly displayed as in Fig. 13.9. The stability of the syndesmosis in both such cases, however, will be checked carefully during the open surgical refixation

Stage 2 (PA-2): + rupture of the anterior and posterior tibiofibular ligaments, possibly with a fracture of the posterior lip of the tibia (the interosseous membrane remains intact)

Stage 3 (PA-3): + an oblique fracture of the fibula just above the level of the syndesmosis

In pronation, the medial structures are the most vulnerable. Either the deltoid ligament or the medial malleolus is damaged first. Thereafter, both tibiofibular ligaments rupture. Finally, the hallmark is a supramalleolar oblique fracture of the fibula. Note that the interosseous membrane remains intact.

13.3.1.4 Pronation-External Rotation (Figs. 13.10, 13.11)

Stage 1 (PE-1): Transverse fracture of the medial malleolus or tear of the deltoid ligament (see Fig. 13.25b; same as PA-1)

Stage 2 (PE-2): + rupture of the anterior tibiofibular and interosseous ligaments

Stage 3 (PE-3): + short spiral fracture of the fibula, typically 6–8 cm above the ankle joint, i.e., higher than PA-2, indicating a rupture of the interosseous membrane

Stage 4 (PE-3): + avulsion fracture of the posterior lip of the fibula or tear of the posterior tibiofibular ligament

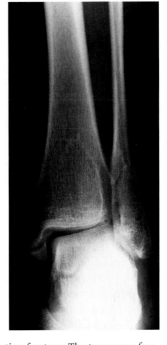

Fig. 13.9. Pronation-abduction fracture: The transverse fracture of the medial malleolus (PA-1) and the steeply oblique fibular fracture (PA-3) indicate the rupture of the anterior and posterior tibiofibular ligament. The intactness of the interosseous ligament and membrane is likely due to the normal distance of the medial aspect of the fibula from the fibular groove of the tibia

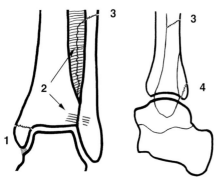

Fig. 13.10. Pronation-external rotation: Initially, the tension stress leads either to a transverse fracture of the medial malleolus or to a tear of the deltoid ligament (PE-1). Then, the anterior tibiofibular and interosseous ligaments and membrane rupture (PE-2). The third stage is a short spiral fracture of the fibula, often located 8–10 cm above the joint. Further rotation leads to a fracture of the posterior margin of the tibia or, as an equivalent, a rupture of the posterior tibiofibular ligament (PE-4). The fibular fracture occasionally may be located much more proximally, and then can be missed on the initial radiographs

Just as in pronation-abduction, one of the medial structures suffers first. With further movement – lateral rotation of the foot or internal rotation of the leg – the talus, no longer being fixed medially, presses upon the lateral malleolus and thus tension is exerted on the anterior inferior tibiofibular and interosseous ligaments. Should the force continue, the fibula fractures typically 6–8 cm above the ankle joint, a so-called Dupuytren fracture (DUPUYTREN 1839) (Fig. 13.12). Occasionally, however, the fracture may be located much more proximally in the fibula (Fig. 13.11), representing an injury that, among others, was originally described by MAISSONEUVE (1840). Further lateral rotation will exert force on the posterior lip of the tibia, resulting either in its fracture or in a rupture of the posterior tibiofibular ligament.

13.3.2 Weber's Classification

While Lauge-Hansen's classification of ankle trauma is very useful for understanding the biomechanics involved, in times of osteosynthesis Weber's classification (WEBER 1972) has become more widely accepted since it is more practical and appears to be clinically sufficient (ZWIPP 1991). Weber focuses on the most important structures, i.e., the syndesmosis and the interosseous membrane between the tibia and fibula, and relates their stability to the height of the fibular fracture.

Type A is characterized by a transverse fracture of the distal fibula, usually at the level of or below the joint space. Just as in Lauge-Hansen's supination-adduction trauma, the equivalent would be a tear of the anterior fibulotalar ligament. There may be an accompanying fracture of the medial malleolus (Figs. 13.5, 13.13).

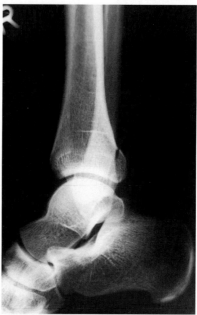

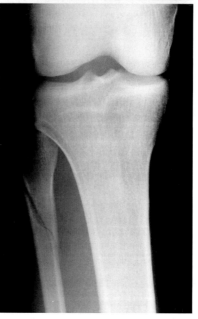

Fig. 13.11a,b. The avulsion fracture of the posterior lip of the tibia suggests the possibility of a pronation-external rotation injury. In such cases a proximal fibular fracture must be excluded at least clinically and preferably also by x-ray. The presence of this very high fibular fracture (PE-3) makes this a complete stage 4 PE injury, often referred to as a Maissoneuve fracture

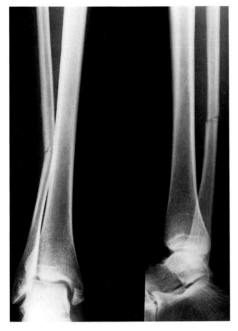

Fig. 13.12. Pronation-external rotation fracture (PE-1). The initial injury is fracture of the medial malleolus followed by a tear of the tibiofibular ligament (PE-2). The next step is a fracture of the distal shaft of the fibula (PE-3), indicating a rupture of the interosseous membrane. PE-4, an avulsion fracture of the posterior lip of the fibula, is not present

Type C has as its hallmark a fibular fracture above the level of the ankle joint associated with a rupture of the posterior fibulotalar ligament and the syndesmosis, thus resulting in lateral instability. In the case of a high fibular fracture (Maissoneuve fracture), the interosseous membrane is ruptured up to that level (Figs. 13.12, 13.15).

13.3.3 Distal Tibial Fractures

Distal tibial fractures, also referred to as pilon tibial fractures, result from direct axial compression

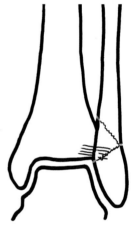

Fig. 13.14. Weber type B: The fibular fracture begins at the level of the joint space and extends as an oblique or spiral fracture proximally. The syndesmosis is partially or completely ruptured. Medially, a ruptured deltoid ligament or a transverse malleolar fracture may be present

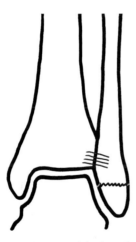

Fig. 13.13. Weber type A: A transverse fracture of the lateral malleolus or a rupture of the lateral collateral ligaments is classified as Weber type A. The syndesmosis usually remains unaffected. Medial involvement would result in an oblique malleolar fracture or rupture of the deltoid ligament

Type B is defined as a spiral or oblique fracture of the fibula at the height of the joint space with partial or questionable destruction of the tibiofibular syndesmosis. It may be accompanied by an avulsion fracture of the medial malleolus or a rupture of the deltoid ligament (Figs. 13.8, 13.9, 13.14).

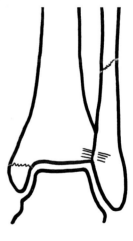

Fig. 13.15. Weber type C: The fibular fracture usually occurs 6–8 cm above the tibial plafond, indicating a complete rupture of the syndesmosis up to that level. The medial injuries would be similar to those in Weber type B. In addition there may be a fracture of the posterior tibial lip

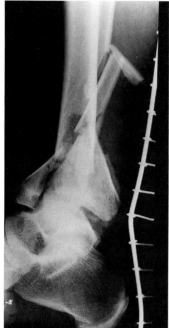

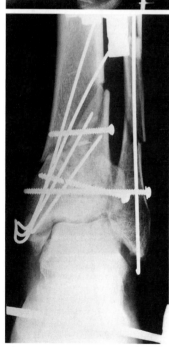

a

b

Fig. 13.16a,b. Complex, comminuted pilon tibial fracture. Note that the talus was driven into the tibia and remained intact. The fragments of the distal tibia and fibula are widely displaced. Even after open surgical repositioning and refixation, limitations in movement and early arthritis must be expected. (Case by courtesy of H. Drews, MD)

trauma: the talus is driven into the mortise and fractures the distal tibia (Fig. 13.16). The usual accident is a fall from a great height. Several classifications exist that describe the various degrees of displace-

ment of bone fragments and the joint surface involvement (RUEDL and ALLGÖWER 1979; OVADIA and BEALS 1986; MÜLLER et al. 1991).

Due to the immense forces exerted on the distal tibial joint surface – the so-called tibial plafond – even minimal incongruencies can lead to rapidly progressing arthrotic changes. Therefore, almost all pilon tibial fractures require open surgical repositioning and osteosynthesis. Even after optimal repositioning, there remains a high risk of partial or even total necrosis of the talus as a result of the initial severe trauma, and premature degenerative changes are likely to occur in most cases. Complex comminuted fractures like that in Fig. 13.16 are further complicated by extensive soft tissue damage and perfusion deficits which often slow down convalescence considerably.

13.3.4 Osteochondral or Flake Fractures and Bone Bruises

Direct trauma as well as luxation injuries can produce small osteochondral flakes that may be difficult to detect on conventional x-ray films. In cases of persisting pain and joint effusion, tomography – conventional or computed – is often the next step to detect small flakes. The most likely locations for osteochondral flakes are the medial and lateral joint face of the talus (Fig. 13.17). Since bone bruises without a fracture may go undetected, a STIR sequence in MRI may be the better diagnostic tool.

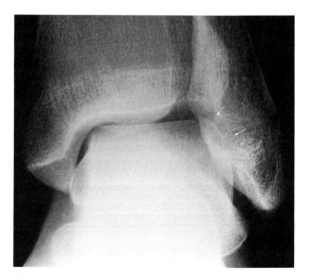

Fig. 13.17. Please note the flake fracture at the lateral aspect of the talus dome (arrows)

13.4 Ankle Trauma in Children and Adolescents

There is a notable difference in ankle trauma between children and adults: In children, the ligaments are stronger than the physis. Thus, it is much more likely for a child to suffer from an epiphyseal injury than an osseous fracture or ligamental tear. In fact, the distal tibial epiphysis is the second most common site (the most common is the radius) of an epiphyseal injury in the entire skeleton (DINGEMANN and SHAVER 1978; SALTER 1974). The classifications of SALTER and HARRIS (1963) are appropriate for the description of these fractures.

Widening and displacement of the epiphysis are the key indicators in the radiological evaluation of an injured ankle. The amount of displacement may be minimal, so comparative views of the opposite site or MRI may become necessary for an adequate diagnosis. Due to the relative strength of the ligaments, small avulsion fractures that are sometimes very hard to detect are much more common in children than in adults and must be searched for (ROGERS 1992).

In epiphyseal fractures, the chondral cells responsible for the growth remain attached to the dislocated fragment so that exact repositioning is very important for the further development of the joint. In order to avoid additional damage to the injured joint, stress examinations should only be done manually under x-ray control (ERLEMANN et al. 1991).

The distal tibial physis usually closes between the 12th and the 15th year. The closure begins at a medial "bump" in the medial physis pointing proximally and progresses first medially and then laterally (ERLEMANN et al. 1991). Thus, after the age of 10 years, injuries to the physis are usually combined with fractures (Fig. 13.18).

13.5 Achilles Tendon

Complete ruptures of the Achilles tendon present with distinct clinical findings and are usually straightforward to diagnose. Typically, men between the ages of 30 and 50 are affected during some sports activity. They often describe a sensation of having been kicked in the back of their leg. Complete tears, of course, result in an inability to stand on one's toes, and the gap just above the calcaneus can be felt easily. The clinical findings are then confirmed with ultrasonography. Plain x-ray films are acquired to exclude other injuries.

Incomplete tears are also visible on ultrasonography and, of course, can be displayed excellently by means of MRI.

13.6 Examination Methods

It is common practice at many institutions to use a "standard ankle" examination, i.e., anteroposterior, lateral, and mortise views (the anteroposterior view being acquired with the foot rotated internally by 15–20°), in most patients who present at the clinic with ankle trauma. There is growing concern that the radiological evaluation of ankle trauma has superseded the physical examination as the method for detecting fractures. Among the reasons for this development are lack of trust in physical examinations, the desire to prove even the absence of fractures, the expectations of patients ("...they didn't even take an x-ray..."), medicolegal reasons, and simply the understandable desire to be on the safe side. Several authors have suggested that a brief – less than 5 min (AULETTA et al. 1991) or even less than 1 min (HALL 1992) – but thorough physical examination can eliminate the need for a large percentage of radiographs ordered in patients with acute ankle trauma. In the 50% of the radiological studies that AULETTA et al. (1991) found not to be indicated, they missed

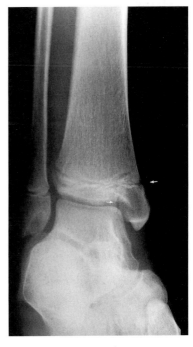

Fig. 13.18. Aitken 2 or Salter-Harris 3 fracture (*arrows*) in the medial aspect of the distal tibia with minimal widening of the medial margin of the growth plate

only one small avulsion fracture of the dorsal aspect of the talus that was clinically insignificant, i.e., no cast or surgery was required.

13.6.1 Clinical Examination

Although we are well aware of the fact that a thorough physical examination of every patient referred for ankle radiographs is impractical or simply impossible in everyday routine work, it cannot be sufficiently emphasized that a brief look at, and a short talk with, the patient can yield very important information far beyond the often minimal or even completely lacking information given on the referral form. The doubts over whether or not a suspicious line seen on the radiograph represents a fracture can often be resolved by a very quick physical examination: if it doesn't hurt, it won't be an acute fracture. It would be very beneficial to convince the referring clinicians to give at least two pieces of information on the referral form – (a) how the injury happened and (b) where it hurts – and then to ask a specific question.

The clinical examination itself is a fairly straightforward exercise (the following list is adopted from AULETTA et al. 1991):

1. Check for gross deformity, instability, or crepitation
2. Palpate all medial and lateral ligaments
3. Palpate the medial and lateral malleolus
4. Try to distinguish between bony and soft tissue tenderness
5. Palpate the fifth metatarsal, the dorsal tibia, and the dorsal talus

Then, one should try to reach one of four conclusions:

1. A clinically significant injury is not suspected.
2. It remains unclear whether or not there is a clinically significant injury.
3. There is sufficient evidence to suspect a clinically significant soft tissue injury.
4. There is sufficient evidence to suspect a clinically significant bone injury.

An injury is considered clinically significant if it requires open surgery or closed manipulation or a long period of immobilization in a cast. Clinically insignificant injuries are those that are treated conservatively, that is, with weight bearing as tolerated, elevation, nonsteroid inflammatory drugs, and/or an elastic wrap.

Last but not least we would like to quote DeLacey and Bradbrooke (1979), whose approach was designed to restrict the use of radiographs to the bare minimum. They stated that the number of radiographs of the ankle could be reduced by two-thirds if one were to apply the following simple rule: "No swelling, no radiograph." Of course, the immediate posttraumatic hours, when a swelling may not yet have developed, are exempt from this rule.

13.6.2 Standard Radiographs

The standard views to be taken in order to examine the ankle are a plain film mortise view (see below) and a lateral projection. The strict anteroposterior view is often requested as a standard examination for ankle trauma although it does not fully take into account the anatomical peculiarities of the ankle joint. Since the axis of plantar and dorsal flexion which runs through both malleoli is not parallel to the film but angled by about 15–20°, both malleoli will overlap the medial and lateral joint surface of the talus. In this way, flake fractures of the talus dome, which are usually located at the medial and lateral aspects of the talus plateau, the width of the syndesmosis, and the width of the medial and lateral joint space, cannot be sufficiently well judged.

Consequently, the diagnostically better view is a modified anteroposterior projection with the ankle rotated inwardly by about 15–20°, the so-called mortise view (Fig. 13.19a). The malleoli should have equal distances to the film. In this way the medial and lateral joint spaces of the malleolar fork and the talus plateau can be seen unobstructed. The central beam should be aimed at the joint space above the talus plateau. One should pay close attention to the cortical outline, as flake fractures within the joint are easily overlooked. Also, avulsion fractures with only tiny bony fragments are common, particularly in children and adolescents. The width of the joint spaces should be 3–4 mm medially and less than 5 mm laterally. When the distance between the tibia and fibula exceeds 4 mm (Rogers 1992), one should become suspicious and proceed to further investigations such as stress examinations or MRI. Of course, slightly "off" projections may render these values unusable.

For the lateral view (Fig. 13.19b) the foot is placed in neutral position with the fibula resting on the film and the beam is centered on the medial malleolus.

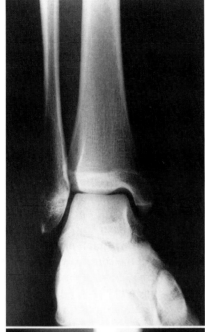

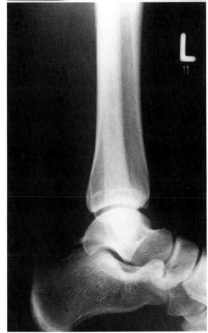

Fig. 13.19. a Mortise view. Through internal rotation both malleoli are positioned parallel to the film. Thus, the medial and lateral joint spaces as well as the talus dome are depicted freely. **b** Lateral view: The joint space can be seen clearly. If the base of the fifth metatarsal is not included, a fracture must be excluded clinically

The reverse position with the lateral malleolus being near the film is also acceptable. The lateral view is more difficult to read since most structures overlap with others. The medial and lateral malleolus should

be checked for integrity. It is advisable to include the base of the metatarsals in this projection since avulsion fractures, in particular of the fifth metatarsal, are not uncommon. Care should be taken, however, not to interpret accessory bones as fractures (see Chap. 14 for an overview of accessory bones). MANDELL (1971) points out that a slight "off" lateral projection can depict the dorsal angle of the tibia, i.e., the insertion of the posterior tibiofibular ligament, better than a strictly lateral projection.

13.6.3 Special Projections

Every radiologist will be aware, through practical experience, that certain fractures are not visible on standard projections. Therefore, if there is convincing clinical evidence of substantial trauma, additional projections should be obtained, either to search for as yet undetected fractures or to visualize already recognized fractures better.

The 45° internal oblique view improves the visualization of the medial malleolus and the posterior facet of the talocalcaneal joint. The 45° external oblique view shows the contour of the anterior tubercle of the tibia. The lateral malleolus is seen from a different angle but is obstructed by the tibia.

An isolated fracture of the dorsal lip of the tibia or a widened syndesmosis may indicate the presence of a Maissoneuve fracture and requires a full view of the fibula up to the knee (Fig. 13.11b).

13.6.4 Stress Examinations

When osseous lesions have been ruled out and clinical evidence is suggestive of a significant injury, stress examinations have to be taken into consideration. They should, if possible, be obtained within the first 2 h after the trauma. Later, swelling and pain will be likely to influence the measurements and local anesthesia is often required to arrive at meaningful results.

To examine the anterior fibulotalar ligament, the foot is positioned laterally with the knee bent about 30°. The foot and lower tibia are fixed. Then, pressure is exerted on the frontal tibia and a lateral film is taken. The distance between the most distal part of the tibial joint surface and the closest point on the talar joint surface is measured (Fig. 13.20). A distance of up to 5 mm is considered normal; 6–10 mm is doubtful (indicating a partial tear or ligamentous laxity, requiring comparison with the unaffected

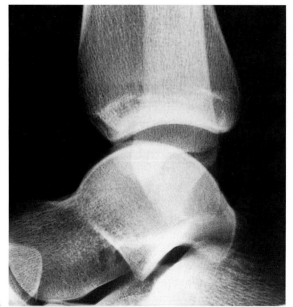

a

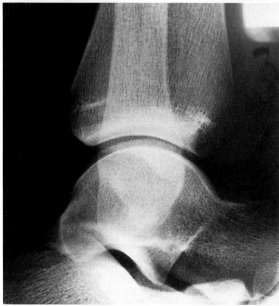

b

Fig. 13.20a,b. Stress examination shows an increase in the tibiotalar distance, indicating a tear of the anterior fibulotalar ligament. See uninjured side for comparison

side), and more than 10 mm is interpreted as a complete rupture.

For testing of the lateral ligaments, i.e., the fibulocalcanear and deltoid ligaments, the patient is positioned sitting upright or supine with the knee bent to about 20°. The foot and proximal lower limb are then affixed. Stress is applied to the medial or lateral side of the tibia and an attempt is made to force the talus into medial or lateral subluxation out

of the mortise (Fig. 13.21). The talus may normally tilt to about 6° or 7°, though in some people with ligamentous laxity it may tilt up to 10° or even 15°. At our institution less than 6° is considered normal; 7–10° is regarded as doubtful, requiring comparison with the unaffected foot, and more than 10° is seen as indicative of a significant ligamentous injury. Stress examinations can depict the extent of the damage to the invisible joint but in many cases do not allow precise predictions of which structures are injured. Recently, MRI has been able to show ligamentous injuries to be much more severe than originally suspected after stress examinations (BREITENSEHER et al. 1995).

Below the age of 10 years the ligamentous structures are less tight than in adolescents, so that comparison with the contralateral side is often required. A difference of more than 5° usually indicates a significant injury.

Stress examinations in general and the above-mentioned values in particular are, however, subject to much controversy among radiologists and surgeons; the cited values are by no means unilaterally accepted and may vary from clinic to clinic. Also, personal experience, judgment, and different preferences regarding surgery versus a conservative treatment approach may lead to different interpretations of the results. The more or less liberal use of anesthesia or manually applied force will add to the differences in criteria.

Efforts have been made to standardize the procedure employed in stress examinations. Rather than having the radiologist or surgeon exerting pressure on the foot, automatic devices are used that allow application of a standardized force. A value often used, but by no means universally accepted, is 15 kp. Simply applying 15 kp, however, does not necessarily mean that a precise measurement can be taken in a reproducible manner; e.g., the position of the lever may differ so that the resulting force will not be the nominally applied 15 kp. Chandani and co-workers found that there seems to be only a slight degree of standardization among radiologists and orthopedic surgeons regarding stress examinations (CHANDANI 1994; CHANDANI et al. 1994). In addition, size, physical strength, positioning, and degree of pain vary considerably among patients and will yield results that cannot necessarily be assumed to be comparable. Even the right/left comparison obviously can be influenced by a previous injury to the contralateral side if it resulted in ligamentous laxity.

Fig. 13.21. Stress examination shows an increase in talar tilt, indicating a rupture of the fibulocalcanear ligament. See uninjured side for comparison

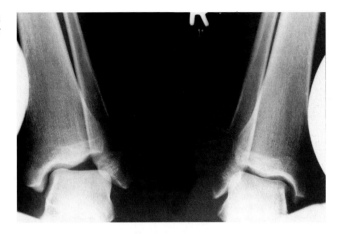

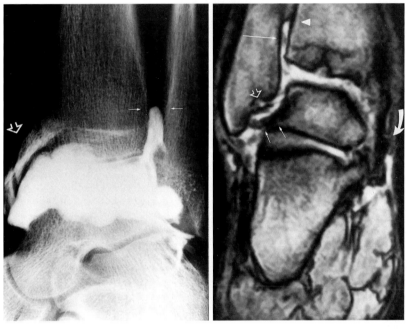

a   b

Fig. 13.22. a Arthrography demonstrates an intact syndesmosis. The contrast medium fills the tibiofibular recess which ends about 2 cm proximal to the joint surface (*arrows*). There is a minor injury to the medial joint capsule and possibly parts of the deltoid ligament, as indicated by the contrast medium escaping to the medial soft tissue (*open arrow*). **b** T2*-weighted MRI indicates that the joint fluid reaches to the same level (*arrowhead*) as the contrast medium in **a**. Traversing the lateral joint space are the posterior fibulotalar (*arrows*) and intermalleolar ligaments (*open arrow*), the dorsal syndesmosis (*long arrow*), the interosseous membrane (*arrowhead*), and the deltoid ligament (*curved arrow*)

13.6.5 Arthrography

Arthrography (Fig. 13.22a) of the ankle joint is a reliable method to prove, but not necessarily to exclude significant injuries of the ligaments. The correlation between the findings of arthrography and intraoperative results ranges from 62.5% (KARL and WRAZIDLO 1987) to 100% (!) (FRANKE et al. 1986). The sensitivity of arthrography for detecting an isolated rupture of the syndesmosis is about 90%, and the accuracy about 78% (WRAZIDLO 1988). However, it is a more invasive technique than stress examination and bears a small risk of infection. Reliable results can only be expected within the first 48 h after the trauma since adhesions of the joint capsule can mask ruptures thereafter. A disadvantage of this technique is that although it can demonstrate the damage to the ligaments and the syndesmosis, it often fails to show the extent of the damage. Despite some drawbacks, this remains the stronghold of

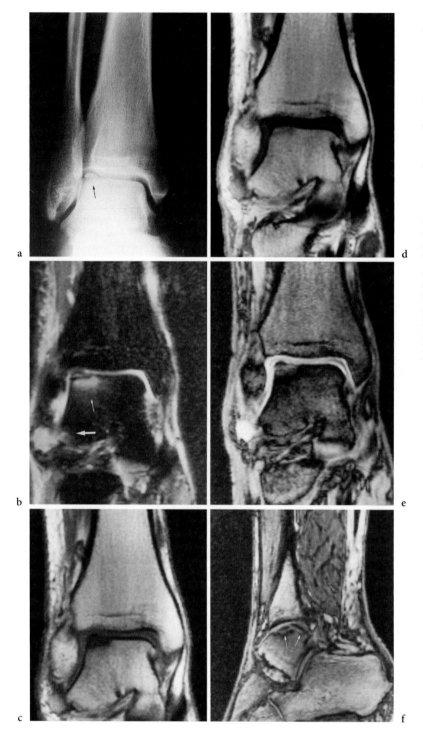

Fig. 13.23. a Note the flake fracture at the lateral aspect of the talus dome (*arrow*). It was suspected to have resulted from an old injury aggravated by a 2-week-old trauma which also caused a lateral ligamentous injury. **b** The STIR sequence shows a small bone edema below the flake (*small arrow*), a small joint effusion, and a fluid-like signal below the fibula (*large arrow*). **c, d** (T1 SE and T1 SE + gadolinium): There is enhancement of the osteochondral bed but not of the flake itself. **e** Flash three-dimensional (flip 60°, TR 60, TE 11) T1-weighted sequence visualizing a thinned chondral surface above the flake and the presence of fibrous tissue in the bed. **f** A sagittal multiplanar reconstruction [(TR 11.4 ms, T2 4.4 ms, TA 4.31 min, SL 1.2 mm) three-dimensional data acquisition, allowing for reconstruction of images in any plane] indicates the presence of two flakes (*arrows*). The different signal characteristics of the fluid-filled space below the fibula are notably different from joint fluid (which has a water-like signal) due to the presence of blood

stress examinations and is one of the reasons why arthrography is less and less often performed in many institutions. Furthermore, MRI is able to depict the "invisible joint" much better than radiographs or CT and will probably largely supersede arthrography (Fig. 13.22).

13.6.6 Magnetic Resonance Imaging

Magnetic resonance imaging seems to be able to combine most of the advantages of stress examinations, arthrography, and CT and in addition supplies excellent soft tissue contrast (Fig. 13.23). It has a

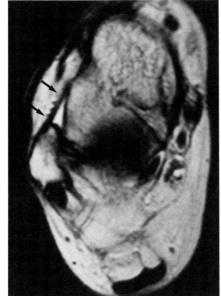

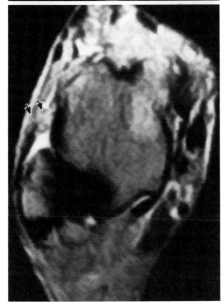

Fig. 13.24. a Intact anterior fibulotalar ligament of a healthy volunteer viewed in slight plantar flexion of the foot in order to achieve stretching of the ligament (*arrows*). **b** *Arrows* indicate a ruptured anterior fibulotalar ligament and joint effusion

with previous examinations. If radiologists want MRI to be accepted by surgeons, they have to use standardized imaging protocols and patient positioning; "fancy stuff" is allowed only after the standard images are in the box. Then, initial and follow-up examinations can be compared easily.

Positioning not only should allow for optimal visualization of the most important and most commonly injured anatomical structures but also should be comfortable for the patient in order to minimize motion artifacts. A convenient position for the foot and in particular for an injured joint is in slight plantar flexion. Due to the talar shape this position allows for small movements in the ankle joint and thus takes some pressure off the effused joint capsule. An additional benefit of this position is the better visualization of the fibulotalar ligament. In slight plantar flexion, this most commonly injured ligament is placed under slight tension (Fig. 13.24), thus reducing the likelihood of a potential pitfall, i.e., of having a bowed ligament running in and out of the slice volume (see also the recommendations regarding slice thickness below). One should watch for joint effusion and signal increases in the STIR sequence and let them be the guide to the injuries (Fig. 13.23b, 13.25b).

In imaging ligaments, it is important to be aware of the "magic angle" phenomenon (TIMINS et al. 1994). This artifact can lead to a signal increase in fibrous structures which are crossing the vector of the magnetic field at an angle of about 55°. Sequences with a short echo time (TE) are most vulnerable to this phenomenon while sequences with a long TE, i.e., a T2-weighted spin echo (SE) or turbo spin echo (TSE), help to avoid it.

The most important plane able to depict the majority of the ligaments is an axial one (Fig. 13.26). It allows the evaluation of the anterior and posterior fibulotalar, intermalleolar, and anterior and posterior tibiofibular ligaments as well as the anterior and posterior syndesmosis and to a lesser extent the deltoid ligament. In very rare cases the fibulocalcanear ligament also can be visualized. For optimal results this plane should be angulated in a sagittal scout view in the direction of the deep flexor muscles of the foot (Fig. 13.27a) – this is the direction of the anterior fibulotalar ligament. To improve the visualization of the syndesmosis, the anterior tibiofibular ligament, and the intermalleolar ligament, a second angulation of the axial plane, i.e., to raise it medially by 10–15°, is useful (Fig. 13.27b). A T2 SE sequence in this angulation provides a lot of

good chance of replacing the aforementioned examinations to a large extent. Already it should complement doubtful stress examinations in young and active patients (BREITENSEHER et al. 1995). One of MRI's biggest advantages, however, is also its greatest hindrance in achieving general acceptance: the absolutely free choice of orientation and the innumerable sequences make the images difficult to understand and not infrequently preclude comparison

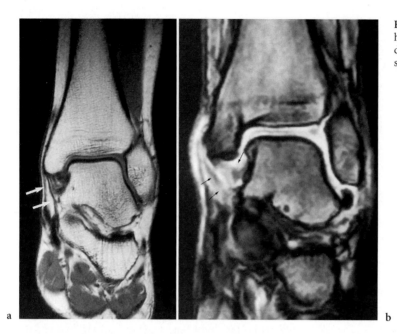

Fig. 13.25. a Normal deltoid ligament in a healthy volunteer (*arrows*). **b** A ruptured deltoid ligament has flipped into the joint space (*arrows*); note, also, the joint effusion

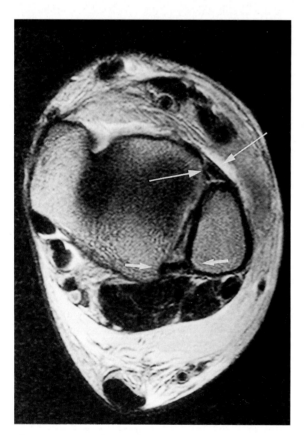

Fig. 13.26. T1 SE shows normal posterior tibiofibular (*short arrows*), anterior tibiofibular, and (partially) anterior fibulotalar ligaments (*long arrows*)

information about tendons, nerves, soft tissue, and vessels and it is sometimes useful to have it in T1 weighting as well.

A T1-weighted sequence in the sagittal plane gives a good overview of the bone structures and a first impression about the cartilage and subchondral bone. It should be angulated using an axial view perpendicular to the line connecting the malleoli or the anterior margin of the talus (Fig. 13.27c).

The third important plane is the coronal view angulated parallel to the intermalleolar line using the axial view and following the course of the tibia in the sagittal view (Fig. 13.27d). This again serves to visualize the cartilage and bone structures, especially the lateral and medial aspect of the talar dome, where cartilage defects are mostly located (Fig. 13.23e). The syndesmosis and the posterior fibulotalar, intermalleolar, posterior tibiofibular, anterior tibiofibular, deltoid, and (to a limited extent) fibulocalcanear ligaments can also be evaluated in most cases. An angulation of 15–20° towards the calcaneus (Fig. 13.27e) can help to yield a better view of the cartilage of the anterior part of the talus due to the shape of the talar dome and in some cases also of the fibulocalcanear ligament. It bears the disadvantage of losing the ease of anatomical orientation of the straight coronal view (Fig. 13.27d). In order to improve the evaluation of the cartilage, one should use a gradient echo (GRE) T2*-weighted (small flip angle) sequence. The T2* effect allows for the visualization of joint and soft tissue effusion and

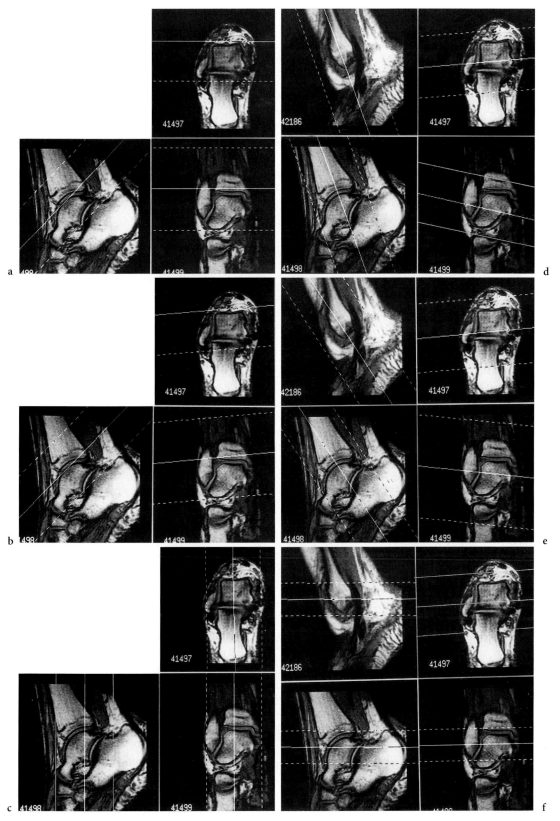

Fig. 13.27. a–f Three-dimensional scout film demonstrating the angulation of the MR imaging as described in Table 13.1. The resulting changes in one plane are immediately displayed in the other two planes. *Upper right image*: transversal scout view; *lower right image*: coronal scout view; *lower left image*: sagittal scout view; *upper left image*: supplemental view to simplify angulation

Table 13.1. Standard MRI sequences

Sequence	Direction/extension	Important structures
SE T2/PD 3.5 mm, 13–15 slices	Axial: parallel to the deep flexor muscles (Fig. 13.27a), raised medially by 10° (Fig. 13.27b) From about 2 cm above the tibiotalar joint gap down to the region of the collum tali/below the the tip of the fibula	Ligaments: anterior fibulotalar, posterior fibulotalar, intermalleolar, posterior tibiofibular, anterior tibiofibular; (deltoid, fibulocalcanear) Syndesmosis
GRE/SE T1 3–3.5 mm 15–17 slices	Sagittal: angulated perpendicular to a line connecting both malleoli or a line anterior to the talar dome (Fig. 13.27c) From the lateral part of the fibula to the medial part of the medial malleolus	Cartilage Subchondral bone, bone Soft tissue
GRE T2, 3.5 mm, 15–17 slices	Coronal: parallel to a line connecting both malleoli (or a line anterior to the talar dome) (Fig. 13.27d), if possible angulated perpendicular to the long axis of the talus (Fig. 13.27e) From the collum tali to the medial third of the tuber of the calcaneus	Cartilage Subchondral bone, bone Ligaments: posterior fibulotalar, intermalleolar, posterior tibiofibular, syndesmosis, anterior tibiofibular, deltoid (fibulocalcanear ligament)
SE T2 3.5 mm 9 slices	Axial: perpendicular to a line between the anterior tip of the tibia and the upper rim of the caput tali (Fig. 13.27f) From below the tip of the fibula 30 mm upwards	Fibulocalcanear ligament Soft tissue
SE/GRE T1, 3.5 mm, 13–15 slices	Axial: parallel to the deep flexor muscles (Fig. 13.27a), raised medially by 10° (Fig. 13.27b) From about 2 cm above the fibulotalar joint gap down to the region of the collum tali/below the tip of the fibula	In addition to SE T2 axial. It helps to distinguish between fat/effusion, vessels/tendons/nerves, and ligaments
STIR 4 mm	Sagittal and/or coronal	Bone edema, osteomyelitis fracture

ligamental edema (pitfall: magic angle). Alternatively, a T1-weighted flash sequence with fat suppression may provide similar information (Fig. 13.23e)

The fibulocalcanear ligament can sometimes be evaluated more easily in a paraxial plane, i.e., parallel to the ligament, perpendicular to a line between the anterior tip of the tibia and the upper rim of the caput tali (Fig. 13.27f).

For acquisition of detailed anatomical information without the risk of partial volume artifacts, e.g., a slightly bowed ligament that runs in and out of a slice and thus possibly looks partially torn, a slice thickness of 3.5 mm is very practical for all sequences. If possible, the scout view should be performed as a multiplanar scout, thus being able to angulate all sequences rapidly and effectively. If this is not possible, one should start with an axial multislice scout and begin with the sagittal sequence. Then Coronal and subsequently axial sequences can be planned using the previous sequences.

To answer specific questions, e.g., regarding the presence of osteomyelitis or fracture, usually a short T1 inversion recovery (STIR) sequence is recommended. It also serves as an excellent screening device to detect small injuries or to differentiate between old and acute injuries. As a general rule, one should become familiar with a set of four or five standard sequences and their angulation and then add additional examinations as deemed necessary (Table 13.1).

13.7 Diagnostic Algorithm

A diagnostic algorithm in respect of ankle trauma is shown in Fig. 13.28.

Acknowledgments. We would like to thank Heidi Schnepel, Regina Träger, and Tine Neumann for searching (and finding!) most of the radiographs in our archives and Gabi Klotz for preparing the photographs. Gesa Mester and Sabine Kröger lent us their ankles for the MRI anatomy.

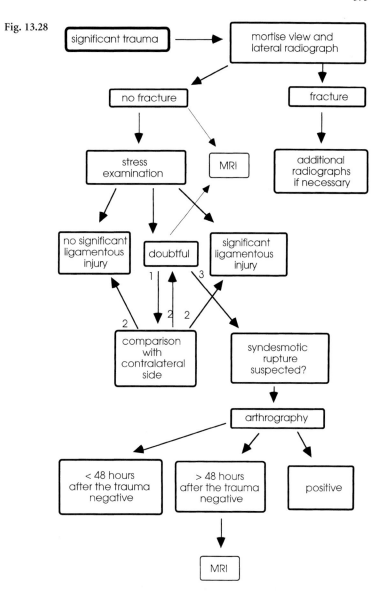

Fig. 13.28

References

Arimoto HK, Forrester DM (1980) Classification of ankle fractures: an algorithm. AJR 135:1057–1063

Auletta AG, Conway WF, Hayes CW, Guisto DF, Gervin AS (1991) Indications for radiography in patients with acute ankle injuries: role of the physical examination. AJR 157:789–701

Blei CL, Nirschi RP, Grant EG (1986) Achilles tendon: US diagnosis and pathologic conditions. Radiology 159:765

Breitenseher MJ, Trattnig S, Kukla C, Gabler C, Haller J, Imhoff H (1995) Injured lateral ankle ligaments. MR imaging compared with stress radiography. Radiology 197(P)(Suppl):166

Chandani VP (1994) Response to Rijke AM. Radiology 196:580

Chandani VP, Harper MT, Ficke JR, Gagliardi JA, Rolling L, Christensen KP, Hansen MF (1994) Chronic ankle instability: evaluation with MR arthrography, MR imaging, and stress radiography. Radiology 192:189–194

DeLacey GJ, Bradbrooke S (1979) Rationalizing the requests for x-ray examination of acute ankle injury. BMJ 1:1597–1598

Dupuytren G (1839) Of fractures of the lower extremity of the fibula, and luxations of the foot. (From: Clinical Lectures on Surgery, delivered at Hotel Dieu in 1832.) Med Class 4:151. Quoted from: Rogers (1992)

Dingemann RD, Shaver GD (1978) Operative treatment of displaced Salter-Harris III distal tibial fractures. Clin Orthop 135:101

Erlemann R, Wuismann P, Just A, Peters PE (1991) Mißbildungen und Traumafolgen des kindlichen und jugendlichen Sprunggelenks. Radiologe 31:601–608

Frahm R, Wimmer B, Bonnaire F (1991) Computertomographie des oberen und unteren Sprunggelenks. Radiologe 31:609–615

Franke D, Weiher U, Sossinka NP, Fenn K (1986) Die Wertigkeit der Arthrographie im Vergleich zur gehaltenen Aufnahme in der Diagnostik von Kapselbandläsionen am oberen Sprunggelenk. Röntgenpraxis 39:41

Gebing R, Fiedler V (1991) Röntgendiagnostik der Bandläsionen des oberen Sprunggelenks. Radiologe 31:594–600

Hall FM (1992) Indications for radiography in acute ankle injuries. AJR 158:141

Hamilton WG (1993) Foot and ankle injuries in dancers. In: Mann RA, Coughlin MJ (eds) Surgery of the foot and ankle, 6th edn. Mosby, St. Louis, pp 1241–1276

Jend HH, Daase M, Heller M, Holzrichter D (1983) Zur Diagnostik von Bandverletzungen des oberen Sprungngelenks mit gedrückten Aufnahmen. Fortschr Röntgenstr 139:540

Karl EL, Wrazidlo W (1987) Die frische Syndesmosenruptur am oberen Sprunggelenk. Klinische Bedeutung und arthrographische Diagnostik. Unfallchirurg 90:92–96

Lauge-Hansen N (1953) Fractures of the ankle. V. Pronation-dorsiflexion fracture. Arch Surg: 67:813

Lauge-Hansen N (1954) Fractures of the ankle. III. Genetic Roentgenologic diagnosis of fractures of the ankle. AJR 71:456

Mainwaring BL, Daffner RH, Riemer BL (1988) Pylon fractures of the ankle: a distinct clinical and radiologic entity. Radiology 168:215

Maissoneuve JGT (1840) Recherches sur la fracture du péronè. Arch Gen Med 7:165 quoted from: Rogers (1992)

Mandell J (1971) Isolated fractures of the posterior tibial lip at the ankle as demonstrated by an additional projection, the "poor" lateral view. Radiology 101:319

Müller ME, Allgöwer M, Schneider R, Willenegger H (1991) Manual of internal fixation. Techniques recommended by the AO-ASIF Group, 3rd edn. Springer, Berlin Heidelberg New York

Oesterreich FU, Heller M, Maas R, Langkowski JH, Hemker T (1988) Magnetresonanztomographie der Füße und oberen Sprunggelenke. Fortschr Röntgenstr 148:169

Ovadia DN, Beals RK (1986) Fractures of the tibial plafond. J Bone Joint Surg [Am] 68:543

Rijke AM (1994) Comment to Chandani et al. Radiology 196:580

Rogers LF (1992) with contributions by Hendrix RW. Radiology of skeletal trauma, 2nd edn. Churchill Livingstone, Edinburgh

Rosenberg ZS, Cheung YY, Beltran J, Sheskier S, Leong M, Jahss M (1995) Posterior intermalleolar ligament of the ankle. AJR 165:387–390

Ruedi TP, Allgöwer M (1979) The operative treatment of intra-articular fractures of the lower end of the tibia. Clin Orthop 138:105

Salter RB (1974) Injuries of the ankle in children. Orthop Clin North Am 5:147

Salter RB, Harris WR (1963) Injuries involving the epiphyseal plate. J Bone Joint Surg [Am] 45:587

Thelen M, Ritter G, Bücheler E (1993) Radiologische Diagnostik der Verletzungen von Knochen und Gelenken. Thieme, Stuttgart

Timins ME, Erickson SJ, Estkowski LD, Carrera GF, Komorowski RA (1994) Increased signal in the normal supraspinatus tendon on MR imaging: diagnostic pitfall caused by the magic angle effect. AJR 165:109–114

Töndury (1981) Agewandte und topographische Anatomie, 5th edn. Thieme, Stuttgart

Vestring T, Bongartz G, Erlemann R, et al. (1991) Magnetresonanztomographie des Sprunggelenks. Radiologe 31:616–623

Weber BG (1972) Die Verletzungen des oberen Sprunggelenks. Huber, Bern

Wrazidlo W, Karl EL, Koch K (1988) Die arthrographische Diagnostik der vorderen Syndesmosenruptur am oberen Sprunggelenk. Fortschr Röntgenstr 148:492

Zwipp H (1991) Verletzungen des oberen Sprunggelenkes aus unfallchirurgischer Sicht. Radiologe 31:585–593

14 Foot

M. FREUND and M. HELLER

14.1 General Considerations

Trauma to the feet is common and is often followed by fractures, so that approximately 10% of all fractures occur in the pedal skeleton (ROGERS 1992). Often the patient's history is difficult to evaluate because the patient is not able to describe the mechanism of the accident. In most cases the patient complains only of a "twisted foot." Therefore, it is not easy to differentiate between lesions of the ankle and lesions of the foot.

M. FREUND, MD, Klinik für Radiologische Diagnostik, Klinikum der Christian-Albrechts-Universität zu Kiel, Arnold-Heller-Straße 9, 24105 Kiel, Germany
M. HELLER, MD, PhD, Professor and Direktor der Klinik für Radiologische Diagnostik, Klinikum der Christian-Albrechts-Universität zu Kiel, Arnold-Heller-Straße 9, 24105 Kiel, Germany

Ankle injuries may be associated with lesions of the foot, especially osteochondral fractures of the dome of the talus. Traumatic luxations are less frequent and are usually combined with bony fractures. Most bony lesions of the foot following an acute trauma are not difficult to detect, but some subtle fractures may cause diagnostic problems. Sometimes soft tissue changes like swelling or obliteration and dislocation of fat planes are the only clue to a fracture, and should be observed closely.

14.2 Pathogenic Mechanisms and Anatomy

14.2.1 Pathogenic Mechanisms

Most injuries of the foot are due to direct trauma, e.g., heavy objects falling on the foot or falling from a height; less frequently they result from striking objects with the foot during walking. Especially after falling from a height, a thorough examination of the patient is necessary, since associated lesions such as fractures of the spine, the tibia, or the femur and bilateral foot lesions are not uncommon.

Excessive torsional movements and avulsion by tendinous and fibrous articular capsule cause indirect injuries, which occur less often than direct trauma.

Rarely, pathological fractures of the foot are a consequence of metastatic disease or other causes. In most cases pathological fractures of the foot, especially of the tarsometatarsal joints and tarsal bones, are caused by diabetic neurotrophic osteopathy.

Mechanical overstrain and lack of exercise can be a cause of stress fractures, which are sometimes difficult to diagnose because of only small pathomorphological changes and minimal radiographic findings.

A systematic approach should be used in describing the radiological findings after a trauma to the foot, and it is also very important to have all the clinical information available.

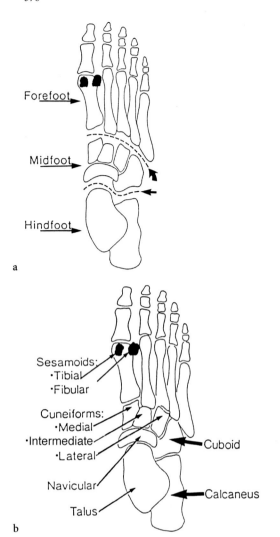

Fig. 14.1a,b. Anatomy. **a** Three main segments of the pedal skeleton: hindfoot, midfoot, and forefoot. *Straight arrow proximally*: Chopart's joint; *curved arrow distally*: Lisfranc's joint. Dark bony structures at the head of the first metatarsal bone: sesamoids. **b** Hindfoot: talus and calcaneus. Midfoot: navicular, cuboid, and cuneiforms. Forefoot: five metatarsal bones and five phalanges. Typical location of the tibial and fibular sesamoids

14.2.2 Anatomy

The foot has two major functions. The first is to support the body in standing and progression; therefore the pedal skeleton must be able to spread forces of moving and standing and be pliable enough for uneven and sloping surfaces. The second function is to lever the body forwards in walking, running, and jumping; therefore the pedal platform must be transformable into a strong adjustable lever. Anatomically, clinically, and radiologically the pedal skeleton can be divided into three segments: the hindfoot,

midfoot, and forefoot (Fig. 14.1a). The joint between the hindfoot and the midfoot is called Chopart's joint, while that between the midfoot and the forefoot is termed Lisfranc's joint or the tarsometatarsal joint (Fig. 14.1a) (GREENSPAN 1990; GRAY 1989).

14.2.2.1 Hindfoot

The hindfoot includes the two largest tarsal bones: the talus and the calcaneus. The talus articulates with the tibia, medial and lateral malleoli, the navicular, and the calcaneus. The calcaneus articulates with the talus and the cuboid (Fig. 14.1b). Chopart's joint separates the talus and calcaneus from the navicular and cuboid bone. Movements between the talus and calcaneus are complex and always involve the talocalcaneonavicular joint, knowledge of which is important for therapy planning and to prevent complications like posttraumatic arthritis.

Knowledge of the normal radiographic appearance of the apophysis of the dorsal os calcis is important, since it is often denser than the rest of the bone. However, the typical location and radiological findings usually render differentiation from pathology easy.

14.2.2.2 Midfoot

The midfoot includes the navicular, the cuboid, the medial, the intermediate and lateral cuneiforms. The navicular articulates with the talus and the cuneiforms, the cuboid with the calcaneus, and the two lateral metatarsals and the medial cuneiform with the lateral cuneiform (Fig. 14.1b). The cuneiforms articulate with the navicular and the first to fourth metatarsals and with each other.

14.2.2.3 Forefoot

The forefoot includes the five metatarsals and phalanges. Proximally the metatarsals articulate with the cuneiforms and distally with the phalanges. Each of the toes comprises three phalanges, except for the hallux, which consists of only two (Fig. 14.1b).

As in the case of the calcaneal apophysis, one should be familiar with the normal radiographic findings of the apophysis at the base of the fifth metatarsal bone. The apophysis runs more or less parallel to the metatarsal shaft. A fracture line representing an avulsion fracture of the base of the fifth metatarsal

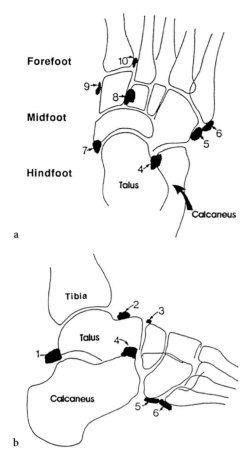

Fig. 14.2a,b. Physiological variations. a Typical location of accessory centers of ossification in an anterior-posterior projection: *4*, os calcaneus secondarius; *5*, os fibulare (os peroneum); *6*; os vesalianum pedis; *7*, os tibiale externum; *8*, os intercuneiforme; *9*, sesamoid; *10*, os intermetatarseum. b Typical location of accessory centers of ossification in a lateral projection: *1*, os trigonum tarsi; *2*, os supratalare; *3*, os supranaviculare; *4*, os calcaneus secundarius; *5*, os fibulare (os peroneum); *6*, os vesalianum pedis

runs transversely in most cases. Physiologically the epiphyses of the phalanges and the first metatarsal bone are located proximally, while the epiphyses of the second to fifth metatarsals are located distally (GRAY 1989).

14.2.2.4 Physiological Variations

The normal pedal skeleton can include a large number of accessory centers of ossification that can mimic traumatic pathology. Therefore, the location and shape of these common sesamoid bones should be known. In general these nodular structures are only a few millimeters in size, but there is a broad variation in shape and size. They are typically located

close to articular joints, partly ossified and embedded in tendons.

It is very common for there to be a pair of sesamoid bones at the head of the first metatarsal, usually bilaterally (Fig. 14.1b). Sometimes the sesamoid bones are bipartite, but if they appear with a sclerotic, plane and intact surface, they can be distinguished from a sequel caused by trauma.

Other common structures are the os trigonum, os tibiale externum, and os peroneum; occasionally accessory bones are found at the metatarsophalangeal joint of the second and fifth phalanges (Fig. 14.2) (GRAY 1989; GREENSPAN 1990). The os trigonum is located posterior to the lateral tubercle of the posterior process of the talus and is found in nearly every other individual.

14.2.2.5 Terminology

A certain terminology has been established to describe the complex mechanisms of foot movements. For a detailed description and correct reporting of findings it is important to be familiar with the following eight terms: *Supination* describes the elevation of the medial border of the foot, and *pronation* the elevation of the lateral border of the foot. *Abduction* describes external rotation, while *adduction* is the opposite; both movements are rotations of the foot about the vertical axis. Rotation about the long axis is described as *eversion* for outward rotation and *inversion* for inward rotation. Finally, *Plantar flexion* is movement toward the plantar side of the foot, while *dorsiflexion* is motion towards the foreleg.

14.3 Classifications of Trauma

14.3.1 Talus

Fractures of the talus are not very frequent. Only 6% of all traumatic lesions of the foot are talar injuries. Most fractures are avulsion factures and fractures of the neck and body. Compression fractures occur less frequently.

The most common and widely accepted classification of talar fractures is that established by HAWKINS, defining three categories (Table 14.1). This classification was subsequently modified to include four types (CANALE and KELLY 1978).

A fracture of the talar neck without luxation or subluxation is defined as type I; subluxation or dislocation of the subtalar joint without luxation of the

Table 14.1. Differentiation of talar lesions and classification of talar neck lesions by Hawkins (modified by Canale and Kelly)

Isolated fractures	Fractures with dislocation
1. Avulsion fracture	1. Body fracture with subtalar
2. Compression fracture	dislocation
3. Body fracture	2. Complete dislocation

Talar neck lesions
1. Type I: Vertical neck fracture without dislocation
2. Type II: Vertical neck fracture with subtalar dislocation
3. Type III: Vertical neck fracture with subtalar and tibiotalar dislocation
4. Type IV: Vertical fracture of the talus with subtalar or tibiotalar dislocation and dislocation of the talonavicular articulation

Table 14.2. Classification of calcaneal fractures by Essex-Lopresti

Subtalar joint not involved	Subtalar joint involved
A. *Extra-articular fractures*	
1. Beak type (Boyer)	A. Undisplaced lesion
2. Avulsion of the medial border	B. Displaced lesion
3. Vertical	C. With gross
4. Horizontal	comminution
B. *Calcaneocuboidal joint involved*	

ankle joint is typical of a type II fracture, and type III is defined as a lesion with complete luxation of the body of the talus from the ankle joint as well as from the subtalar joint (HAWKINS 1970). A type IV fracture is associated with a dislocation of the talonavicular joint. Severe complications may occur in types III and IV, in which interruption of the blood supply to the talus can cause acute vascular necrosis (see Sect. 14.5.1.1).

14.3.2 Calcaneus

The most popular classification of fractures of the os calcis is that proposed by ESSEX-LOPRESTI in 1952. This classification distinguishes between fractures with and fractures without involvement of the subtalar joint. Each group is divided into different subtypes (Table 14.2).

In the group of intra-articular fractures two types need to be differentiated: the "joint depression" and the "tongue" type. The more common joint depression type is characterized by a lateralization of the central fragment which carries the posterior facet of the subtalar joint and by a second fracture line run-

ning dorsal to the posterior facet (see Fig. 14.14). The tongue type shows a tongue-like fragment in the lateral view and a straight fracture line running to the posterior margin of the calcaneus (see Fig. 14.12).

The extra-articular fractures are mostly avulsions and are classified into the "beak" type, vertical and horizontal types, and medial avulsion (Table 14.2).

Another classification of calcaneus fractures was established by ROWE et al. (1963). This classification consists of five types; types I and II are defined as results of avulsion mechanisms, while the other types are more complex lesions. The Essex-Lopresti classification is more commonly used.

With the introduction of computed tomography (CT) for the imaging of fractures of the calcaneus, several modified classifications have been suggested, based on the various CT findings; however, none has become widely accepted. Most of these have derived from Essex-Lopresti's classification (HÄBERLE et al. 1993).

14.4 Imaging Techniques

14.4.1 Radiographic Examination

Radiographic studies of the foot after trauma are based on examinations of the pedal skeleton. Only rarely are lesions of the ligaments and tendons examined. Radiographic studies of the foot are difficult because a large number of small bones lie closely together and articulate in a complex manner.

Routinely anteroposterior, lateral, and oblique views should be included when a radiographic evaluation of the foot is requested. Plain film examination of the calcaneus requires an axial as well as a lateral projection and different oblique views of the ankle (BERQUIST et al. 1992). The anteroposterior projection usually visualizes parts of the tarsometatarsal and phalangeal joints, the head of the talus, and the distal parts of the metatarsals. The phalanges are clearly identified on the anteroposterior views, and traumatic lesions are usually revealed without difficulties.

The bases of the second to fourth metatarsals are difficult to identify since they overlap with the distal portion of the intermediate and lateral cuneiform. However, oblique views, for instance elevating the lateral border of the foot, are able to separate the structures.

Lateral radiographs show overlapping of all tarsal and metatarsal bones. The phalanges, including the

Fig. 14.3. Medial view of the right os calcis showing the Böhler's angle, subtalar joint, and calcaneocuboid joint

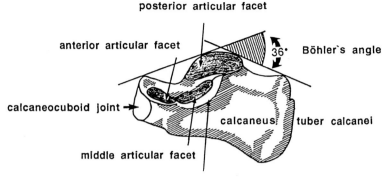

interphalangeal joints, can be clearly visualized on lateral views.

Böhler's angle, formed by the intersection of two lines, one drawn from the posterior facet to the anterior superior calcaneus, the other drawn along the tuberosity and posterior facet, ranges between 20° and 40° (Fig. 14.3) (BERQUIST et al. 1992; TRIEBEL and AHLERS 1993).

Oblique projections demonstrate Chopart's joint, the midfoot, and the bases of the metatarsals.

A number of special projections may be required to answer certain demands. Usually there is no use for stress views in the evaluation of ligamentous lesions of the foot after trauma: only in ankle lesions may stress views be useful.

Conventional tomography can be a useful additional diagnostic tool if more information is needed or subtle skeletal changes have to be identified. The tomograms are obtained in anteroposterior or lateral planes or in both. WHITBY and BARRINGTON (1995) recommend lateral tomography of the lateral process of the talus for all patients with clinically suspected fracture and no findings on the initial standard plain films. Conventional tomography can also be very helpful after surgical treatment and osteosynthesis.

14.4.2 Computed Tomography

Since CT developed into a widespread technique, CT examinations of the hindfoot have become common and have proved very helpful, since they are able to show the complex anatomy and pathomorphological changes after injuries of the tarsus. CT is particularly useful for evaluation of lesions of the calcaneus; less frequently it is used to evaluate the talus.

Computed tomography clearly demonstrates intra-articular lesions, comminution, and changes in the shape of the hindfoot shape without overlapping structures. Fragment displacement can be visualized better than on conventional radiographs. Another advantage of CT is its ability to detect soft tissue abnormalities, although it does not do so as well as MRI. Nowadays CT is the technique of choice for tarsal and subtalar joint trauma. It helps to decide between conservative treatment and surgery and assists in planning the surgical reconstruction (HEGER et al. 1985; HEUCHEMER et al. 1992; KERR et al. 1994).

One other aspect of CT is its 3D capability. Many authors have reported on the usefulness of 3D reformations in treatment planning (ALLON and MEARS 1991; CARR et al. 1990; TANYÜ et al. 1994). "Electronic disarticulation" of the calcaneus from the talus and cuboid in order to visualize the articular facets in 3D reformations without overlapping bony structures might be another means to demonstrate the full extent of trauma (FREUND et al. 1996).

Under normal circumstances there is no routine use for CT examinations in the evaluation of isolated metatarsal or phalangeal injuries. However, they may serve as an adjunct in the assessment of complex soft tissue injuries.

14.4.3 Ultrasound

Ultrasound (US) is inexpensive, quickly performed, and usually used to examine soft tissue structures such as hematomas, tendons, ligaments, and vessels. It is also preferred in the examination of newborns, infants, and smaller children. In the lower extremity US is routinely used to examine lesions of the Achilles tendon (BLEI et al. 1986; KAINBERGER et al. 1990). In general US is not used to examine fractures due to the limited ability of sound waves to penetrate bones (BLUTH et al. 1982).

14.4.4 Magnetic Resonance Imaging

Magnetic resonance imaging is a very suitable method for the examination of musculoskeletal disorders of the foot. It is especially helpful in detecting lesions of tendons, ligaments, and muscles and post-traumatic complications such as avascular necrosis. Subtle traumatic changes, e.g., osteochondral fractures and osteochondrosis dissecans, and also indications for MRI.

One limitation of MRI is its inability to visualize cortical bone directly; however, it is highly superior to other imaging techniques in the differentiation of muscle, tendons, ligaments, fat, cartilage, and fluid (ERICKSON et al. 1990; SIERRA et al. 1986). Today MRI is not generally accepted as a technique used to evaluate acute foot trauma, but this might change in the future (DAFFNER et al. 1986).

14.4.5 Nuclear Medicine

Radionuclide studies are a very helpful diagnostic tool when radiographs are negative in patients with a history of trauma and clinical signs of a traumatic lesion. They are also useful in patients suspected of having stress fractures and in detecting bone infections (BROWN et al. 1986; GESLIAN et al. 1976).

Bone scans are also able to detect more bony lesions in other areas of the skeleton. Occasionally the bone scan indicates the presence of systemic disease, for instance metastatic or inflammatory disease, which one would not have suspected only by looking at the foot.

14.5 Radiographic Findings of Trauma

14.5.1 Hindfoot

14.5.1.1 Talar Lesions

The talus is the link between the lower leg and the foot through the ankle joint. It consists of three parts: head, neck, and body (GRAY 1989). The blood supply of the talus is vulnerable and may be easily disrupted by fractures, especially those of the neck associated with dislocations. Therefore, traumatic lesions of the talus can cause aseptic necrosis of the body of the talus. The reason for this vulnerability is that the talus is free of any direct attachment of muscles or tendons and that 60% of the talar surface is covered

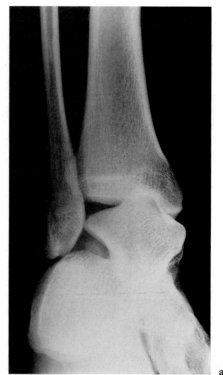

a

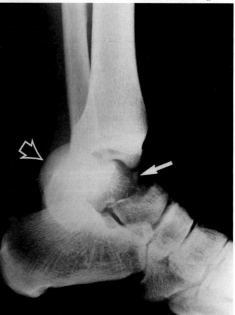

b

Fig. 14.4. a AP view of the ankle showing tibiotalar and subtalar dislocation (Hawkins type III). The talar dome is directed medially. **b** Lateral radiograph of the ankle showing vertical talar neck fracture (*arrow*) and dislocation of the talus (*open arrow*)

with articular cartilage (MULFINGER and TRUETA 1970; PETERSON et al. 1974).

Fractures of the talus are not very common, accounting for about 0.3% of all fractures. In general

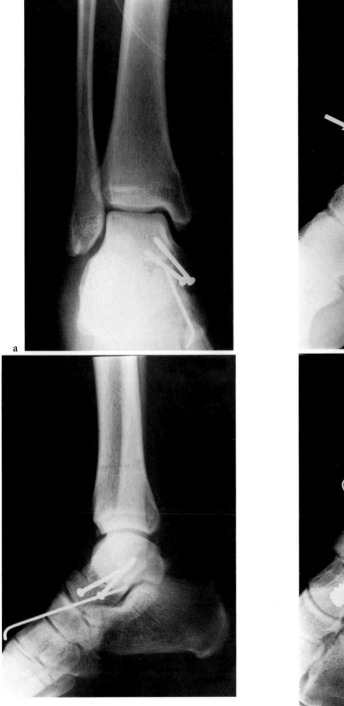

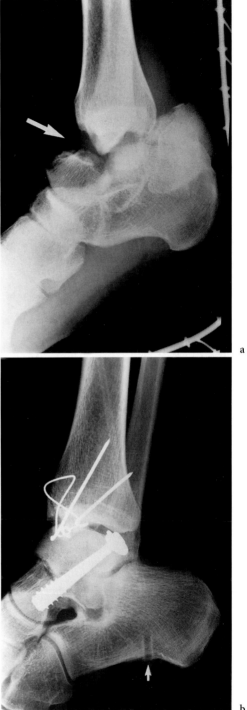

Fig. 14.5a,b. Same patient as in Fig. 14.4: Following closed reduction and screw and K-wire fixation, the talus is in a normal position on the AP and lateral views

Fig. 14.6. a Lateral radiograph showing a talar neck fracture (*arrow*) and dorsally directed dislocation of the talus body. **b** Lateral radiograph after treatment showing a medial ankle fracture treated with K-wire and screw fixation of the talus with residual displacement of the talar neck fracture. The *arrow* indicates a bur hole after temporary external arthrodesis

they are caused by accidents like aircraft crashes or car collisions (TRIEBEL and AHLERS 1993). Fractures of the head of the talus are also infrequent and usually associated with lesions of the talonavicular joint or fractures of the navicular.

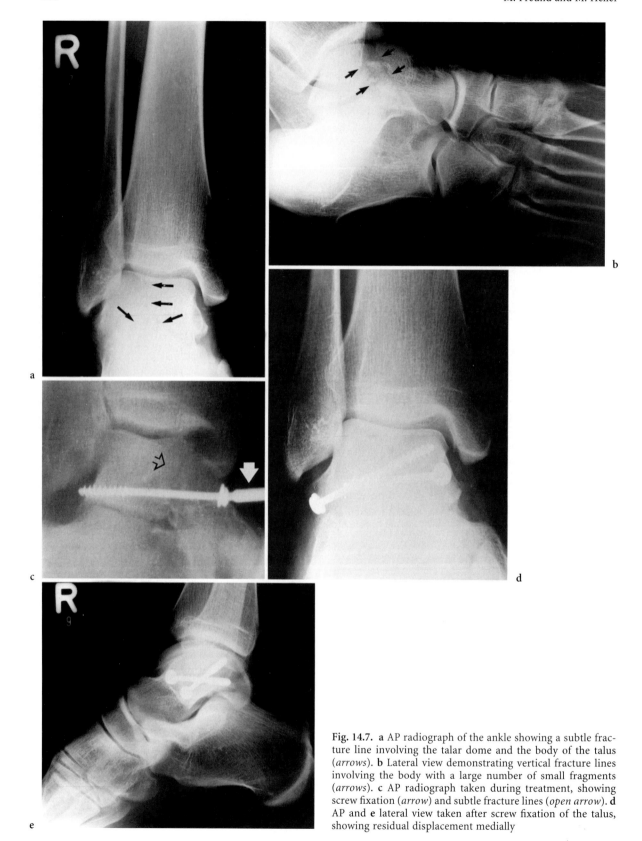

Fig. 14.7. a AP radiograph of the ankle showing a subtle fracture line involving the talar dome and the body of the talus (*arrows*). **b** Lateral view demonstrating vertical fracture lines involving the body with a large number of small fragments (*arrows*). **c** AP radiograph taken during treatment, showing screw fixation (*arrow*) and subtle fracture lines (*open arrow*). **d** AP and **e** lateral view taken after screw fixation of the talus, showing residual displacement medially

Often the neck of the talus is involved in fractures. One particular type is called aviator's astragalus, because this fracture occurred during crash landings of fighter pilots in World War I. The same mechanism is found in car accidents: a strong force from the plantar side of the fore- and midfoot pushes the neck of the talus against the anterior lip of the tibia. If the force is strong enough, the body of the talus can be locked in the ankle mortise and anterior subtalar subluxation and posterior dislocation of the body can result (COLTART 1952; KLEIGER and AHMED 1976).

The incidence of fractures of the talar body and the lateral and posterior processes is lower than that of talar neck fractures. They also bear the risk of avascular necrosis (BERQUIST et al. 1992), and in general are caused by accidents. Fracture fragments of lateral process fractures are not easy to detect because they are small and often overlapped by other bony structures. Early clinical studies showed that close to 50% of these fractures were overlooked on the initial x-ray films (MUKHERJEE et al. 1974; HAWKINS 1965).

Due to the fact that nearly half of the neck and body fractures are associated with subtalar subluxation or posterior dislocation of the body, this possibility must be excluded by looking at the position of the calcaneus and the posterior facet of the subtalar joint (Figs. 14.4–14.7). It is also important to exclude osteochondral lesions of the dome of the talus, which are often associated with fractures of the ankle (Fig. 14.8).

14.5.1.2 Calcaneal Lesions

The calcaneus is the largest bone of the foot and is the most commonly fractured tarsal bone, accounting for approximately 1%–2% of all fractures (BERQUIST et al. 1992). In most cases the mechanism is a fall from a height onto the heels or a car accident with strong axial loading of the calcaneus (CARR 1993).

Extra-articular fractures are usually easy to identify on conventional x-rays and in most cases do not cause therapeutic problems (Figs. 14.9, 14.10).

Most fractures of the os calcis are intra-articular fractures with involvement of the subtalar joint. These fractures are a diagnostic and therapeutic challenge, requiring experience in both. The most important information required by the surgeon in order to decide whether to perform surgery or to recommend conservation treatment concerns the

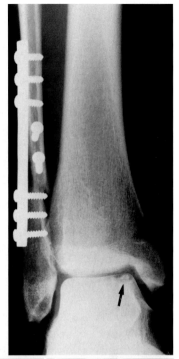

a

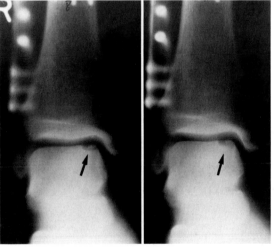

b

Fig. 14.8. a AP view of the ankle showing a medial osteochondritis dissecans (*arrow*) after ankle injury and reduction of the fibular fracture with a six-whole compression plate and additional screw fixation. b AP tomography demonstrating clearly the whole expansion of the osteochondritis dissecans (*arrows*) and the osteochondral lesion

comminution of the posterior facet of the subtalar joint and hindfoot alterations such as increased width and decreased height of the fractured os calcis. Additionally, information on the number and location of fragments and on soft tissue lesions is of importance.

Usually lateral, axial, and oblique radiographs allow diagnosis of an intra-articular calcaneal fracture

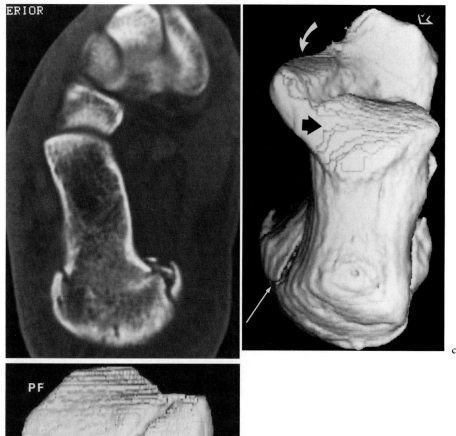

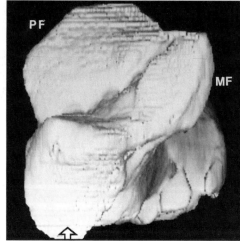

Fig. 14.9. a Extra-articular fracture of the calcaneus examined by thin-section (2 mm) CT in the longitudinal plane. A fracture of the tuber calcanei is present. b Frontal view of a three-dimensional reconstruction after electronic disarticulation showing the posterior facet (*PF*) and the medial facet (*MF*) of the subtalar joint and the calcaneocuboid joint (*open arrow*): no bony lesion is seen. c Cranial view of a three-dimensional reconstruction after electronic disarticulation demonstrating the medial fracture of the tuber calcanei (*long arrow*). There is no involvement of the posterior facet (*short arrow*), the medial facet (*curved arrow*), or the calcaneocuboid joint (*open arrow*)

(Figs. 14.11–14.13). However, it is impossible to obtain all the information needed for exact treatment planning just from the standard x-rays because most of the pathological anatomy is obscured by overlapping bony structures. Therefore CT is the method of choice in the examination of intra-articular calcaneal fractures, given that it clearly visualizes the pathological anatomy (Figs. 14.14–14.16) (KERR et al. 1994; SEGAL et al. 1985).

Most calcaneal fractures involve the body of the os calcis after a fall from a height onto the heels. This mechanism forces the body weight through the tibia and the talus right to the calcaneus. The result is

usually a crushed os calcis with depression of the posterior facet of the subtalar joint and comminution of the calcaneus.

Essex-Lopresti differentiated two major types of intra-articular fractures according to their secondary fracture line: first, the "tongue-type fracture" with the secondary fracture line running straight to the posterior border of the tuberosity (Fig. 14.12) and second, the more common "joint depression fracture" (Fig. 14.14). In this type the secondary fracture line runs across the body just behind the subtalar joint (ESSEX-LOPRESTI 1952). Bony lesions not involving the subtalar articular

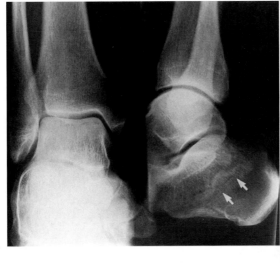
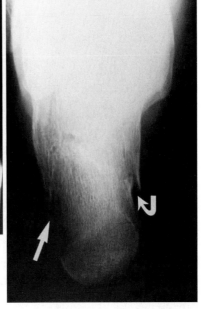

Fig. 14.10. a AP and lateral radiographs of the os calcis showing a "joint depression type" of calcaneal fracture. b In the axial projection of the fracture is apparent at the medial margin (*curved arrow*) and the lateral border (*straight arrow*)

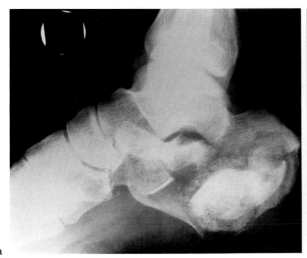
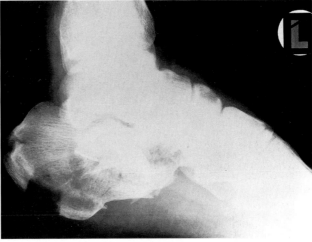

Fig. 14.11a,b. Bilateral fractures of the calcaneus. Approximately 10% of calcaneal fractures are bilateral and such fractures are also often associated with fracture of the spine, usually the thoracolumbar spine. a Lateral view of the right os calcis, showing a comminuted depressed fracture of the calcaneus. b Lateral view of the left os calcis, showing a comminuted depressed fracture of the calcaneus

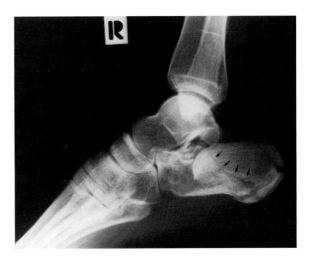

Fig. 14.12. Lateral view of the right os calcis, demonstrating a "tongue-type" comminuted fracture of the calcaneus (*arrows*). Böhler's angle measures approximately 0°. The largest fragment consists of the superior portion of the tuberosity and contains a portion of the posterior facet. This is the typical appearance of a "tongue-type" fracture

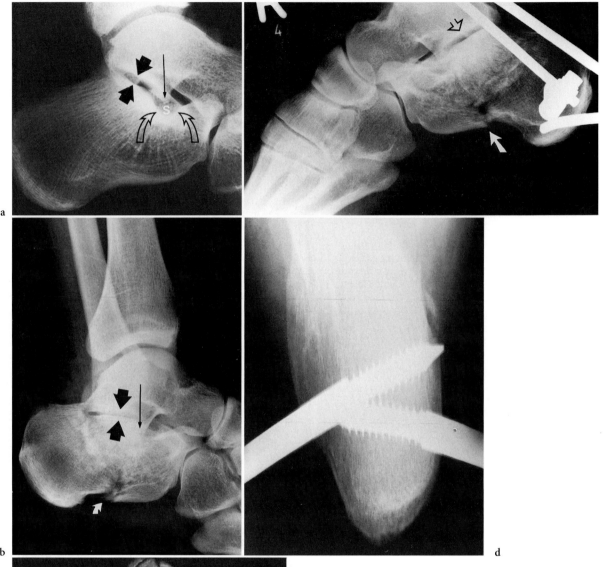

Fig. 14.13. a Lateral radiograph of a normal hindfoot demonstrating the the tuber angle of the calcaneus formed by the anterior process of the os calcis and the posterior facet (*curved arrows*) into which projects the lateral portion of the talus (*long arrow*). Usually in this projection the sustentaculum tali (*S*) is demonstrated anterior to the posterior facet (*short arrows*). **b** Lateral projection of the ankle demonstrating a severely comminuted fracture of the calcaneus (*curved arrow*). Böhler's angle is frankly reversed. The posterior facet still appears with parallel margins but is depressed (*short arrows*). The lateral portion of the talus is also depressed deep into the calcaneus (*long arrow*). **c** Lateral view after treatment with temporary external arthrodesis showing the fracture line (*arrow*) and an uprighted posterior facet (*open arrow*). **d** Axial view demonstrating the lower screws of the external arthrodesis. **e** Cranial view of a three-dimensional reconstruction of a CT examination for therapy control purposes showing an oblique fracture line and metal artifacts

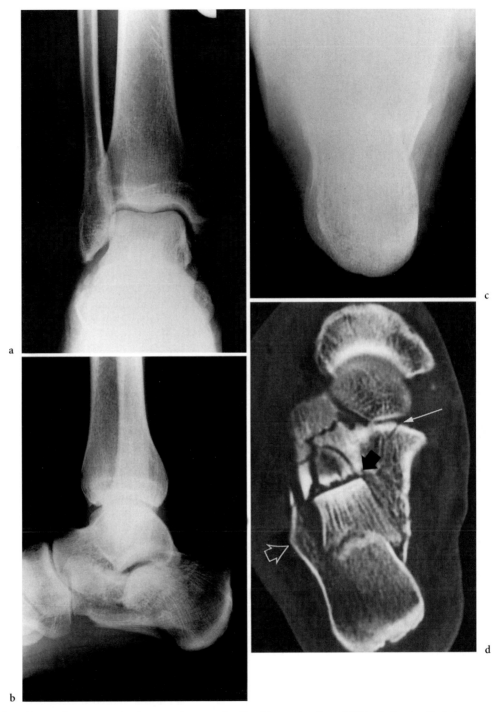

Fig. 14.14. a AP and **b** lateral view of a compression fracture of the calcaneus demonstrating depression of the posterior facet. **c** Axial projection showing the involvement of the medial margin of the calcaneus. **d** Intra-articular fracture of the calcaneus examined by thin-section (2 mm) CT in the longitudinal plane. Axial slice demonstrating depression of the posterior facet (*short arrow*) and fracture of the medial facet (*long arrow*). Typical lateral bulge (*open arrow*)

facets are usually avulsion type fractures of the tuberosity at the insertion of the Achilles tendon, fractures of the anterior process, fractures of the sustentaculum tali, and beak fractures (ROWE et al. 1963). Fractures of the anterior process are easily missed on standard radiographs because the fragments are only minimally dislocated and projected onto other bones. Oblique views show the

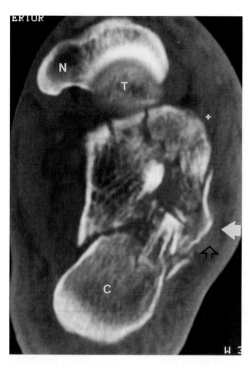

Fig. 14.15. Intra-articular fracture of the calcaneus examined by thin-section (2 mm) CT in the longitudinal plane. Axial slice demonstrating a typical lateral bulge (*arrow*) with impingement of the peroneal tendons. *C*, Calcaneus; *T*, talus; *N*, navicular

anterior process without overlapping structures and allow a diagnosis.

A reduction of Böhler's angle in the lateral radiograph (Fig. 14.12) may suggest a subtle intra-articular calcaneal fracture, but a normal Böhler's angle does not exclude the possibility of a fracture since the fragments may rebound and mimic a normal Böhler's angle in the lateral projection (ROGERS 1992).

A large number of undisplaced fractures not involving the subtalar joint are easily overlooked on plain films but can be detected on conventional tomograms or computed tomography.

14.5.2 Midfoot

14.5.2.1 Navicular Lesions

Isolated fractures of the navicular bone are relatively uncommon. In a study by EICHENHOLTZ and LEVENE (1964), 47% of them were avulsions (Fig. 14.17), 29% involved the body, and 24% were tuberosity fractures (Fig. 14.18) (EICHENHOLTZ and LEVENE 1964).

Usually the avulsion fracture is located dorsally and close to the talonavicular joint. The supranavicular bone can be distinguished from an avulsion fracture by its sharp margins. Another secondary center of ossification is the os tibiale externum, which has to be differentiated from tuberosity fractures.

Vertical fractures of the body of the navicular bone may be associated with medial dislocation of the medial fragment while horizontal lesions are associated with dorsal dislocation of the anterior fragment (SANGEORZAN et al. 1989).

14.5.2.2 Cuboid Lesions

Isolated lesions of the cuboid are rare and usually caused by direct trauma to the bone. Like the navicular bone, the cuboid is in close contact with some secondary centers of ossification, which have to be differentiated from bony fragments. These accessory bones are the os vesalianum and the os peroneum. Fractures of the os peroneum in combination with rupture of the peroneus longus tendon have been reported (PEACOCK et al. 1986).

14.5.2.3 Lesions of the Cuneiform Bones

Traumatic lesions of the cuneiform bones are in general combined with tarsometatarsal luxations. Sole fractures of one or two cuneiform bones are very rare. For this reason a tarsometatarsal lesion has to be excluded after identifying a fracture of a cuneiform bone on a radiograph.

14.5.3 Forefoot

14.5.3.1 Lesions of the Metatarsal Bones

Traumatic lesions of the metatarsal bones are frequent and usually caused by direct trauma due to heavy objects striking the foot. However, shearing and twisting mechanisms also may be followed by fractures (ANDERSON 1977; HECKMANN 1984).

Transverse fractures of the proximal part of the fifth metatarsal are relatively common. These fractures occur as two distinct types: (a) Jones fracture and (b) avulsion fracture of the tip of the proximal tuberosity. The latter is the more frequent and is the result of an abrupt pull of the

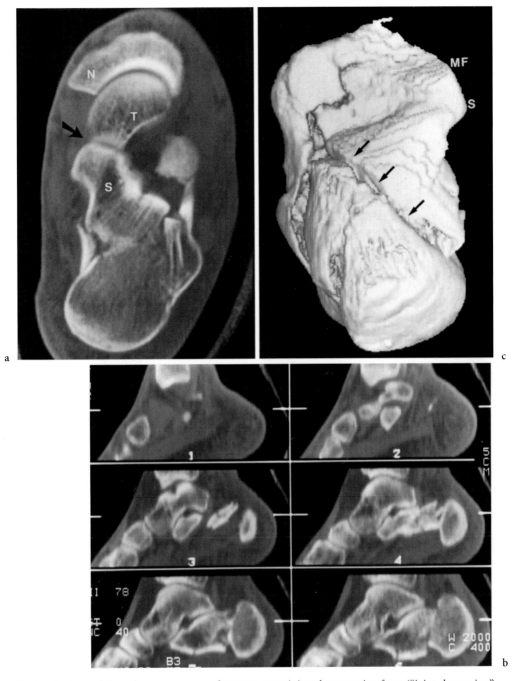

Fig. 14.16. a Intra-articular fracture of the calcaneus examined by thin-section (2 mm) CT in the longitudinal plane. Axial slice demonstrating a normal medial facet (*arrow*), a lateral bulge, and involvement of the medial margin of the calcaneus. *S,* Sustentaculum tali; *T,* talus; *N,* navicular bone. **b** Sagittal reconstructions demonstrating the depression of the fragment containing the posterior facet ("joint depression" type). **c** Cranial view of a three-dimensional reconstruction after electronic disarticulation demonstrating posterior facet involvement (*arrows*). The medial facet (*MF*) appears normal. *S,* Sustentaculum tali

peroneus brevis tendon or the lateral part of the aponeurosis, both of which are attached to the proximal tuberosity. The Jones fracture is usually located 2 cm distal from the proximal tuberosity and is due to inversion of the foot (Fig. 14.19) (JONES 1902). The remaining isolated fractures of the metatarsal bones are usually the result of heavy objects falling on the foot (Fig. 14.20).

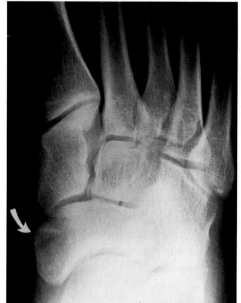

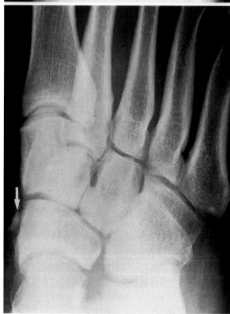

Fig. 14.17. a Oblique view of the midfoot showing a subtle lesion at the medial margin of the navicular bone representing an avulsion fracture (*arrow*). **b** AP projection clearly demonstrating the fracture (*arrow*)

14.5.3.2 Lesions of the Phalanges

Fractures of the phalanges are commonly caused by striking objects with the foot during walking or due to heavy objects falling on the toes (ANDERSON 1977). One of the most common fractures of the foot is the traumatic lesion of the distal phalanx of the first toe (Figs. 14.21, 14.22). Usually fractures of the

phalanges are minimally displaced and sometimes they are not easy to differentiate from skin folds simulating fractures (Figs. 14.23, 14.24). A major role of the radiographic examination is to detect or exclude articular involvement, because this usually requires changes in treatment (Figs. 14.25, 14.26).

Dislocations of the interphalangeal or the metatarsophalangeal joint, whether or not combined with fractures, are commonly due to hyperextension. The direction of the dislocation is either volar or dorsal; lateral and medial dislocations are less common.

14.5.4 Lesions of Sesamoid Bones

Excluding a traumatic lesion of a sesamoid bone can be very difficult or even impossible since the sesamoids can be bipartite and mimic a fracture. Apart from clinical findings, a radiograph of the opposite side can help to solve the problem, given that bipartite sesamoid bones are often found bilaterally.

The medial sesamoid bone of the great toe is more often fractured than the lateral one. Usually these

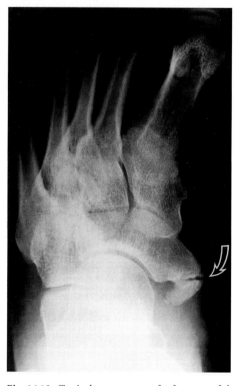

Fig. 14.18. Typical appearance of a fracture of the tuberosity of the navicular bone (*open arrow*), which is usually caused by an abduction mechanism. These fractures may be associated with fractures of the calcaneocuboid joint. Generally there is no fragment displacement

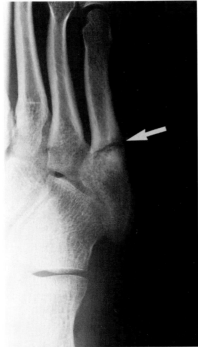

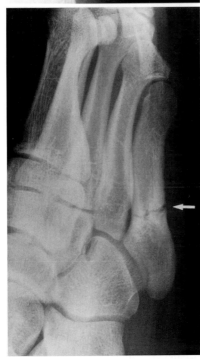

Fig. 14.19. a Oblique view of the forefoot demonstrating a complete transverse fracture (Jones fracture) at the base of the fifth metatarsal bone (*arrow*). Typically such lesions occur without displacement of the fracture fragment; clinically they may mimic ankle injuries. **b** Three weeks later: reactive sclerosis of the margins (*arrow*) is demonstrated

fractures are transverse or oblique (ZINMAN et al. 1981).

14.5.5 Stress Fractures

In general two types of stress fractures are to be differentiated: the "fatigue fracture" and the "insufficiency fracture." The metatarsal bones are the site of the more frequent fatigue fracture, which is caused by abnormal stress to a bone with normal elastic resistance and is common in military training. Most frequently the shaft of the second or third metatarsal bone is involved (Figs. 14.27, 14.28). The first radiographic sign is a sclerotic line; with increased or ongoing stress a frank fracture will result (TRIEBEL and AHLERS 1993; ROGERS 1992). The second type of stress fracture (insufficiency fracture) is caused by normal stress to a bone with deficient elastic resistance.

Stress fractures of a sesamoid bone may be difficult to differentiate from a bipartite sesamoid, but again, clinical examination and radiographs of the opposite side may help.

14.5.6 Midtarsal Dislocation (Chopart's Dislocation)

A complete and sole dislocation of the talonavicular and calcaneocuboid joints is rare. Usually these lesions are combined with avulsion fractures and fractures close to the articular facets or fractures of the facets (SUHREN and ZWIPP 1989). In most cases the foot is displaced medially; less often it is displaced laterally. Instead of involving the talonavicular joint, a midtarsal dislocation may involve the cuneonavicular joint (ROGERS 1992).

Chopart's dislocation has to be differentiated from the subtalar dislocation involving the talonavicular and the subtalar joints. This distinction should be possible by close evaluation of the radiographs.

14.5.7 Tarsometatarsal Fracture-Dislocation (Lisfranc's Dislocation)

Tarsometatarsal fracture-dislocation does not occur very often and accounts for less than 1% of all fracture-dislocations involving the tarsometarsal joint (AITKEN and PAULSEN 1963; ENGLISH 1964). In general the mechanism is a forced plantar flexion of

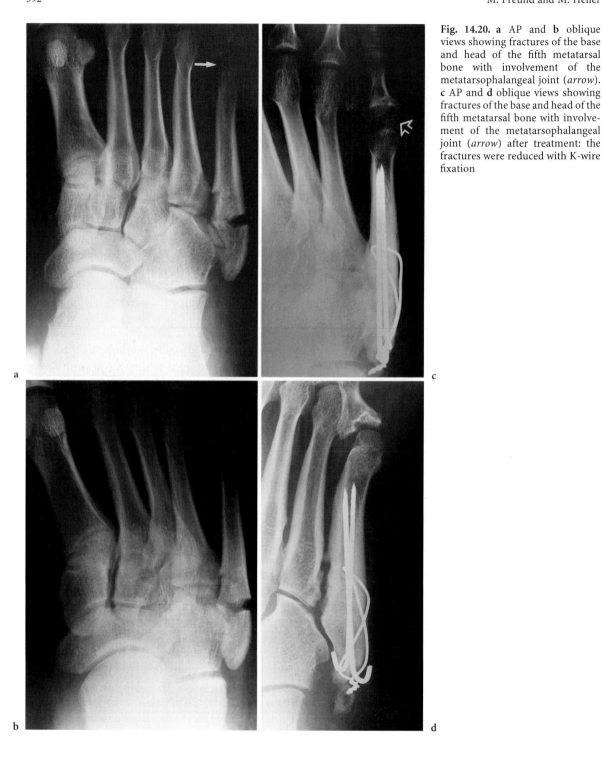

Fig. 14.20. a AP and **b** oblique views showing fractures of the base and head of the fifth metatarsal bone with involvement of the metatarsophalangeal joint (*arrow*). **c** AP and **d** oblique views showing fractures of the base and head of the fifth metatarsal bone with involvement of the metatarsophalangeal joint (*arrow*) after treatment: the fractures were reduced with K-wire fixation

the forefoot with or without a rotational component (WILEY 1971). Nowadays in most cases the lesion is the result of severe traffic accidents when the car driver's foot is caught under the clutch or break pedal. But the dislocation can also occur after a fall from a height.

Unlike the bases of the second to fifth metatarsals, the first and second metatarsal bones are not connected by a ligament.

The classification of these injuries differentiates between homolateral and divergent types, based on the direction of the metatarsal dislocation. The

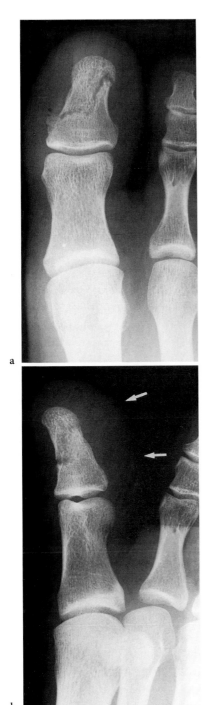

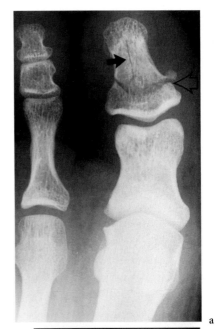

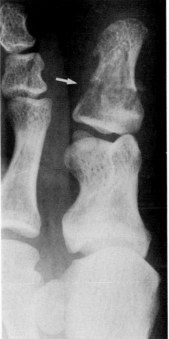

Fig. 14.21. a AP radiograph of the first toe demonstrating a clear fracture line of the shaft of the distal phalanx, without articular involvement. **b** Lateral projection showing an impressive soft tissue swelling (*arrows*) which represents strong supportive evidence for a bony lesion

Fig. 14.22. a AP projection demonstrating an incomplete longitudinal fracture (*arrow*) and a complete undisplaced transverse fracture (*open arrow*) of the distal phalanx of the first toe. **b** Lateral view showing the transverse fracture of the base of the distal phalanx of the first toe (*arrow*)

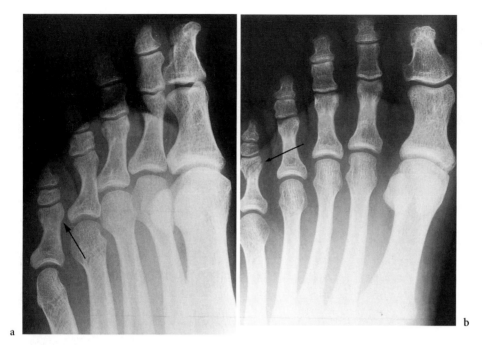

Fig. 14.23. a Subtle cortical lesion of the head of the proximal phalanx of the fifth toe on the oblique radiograph (*arrow*). b AP view clearly demonstrating the complete oblique fracture (*arrow*)

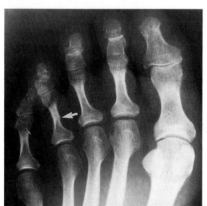

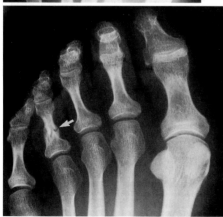

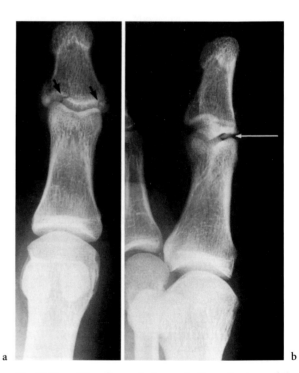

Fig. 14.25. a AP radiograph demonstrating a fracture of the base of the distal phalanx of the first toe with involvement of the articular facet (*arrows*). b Lateral view showing fragment displacement (*arrow*)

Fig. 14.24. a AP projection showing a complete transverse fracture of the shaft of the proximal phalanx of the fourth toe (*arrow*). b AP projection showing malunion after 3 months

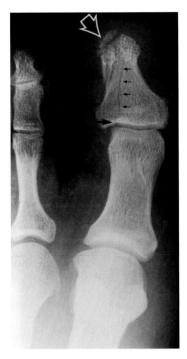

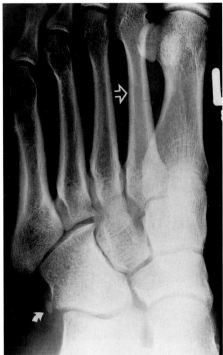

Fig. 14.26. AP projection demonstrating an incomplete longitudinal fracture (*small arrows*), involvement of the articular facet, and a comminuted minimally displaced fracture of the subungual tuft of the great toe (*open arrow*)

homolateral type is more common than the divergent one. If the first metatarsal bone still has its normal relationship to the medial cuneiform and the four lateral metatarsals are dislocated laterally, these findings are described as a homolateral Lisfranc dislocation. If the first metatarsal bone is displaced medially and the four lateral metatarsals are dislocated laterally, these findings are described as a divergent Lisfranc dislocation (ROGERS and CAMPBELL 1978). Both types are usually associated with fractures of the base of the metatarsal and tarsal bones, but such fractures are especially frequent in conjunction with the divergent type.

Significant arterial injury may occur because the dorsalis pedis artery passes between the first and second metatarsal bones, forming the plantar arterial arch (HECKMANN 1984).

14.6 Traumatic Lesions of the Foot in Children

Fractures of the pedal skeleton in childhood and adolescence are not very common. Usually these lesions are of the greenstick variety or epiphyseal fractures. Torus fractures may be subtle and may not be initially apparent. On follow-up a line of sclerosis is

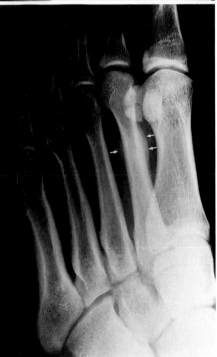

Fig. 14.27. a *Arrow*: os tibiale externum. A Fracture line of the midshaft of the second metatarsal bone is barely perceptible (*open arrow*). **b** Six weeks later a solid callus formation of the entire metatarsal shaft of the second metatarsal bone is visible, indicating a stress fracture (*arrows*)

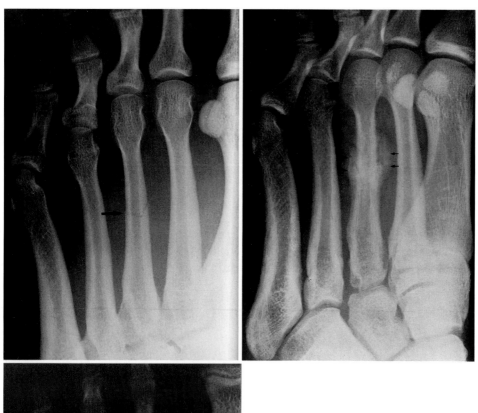

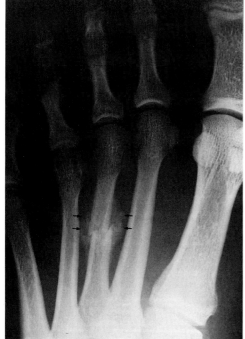

Fig. 14.28. a Stress lesion of the shaft of the third metatarsal bone; there is a V-shaped fracture line (*arrow*). **b** Six weeks later after trauma a solid callus formation (*arrows*) is visible as well as fragment displacement. **c** Twelve weeks after trauma an extensive and solid callus formation is visible (*arrows*); the fracture line is barely perceptible

seen across the bone, proving that the fracture has affected the entire bone (POZNANSKI 1995).

In young children most fractures of the os calcis are extra-articular and they are often overlooked because of their subtle radiographic findings. Intra-articular calcaneal fractures may be associated with other lesions, such as spinal fractures, caused by the trauma mechanism, but SCHMIDT and WEINER

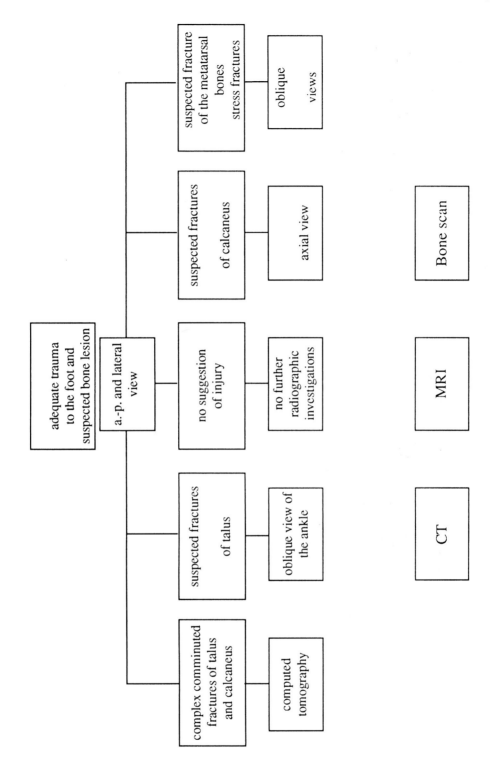

Fig. 14.29. Diagnostic algorithm indicating procedures to be used following adequate trauma to the foot

(1982) found them to be less frequent compared with such lesions in adults.

Knowledge of the exact time of the appearance of the different ossification centers of the pedal skeleton in childhood is important (TRIEBEL and AHLERS 1993). Usually the ossification of the talus starts in the 6th fetal month, the ossification of the calcaneus starts in the 3rd to 4th fetal month, and the epiphysis of the posterior part of the calcaneus appears in the 6th to the 8th year and will unite with the anterior os calcis in the 14th to 16th year. The ossification of the cuboid starts in the 9th fetal month, while that of the other midfoot bones starts between the 1st and the 3rd year. The ossification of the forefoot starts at the age of 9 weeks and is completed at 17–20 years (GRAY 1989).

The apophysis at the base of the fifth metatarsal bone during childhood should be differentiated from a fracture fragment.

If multiple metaphyseal corner fractures and other more traumatic lesions of different ages are present, child abuse should be suspected. In that case, after excluding other reasons for the lesions, e.g., osteogenesis imperfecta, further studies should be obtained (POZNANSKI 1995).

14.7 Complications

In general post-traumatic arthritis with early degenerative changes, persistent pain, and malunion or pseudarthrosis are the main complications after fractures of the pedal skeleton. Avascular necrosis of the talus is a common complication after displaced talar neck fractures (CANALE and BELDING 1980; HAWKINS 1970).

The main problem of calcaneal fractures is prolonged pain and loss of motion even years after the injury. During the acute phase there is also always the danger of a compartment syndrome, rupture of tendons, and iatrogenic complications after treatment, e.g., skin infection and osteomyelitis (BERQUIST et al. 1992). Calcaneal fractures are frequently bilateral and often combined with fractures of the thoracolumbar spine. If patients complain of back pain, the spine should be examined immediately. Vascular complications of the metatarsal bones have been reported, but these complications are not very frequent. Sometimes posttraumatic soft tissue calcifications will cause problems, especially if they are located close to articular facets.

14.8 Diagnostic Algorithm

A diagnostic algorithm relating to trauma of the foot is shown in Fig. 14.29.

References

Aitken AP, Paulsen D (1963) Dislocation of the tarsometatarsal joints. J Bone Joint Surg [Am] 45:246–260

Allon SM, Mears DC (1991) Three dimensional analysis calcaneal fractures. Foot Ankle 11:254–263

Anderson LD (1977) Injuries of the forefoot. Clin Orthop 122:18–27

Berquist TH, Morrey BF, Cass JR, Johnson KA (1992) The foot and ankle. In: Berquist TH (ed) Imaging of orthopedic trauma. Raven Press, New York, pp 462–467, 475–492, 525–570

Blei CL, Nirschl RP, Grant EG (1986) Achilles tendon: US diagnosis of pathologic conditions. Radiology 159:765–767

Bluth EI, Merrit CR, Sullivan MA (1982) Grey scale ultrasound evaluation of the lower extremities. JAMA 247:3127–3129

Brown ML, Swee RG, Johnson KA (1986) Bone scintigraphy of the calcaneus. Clin Nucl Med 11:530–536

Canale ST, Kelly FB (1978) Fractures of the neck of the talus. J Bone Joint Surg [Am] 60:143–156

Canale ST, Belding RH (1980) Fractures of the neck and talus. J Bone Joint Surg [Am] 62:97–102

Carr JB (1993) Mechanism and pathoanatomy of the intraarticular calcaneal fracture. Clin Orthop 290:36–40

Carr JB, Noto AM, Stevenson S (1990) Volumetric three-dimensional computed tomography for acute calcaneus fractures: preliminary report. J Orthop Trauma 4:346–348

Coltart WD (1952) Aviators astragalus. J Bone Joint Surg [Am] 62:143–156

Daffner RH, Reimer BL, Lupetin AR, Dash N (1986) Magnetic resonance imaging of acute tendon ruptures. Skeletal Radiol 15:291–294

Eichenholtz SN, Levene DB (1964) Fracture of the tarsal navicular bone. Clin Orthop 34:142–157

English TA (1964) Dislocation of the metarsal bone and adjacent toe. J Bone Joint Surg [Br] 46:700–704

Erickson SJ, Quinn SF, Kneeland JB et al. (1990) MR imaging of the tarsal tunnel and related spaces. AJR 155:323–328

Essex-Lopresti P (1952) The mechanism, reduction technique, and results in fractures of the os calcis. Br J Surg 39:395–419

Freund M, Hohendorff B, Zenker W, Hutzelmann A, Heller M (1996) CT von Kalkaneusfrakturen: 3D-Rekonstruktionen mit elektronischer Desartikulation. Fortschr Röntgenstr 164:189–195

Geslian JE, Thrall JH, Espenosa JL, Older RA (1976) Early detection of stress fractures using Tc-99m polyphosphate. Radiology 121:683–687

Gray H (1989) Gray's anatomy, 37th edn. Churchill Livingstone, London, pp 447–458, 535–541

Greespan A (1990) Skelettradiologie. Edition Medizin, Weinheim, pp 162–173, 187–194

Häberle HJ, Minholz R, Bader C et al. (1993) CT-Klassifikation intraartikulärer Kalkaneusfrakturen. Fortschr Röntgenstr 159:548–554

Hawkins LG (1965) Fractures of the lateral process of the talus. J Bone Joint Surg [Am] 47:1170–1175

Hawkins LG (1970) Fractures of the neck of the talus. J Bone Joint Surg [Am] 52:991–1002

Heckmann JD (1984) Fractures of the foot and ankle. In: Rockwood CA, Green DP (eds) Fractures. Lippincott, Philadelphia, p 1703

Heger L, Wulff K, Seddiqi MSA (1985) Computed tomography of calcaneal fractures. AJR 145:131–137

Heuchemer T, Bargon G, Bauer G, Mutschler W (1992) Computertomographie nach intraartikulärer kalkaneusfraktur. Unfallchirurg 95:31–36

Jones R (1902) Fractures of the base of the fifth metatarsal bone by indirect violence. Am J Surg 35:697–700

Kainberger FM, Engel A, Barton P, Huebsch P, Newbold A, Salomonowitz E (1990) Injury to the Achilles tendon: diagnosis with sonography. 155:1031–1036

Kerr PS, Cole AS, Atkins RM (1994) The use of the axial CT scan in intra-articular fractures of the calcaneum. Injury 25:359–363

Kleiger B, Ahmed M (1976) Injuries of the talus and its joints. Clin Orthop 121:243–262

Mukherjee SK, Pringle RM, Baxter AD (1974) Fracture of the lateral process of the talus. J Bone Joint Surg [Br] 56:263–273

Mulfinger GL, Trueta JC (1970) The blood supply of the talus. J Bone Joint Surg [Br] 52:160–167

Peacock KC, Resnick EJ, Thoder JJ (1986) Fracture of the os peroneum with rupture of the peroneus longus tendon. Clin Orthop 202:223–225

Peterson L, Goldie IF, Lindell D (1974) The arterial supply of the talus. Acta Orthop Scand 48:696–707

Poznanski AK (1995) Pediatric musculoskeletal radiology. In: Pettersson H (ed) A global textbook of radiology. Nicer, Oslo, p 476

Rogers LF (1992) Radiology of skeletal trauma, vol 2, 2nd edn. Churchill Livingstone, New York, pp 1429–1516

Rogers LF, Campbell RE (1978) Fractures and dislocations of the foot. Semin Roentgenol 13:157

Rowe CR, Sakillarides HT, Freeman PA (1963) Fractures of the os calcis. A long term follow-up study in 146 patients. JAMA 184:920–924

Sangeorzan BJ, Benirschke SK, Mosca V et al. (1989) Displaced intra-articular fractures of the tarsal navicular. J Bone Joint Surgery [Am] 71:1504–1509

Segal D, Marsh JL, Leiter B (1985) Clinical application of computerized axial scanning of calcaneus fractures. Clin Orthop 199:114–123

Schmidt TL, Weiner DS (1982) Calcaneal fractures in children. An evaluation of the nature of injury in 56 children. Clin Orthop 171:150–155

Sierra A, Potchen EJ, Moore J, Smith HG (1986) High-field magnetic resonance imaging of aseptic necrosis of the talus. J Bone Joint Surg [Am] 68:927–928

Suhren EG, Zwipp H (1989) Luxationsfrakturen im Chopart- und Lisfranc-Gelenk. Unfallchirurg 92:130–137

Tanyü MO, Vinée P, Wimmer B (1994) Value of 3D CT imaging in fractured os calcis. Comput Med Imaging Graph 18:137–143

Triebel HJ, Ahlers J (1993) Sprungelenk und Fuß. In: Thelen M (ed) Radiologische diagnostik der verletzungen von knochen und gelenken. Thieme, Stuttgart, p 540

Whitby EH, Barrington NA (1995) Fractures of the lateral process of the talus – the value of lateral tomography. Br J Radiol 68:583–586

Wiley JJ (1971) The mechanism of tarsometatarsal joint injuries. J Bone Joint Surg [Br] 53:474–482

Zinman H, Keret Q, Reis ND (1981) Fracture of the medial sesamoid bone of the hallux. J Trauma 21:581–582

Subject Index

List of Contributors

ALBERT L. BAERT, MD, PhD
Professor and Chairman
Department of Radiology
University Hospital K.U. Leuven
Herestraat 49
3000 Leuven
Belgium

JOACHIM BROSSMANN, MD
Klinik für Radiologische Diagnostik
Klinikum der Christian-Albrechts-Universität
zu Kiel
Arnold-Heller-Str. 9
24105 Kiel
Germany

CARLOS H. BUITRAGO-TÉLLEZ, MD
Abteilung Röntgendiagnostik
Radiologische Universitätsklinik
Klinikum der Albert-Ludwigs-Universität Freiburg
Hugstetterstr. 55
79106 Freiburg
Germany

AJAY CHAVAN, MD
Abteilung Diagnostische Radiologie I
der Medizinischen Hochschule Hannover
Konstanty-Gutschow-Str. 8
30635 Hannover
Germany

U. Dietrich, MD
Klinik für Neuroradiologie
Universitätsklinikum Essen
Hufelandstr. 55
45122 Essen
Germany

F.J. FERSTL, MD
Abteilung Röntgendiagnostik
Radiologische Universitätsklinik
Klinikum der Albert-Ludwigs-Universität Freiburg
Hugstetterstr. 55
79106 Freiburg
Germany

A. FINK, MD
Klinik für Radiologische Diagnostik
Klinikum der Christian-Albrechts-Universität
zu Kiel
Arnold-Heller-Str. 9
24105 Kiel
Germany

MICHAEL FREUND, MD
Klinik für Radiologische Diagnostik
Klinikum der Christian-Albrechts-Universität
zu Kiel
Arnold-Heller-Str. 9
24105 Kiel
Germany

MICHAEL GALANSKI, MD, PhD
Professor and Direktor
der Abteilung Diagnostische
Radiologie I der Medizinischen Hochschule
Hannover
Konstanty-Gutschow-Str. 8
30635 Hannover
Germany

S. GRYSPEERDT, MD
Department of Radiology
University Hospitals K.U. Leuven
Herestraat 49
3000 Leuven
Belgium

FRANZ HÄCKL, MD
Department of Radiology
University of California
San Francisco, CA 94143
USA

KLAUS D. HAGSPIEL, MD
Division of Cardiovascular
and Interventional Radiology
Department of Radiology
Brigham and Women's Hospital
Harvard Medical School
75 Francis Street
Boston, MA 02115
USA

MARTIN HELLER, MD, PhD
Professor and Direktor der
Klinik für Radiologische Diagnostik
Klinikum der Christian-Albrechts-Universität
zu Kiel
Arnold-Heller-Str. 9
24105 Kiel
Germany

KARL-FRIEDRICH KREITNER, MD
Klinik und Poliklinik für Radiologie
Johannes-Gutenberg-Universität Mainz
Langenbeckstr. 1
55131 Mainz
Germany

M. LANGER, MD, FICA
Professor and Direktor
Abteilung Röntgendiagnostik
Radiologische Universitätsklinik
Klinikum der Albert-Ludwigs-Universität Freiburg
Hugstetterstr. 55
79106 Freiburg
Germany

ROLAND LÖW, MD
Klinik und Poliklinik für Radiologie
Johannes-Gutenberg-Universität Mainz
Langenbeckstr. 1
55131 Mainz
Germany

V.M. METZ, MD, PhD
Associate Professor
Universitätsklinik für Radiodiagnostik
Allg. Krankenhaus Wien
Währinger Gürtel 18–20
1090 Wien
Austria

C. MUHLE, MD
Klinik für Radiologische Diagnostik
Klinikum der Christian-Albrechts-Universität
zu Kiel
Arnold-Heller-Str. 9
24105 Kiel
Germany

RAYMOND H. OYEN, MD, PhD
Professor, Adjunct Clinic Head
Department of Radiology
University Hospitals K.U. Leuven
Herestraat 49
3000 Leuven
Belgium

S. PALMIÉ, MD
Klinik für Radiologische Diagnostik
Klinikum der Christian-Albrechts-Universität
zu Kiel
Arnold-Heller-Str. 9
24105 Kiel
Germany

M. REUTER, MD
Klinik für Radiologische Diagnostik
Klinikum der Christian-Albrechts-Universität
zu Kiel
Arnold-Heller-Str. 9
24105 Kiel
Germany

HELMUT SCHWARZENBERG, MD
Klinik für Radiologische Diagnostik
Klinikum der Christian-Albrechts-Universität
zu Kiel
Arnold-Heller-Str. 9
24105 Kiel
Germany

L. VAN HOE, MD
Department of Radiology
University Hospitals K.U. Leuven
Herestraat 49
3000 Leuven
Belgium

Friedhelm E. ZANELLA, MD, PhD
Professor and Direktor
des Instituts für Neuroradiologie
am Klinikum der J.W. Goethe-Universität
Schleusenweg 7–10
60528 Frankfurt
Germany

MEDICAL RADIOLOGY – Diagnostic Imaging and Radiation Oncology

Titles in the series already published

Diagnostic Imaging

Innovations in Diagnostic Imaging   Edited by J.H. ANDERSON

Radiology of the Upper Urinary Tract   Edited by E.K. LANG

The Thymus – Diagnostic Imaging, Functions, and Pathologic Anatomy
Edited by E. WALTER, E. WILLICH, and W.R. WEBB

Interventional Neuroradiology   Edited by A. VALAVANIS

Radiology of the Pancreas   Edited by A.L. BAERT, co-edited by G. DELORME

Radiology of the Lower Urinary Tract   Edited by E.K. LANG

Magnetic Resonance Angiography   Edited by I.P. ARLART, G.M. BONGARTZ, and
G. MARCHAL

Contrast-Enhanced MRI of the Breast   S. HEYWANG-KÖBRUNNER and R. BECK

Spiral CT of the Chest   Edited by M. RÉMY-JARDIN and J. RÉMY

Radiological Diagnosis of Breast Diseases   Edited by M. FRIEDRICH and E.A. SICKLES

Radiology of the Trauma   Edited by M. HELLER and A. FINK

Biliary Tract Radiology   Edited by P. ROSSI, co-edited by M. BEZZI

Radiation Oncology

Lung Cancer   Edited by C.W. SCARANTINO

Innovations in Radiation Oncology   Edited by H.R. WITHERS and L.J. PETERS

Radiation Therapy of Head and Neck Cancer   Edited by G.E. LARAMORE

Gastrointestinal Cancer – Radiation Therapy   Edited by R.R. DOBELBOWER, Jr.

Radiation Exposure and Occupational Risks   Edited by E. SCHERER, C. STREFFER, and
K.-R. TROTT

Radiation Therapy of Benign Diseases – A Clinical Guide   S.E. ORDER and
S.S. DONALDSON

Interventional Radiation Therapy Techniques – Brachytherapy   Edited by R. SAUER

Radiopathology of Organs and Tissues   Edited by E. SCHERER, C. STREFFER, and
K.-R. TROTT

Concomitant Continuous Infusion Chemotherapy and Radiation   Edited by M. ROTMAN
and C.J. ROSENTHAL

Intraoperative Radiotherapy – Clinical Experiences and Results   Edited by F.A. CALVO,
M. SANTOS, and L.W. BRADY

Radiotherapy of Intraocular and Orbital Tumors   Edited by W.E. ALBERTI and
R.H. SAGERMAN

Interstitial and Intracavitary Thermoradiotherapy   Edited by M.H. SEEGENSCHMIEDT
and R. SAUER

Non-Disseminated Breast Cancer   Controversial Issues in Management   Edited by
G.H. Fletcher and S.H. Levitt

Current Topics in Clinical Radiobiology of Tumors   Edited by H.-P. Beck-Bornholdt

Practical Approaches to Cancer Invasion and Metastases
A Compendium of Radiation Oncologists' Responses to 40 Histories   Edited by
A.R. Kagan with the Assistance of R.J. Steckel

Radiation Therapy in Pediatric Oncology   Edited by J.R. Cassady

Radiation Therapy Physics   Edited by A.R. Smith

Late Sequelae in Oncology   Edited by J. Dunst and R. Sauer

Mediastinal Tumors. Update 1995   Edited by D.E. Wood and C.R. Thomas, Jr.

Thermoradiotherapy and Thermochemotherapy
Volume 1: Biology, Physiology, and Physics
Volume 2: Clinical Applications
Edited by M.H. Seegenschmiedt, P. Fessenden, and C.C. Vernon

Carcinoma of the Prostate.   Innovations in Management   Edited by Z. Petrovich,
L. Baert, and L.W. Brady

Springer
and the
environment

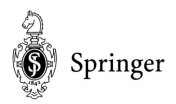

Druck- und Bindearbeiten: Universitätsdruckerei H. Stürtz AG, Würzburg